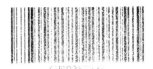

ASPARTAME DISEASE
AN IGNORED EPIDEMIC

H. J. ROBERTS, M.D., F.A.C.P., F.C.C.P.

Staff, Good Samaritan Hospital and St. Mary's Hospital, West Palm Beach, Florida; Director, Palm Beach Institute for Medical Research, West Palm Beach; Diplomate, American Board of Internal Medicine (recertified); Member or Fellow – American College of Physicians, American College of Chest Physicians, The Endocrine Society, American Academy of Neurology, American Federation for Clinical Research, New York Academy of Sciences, American Association for the Advancement of Science, Sigma Xi (honor scientific research society), Alpha Omega Alpha (honor medical society); Listed in *The Best Doctors In The U.S., Who's Who in America, Who's Who In The World, Who's Who In Science and Technology, Who's Who in Medicine and Healthcare*.

Copyright © 2001 by H. J. Roberts, M.D.
Library of Congress Control Number 2001116889

ISBN 1-884243-17-7

Publisher's Cataloging-in-Publication
(*Provided by Quality Books Inc.*)

Roberts, H. J. (Hyman Jacob), 1924-
    Aspartame disease: an ignored epidemic / H. J.
Roberts. – 1st ed.
    p. cm.
    Includes bibliographical references and index.
    IBSN: 1-884243-177

    1. Aspartame –Health aspects. 2. Aspartame –
Toxicology. 3. Food additives – Toxicology.   I. Title.

    RA1242.A73R63 2001   615.9'54
                                          QB101-200457

Physicians and health professionals should be consulted for
advice about questions or problems relating to any of the
matters considered.

Printed in the United States of America.

        Sunshine Sentinel Press, Inc.
        P.O. Box 17799
        West Palm Beach, FL 33416
        FAX   (561) 547-8008

CONTENTS

OTHER TITLES BY THE AUTHOR

Difficult Diagnosis: A Guide to the Interpretation of Obscure Illness
W. B. Saunders, Philadelphia, 1958

The Causes, Ecology and Prevention of Traffic Accidents
Charles C Thomas, Springfield, 1971

Is Vasectomy Safe? Medical, Public Health and Legal Implications
Sunshine Academic Press, West Palm Beach, 1979

Aspartame (NutraSweet®): Is It Safe?
The Charles Press, Philadelphia, 1990

Sweet'ner Dearest: Bittersweet Vignettes About Aspartame (NutraSweet®)
Sunshine Sentinel Press, West Palm Beach, 1992

Is Vasectomy Worth the Risk? A Physician's Case Against Vasectomania
Sunshine Sentinel Press, West Palm Beach, 1993

A Guide to Personal Peace: The Control of Stress, Depression and Anxiety
(Set of three cassettes) Sunshine Sentinel Press, West Palm Beach, 1993

Mega Vitamin E: Is It Safe?
Sunshine Sentinel Press, West Palm Beach, 1994

West Palm Beach: Centennial Reflections
Sunshine Sentinel Press, West Palm Beach, 1994

Defense Against Alzheimer's Disease: A Rational Blueprint for Prevention
Sunshine Sentinel Press, West Palm Beach, 1995

Health and Wealth, Palm Beach Style: Diseases, Behavior and Sexuality of the Rich
Sunshine Sentinel Press, West Palm Beach, 1997

Ignored Health Hazards For Pilots and Drivers: The A-B-C-D-E-F-G-H File
(Set of two cassettes) Sunshine Sentinel Press, West Palm Beach, 1998

*Princess Diana, The House of Windsor and Palm Beach: America's Fascination with
the "Touch of Royalty"*
Sunshine Sentinel Press, West Palm Beach, 1998

The CACOF Conspiracy: Lessons for the New Millennium
Sunshine Sentinel Press, West Palm Beach, 1997

*Breast Implants or Aspartame (NutraSweet®) Disease? The Suppressed Opinion
About a Perceived Medicolegal Travesty*
Sunshine Sentinel Press, West Palm Beach, 1999

DEDICATION

This book is dedicated to

Betty Martini

and the many worldwide members of

Mission Possible

for their valuable input and inspiring encouragement

ACKNOWLEDGMENTS

I acknowledge with gratitude the following persons whose energies and talents enabled the completion of this book.

Carolyn Baldas Gray, Shirley Brightwell and Kathleen Brightwell for typing the manuscript.

Betty Martini of Mission Possible, Mary Stoddard of Aspartame Consumer Network, Barbara Mullarkey, and many "Roberts' Angels."

Kellie McDaniel, Lillian Capote, George Leavitt and Jane Scotto of the Data Information Services Department at Good Samaritan Hospital (West Palm Beach) for assistance with the initial survey questionnaire.

Rebecca Ephraim for assistance in compiling the data.

Esther Sokol and Rabbi Stephen Roberts for their perceptive comments.

Jackie Taylor, Linda O'Callahan, Barbara Burke and Claire Searl for bibliographic assistance.

Carla Santiago for the aspartame formula figure.

Sandra Thomas for the cover design.

Special thanks go to aspartame reactors and their relatives/friends who completed and amplified the ten-page questionnaire. Excerpts of their correspondence generally appear verbatim. A minimum of editing was required for clarity and the avoidance of trade names.

Dr. David G. Hattan, Chief of the Regulatory Affairs Staff of the FDA Office of Nutrition and Food Sciences, and Dr. Linda Tollefson furnished early FDA data submitted by consumers with reactions to aspartame products.

The following individuals, companies, institutions, journals, editors and publishers granted permission to reproduce pertinent data, excerpts, figures, tables and other material. The original sources appear in the text and bibliography.

Fredrick R. Abrams, M.D.
Annual Review of Nutrition
Jeffrey L. Bada, Ph.D.
Blackwell Scientific Publications Limited
Mr. William H. Boserman
British Medical Journal
Curtis Publishing Company, *Clinical Symposia* (Plates 6 and 7, Volume 30, 1980)
Diabetes

Elsevier Science
The Evening Times of West Palm Beach
John C. Floyd, M.D.
Clifford Grobstein, M.D.
International Life Sciences Institute-Nutrition Foundation
  (*Nutrition Reviews*)
Journal of the American Medical Association
Journal of Applied Nutrition
Journal of Clinical Endocrinology and Metabolism
Journal of Chromatography
Journal of the Florida Medical Association
Journal of Pesticide Reform
Journal of Toxicology and Environmental Health
The Lancet
Mr. Rodney E. Leonard
Rodger A. Liddle, M.D.
Walter M. Lovenberg, Ph.D.
Marcel Dekker, Inc. (publisher of *Aspartame: Physiology and Biochemistry* by L. Stegink and L. J. Filer, Jr., 1984)
Medical Tribune
Medical World News
Modern Medicine
Woodrow C. Monte, Ph.D.
Mrs. Barbara Mullarkey
New England Journal of Medicine
The News/Sun-Sentinel of Fort Lauderdale
William M. Pardridge, M.D.
The Palm Beach Post
Professor Darden Asbury Pyron
Scandinavian Journal of Clinical and Laboratory Investigation
Southern Medical Journal
Charles C Thomas (publisher of *Disease of Medical Progress: A Study of Iatrogenic Disease* by R. H. Moser, M.D., 3rd edition, 1969)
John B. Thomison, M.D. (Editor, *Southern Medical Journal*)
Transactions of the Association of American Physicians
James S. Turner, Esquire
Richard J. Wurtman, M.D.

DISCLAIMERS

PREFACE

"The beginning of wisdom is to call things
by the right names."
Chinese Proverb

"When we sit back and look at it, we live in a
sea of nutrition misinformation directed to the
general public."
Allen L. Forbes, M.D. (1986)
(former Director of Nutrition and
Food Sciences, Food and
Drug Administration)

"The scientist...must be free to ask any question,
to doubt any assertion, to seek for any evidence,
to correct any errors."
J. Robert Oppenheimer

Aspartame is the generic name of a chemical sweetener currently being consumed by over half the population. The serious reactions to aspartame previously described by me are amplified in this book; some are cited for the first time.

Aspartame disease, a term I coined, is a medical and public health problem that continues to escalate. The fact that my own database exceeds 1,200 aspartame "victims" suggests its magnitude, and validates "**epidemic**" in the title. Its use is consistent with Hippocratic writings: "When a large number of people all catch the same disease at the same time, the cause must be ascribed to something common to all" (Rosenberg 1992).

Persons justifiably regard the word epidemic with skepticism, especially when uttered by public health officials having biased agendas. Although Dr. Flexner was referring to the epidemic of viral encephalitis lethargica between 1918 and 1930, his comment also could apply to aspartame disease: "The disease in spite of all barriers penetrated into England and Wales *in advance of the literature concerning it*" (cited by *The Lancet* 2000; Volume 355:509) (italics by the author).

The attitude of both the medical profession and the Food and Drug Administration (FDA) remains one of virtual denial. Indeed, the November/December 1999 issue of *FDA Consumer Magazine* stressed, "FDA stands behind its original approval of aspartame, and subsequent evaluations have shown that the product is safe." This is remarkable in view of the literal flood of complaints **volunteered** by irate consumers to this agency.

I continue to be inundated with requests for **specific** details about aspartame disease from patients, concerned relatives and friends of these sufferees, health professionals, the media, and various consumer groups. Hundreds of such letters, calls and e-mail messages are received monthly. Additionally, some were from high school and college students who selected aspartame disease as the topic for their research projects... often when a relative had been afflicted.

Another plea that stimulated completion of this volume pertained to requests for **updated** material when individuals realized the relevance of aspartame disease to problems confronting them or their families. Examples are its causative or aggravating role in headache, depression, convulsions, impaired vision, obesity, diabetes mellitus, hypoglycemia, multiple sclerosis, addiction, arthritis, Alzheimer's disease, and even brain tumors.

More Factors Influencing the Decision

I procrastinated completing this book in the face of mounting incriminatory evidence, anticipating that aspartame products would be declared an "imminent public health hazard" and removed from the market. But this scenario failed to materialize... and remains unlikely. In effect, powerful corporate interests emasculated earlier conservative cautions about aspartame use, and intimidated the FDA and other organizations with this economic/political hot potato. Furthermore, they are now launching programs to incorporate analogs of aspartame in "nutraceutical" foods. (PR agencies favor this term because "nutra" sounds better than "nutri.")

Two aspects involving my conscience as a doctor and citizen reinforced this commitment. One was failure to stimulate a new Congressional hearing aimed at clarifying the nature and extent of aspartame disease despite much personal correspondence. The other was FDA approval of aspartame as a general purpose sweetener in June 1996. This meant that the chemical could be added to virtually every category of food and beverage.

Another incentive for completing this volume has been the revolutionary role of the Internet in exposing societal health threats. It is a corporate-neutral, worldwide forum for constructive dialogue used by intelligent individuals to clarify perceived evolving problems – in this instance, aspartame disease – and to bypass professional/bureaucratic bias and self-serving business interests.

WHAT KIND OF BOOK?

I debated the nature of this manuscript relative to content and likely readership. For proper presentation, the amount of clinical and scientific data would necessitate many pages. As the author of previous large texts, I realized that a costly tome might discourage potential readers. When daunted by its projected size, however, I was consoled by this unappreciative response of the Duke of Gloucester in 1781 on receiving Edward Gibbon's *The History of the Decline and Fall of the Roman Empire*: "Another damned, thick, square book!"

The compromise involved a distillate aimed at **both** professional and general readers. It attempts consilience, a term that denotes the linking of facts and fact-based theory from various disciplines. This reflects a remarkable paradox: concerned "non-medical" persons often are as interested in the details as doctors and dietitians. Indeed, many invited medicalese in their correspondence.

The decision to use *Aspartame Disease* as the title was made after prolonged reflection. It **is** appropriate because this affliction fulfills these four Koch-like postulates:

- There is an identifiable cause.
- Symptoms and signs follow such exposure, and are reproducible in a given individual.
- Improvement occurs after avoiding aspartame products (not always an easy feat).
- The same complaints usually promptly recur on challenge.

I had to consider another criticism: some might equate this opus with the Pygmalion effect – that is, an author infatuated with his subject. If my effort convinces doubting Thomases who repeatedly insist on more medical data and scientific evidence in order to come to grips with the aspartame epidemic, I accept the implication.

I have omitted the names of trademarked products containing aspartame except where they appear in official documents within the public domain. This is consistent with **the scientific nature and corporate neutrality of my inquiry**. I frequently refer to aspartame products by several acronyms – notably, ACB for aspartame cola beverages, ASD for aspartame soft drinks, and ATS for aspartame tabletop sweetener.

The **bibliography** contains many references to the pertinent clinical and scientific literature, as well as my earlier publications.

SOME RELEVANT QUESTIONS

The following questions orient readers to the perceived enormity and serious nature of aspartame disease:

- Did you know that at least two-thirds of the adult population currently consumes products containing aspartame, as do an estimated 40 percent of children?
- Did you know that FDA in-house scientists, consultants for the General Accounting Office, and a Public Board of Inquiry urged this agency **NOT** to approve aspartame for human use?
- Did you know that the approving FDA Commissioner ignored (a) impressive evidence in animals indicating the induction of brain tumors by this neurotoxic chemical, and (b) an important law (the Delaney Clause) aimed at preventing the approval for human consumption of any substance shown to cause experimental cancer?

- Did you know that the FDA continues to condone the sale of this chemical in thousands of products despite numerous complaints **volunteered** by outraged consumers who suffered severe reactions, often with considerable personal and economic loss?
- Did you know that the FDA regards serious reactions (such as convulsions) to products containing aspartame as "only anecdotal idiosyncrasies" that do **not** have to be reported because of its "Generally Recognized As Safe" (GRAS) classification?
- Did you know that most physicians remain ignorant of aspartame disease, or adamantly refuse to accept its legitimacy? This reflects a virtual blackout of information for doctors and consumer groups about the adverse effects of aspartame, and apathy/resistance by professional organizations and publications receiving corporate largesse.
- Did you know that the successful public relations barrage aimed at promoting aspartame products includes much troubling disinformation – most notably, its purported safety for pregnant women?
- Did you know that the majority of flawed "scientific" studies being used to defuse concern about the safety of aspartame products were funded by industry? The shortcomings variously pertain to the materials used, the amounts and methods of administration, the nature of control subjects, the duration of such studies, the contents of presumed placebos, and arbitrary interpretation of the results.

IMPLICATIONS OF ASPARTAME DISEASE

It is my opinion that hundreds of thousands of consumers in the United States, more likely millions, currently suffer major reactions to products containing aspartame. Corporate-sponsored academics arrogantly ridicule their diversity by calling them "a textbook of medicine."

I coined the neologism "aspartame disease" to encompass its symptoms, complications, public health implications, and medicolegal ramifications. The basic issue, however, is contained in an observation by philosopher J. L. Austen that it does not matter what name is used as long as the reference is valid.

Even after nearly two decades of interest in this realm, I encounter unanticipated revelations, some alarming. Examples are eating and memory disorders, chronic refractory fatigue, aspartame addiction, "fibromyalgia," hyperthyroidism, unexplained retinal changes (including pseudotumor cerebri), carpal tunnel syndrome, the simulation or precipitation of multiple sclerosis and systemic lupus erythematosus, dual sensitivity to aspartame and monosodium glutamate (MSG), brain cancer, and the profound effects of chronic methanol poisoning.

These serendipitous insights generated novel concepts about the nature of many important diseases. In turn, they necessitated probing and rethinking pertinent aspects in such disciplines as biochemistry, neurophysiology, food technology, epidemiology and toxicology. This "experiment of nature" created by aspartame use reminded me of the need to rethink (re-search) most diseases after the introduction of cortisone in medical practice. In this sense, *Aspartame Disease: An Ignored Epidemic* could be regarded as a new commentary on contemporary medicine.

None of the conclusions and projections from this agonizing reappraisal are casual. The "Alzheimer connection" provides an example. Alzheimer's disease obviously existed long before the availability of aspartame. But its simulation by the confusion and memory loss suffered by scores of aspartame victims in their 30s and 40s had led neurologists to diagnose "probable early Alzheimer's disease" before the correct diagnosis was fortuitously made. As dementia continues to escalate in younger persons, these and other important leads – elaborated in *Defense Against Alzheimer's Disease* (Roberts 1995b) – cannot be ignored.

This experience teaches another vital lesson: *vast harm can result when products created in the ongoing drug and food technology revolution are released prematurely.* The absence of <u>premarketing long-term studies in humans</u> by <u>corporate-neutral investigators</u> using <u>"real world" products</u> compounds the danger.

I have engaged in independent patient-based clinical research involving various realms for more than four decades. They include pesticides (notably pentachlorophenol), products contaminated with toxic metals, arbitrary severe caloric restriction, megadoses of vitamin E, antistatic clothes softeners, fluoridation of water, and even vasectomy. I repeatedly stressed two pertinent issues. First, a long time may be required to identify the hazards of new products and medical interventions, particularly drugs and industrial chemicals. Second, it may take even longer for these risks to be acknowledged by physicians and public health officials.

ADDITIONAL COMMENTS

Several added points deserve <u>clarification for critical readers</u>.

ITEM 1. I wrote this book myself. (The term "authentic" comes from a Greek word meaning "one who does things with his own hands.") There were no collaborators, "ghost writers," or editors.

ITEM 2. I am not an anti-corporate technophobe whose aim is to conjure up phantom risks.

ITEM 3. The many case histories presented are a representative sampling. Inasmuch as numerous other aspartame reactors gave convincing accounts of comparable and reproducible afflictions, the process of selection proved challenging.

ITEM 4. Use of term "aspartame" in the case reports and elsewhere is usually synonymous with "aspartame products."

ITEM 5. The considerable cross-referencing of complaints is justified because most persons with aspartame disease suffer multiple reactions.

ITEM 6. There has been no intent of bias or malice to any manufacturers, physicians or researchers who may disagree with my data or projections.

Publication of this extensive work reflects several <u>other considerations</u>. First, it enables an in-depth presentation of the clinical experience and scientific validation for aspartame disease. Such detail counters the repetitious criticism about "only anecdotal evidence."

Second, the reader is provided with insights and adequate discussions about related major public health issues.

Third, an array of corporate/bureaucratic/legal obstacles to information and regulation, and commentaries thereon, are relevant not only to aspartame but also future analogs of this chemical and other "supplements."

Fourth, valuable pointers, precautions and options are summarized for both consumers and doctors.

8

Fifth, the volume enables access to considerable cross-referenced material, the inclusion of a number of "position papers" that concisely address basic issues or questions directed to me, and an extensive bibliography.

Corporate Neutrality

I take pride in my corporate neutrality. No grants or salary were received for this effort, which originated in clinical practice.

My sense of the need to maintain both autonomy and reputation dates back to antiquity. An interpretation of the statement by Moses, "Respect not Thou their offering. I have not taken one donkey from them" (*Numbers* 16:15), avers that a leader who receives considerable material benefit becomes tainted with the perception of opportunism.

Personal Nonmonetary Rewards

A physician who reports observations in an area as controversial as aspartame disease at times may wonder if such an unorthodox effort is worthwhile. When asked during a 1954 interview, "What about the risk of pursuing a theory for years and having it lead nowhere?", Albert Einstein aptly replied, "That is no risk. That is the fun" (*Sun-Sentinel* March 20, 1999, p. A-13).

Unsolicited correspondence from aspartame victims who expressed appreciation constituted profound personal rewards. A similar motif appeared as the title of a feature in *The Wall Street Journal* (February 28, 1994, p. B-1), "Dear Author: Your Book Has Changed My Life."

- Statements of gratitude appear in many of the excerpted letters.
- Unbeknown to me, dozens of grateful aspartame victims began calling themselves "Roberts' Angels." Some even named their babies Robert and Roberta!
- I discouraged the designation of "Roberts' disease" by anti-aspartame activists. It has been suggested that the naming of diseases after persons who discovered them is an important, nonmonetary reward for intellectual achievement in clinical research (Schafer 2000). Richard Asher (*Transactions of*

Medical Society of London 1959; Volume 79:66-72) allayed apprehension thereon with these comments: "The bestowal of a name upon a concept, whether real or imaginary, brings it into clinical existence"; and "A rose without a name may smell as sweet, but it has far less chance of being smelled."

I recognize that this exposition of aspartame disease will generate hostile criticism from corporate interests. Salman Rushdie, who had been condemned for alleged blasphemy, provided this comforting observation, "A writer's injuries are his strengths, and from his wounds will flow his sweetest, most startling dreams" (*The Miami Herald* February 9, 1999, p. A-2).

West Palm Beach, Florida   H. J. Roberts, M.D., F.A.C.P., F.C.C.P.

OVERVIEW

"If anything can go wrong, it will."
    Murphy's Law

"Human history becomes more and more a race
between education and catastrophe."
    H. G. Wells

"The fight against future plagues is fought as much
by education, economics, equity, justice, and fairness
to all people, as by science and technology."
    Professor P. J. John (1999)

This overview of aspartame disease considers some basic issues: the nature of the chemical aspartame; its approval for human use as a safe substance; the magnitude of aspartame consumption; and reasons for escalating concern. One anti-aspartame activist estimated that $60 billion are spent annually on medical procedures relating to unrecognized aspartame disease... exclusive of loss in productivity. The public health and societal implications are also profound.

A. ASPARTAME

Aspartame was approved as a sweetener by the Food and Drug Administration (FDA) in dry form in July 1981, in carbonated beverages in July 1983, as an additive to multivitamins in May 1984, and as a general all-purpose sweetener in June 1996. Two key official rulings were published by the FDA on July 15, 1981 and July 8, 1983 (see References).

Aspartame is 180-200 times more sweet than table sugar (sucrose). It has been marketed under a variety of popular brand names, most notably NutraSweet® and Equal®.

Aspartame is a synthetic substance manufactured by combining the amino acids L-phenylalanine and L-aspartic acid with the ester of methyl alcohol (Figure 5-1). Methyl alcohol is also referred to as methanol and wood alcohol. The scientific literature refers to this compound as "aspartylphenylalanine-methylester" and "a phenylalanine-containing dipeptide."

The patent protection enjoyed by The NutraSweet Company expired on December 14, 1992. The firm, however, had 70 additional production process and distribution patents.

B. THE ALLEGED SAFETY OF ASPARTAME

The FDA Commissioner who approved aspartame for human use asserted that "few compounds have withstood such detailed testing and repeated close scrutiny" (46 *Federal Register* p. 38289, July 24, 1981). The agency still maintains this position.

- Dr. Sanford Miller, Chief of the FDA Bureau of Foods, stated, "I don't know of any substance in recent years that has been looked at with the intensity of aspartame. No one has yet come up with the slightest evidence to show that we were wrong in approving it" (*Congressional Record* 1985a, p.S 5493).

- Dr. Frank E. Young, a subsequent FDA Commissioner, testified before a Senate hearing on November 3, 1987:

  > "In conclusion, we do not have any medical or scientific evidence that undermines our confidence in the safety of aspartame. This confidence is based on years of study, analysis of adverse reactions, and research in the scientific community, including studies supported by the FDA."

- Once the FDA approved aspartame as a general all-purpose sweetener, it could be added to virtually all products – including baking goods. The only remaining limitation was that baked goods not contain more than a 0.5 percent aspartame.

The Public's Perception

A manufacturer of aspartame asserts that its "two building blocks of protein" are contained in "over half the food you eat today," and the body "treats them no differently than if they came from a peach or a string bean or a glass of milk" (*Newsweek* June 30, 1986, p. 25). Television ads infer aspartame to be as natural as bananas and cows, causing most viewers to conclude that it comes from "natural sources" or is "organic."

A "natural" attribute, however, does not preclude toxicity of that substance when consumed in excessive amounts. This applies, for example, to amino acids – "the building blocks of protein". Paracelsus, a famous physician in medical history, declared in his third "defection" (August 19, 1538): "Everything is a poison; the dose alone makes a thing not a poison."

Professional Perceptions

The safety of aspartame products has been repeatedly stressed to the medical and dietetic professions.

- The Council on Scientific Affairs of the American Medical Association (1985) issued such a favorable report.
- Physicians routinely recommend aspartame to diabetic patients as "a safe low-calorie sweetener with no undesirable aftertaste" (Horwitz 1983).

- The American Dietetic Association continues to assert that aspartame is innocuous for most persons. Furthermore, when reduced calories and carbohydrates are desired, dietitians tend to recommend the use of a widely-advertised aspartame tabletop sweetener. Their enthusiasm is heightened by the absence of both saccharin and sodium.

- A position statement by the American Diabetes Association (1987) emphasized that "...aspartame has been determined to be safe for the general population as well as for people with diabetes." It approved the consumption of an aspartame tabletop sweetener by diabetics as a "free exchange" – that is, containing less than one gram (gm) carbohydrate and only four calories per packet – and because it has the "clean sweet taste" of two teaspoons of sugar.

- The Centers for Disease Control (CDC) (1984) officially interpreted the majority of adverse effects that had been voluntarily reported by consumers as an infrequent "unusual sensitivity to the product."

- An ad appearing in the July 4, 1986 issue of the *Journal of the American Medical Association* emphasized that aspartame "is metabolized by the body as protein."

- Dr. Gerald E. Gaull (1986), representing the NutraSweet Company, asserted in the *New England Journal of Medicine*: "Aspartame is used by over 100 million people in the United States, and it is remarkable that the product has been associated with so few idiosyncratic reactions, even at the anecdotal level."

- Noted nutritionists provided their approval. Dr. Frederick J. Stare (1986), Harvard University Department of Nutrition, maintained: "In general, aspartame is safe for use by everyone, with the exception of those individuals who have the metabolic disorder called phenylketonuria."

- Apparently unaware of its severe systemic effects (Chapter II-E), the British Dental Association recommended aspartame chewing gum to help prevent tooth decay.

Producers emphasize the unprecedented research concerning the safety of aspartame relative to its metabolism, pharmacology, toxicology, teratology (birth defects), and mutagenicity (genetic changes). Inquiring professionals are furnished many reprints and an impressive bibliography of studies done at leading medical centers. (The vast majority were funded by this industry.)

As a result, most physicians and dietitians routinely recommend aspartame products "to avoid sugar" for patients with diabetes, hypoglycemia and weight problems. *The Equal®Times* (March 8, 1987) alleged that the use of a popular aspartame tabletop sweetener facilitates weight loss. It indicated that 2,262 calories of this product is equivalent to ten pounds of sugar (18,080 calories), a reduction of 15,820 calories.

There is the concomitant inference that coronary heart disease might be prevented by avoiding sugar and extra calories.

International Authorities and Regulatory Agencies

The aspartame industry stresses that regulatory authorities around the world concur aspartame has passed one of the most comprehensive testing programs ever undertaken for a food additive. As of October 1986, the following list of organizations definitively "reviewed studies pertaining to aspartame," and were satisfied with the safety data they received.

Regulatory

- The World Health Organization of the United Nations, December 1980
- Food and Agricultural Organization, December 1980
- The Canadian Health Protection Branch, August 1981
- The Food and Drug Administration, July 1981 for dry foods, and July 1983 for carbonated beverages
- The United Kingdom Committee on Toxicity of Chemicals in Food Consumer Products and the Environment, October 1983

Scientific

- British Toxicology Committee, October 1983
- Centers for Disease Control, November 1984
- American Medical Association, July 1985
- Epilepsy Institute, March 1986
- American Diabetes Association, June 1986

Legal

- District Court, April 1984
- Court of Appeals, September 1985
- U.S. Supreme Court, April 1986

Regulatory authorities in more than 100 countries have approved the use of aspartame products – along with the Joint Expert Committee on Food Additives of the World Health Organization, the United Nations Food Agriculture Organization, the Scientific Committee on Foods of the European Commission, and the European Parliament. Other organizations and agencies that endorse the safety of aspartame include the American Dietetic Association (July 1993), the American Cancer Society (1996), the American Dental Association (July 1981), and the American Council on Science and Health (March 1993).

There is a major problem with the foregoing stamps of approval. These organizations did **not** insist upon independent confirmatory studies by corporate-neutral investigators.

C. ASPARTAME CONSUMPTION

It is conservatively estimated by the <u>National Center for Health Statistics</u> that *two-thirds of adults in the United States consume aspartame products, and nearly 40 percent of children up to the age of nine regularly drink soft drinks containing artificial sweeteners.*

A March 1998 survey by the <u>Caloric Control Council</u> indicated that about 73 percent of adults in the United States currently use "light" foods and soft drinks. (Booth Research Services, Inc. sampled 1,163 persons 18 years and older.) The CCC study further revealed that consumers regularly partake of <u>at least four</u> different types of low-calorie products – notably diet soft drinks, sugar-free gum, and substitutes.

- The most popular were diet soft drinks, being taken by 60 percent of low-calorie product consumers.
- Low-calorie products were used by 78 percent of women, compared to 67 percent of men.
- In recent years, the popularity of sugar-free frozen dessert, ice cream and frozen yogurt has soared.

An estimated 800 million pounds of aspartame have been consumed since its approval for human use. Even in 1985, the consumption averaged 5.8 pounds per person. (This is the equivalent of 1.6 <u>billion</u> pounds of sugar.) Americans drink more soda beverages than coffee and tap water <u>combined</u> (*The Wall Street Journal* June 8, 1999, p. B-1)!

These are some of the more than 9,000 products containing aspartame:

16

- cola beverages
- soft drinks
- tabletop sweeteners
- hot chocolate
- diet pudding/diet gelatin
- chewing gum
- presweetened tea
- presweetened cereals
- mouth washes
- toothpaste
- bulk laxatives
- numerous drug and vitamin preparations, especially for children
  – for example, chewable acetaminophen, a non-aspirin analgesic
- "diet water"

Joking that "aspartame is everywhere," a patient quipped, "If it's not on your right in a market, it's on your left."

Many reactors were reluctant to admit the amount of aspartame products they used in anticipation of an amazed response (see Chapter II-C). Such reluctance was striking among persons with aspartame addiction (Chapter VII-G). For example, a recently-diagnosed diabetic woman who suffered headaches, dizziness and palpitations over a seven-year period wrote, "I average about 101 ounces of diet cola a day... yes, you read it right."

Extended Uses

The escalation of aspartame production and consumption seems limited only by the imagination of producers and their advertising consultants, and the time required for FDA approval.

- The FDA approved the extended use of aspartame in juice drinks, frozen novelties, tea beverages and breath mints in 1986. These were envisioned to generate total annual commercial sales of $6 billion (*The Wall Street Journal* November 26, 1986, p.9).
- Aspartame sprays have been used as an aid to dieting, presumably by saturating tongue receptors and inducing satiety. Their flavors include chocolate, apple cinnamon, and peanut butter and jelly. My reservations for these products are similar to those for gum (Chapter II-E).

- Reports of lowered serum cholesterol with the use of psyllium hydrophilic mucilloid preparations containing aspartame by hypercholesterolemic patients (Anderson 1988) increased their intake.
- There has been an increasing tendency for adults to replace coffee with aspartame-sweetened cola beverages. This phenomenon was triggered by sophisticated ads aimed at persons desiring "a cool refreshing drink to come alive."
- Drug companies continually market "sugar free" variations of conventional products. Their aspartame content, however, may not be known either to the consumer or prescribing doctor, as in the case of a popular calcium carbonate supplement. Repeated encounters of this problem necessitated trips for verification to drug stores by the author.
- The owner of a "sex toy store" indicated that edible lotions containing aspartame are available for his clientele.
- An adhesive applications firm apparently embarked on a project aimed at including aspartame on the back of Postal Service stamps to improve their taste.
- At least one "lubricating gel" contains aspartame.
- Personal fitness trainers have noted the considerable consumption of aspartame products by "bodybuilders."

A Marketing Miracle

Businessmen refer to aspartame products as "the marketing miracle of the 1980s." In the United States, sales exceeded $750 million during 1986, indicating that this "sweet taste of success" had captured the taste buds of the American public. The United States currently accounts for 83 percent of world aspartame consumption – an estimated 151 million adults using low-calorie, sugar-free foods and beverages according to the Calorie Control Council. Negative attitudes to both sugar and saccharin contributed to this phenomenon. An impressed Ted Koppel asked on the May 29, 1985 edition of *Nightline*, "Is it (aspartame) too late – and too big – to be challenged?"

The demand for aspartame products in the United States, Western Europe and Japan is expected to increase about 5.5 percent annually.

The following statistics about **United States** consumption are relevant.

- "Diet" beverages represent the greatest growth in the soft drink market. Even a decade ago, consumers drank up to six times more diet drinks as sugared sodas (*The Wall Street Journal* June 27, 1988, p. 20).

- Once a popular aspartame-sweetener cola beverage was marketed, other manufacturers hastily introduced their "diet" soft drinks as consumers sought "the fizz without the sugar and calories."

- Aspartame products deeply penetrated major fast-food chains and eating establishments.

- The incorporation of aspartame in chewing gum revitalized the profits of several gum producers, in part because its sweetness lasts up to five times longer than regular gum. (Its unique hazards are amplified in Chapter II-E.)

- Consumption of the two leading brands of aspartame colas rank them #3 and #6 among beverages consumed in the United States. In effect, they have become mainstream soft drinks.

- According to the Department of Agriculture, the per capita consumption of aspartame rose from zero pounds in 1980 to 14 pounds in 1990, while that of saccharin fell from 7.7 to 6.0 pounds. These dramatic changes appear in Table OV-1.

U.S. per capita consumption of caloric and low-calorie sweeteners

Calendar year	Refined sugar	Corn sweeteners 1/				Total of all caloric sweeteners 2/3/	Sac-charin	Aspar-tame	Total of low-calorie sweeteners 4/	Total of all sweeteners	Population
		HFCS	Glucose	Dextrose	Total 2/						
				Pounds per capita							Millions
1970	101.8	0.7	14.0	4.6	19.3	122.6	5.8	0.0	5.8	128.4	205.1
1971	102.1	0.9	14.9	5.0	20.8	124.3	5.1	0.0	5.1	129.4	207.6
1972	102.3	1.3	15.4	4.4	21.1	124.9	5.1	0.0	5.1	130.0	209.9
1973	100.8	2.1	16.5	4.8	23.4	125.6	5.1	0.0	5.1	130.7	211.9
1974	95.7	3.0	17.2	4.9	25.1	121.9	5.9	0.0	5.9	127.8	213.9
1975	89.2	5.0	17.5	5.0	27.5	118.1	6.1	0.0	6.1	124.2	216.0
1976	93.4	7.2	17.5	5.0	29.7	124.4	6.1	0.0	6.1	130.5	218.0
1977	94.2	9.5	17.6	4.1	31.2	126.8	6.6	0.0	6.6	133.4	220.2
1978	91.4	12.1	17.8	3.8	33.7	126.6	6.9	0.0	6.9	133.5	222.6
1979	89.3	14.9	17.9	3.6	36.3	127.1	7.3	0.0	7.3	134.4	225.0
1980	83.6	19.1	17.6	3.5	40.2	125.1	7.7	0.0	7.7	132.8	227.7
1981	79.4	23.2	17.8	3.5	44.5	125.1	8.0	0.2	8.2	133.3	230.0
1982	73.7	26.7	18.0	3.5	48.2	123.2	8.4	1.0	9.4	132.6	232.3
1983	71.1	30.7	18.0	3.5	52.2	124.6	9.5	3.5	13.0	137.6	234.5
1984	67.4	36.3	18.0	3.5	57.8	126.6	10.0	5.8	15.8	142.5	237.0
1985	63.0	45.0	18.0	3.5	66.5	130.9	6.0	12.0	18.0	142.4	239.3
1986	60.2	45.6	18.0	3.5	67.1	128.7	5.5	13.0	18.5	148.9	241.6
1987	62.2	47.3	18.0	3.5	68.8	132.4	5.5	13.5	19.0	147.2	243.9
1988 5/	62.6	48.0	17.9	3.6	69.5	133.5	6.0	14.0	20.0	152.4	246.1

1/ Dry basis. 2/ May not precisely add to total of individual items because of rounding. 3/ Includes honey and edible syrups.
4/ Sugar sweetness equivalent. Assumes saccharin is 300 times as sweet as sugar and aspartame is 200 times as sweet as sugar.
5/ Forecast

SOURCE: ERS, USDA estimates.

Sugar and Sweetener, Situation and Outlook Yearbook
USDA Economic Research Service, June 1988
Table OV-1

- Thayer (1991) listed the increased use of aspartame by 1990, compared to other food additives.

	1990 sales $ millions	Function
Aspartame	$ 750	Sweetener
Vanillin ethyl vanillin	160	Flavoring
Citric acid	160	Acidulant
Monosodium glutamate	75	Flavor enhancer
Xanthan gum	50	Thickener
Sorbates	55	Preservative
Carrageenan	45	Thickener
Caramel	40	Colorant

- The average American consumer used an estimated 134.6 pounds of caloric sweeteners and 20 pounds of non-caloric sweeteners in 1990.
- By 1991, the aspartame-created revolution in the dairy industry resulted in more than 100 frozen novelties, 50 frozen yogurts, and 80 frozen daily desserts containing this sweetener (*Prepared Foods* May 1991, p. 123).
- Many "New Age" beverages – including flavored and essenced waters, gourmet and natural soft drinks, and carbonated juice drinks – are sweetened with aspartame.
- *Food Engineering* (August 1993, p. 26) reported that the aspartame industry was a $4.1 billion business in 1993.
- U.S. consumers spent $54 billion on sodas in one year, more than double the amount for books (*Centers for Science in the Public Interest Newsletter* October 21, 1998).
- The ongoing expansion of "smart" vending machines enables cashless buying – either with a credit or debit card, or by charging a cellular phone account.

The **worldwide** consumption of aspartame also increased dramatically.

- The consumption of aspartame cola beverages during 1986 grew 27 percent in 70 markets worldwide.
- An estimated 300 metric tons of aspartame were being consumed annually in Canada during 1987, with estimated sales of $30 million

(*The Wall Street Journal* July 8, 1987.) The heavy use of a popular aspartame cola by Canadians in 1986 caused it to capture eight percent of that country's overall soft drink market.

- India amended its Food Products Order to allow the use of aspartame in fruit juices and jams, effective June 15, 1997.

- Virtually all other sugar substitutes were replaced by aspartame-containing products in stores abroad. The author confirmed this in several countries when attempting to buy a standard brand of saccharin tablets (marketed internationally as Hermesetas®). Stores and pharmacies no longer stocked it, but had large stocks of an aspartame tabletop sweetener.

- Britons consume more than *nine billion* cans or bottles of soft drinks a year, of which about half contain aspartame (*Sunday Times* of London, February 27, 2000).

With the overt promotion of "high-quality and cheap" aspartame by a major Chinese chemical company in August 2000, its international consumption seems destined to increase drastically. A concerned resident of Hong Kong equated plans to sell aspartame products to at least 80 million Chinese as "handwriting on the Great Wall."

D. ADVERTISEMENT OF ASPARTAME

Exposure to media hype promoting aspartame products has become enormous. Consumers are exposed to such ad images daily in newspapers, television, road signs, and elsewhere. This has contributed to the widespread "fear of fat," especially among women with eating disorders (Chapter IX-B).

The PR Siege

The American public and its health professionals continue to be bombarded with campaigns promoting aspartame products. Their success confirms Oscar Wilde's remark, "The only way to get rid of the temptation is to yield to it." Others have joked on the matter in more specific terms.

- The extensive incorporation of aspartame in desserts has been termed "sweet abandon."

- The seductive nature of aspartame-sweetened products is variously described as "hedonic sweetness" and "Eve's apple."
- The phrase, "La Cuisine du Diable Lite" ("the Devil's lite recipe"), appeared in an influential French magazine.

The amounts spent for advertising were impressive even 15 years ago.

- The producers of several popular aspartame colas spent $34.4 million and $10.1 million in ads during 1986, exclusive of the advertising campaigns by bottlers (*The Wall Street Journal* June 3, 1987, p. 33). These costs were slightly less than for their "regular" cola beverages.
- Three of Video Storyboard's ten most popular television ad campaigns at the time were for aspartame products (*The Miami Herald* February 27, 1987, p. E-1).
- The number of expensive ads for two aspartame products in selected medical, pharmaceutical and nursing journals tripled between August 1985 and August 1986.

Some regarded this aspartame blitz – costing more than $100 million a year – as the largest advertising campaign designed around a product ingredient. The celebrities paid to make pitches for these products including Bill Cosby, Raquel Welch, Tony Bennet, Billy Crystal, Joe Montana, Dan Marino, Marvin Hagler, and Geraldine Ferraro (former Democratic Vice-Presidential candidate). New media stars were hastily solicited to promote diet drinks and other aspartame products, including Roger Rabbit (the animated movie character).

Additionally, the package designs of aspartame products, especially diet sodas, were devised to make them objects of desire. Ellen Ruppel Shell described such "silent salesmen" as generating customers "hungry for things they don't need, even for things they don't want" (*Smithsonian* April 1996, p. 55).

Targeted Youth

Children are targeted in this campaign. Even concerned parents cannot counter the sophisticated child-oriented promos for famous-brand gelatins and puddings. Their appeal is enhanced through enthusiastic promotions by stars identified with family-oriented humor. In one television commercial, a boy referred to aspartame as "the good stuff."

Consumption of diet sodas by one- to three-year-old children predictably escalated. A survey for the Department of Agriculture by National Analysis Inc. estimated the mean to be **seven** fluid ounces daily.

The massive promotion oriented to figure-conscious teenagers and young adults surpassed that of cigarette advertisements in previous decades. There is one notable difference: aspartame products do <u>not</u> carry health warnings comparable to those mandated for cigarettes by the Surgeon General... with the now-arbitrary exception of reference to phenylketonuria (PKU). Most persons, however, have no inkling about the nature or prevalence of PKU.

Furthermore, diet soft drinks have become a primary source of caffeine among young persons. Wiedner and Istvan (1985) reported that soft drinks accounted for half the caffeine intake by persons 18-24 years a decade ago.

Targeted Health- and Weight-Conscious Persons

Advertising agencies promote aspartame products to a health-conscious public by exploiting fear and insecurity in our fear-of-fat culture.

- A six-page insert in a national television magazine titled, "Guide to Health & Fitness," emphasized the value of a popular tabletop sweetener in "slimming down" and "the difference it can make on your waistline!"
- A "fitness water" containing aspartame (appearing only in the label's fine print) is promoted to health-conscious women.

A promotional tactic used at the U.S. 1988 Figure Skating Olympic Finals illustrates the matter. The sign of this event for television audiences was flanked on either side by ads of comparable size for NutraSweet®. The subliminal inference while watching graceful and skaters was as convincing as the beautiful bodies who emerge from the ocean smiling as they purportedly rejoice with aspartame sodas.

The extraordinary paradox of aspartame-associated <u>weight gain</u> is detailed in Chapter IX-B. It recalls a definition for foxhunting: "Pursuit of the inevitable for the inedible."

E. THE ECONOMIC IMPACT

The "diet" food and soft drink industries using sugar substitutes generate over $7 billion in retail sales annually according to the Calorie Control Council, a trade group. Pardridge (1986) once projected that aspartame consumption would approach 25 percent the overall consumption of sugar during the 1990s.

The *negative impact on the sugar cane industry* underscores this economic achievement. (The author has received NO grant or support from the sugar industry.) It became coupled with a reduction of price supports for domestic sugar cane and sugar beet crops, and the intense protection afforded major exporters in other countries. The European Economic Community went from being a major importer of sugar to a net exporter, shipping 4-5 million tons annually.

- From 1981 to 1987, eight U.S. sugar refineries closed and five companies went out of business according to Senator John Breaux (*The Miami Herald* July 19, 1987, p. PB-5).
- The reduction in sugar consumption after aspartame approval, with a concomitant increase of corn sweeteners and total caloric intake, is indicated by these per capita figures (in pounds) compiled by the Economic Research Service and the U.S. Department of Agriculture. (Aspartame was licensed during July 1981, and for soft drinks during July 1983.)

Year	Refined Sugar	Corn Sweeteners	Total Caloric Sweeteners
1975	89.2	27.5	118.1
1976	93.4	29.7	124.4
1977	94.2	31.2	126.8
1978	91.4	33.7	126.6
1979	89.3	36.4	127.1
1980	83.6	40.2	125.1
1981	79.4	44.5	125.1
1982	73.7	48.2	123.2
1983	71.1	52.2	124.6
1984	67.6	57.8	126.7
1985	63.3	66.6	131.4
1986	60.8	67.3	129.5
1987	62.1	67.8	131.3

- In response, sugar cane growers, refiners and processors throughout the country launched a $4 million campaign to focus on the "sweet, pure and natural" aspects of sugar (*News/Sun-Sentinel*, February 21, 1988, D-1).
- Due to loan forfeitures, sugar processors were forced to surrender over 300,000 tons to the government during 1985 (*News/Sun-Sentinel* of Fort Lauderdale, August 31, 1986, p. F-1). (Specifically, the sugar had been pledged as collateral for a Department of Agriculture loan equivalent to 17.97 cents per pound raw sugar, being due and payable before the end of the fiscal year. Even though sugar imports were restricted, the low market price forced some processors to forfeit part or all of their crop to the government in lieu of repaying the loans.)
- At an International Sugar Symposium, officials of this industry emphasized that cane refiners could be ruined, and beet producers forced to find other crops by the time the sugar program expired in September 1991 (*The Palm Beach Post* August 2, 1987, p. D-1).
- The bleak future projected for the sugar industry, coupled with changes in federal price supports and quotas, stimulated the replacement of sugar with other crops in the Florida Everglades.

The consumption of aspartame accelerated when patent rights expired on December 14, 1992 – with a decline in price. (As a point of reference, a 25 percent decline in the price of sugar tends to increase consumption by about 2.5 percent.) Within days after going off patent in Canada during July 1987, a Toronto firm began arrangements to import Japanese-manufactured aspartame.

Table OV-2 projected the increased use of aspartame and other food additives to 2000.

PROJECTED INCREASED USE OF FOOD ADDITIVES

(million dollars)

Item	1982	1989	1994	2000	% Annual Growth 89/82	94/89
Food Industry Shipments (bil $)	281	352	430	530	3.3	4.1
additives/000$ shpts	4.8	7.3	9.1	11.2	--	--
Food Additives by Type	1341	2563	3900	5930	9.7	8.8
Artificial Sweeteners	58	703	1395	2360	42.8	14.7
Flavors & Enhancers	332	463	630	865	4.9	6.4
Emulsifiers	207	276	350	465	4.2	4.9
Acidulants	171	275	350	450	7.0	4.9
Thickeners & Stabilizers	159	208	275	365	3.9	5.7
Antioxidants	85	149	205	275	8.3	6.6
Enzymes	94	139	177	235	5.7	5.0
Microbial Preservatives	66	90	120	165	4.5	5.9
Coloring Agents	45	61	85	123	4.4	6.9
Leavening Agents	12	15	18	22	3.4	3.7
Other Food Additives	112	184	295	605	7.3	9.9
Food Additives by Market	1341	2563	3900	5930	9.7	8.8
Soft Drinks	205	728	1170	1800	19.8	10.0
Sauces, Dressings, Oils	272	432	675	1090	6.8	9.3
Meat, Poultry, Seafood	211	330	455	630	6.6	6.6
Dairy Products	187	285	415	590	6.2	7.8
Baked Goods	159	273	395	610	8.0	7.7
Processed & Frozen Foods	82	148	220	330	8.8	8.3
Grain Mill Products	68	108	150	215	6.8	6.8
Alcoholic Beverages	34	53	70	95	6.5	5.7
Other Food Markets	123	206	350	570	7.6	11.2
Price Index (1982=100)	100.0	140.7	167.0	198.3	5.0	3.5
Food Additive Markets (bil 1982$)	1341	1822	2335	2990	4.5	5.1

Table OV-2

The success of aspartame also served to delay incentives by firms and researchers seeking new sugar substitutes, and FDA approval of Stevia as a "natural" sweetener.

The bias against saccharin proved an enormous advantage for this industry. It was largely based on urinary bladder tumors attributed to saccharin in limited rat studies. The President of the NutraSweet Company asserted that saccharin "had no reason for existence the instant there was another low-calorie sweetener" (cited by *The Argus* [Rock Island, Illinois], May 7, 1986). The scientific validity of these studies, and their significance for humans, has been challenged, culminating with the delisting of saccharin as a human carcinogen (Chapter XXVII-G).

F. EVOLVING DOUBTS: "GOING PUBLIC"

Like most physicians, the author had no reason to doubt the scientific basis for its safety when aspartame was approved by the FDA. My attitude changed, however, after repeatedly encountering serious reactions in my patients (Section 2) that seemed justifiably linked to use of such products.

These doubts increased after learning by mid-1986 that over 10,000 consumers had sent complaints to the FDA, the Centers for Disease Control (CDC), the manufacturer, interested investigators, and consumer organizations. It later became apparent that this number grossly underestimated the problem because most consumers are not inclined to submit reports of adverse reactions once they suspect the cause. Senator Howard Metzenbaum told a Senate hearing as far back as November 3, 1987 that the FDA had received "close to 4,000 consumer complaints ranging from seizures to headaches to mood alterations." Similarly, physicians are not required to do so for a GRAS (generally recognized as safe) additive.

Self-Diagnosis By Patients

Other patients in my practice had reached the same conclusion, and avoided aspartame-containing products. Ironically, they didn't mention it to me for fear of being labeled "a hypochondriac" (Chapter VII-A).

The ways in which these persons had deduced that aspartame products were **the** major cause of their difficulties evoked my admiration as a clinical researcher. Such insight often surfaced when they broke their routine (as while vacationing abroad) and did not have ready access to aspartame products, as in Cases III-12 and IV-13C.

- A 48-year-old woman with severe impairment of vision later attributed to aspartame sodas made this association while visiting Mexico. Her vision improved when she could obtain only regular sodas.
- A secretary experienced extreme fatigue, a recurrent rash, abdominal pains, and unexplained shortness of breath while drinking considerable diet sodas in an attempt to lose weight. Even though feeling ill, she agreed to accompany her husband to Switzerland for a trip he had won. She described her ensuing experience.

> "On the flight over, I felt terrible. I had a hard time breathing and felt my throat was closing up. After being there for ten days, I began to feel better. At the time, there was no aspartame in soda in Europe. I still had no idea then that aspartame was causing my problem."

Case Overview-1

A 42-year-old prominent business executive described his tribulations with recent severe headaches and visual difficulty. He had tried ibuprofen and new prescription glasses without benefit.

This patient then embarked on an effort to nail down the cause, chiefly at the insistence of a wise mother who firmly insisted, "It must be something in your diet, or some medicine you're taking." Over the ensuing months, he excluded most of the possibilities.

The breakthrough came when he vacationed in Europe and could not purchase aspartame products. His headaches and visual symptoms disappeared. They recurred when he resumed these drinks after returning home. His symptoms totally and permanently subsided over the ensuing seven months of aspartame abstinence.

More On the Author's Background

The reader is entitled to specifics about the author's interest and credentials.

At the time my observations on aspartame disease first evolved, I was a primary-care internist, medical consultant, and director of a corporate-neutral medical research organization. Patients with a broad spectrum of diagnostic and therapeutic difficulties were seen, generally after having consulted a number of physicians and clinics. This unique role stemmed from having authored many scientific articles and books. The first, *Difficult Diagnosis: A Guide To The Interpretation of Obscure Illness* (W. B. Saunders Company, 1958), had been used by more than 60,000 physicians in the United States.

In the mid-1980s, I became aware of subtle changes and challenges pertaining to both the diagnosis and management of patients whose difficulties later could be related <u>directly</u> to the use of aspartame products.

> A 16-year-old girl (Case III-2) had recurrent seizures that baffled several neurologists. Her convulsions stopped after avoiding aspartame products. An attack was then reproduced within three hours following rechallenge with one small serving of an aspartame pudding.

These insights led to <u>routinely</u> inquiring of "problem patients" about aspartame consumption. Their <u>prompt</u> improvement following abstinence indicated an evolving public health problem... at least within the context of my practice. Numerous persons having "mysterious ailments" came to realize that they were afflicted with aspartame disease when striking improvement occurred after stopping such products. Virtually every day became a learning experience as I delved into the numerous facets of aspartame disease.

The costs for multiple consultations and diagnostic studies confronting patients with unrecognized aspartame reactions – especially neurologic, ocular and allergic – proved equally impressive. The expense of unnecessary invasive testing, hospitalization, and even surgery was staggering in individual cases.

> A 29-year-old businessman suffered repeated seizures four months after he began ingesting aspartame. By the time I saw him, he had been subjected to <u>five</u> CT scans of the head, <u>three</u> magnetic resonance imaging (MRI) studies of the brain (each costing about $750), <u>five</u> electroencephalograms, and several hospitalizations.

Going Public

As my observations and researches continued, they generated professional anxiety as "a majority of one." But how could I remain silent when such a large segment of the population was now consuming aspartame? Furthermore, publication in prestigious medical

30

journals generally entailed a delay at least six months to a year IF the controversial manuscript was accepted <u>after</u> the several months required for peer review. I debated at length about "going public."

Others have faced this dilemma. Drs. Nicole Lurie and Martin Schapiro (1987) discussed, "Is The Pursuit Of Scientific Truth Always The Greatest Good? Ethical Issues In Health Care Research," for members of the American Federation for Clinical Research. One matter posed an enormous conflict – namely, "should scientific publication take precedence over the need for early public disclosure?"

It was easy to anticipate the multitude of arguments that could be leveled at me by physicians, scientists and the industry. Indeed, I could readily conjure up convincing armchair criticisms about the "anecdotal" nature of "idiosyncratic" complaints attributed to aspartame products.

Other motivating forces involving my professional commitment and conscience came into play.

- A poignant statement by Dr. Edmund Pellegrino, Director of Kennedy Institute of Ethics at Georgetown University, had an impact: "As a physician, you can't get off the hook of knowing how to make moral decisions" (*The Miami Herald* February 5, 1987, p. B-1).
- The motto of the British Royal Society is "*mullius in berba*." Historian Daniel J. Borstein provided this translation: "Take no body's word for it; see for yourself." In effect, this is what I had begun preaching to medical colleagues who had been told that aspartame disease is "nonsense."
- In his 1944 book, *Ventures in Science of a Country Surgeon*, Dr. Arthur E. Hertzler asserted, "When one wants to study a disease, one should read the description as recorded by the man first reporting it, if possible. Very often the account given in the old presents a clearer idea of the fundamentals... The calendar is no test."
- Dr. Jan P. Vandenbroucke (2001) emphasized the importance of case reporting and case series for the progress of medical science because they enable "discovery of new diseases and unexpected effects (adverse or beneficial) as well as the study of mechanisms."

Press Conferences and Medical Reports

On July 30, 1986, I presented my data on 100 aspartame reactors at a press conference in West Palm Beach. This summary was coupled with constructive recommendations for physicians, and precautionary information for the public. Acknowledging the limitations of the data in replying to a reporter, I stressed the urgency of researching and confirming my observations.

> "I think it would be a tragedy if this issue is ignored since we could be inviting disastrous medical, psychological and neurological problems. I hope I'm wrong. But let's look at the problem NOW instead of in five or 10 years when we might be having a medical plague on our hands."

The Community Nutrition Institute, a consumer organization, invited me to present my updated findings at a subsequent national press conference in Washington. I did so at the Dirksen Senate Building on October 16, 1986. The ensuing demand for this information proved impressive, including requests for interviews by two Philadelphia television stations.

These conferences and subsequent radio/television interviews served a more valuable function than ego gratification. They provided confirmatory input from a wider spectrum of the general population than I had been previously able to tap. Detailed disclosures about reactions to aspartame inundated my mail, particularly from persons completing the 9-page survey questionnaire (Section 4). Many described serious problems I had not even considered.

> The sister of a 23-year-old man wrote after viewing my interview on Philadelphia's TV Channel 10. He died in a tragic auto accident after apparently developing a seizure at the wheel. He had been consuming up to four gallons of an aspartame cola beverage daily. This and comparable reports later culminated in *Ignored Health Hazards For Pilots and Drivers* (Roberts 1998).

I delivered my first scientific report on 360 aspartame reactors to the Section on Medicine of the Southern Medical Association on November 10, 1986. The first article on 496 aspartame reactors appeared in the January 1987 edition of *On Call*, official publication of the Palm Beach County Medical Society.

The flood of calls and letters from grateful aspartame "victims" and their families dispelled my earlier misgivings about "going public." A husband wrote, "Without someone publishing this information that was so helpful to me, my wife could have died from illness due to this cause."

Important Ironies

My evolving researches on aspartame reactions verified a phenomenon familiar to psychologists: uncritical persons tend to regard statements that are frequently repeated as the truth. This also applies to professionals. Doctors reflexively discounted "minor idiosyncrasies" to products made from "the building blocks of protein" that satisfied one's sweet tooth, and allegedly could avoid dental caries and control weight.

- Despite inferences by television ads showing banana plants and cows, aspartame is **not** an "organic" substance. *It was devised as a drug for treating peptic ulcer.*
- FDA Commissioner Hayes had been in office less than three months when he discounted the objections of FDA scientists, and approved the use of aspartame.
- President Reagan championed "deregulation" when aspartame was approved. There were two subsequent paradoxes. First, he subsequently swore off "all artificial sweeteners" because "we don't know what's in them." Second, he developed Alzheimer's disease which may be accelerated by aspartame products (Chapter XV).
- The cited massive advertising campaign neglected to mention the fact that ten percent of aspartame is metabolized to **free** methyl alcohol (methanol; wood alcohol), a severe poison (Chapter XXI).

The manufacturer's emphasis upon aspartame approval by regulatory bodies around the world was mentioned earlier. Reports by the Joint FAO/WHO Expert Committee on Food Additives (1980, 1981), which reviewed studies published from 1975 to 1981, concluded that aspartame was safe for humans. To my astonishment, however, 79 of the 81 references cited in its 1980 report were "submitted to the World Health Organization by G. D. Searle & Co., Skokie, Illinois, USA"! The other two were authored by investigators who apparently had received grants from this company.

Yet another paradox emerged. Although aspartame is licensed in many countries, their populations tend to avoid such products, especially Europeons. This point was stressed by a German food scientist who served as consultant to major chocolate producers.

G. CORROBORATION

"He will be the physician that should be the patient."
Shakespeare *(Troilus and Cressida)*

Aspartame Victims and Their Friends was a consumer group previously unknown to me. Shannon Roth, its founder, confirmed my preliminary findings and elaborated upon the severity and magnitude of other aspartame reactions (Chapter I).

The Aspartame Consumer Safety Network was organized in August, 1987 to receive complaints from increasing numbers of aspartame reactors.

Betty Martini of Atlanta founded Mission Possible (Chapters I and XXX). This group of volunteers distributed information about aspartame disease, and collected considerable patient data.

A few physicians and biomedical investigators, working in different realms, described problems related to aspartame in clinical case reports and scientific studies.

Other professionals began expressing uneasiness about the safety of aspartame products.

- Dr. Martha Freeman, a former member of the Bureau of Drugs, concluded a 1973 memo: "The information provided is inadequate to permit an evaluation of potential toxicity of aspartame."
- Florence Graves (1984), an editor of *Common Cause Magazine*, stressed that her investigations had uncovered no evidence in the public record that this Bureau or the then-Commissioner ever satisfactorily reconciled approval of aspartame by the FDA relative to questions raised by its Special Task Force concerning "Searle's flawed tests."

Dietitians provided more evidence for aspartame reactions. Several related experiences, both personal and professional. The following correspondence from a dietitian who suffered aspartame-induced headache is representative.

"For over two years now, I have been trying to discourage my clients from using aspartame to sweeten their foods and beverages. I have been expounding on the 'evils' of aspartame since 1983. Without an 'M.D.' or 'Ph.D.' after my name, not many people are likely to take me as seriously about this as they might... So, when dieters complained about depression, insomnia, headaches, or don't see appropriate weight loss (and sometimes we see weight gain), the first thing I ask is, 'How much and what kind of sweeteners or presweetened foods and beverages are you consuming?' Invariably, they're drinking aspartame or lots of coffee with aspartame added."

"Nutritionists" who had suffered severe aspartame reactions warned clients with similar problems about such products.

As aspartame-containing products began to inundate fast-food chains, food markets and restaurants, aspartame reactors in the United States and Canada kept submitting valid observations. For example, a 61-year-old advertising executive suffered a two-hour attack of severe visual difficulty and amnesia after drinking one cup of coffee sweetened with the aspartame tabletop sweetener he obtained at a fast-food outlet. (He had requested a saccharin sweetener, but it was not stocked.)

Further corroboration came from physicians and several professors of food science who *personally* experienced severe reactions to aspartame.

Case Overview-2

A 60-year-old professor of food technology at a major university suffered unexplained recurrent dizziness and nausea. These symptoms disappeared during a six-week visit to China. He drank three diet sodas the day he returned home. Within hours, he experienced an attack of intense "vertigo" and nausea that lasted several days. He could hardly change position without suffering extreme lightheadedness. Aspartame was deduced to be the cause. Learning of my studies shortly thereafter, he called because he was now receiving multiple inquiries about aspartame-associated complaints.

A press release by Senator Howard M. Metzenbaum, dated July 16, 1987, indicated that more than half of the selected scientists surveyed were concerned about the safety of aspartame. This report reflected a two-year investigation by the General Accounting Office (GAO) (1987), the investigative arm of Congress. These researchers expressed particular concern over the neurological reactions to aspartame, and its potential adverse effects on children and pregnant women. The survey indicated that 40 percent requested further research, 32 percent called for new warnings and product labeling, and 15 percent recommended a total ban! The GAO investigations did not wish to "comment on whether important issues surrounding aspartame's safety remain unresolved" because they lacked the scientific expertise to evaluate prior studies.

The initial data base on 3,326 consumers who attributed their complaints to aspartame products, collected by the Food and Drug Administration (Tollefson 1987), confirmed my findings. The details are summarized in Table II-3, and discussed in the sections on epilepsy (Chapter III), visual changes (Chapter IV), and memory loss (Chapter VI).

H. THE NEED FOR PERSPECTIVE AND ACTION

"Where there is no vision, the people perish."
Proverbs (29:18)

Aspartame disease no longer can be ignored as incidental anecdotal reactions. This sobering assertion has been validated by personal observations, those of other physicians, the FDA data, mounting epidemiologic evidence, and a host of experimental studies.

The clinical features are often severe – especially headache, convulsions, impaired vision, dizziness, confusion, profound memory loss, refractory fatigue, intense depression, gross changes in personality or behavior, eating disorders, loss of diabetes control, and the aggravation or simulation of diabetic complications.

Physicians must question ALL patients with the foregoing complaints and other unexplained problems about aspartame use. If these products are being consumed, a brief trial of abstinence should be recommended **before** embarking upon expensive tests, multiple consultations, and various risky interventions.

Education of the public and health professionals about adverse aspartame effects is imperative, particularly for high-risk groups. They include pregnant women, nursing mothers, young children, older persons, families with one or more members known to be aspartame reactors, patients and families at risk for phenylketonuria, and individuals with migraine, hypoglycemia, diabetes mellitus, and histories of alcohol or drug abuse. Failure to do so also incurs the risks of addiction, developmental problems, behavioral abnormalities, suboptimal intelligence, multiple sclerosis, and even accelerated Alzheimer's disease and brain tumors. Unless these concerns are convincingly negated, the current mass consumption of aspartame products could lead to an "aspartame Armageddon."

Severe deficiencies pertaining to the evaluation, licensing, labeling, promotion and surveillance of aspartame and its proposed analogs must be challenged as a potential "recipe for disaster." Senator Howard Metzenbaum correctly warned in the *Congressional Record* (1985b, p.S 10820).

> "We had better be sure that the questions which have been raised about the safety of this product are answered. I must say at the outset, this product was approved by the FDA in circumstances which can only be described as troubling."

SECTION 1

ASPARTAME REACTORS

"This effect defective comes by cause."
Shakespeare (*Hamlet*)

"Disease is very old and nothing about it has changed. It is we who change as we learn to recognize what was formerly imperceptible."
J. M. Charcot

This section reviews the author's observations, those of other physicians and consumers, and the FDA data concerning reactions to aspartame products. They are amplified in Sections 2 and 3.

The role of aspartame products is convincingly predicated upon (1) the <u>prompt</u> relief or disappearance of complaints after such use ceased, and (2) their <u>predictable</u> recurrence, usually within hours or days, following aspartame rechallenge (known or inadvertent) by the individual, or during provocative and double-blind testing. Numerous variations appear in the representative case reports.

An estimated 12 million Americans currently suffer illnesses whose cause cannot be determined despite visits to multiple doctors and clinics, and considerable testing (*Sun-Sentinel* July 25, 1999, p. E-1). To their profound dismay, many end up being regarded as "neurotics" or "hypochondriacs." Others receive a variety of suspected or "wastebasket" diagnoses – including the chronic fatigue syndrome, fibromyalgia, lupus erythematosus, the irritable bowel syndrome, and "some mysterious-whatever disease."

The possibility of aspartame disease in these patients, however, is hardly ever considered, notwithstanding their considerable use of aspartame products. It is pertinent that more than two-thirds of adults indicated that they were trying to lose weight or maintain weight loss in a 1996 survey of 49 states and the District of Columbia by the Centers for Disease Control and Prevention (Serdula 1999).

Having practiced in the trenches of primary care for five decades, I do not accept the explanation that aspartame disease represents a "mass psychogenic illness." Four centuries ago, Michael D. Montage (1533-1592) appropriately observed

> "When a new discovery is reported to the scientific world, they say first, 'It is probably not true.' Thereafter, when the truth of the new proposition has been demonstrated beyond question, they say, 'Yes, it may be true, but it is not important.' Finally, when sufficient time has elapsed to fully evidence its importance, they say, 'Yes, surely it is important, but it is no longer new.' "

I

PATIENT AND CONSUMER EXPERIENCES

"Syndromes are clusters of non-chance associations, and the components of a syndrome can generally be related to a common element."
                    Dr. Ele Ferrannini (2000)

"But the medical profession has a tendency to discard out of hand, and disparagingly, 'anecdotal' information. Digitalis, morphine, quinine, atropine, and the like are chemical derivatives that stem from anecdotal folklore remedies. After all, one anecdote may be a fable, but 1,000 anecdotes can be a biography... A vital function of the medical profession is to sift anecdotes and submit them, if possible, to scientific evaluation. But it all starts as anecdote."*
                    Dr. Charles Harris (1987)

My initial observations concerning reactions to aspartame products were made as a primary-care physician and medical consultant. Once the public began communicating with me, and as consumer groups evolved, the data base expanded. Earlier statistics (Roberts 1988, 1989) are updated in this book, based on 1,200 aspartame reactors. The summarized data appear in Chapter II.

Acronym Legend
      ACB - aspartame cola beverages
      ASD - aspartame soft drink
      ATS - aspartame tabletop sweetener

---

*©1987 *Medical Tribune*. Reproduced with permission.

PRIVATE PATIENTS

The number of aspartame reactors in my practice increased exponentially after I became aware of aspartame disease. Just asking about the consumption of aspartame products proved a revelation, especially in the case of patients with otherwise-unexplained complaints.

The same two criteria – gratifying improvement after aspartame avoidance, and the recurrence of symptoms within hours or days after resuming such products – seemed convincing evidence that aspartame products indeed had been the cause or a prime aggravating factor. The most impressive features were severe headache, seizures (convulsions), marked impairment of vision, atypical pain (especially in the eye, ears, face, neck and chest), dizziness, rashes, extreme fatigue, depression, personality changes, and profound confusion or memory loss. The latter was of sufficient severity for many persons in their 30s and 40s that they expressed this concern: "Doctor, could I possibly be in the early stages of Alzheimer's disease?" (Chapters VI and XV).

As additional complaints were added to the foregoing list, I queried **all** patients about aspartame use. Several (<u>not</u> included in the tabulations) stated that they had stopped using aspartame because "it didn't agree with me" – especially <u>predictable</u> headaches, depression, and gastrointestinal disturbances. For example, a 62-year-old woman with hypothyroidism, reactive hypoglycemia and chronic constipation promptly determined that aspartame caused diarrhea... and therefore avoided it. She related this reaction to me, however, several years later.

DIAGNOSIS BY SELF OR FAMILY

Half the aspartame reactors in this series had deduced by themselves that aspartame products caused their symptoms (Chapter XIX). One-fourth of sufferees did so after reading a newspaper article on the topic. By contrast, the possibility of this association was infrequently raised by physicians.

> The mother of Case VIII-B-19 captured the pathos of her daughter who had severe hives (urticaria) for seven months despite referral to two allergists. "This poor girl had to exchange her wedding gown for one with long sleeves because the hives were so bad." The rash and other symptoms disappeared after <u>one day</u> of abstinence from diet cola!

Some reactors ascertained aspartame to be **the** offender through <u>trial-and-error elimination or retesting</u> (Section 4). Examples are cited throughout this book. The number of rechallenges required to convince them that aspartame products were the culprit is detailed in Chapter XIX. Case II-4 retested herself more than ten times, but several reactors did so <u>over 20 times</u>!

The desperate parents of several children with headache, seizures, learning disabilities and hyperactivity (currently designated attention-deficit disorder) instituted <u>personalized "elimination diets"</u> that provided the convincing conclusion. The mother of Case III-20 wrote

> "Since we were going to try the 'nutrition route,' we decided on our own to take him off the aspartame drink he had been consuming for the past four months (ever since I had been on a diet). He was drinking four to six glasses a day. (Usually one glass was in the form of a frozen popsicle). He has been a healthy little boy since, with absolutely no recurrence of any of the previous problems... It's been five months since the nightmare of the last seizure."

The Eureka Phenomenon

The Eureka ("I have it!") experiences provided by many perceptive individuals who correctly linked the use of aspartame products to their complaints were fascinating. This "hidden agenda of affliction" proved even more impressive when trained skeptics relayed such insights. They included respected authors (Case I-2), health professionals, and members of the media (see below). The objectivity of these seasoned professionals challenges critics who insist that their case histories are "merely anecdotal."

Dozens of aspartame reactors, or their relatives and friends, perceived the association through **serendipity**.

> The fiancé of Case V-3 agonized during her one-year ordeal with extreme headaches. Numerous consultations and multiple therapies (including Percodan®) had not afforded relief. On one

42

occasion, the couple happened to switch their beverages. Her glass contained an ACB, and his a "regular" cola drink. It was the first time the fiancé had tasted an aspartame cola. Feeling "lousy," he urged her to avoid it. Her headaches markedly diminished within a few days, and then disappeared.

Representative Case Reports

Case I-1

A 50-year-old registered nurse experienced a "blotchy, warm and itchy" rash over her chest and arms. It had occurred "at the same beach, at the same time of the year, and for the same length of time" during the summer for over a decade.

She sought out any factor that might have been different. The possibilities included suntan lotions, exposure to plants, and various activities. Her conclusion: "All I could think that I was doing differently was drinking aspartame." She then resumed all previous activities and habits, but avoided aspartame products. The rash did not recur.

Case I-2

A nationally-known 46-year-old writer gave an in-depth account of her severe reactions to aspartame products – and one of its components – shortly after learning of my interest in the matter.

She had experienced numerous symptoms from aspartame products one year previously. They included severe soreness of the jaw and neck (for which she initially saw a dentist), marked stiffness of the neck (to the point of hardly being able to turn her head), "overall" headaches that differed from prior migraine attacks, mental haziness, visual symptoms ("I had to blink in order to focus my eyes"), intense sleepiness, a "clogged head and other allergies," and debilitating depression. All virtually disappeared within four weeks after avoiding aspartame.

More recently, she had felt "the early phase of a depression cycle." Having heard that L-phenylalanine might abort depression, she began taking 500 mg in the morning, and one week later 500 mg before breakfast and bedtime. Her "aspartame symptoms" returned within days, but were far more intense than while consuming aspartame, especially the depression and "muscle spasms." Recognizing this similarity, she requested the <u>exact</u> components of aspartame. Her complaints receded after stopping L-phenylalanine, albeit requiring a longer period.

Case I-3

A 52-year-old housewife experienced numerous symptoms for two weeks while consuming three cans of an ASD, up to four packets of an ATS, three glasses of a presweetened iced tea, and one cup of aspartame-sweetened hot chocolate daily. They included marked ringing in both ears, increased sensitivity to noise, severe headache, inappropriate falling asleep, mental confusion, slurred speech, intense depression, a change in personality, palpitations, great thirst, marked frequency of urination, and joint pains. A son pleaded with her to discontinue the aspartame products. She wrote

> "After experiencing slurred speech, severe headaches, poor coordination and depression, my son suggested a possible aspartame reaction. I stopped it with marked benefit. Thinking that maybe it was psychological, I tried it again two times, and the symptoms returned!"

Case I-4

A 40-year-old artist had suffered more than a score of generalized epileptic seizures. She stated

> "I thought it was strange to have a seizure without anything else having happened for 39 years. Then, in passing, I heard about a possible link between aspartame and brain disorders. So I looked up more information at the library... Now I am fine on medication and off aspartame, but it does not seem wise at present to get off seizure medication. I will never use aspartame again!"

Case I-5

A 62-year-old retired teacher tried one serving of an ASD that had been "sent free through the mail." She suffered severe dizziness, tremors, insomnia, and chills "to the point that I wrapped myself in an electric blanket turned to maximum." The symptoms

44

disappeared within one day after avoiding this product. They recurred within hours after retesting herself with both the same drink and an ACB on <u>four</u> occasions. She observed

> "I could not function fully due to lack of sleep, and the chills made it impossible for me to write or dress normally. As a graduate home economist, I recognized that I was experiencing a reaction to something, so I started checking out the possible sources."

She gave a history of hay fever and asthma. Her husband and son also developed insomnia and "disorientation" after taking aspartame products.

Case I-6 A

A 59-year-old secretary suffered severe headaches, depression, palpitations, atypical chest pain, recurrent unexplained weakness, and joint pains. She drank 4-5 cans of an ACB daily, particularly during the summer. She related the circumstances of self-diagnosis.

> "I have been drinking diet colas since the late 80s. My doctor told me to because I might otherwise upset my insulin balance. No problem before aspartame. I didn't know what was wrong. Got a clean bill of health. Then tried to figure out what I was doing differently. Came up with aspartame. Gave it a week's try – no problem at all. After seven days, I felt like a million."

Case I-6 B

A 42-year-old homemaker suffered severe reactions to a number of products containing aspartame – including diet colas, a tabletop sweetener, presweetened tea, and a weight-reduction preparation. She experienced intense headaches (causing her to quit her job,) blurred vision, difficulty wearing contact lens, severe ringing in the ears with increased sensitivity to noise, marked memory loss, unexplained facial pain, severe anxiety, depression, diarrhea, itching, frequency of urination, intense joint pain, and the loss of her menstrual periods for three months. Many tests failed to uncover the cause. Seeking information on migraine in a library, she chanced to find one of my books. Her symptoms improved within three days after avoiding aspartame, and were essentially gone after several weeks. She wrote, "My dentist and family physician are amazed at my success. I even received an apology from my physician. I truthfully couldn't believe that a food additive could be the cause of my complaints."

INADVERTENT RECHALLENGE

There are many references in this book to inadvertent rechallenge with aspartame products, which the sufferees did not realize contained this chemical. A number faulted themselves for having been so inattentive. This subject is also considered under the survey questionnaire (Chapter XIX).

Several case histories presented in other sections serve as examples of such "trial by illness."

- Case III-14, a 59-year-old forester, suffered violent convulsions on three occasions when he unknowingly consumed aspartame.
- Case VI-B-1, a 30-year-old computer programmer, promptly experienced intense lightheadedness after drinking any soft drink containing aspartame. Dizziness and abdominal pain would recur within minutes whenever he unknowingly drank such products.
- Case IX-D-4 had complained of recurrent unexplained headache, visual problems, and "burning and swelling" of the lips and tongue for months. Although she believed that aspartame products were no longer being consumed, it was found that her ginger ale did contain aspartame.

Reactors kept reiterating, "ASPARTAME IS EVERYWHERE!" At times, health- and nutrition-conscious patients who studiously avoided sugar, took vitamins and minerals, exercised, and regarded additives and drugs with great suspicion failed to realize that some products contained aspartame. They vehemently denied using it when seen in consultation for suggestive aspartame disease. Their intake of aspartame surfaced, however, after mentioning a partial list.

One notable product in this category is a popular powdered laxative sweetened with aspartame. (Its aspartame-free form contains 50 percent dextrose.) Paradoxically, patients who took this "sugar-free effervescent natural-fiber laxative" for gastrointestinal problems, whether constipation or diarrhea, developed more intense symptoms (Chapter IX-D). Their abdominal pain, nausea, and other complaints subsided after shifting to the non-aspartame product.

Aspartame reactors expressed apprehension after having been unknowingly served aspartame in restaurants (Section 4). (Nathan Pritikin used the analogy of entering the enemy's camp when we served as members of a panel discussion on nutrition at a national meeting.) Indeed, severe allergic (anaphylactoid) reactions to aspartame now must be included among "the restaurant syndromes" (Chapter VIII). (This designation refers to acute medical emergencies encountered after ingesting monosodium glutamate or MSG, metabisulfite preservatives, color additives such as tartrazine, scomboidosis due to spoiled fish, and other toxin-containing foods.)

Inadvertent rechallenge became an increasing problem with the inclusion of aspartame in more products that listed this chemical in "the fine print" and without the "swirl" on their labels. It resulted in trial-by-illness for many aspartame reactors who took these presumably "safe" items. Indeed, the author became a label sleuth when managing patients who continued to experience symptoms suggestive of aspartame disease.

A patient with treated hypothyroidism complained of visual difficulty, numbness, fatigue and bladder irritation. Examination of the weight-reducing "nutritional supplement" she had been using five months revealed that the packet mentioned phenylalanine.

Several physicians have also observed that some patients with aspartame disease seem to have more severe reactions when accidentally ingesting aspartame at a later time – including an apparent incident of sudden death under this circumstance.

Representative Case Reports

Case I-7

A 73-year-old retired man had enjoyed a soft drink "because it had no caffeine, which my system will not tolerate." He promptly developed headache, sore eyes, and an "ultra-sick stomach" when the manufacturer started adding aspartame to that soda. He also experienced palpitations, a bad taste in the mouth, and pain in the jaws and both eyes ("my eyeballs felt as though they would burst").

These symptoms abated within three days on two occasions after using, and then stopping, this product. He became convinced of the association after the second trial. ("Thinking I might be wrong, I gave this a second chance several days later, and got the same results.") He expressed gratitude because "the short time I was involved with it may have saved me from more serious problems."

Case I-8

A 51-year-old registered nurse experienced severe itching and an extensive rash that she attributed to aspartame beverages. She wrote

> "I thought about a retest even though I was convinced, but decided against subjecting myself to this discomfort. I went to a pool party a year later. It was hot, and I sat in a lounge chair in the pool from 3-5 PM with three glasses of diet soda. Never gave it a thought. By 10:30 PM, the raised itchy red rash was again present on my chest. I stopped the soda, and used Benadryl and hydrocortisone creme. The rash left."

Case I-9

A 57-year-old woman had violent headaches, dizziness, mental confusion, severe nausea and abdominal pain attributable to aspartame. She would experience nausea within four hours after ingesting any aspartame-containing product.

In view of these attacks after having ingested aspartame unknowingly, she carried plastic bags in her purse and car. One such incident occurred after use of an artificial sweetener while traveling in Europe. Although the ingredients were not listed, she was later informed that the product did contain aspartame.

48

Case I-10 A

A 43-year-old teacher had frequent and excessive menstrual periods while consuming up to four cans of an ASD daily. Her daughter had aspartame-related headaches. She wrote

> "It is becoming increasingly difficult to avoid aspartame. I am constantly irritated by people not being informed when a product containing aspartame is served. This has happened time and again at church suppers and friends' homes. I do not want it foisted on me!"

Case I-10 B

A 49-year-old marketing consultant experienced numerous and incapacitating reactions to aspartame products. Her daily consumption included two cans of a diet cola, two glasses of an aspartame mix, one glass of aspartame hot chocolate, one bowl of an aspartame cereal, and one serving of an aspartame pudding mix. The symptoms consisted of decreased of vision in both eyes, recent "dry eyes," ringing in the ears, impaired hearing, severe dizziness, marked drowsiness, intense tremors, insomnia, mental confusion with memory loss, facial pains, slurred speech, severe depression (with suicidal thoughts), palpitations, abdominal pain, nausea, diarrhea, hives, and cessation of her periods.

Her symptoms twice improved within one week after discontinuing aspartame products, only to recur within two days after "accidental rechallenge." Two daughters also suffered aspartame disease – one having seizures and severe headache.

Concerning her incapacitation, this patient wrote, "I was in such mental and physical pain that my son had to take over the business and work to support me. I was barely able to function."

Case I-11

A patient in her 90s had remained remarkably active and alert. She attributed her vigor to having taken vitamins, minerals and "health foods," and minimizing drugs.

When seen after returning from a summer vacation, she complained of nausea, marked abdominal distress, embarrassing episodes of rectal incontinence, and intense neuropathic discomfort involving the lower extremities. She had been treated with little success by several internists and neurologists. Moreover, her blood pressure remained high notwithstanding a shift to more potent medication for hypertension.

The patient initially denied taking aspartame. On direct questioning, I found that she had begun using a powdered laxative flavored with aspartame. Her symptoms promptly improved when she discontinued this product, and did not recur over the ensuing two years.

Case I-12 A

A 68-year-old woman emphasized the nausea, vomiting and diarrhea after using one tablespoon of an aspartame-flavored powdered laxative twice daily. Other complaints included decreased vision and pain in both eyes, recent "dry eyes" and impaired hearing, sensitivity to noise in both ears, severe headache, dizziness and unsteadiness, marked tremors, extreme depression, irritability and itching. Her symptoms disappeared after avoiding this and other aspartame products.

Case I-12 B

A man with severe aspartame disease wrote in partial jest, "Last night my wife tried to poison me. She says it was unintentional, but she did it anyway with diet ginger ale! There was no aspartame logo on it, but the word diet was there in French as well as English." He elaborated on the episode.

"I had a glass with supper. The effect was almost immediate.
I started to have a general ache all over. My tinnitus increased
about double, and I felt bloated and very tired. All this within
ten minutes! It had been 18 months since I stopped drinking
'diet anything.' How did I ever live through those years when I
was being poisoned every day?"

Case I-13 A

A college student who had suffered "major depression" while drinking 6-8 diet colas daily improved after stopping aspartame products. She then was able to compete with distinction at a speaking competition until inadvertently drinking one diet soda. She promptly became depressed and shaky. Fortunately, there was no severe depressive episode following strict aspartame abstinence thereafter.

Case I-13 B

A 28-year-old customer-relations representative consumed one or two cans of an ACB daily for three weeks. She developed severe abdominal pain that gradually subsided. It recurred "immediately" when she tried another ACB. She described her subsequent experience with a beverage not recognized as containing aspartame.

> "A year after I'd stopped using it, we ordered out lunch at work. I had asked someone to get me a diet cola which did not contain aspartame at the time. They told me that's what they got. (It was in a fountain cup, so I couldn't tell.) It never even crossed my mind that it could contain aspartame until the all-too-familiar cramps returned. So I called the food place and found out I had an aspartame cola. You can't ask for a better test than that!"

Attitudes Concerning Rechallenge

Most persons with severe aspartame reactions vowed "never" to re-expose themselves to aspartame except under specific conditions. An aspartame reactor with multiple sclerosis noted, "My mouth goes weird when I have any aspartame. I don't need to read labels if there is a trace of it. My mouth goes fizzy – in fact, so instantly that I know it, and don't eat or drink it."

Representative Case Reports

Case I-14

A 60-year-old aspartame reactor emphasized she would "never knowingly take it again!" She added, "I would only consume aspartame under a strictly-supervised MEDICAL ENVIRONMENT, and even then I would have to think long and hard before giving permission for same."

Case I-15

A 43-year-old diabetic woman treated with diet and oral medication had violent reactions to aspartame beverages. They included severe headache, dizziness, slurred speech, convulsions (on two occasions), extreme anxiety, palpitations, swelling of the tongue, and difficulty in swallowing. These features did not totally disappear until three months after stopping aspartame. Fearing another attack in public, she commented, "It was the worst and most unusual feeling of my life. I would <u>never</u> want to go through it again."

Case I-16

A 51-year-old woman with multiple severe aspartame reactions asserted, "I might consent to using it a time or two, but I was <u>so sick</u> for <u>so long</u> that it scares me to death."

Case I-17

This letter was received from a Mississippi attorney.

"Dear Dr. Roberts:

"An article by Alan Bavley of the *Fort Lauderdale News & Sun Sentinel* appeared August 7, 1986 in *The Clarion-Ledger*, a Jackson (Mississippi) daily newspaper. (Copy of article enclosed.)

"Immediately after reading the article, I stopped taking into my system any substance known to contain aspartame. By August 11, the physical symptoms of depression that I had been fighting for nearly two years vanished. I averaged the equivalent of ten of the little blue packets of aspartame each day prior to quitting.

"I supposed it would take a test whereby I continued using the little blue packets under a controlled environment, not knowing whether they contained aspartame or powdered sugar or some other substance, and then measure the effect. But I do not desire to experience any more of the symptoms of depression that have gone away since I read the article and stopped ingesting aspartame."

In this context, several grateful persons expressed their willingness to help my researches through an aspartame rechallenge... but <u>only</u> if I was present.

Case I-18

A 63-year-old dentist experienced severe dizziness and unsteadiness after drinking small amounts of aspartame soft drinks. They disappeared within three days. He wrote, "I have not tried aspartame since. I decided it was causing problems. I would be willing to give a test try if this would help in your research."

INPUT FROM OTHERS

The author received a steady stream of letters, calls and e-mail correspondence from aspartame reactors here and abroad. There was no doubt in <u>their</u> minds about my being on the right track regardless of statements to the contrary by others.

The Public

Several communications illustrate the public's increasing perception of aspartame disease.

Case I-20

The following "plain talk" note was received. Her personal physician's intolerance to <u>the same</u> aspartame product (discussed later) is noteworthy.

> "Dear Dr. Roberts:
>
> "I have read your article in the *St. Pete Times* on aspartame sweeteners.
>
> "I too have complained, and was told 'there's no reason for the problem.' This was one year ago. They informed me that I couldn't get dizziness, nausea, severe headaches, and weight gain in just one week of using this product.
>
> "I did a test myself. For one week I drank aspartame products, and used the packets in coffee, iced tea, tea and soft drinks. I used it in cooking as well as in cakes and cookies.
>
> "After using this product, my attitude changed. I became irritable, cranky, and fat.

"Then I contacted my general practice doctor. He said to discontinue its use because <u>he</u> got the same way.

"So, the second week I had everything in regular sugar or none at all. The symptoms disappeared. I also lost weight when I ate the same foods, prepared exactly the same way.

"I wrote letters to the FDA a while back, but no response. So, what do we do about it?"

Case I-21

An outraged Kentucky woman sent this letter to the FDA, dated December 15, 1986. It encompasses the complaints, questions and frustrations of many aspartame reactors.

*   *   *   *   *   *

Department of Health & Human Services
Food and Drug Administration
Rockville, MD 20857
Attention: Mr. Huge C. Cannon, Associate
Commissioner for Legislative Affairs

Gentlemen:

Thank you for your reply to my letter-of-complaint about aspartame. The levity of your reply and of the FDA in general is quite disturbing.

As might be expected, only a small fraction of people who experience problems with aspartame bother to contact the FDA, their congressmen, friends, or anyone else. So don't tell me that you have had only so many complaints. This is only the number of people that have bothered to write. I would estimate that about 90 percent of my female friends have had problems with aspartame, and have quit using diet drinks and other products. Most of their problems have been joint pains (shoulders, sides, chest, hands, ankles), headaches, diarrhea and much more. I also know many men who have problems with headaches, joint pain, and depression.

This may not represent a health problem to the FDA or any other organization, but it certainly has to these people who have been to doctor after doctor, given up their activities, some their jobs – plus the mental and monetary problems. WHAT DOES THE FDA CONSIDER A HEALTH PROBLEM ANYWAY?

Your letter stated, "This sensitivity to aspartame is presumably similar to the adverse response experienced by some individuals to various other food and color additives, as well as to certain foods." Well, somebody presumed wrong! I have never experienced the same problems with anything else in my life, nor have these people with whom I'm familiar. It is very strange how you are trying to rationalize this problem, rather than believing people and removing the problem.

You also stated that aspartame was extensively tested in animals, etc. If I were a mouse, you would not have known about the terrible shoulder and side pains or the other arthritis-like symptoms. You would have known if they had diarrhea or rashes. From what I've heard about the animal tests, the animals were not looked at for a lengthy time, and many questions have not been answered by the FDA about their results. I hope that the clinical studies are underway.

Many people seem to think that the FDA has been paid off. I'm not going that far because I do not know... Two facts I want to strongly state:

(1)   You haven't received millions of complaints because people don't know that aspartame is causing their health problems. Erroneously, they think that the food and drinks they consume are safe.

(2)   Animals cannot speak and tell you how they feel.

By copy of this letter to my interested Congressman Carroll Hubbard, this is to keep you advised of the battle going on to keep our food safe... I am asking Congressman Hubbard to have a thorough investigation into this matter. This health problem is more serious than taxes, arms to Iran or anything else, besides defense.

Sincerely,

Physician-Aspartame Reactors

Several correspondents, as Cases I-20 and I-29, were fortunate in getting positive input from physicians who had suffered aspartame reactions <u>themselves</u>.

Representative Case Report

Case I-22

A 65-year-old woman experienced severe dizziness after drinking aspartame. A cousin had a comparable reaction. She wrote that her surgeon "avoided aspartame because he didn't like the reaction from it."

An Afflicted Media

I was impressed by the extraordinary interest in my work on the part of professionals in the print and electronics media. Furthermore, unsolicited invitations were received from prominent radio and television talk-show hosts. The reason became apparent: most had suffered confusion, memory loss, serious mood swings, and other problems while drinking large amounts of soft drinks, coffee and tea sweetened with aspartame. (Sweating under the hot lights of television studios tended to intensify their aspartame-associated thirst.) Several expressed added concern over the threat that aspartame disease posed to both their health and careers. Nevertheless, some remained reluctant to commit such personal experiences to an outright condemnation of aspartame products (see Case I-24).

Reverend Pat Robertson, former host of *The 700 Club* on the Christian Broadcasting Network, evidenced comparable interest. During a program on August 9, 1985, he told his audience about the marked memory loss he experienced while using aspartame products.

Some aspartame reactors in the media expressed frustration over the indifference to this problem shown by colleagues.

- A television station employee repeatedly experienced headache, nausea and severe fatigue from aspartame products, as did her sisters. She expressed outrage over "the medical reporter's refusal to recognize aspartame reactions as <u>widespread and serious</u>."

- Neil Rogers, a popular South Florida talk-show host, described his multiple reactions to aspartame products during a two-hour personal interview. He suggested to his listeners: "If in doubt, throw it out!"

Representative Case Reports

Case I-23

The 40-year-old manager of a news service fortuitously became aware of <u>his</u> problem with aspartame disease while producing a television program on <u>this</u> subject! He had been consuming two large (two-liter) bottles, and up to ten glasses of aspartame sodas daily. His complaints included severe dizziness, recent "dry eyes," difficulty wearing contact lens, insomnia, nausea, diarrhea, severe itching (without a rash), intense thirst ("the worst of all complaints"), frequent urination at night, "low blood sugar attacks," and "pins and needles" in the arms and legs.

Case I-24

A 31-year-old radio talk-show host had been drinking three cans of diet cola daily in an attempt to avoid gaining weight. He experienced "periodic, uncontrolled outbursts of anger at work, depression, and suicidal thoughts." He also noted his "loss of control over moods," and the feeling of being "pulled down." There was a prior history of migraine and mild depression. The following comment indicated his attempt to remain objective:

> "It's hard to attribute my reactions solely to the use of
> aspartame. However, the most severe reactions appeared as I
> began its use, and lessened considerably – or disappeared – after
> this use was stopped."

Case I-25

A 27-year-old female television producer consumed three cans of aspartame soft drinks and one glass of presweetened iced tea daily over a period of two years. She developed pain in both eyes, trouble wearing contact lens, severe headaches, tingling of the extremities, palpitations, nausea, and marked frequency of urination. (She did not smoke or drink alcohol.) A CT scan of the brain and various eye tests proved normal. A clearcut association of these complaints with aspartame products was deduced when she improved after avoiding them.

Case I-26

A 30-year-old employee for two radio stations suffered severe problems involving memory, confusion, depression (including suicidal thoughts), a change in personality, insomnia and dizziness. She consumed one packet of an ATS in each cup of coffee. Her symptoms improved markedly within three days after stopping it, and did not recur. Refusing to retest herself, she expressed her indignation in these terms:

> "I become angry when I see commercials promoting aspartame.
> How harmless they make it all look. The all-American brown
> & white can and something about bananas. If this product is
> truly harmless, why the marketing aspect?"

Talk Shows

I accepted invitations from radio talk-show hosts as far away as Toronto. One motivating factor was the extraordinary input from aspartame reactors who predictably called. Indeed, these discussions provided my first awareness of several aspartame-related problems.

There were some dramatic and poignant encounters. This anecdote occurred on September 30, 1987 while being interviewed on Radio Station WJNO (West Palm Beach).

> The caller stated that he was still in bed after having had a lumbar puncture for further evaluation of markedly impaired vision. He had become a heavy aspartame consumer since moving to Florida the previous year. Several months later, he began experiencing significant deterioration of his sight for which he consulted several ophthalmologists, both locally and at a university center in Miami. Numerous studies proved normal – including a CT scan and an MRI

study of the brain, an electroencephalogram, and multiple eye tests. A neurologic consultant recommended the lumbar puncture that had been done that morning "for the sake of completeness." Advised to remain in bed for eight hours, he happened to hear my interview. He became indignant over the fact that "no physician ever mentioned the possibility of an aspartame-related eye problem!"

Other talk-show vignettes are offered.

- "Breaks" for commercials are usual during interviews. An occasional commercial caught my attention because of its relevance or contrast. For example, one focused on "properly feeding your lawn before the approaching cold season" during an interview on WWWE (Cleveland). Not having heard this pitch previously, I commented, "There seems to be more interest in feeding lawns properly than feeding people properly."

- The talk-show host of a major radio station expressed extreme interest in interviewing me after receiving an announcement of *Sweet'ner Dearest*. She began by mentioning her reactions, especially severe headaches, hypoglycemia attacks, and an alarming memory loss. When these features promptly subsided after abstaining from aspartame products, she became a "true believer" concerning the validity of aspartame disease.

SUPPORT GROUPS AND INFORMATION NETWORKS

Aspartame sufferees felt no confinement to territorial limits in communicating their personal experiences through support groups, the Internet and newsletters. They imparted various descriptive phases to indicate the inability or unwillingness of physicians and consultants to find the cause of their misery. These included "a mysterious ailment," "a nameless demon," and "the land of no diagnosis."

Aspartame Victims and Their Friends

A major breakthrough in my orientation to the magnitude of aspartame reactions occurred in 1985 when I enlisted the cooperation of Shannon Roth, founder of Aspartame Victims and Their Friends. She attributed her permanent blindness in one eye (Case IV-11) to aspartame use. Extensive testing and prolonged observation had ruled out multiple sclerosis and other causes. Two ophthalmologists finally attributed her problem to excessive aspartame consumption.

This consumer group had already received complaints and other information from more than 800 persons when I called! Learning about Shannon's personal experience, they detailed their own reactions to aspartame products, and the frequent dramatic improvement after stopping them. As in Shannon's case, the most notable exception was persistent visual impairment.

The Community Nutrition Institute, Dr. Woodrow Monte and Mary Stoddard

I also received cooperation from Mr. Rod Leonard of the Community Nutrition Institute, Dr. Woodrow Monte (Chairman, University of Arizona Food Sciences Department), and Mary Stoddard (Aspartame Consumer Safety Network). They provided me with additional names and details of aspartame reactors for my survey questionnaire.

Betty Martini and Mission Possible

Betty Martini of Atlanta and her dedicated colleagues who also had suffered aspartame reactions became ultimate volunteer activists in this realm. They formed "Mission Possible" to inform the world about aspartame disease.

Mission Possible members in many states and abroad distributed "kits" of literature detailing the hazards of aspartame products. Some contained copies of more than a dozen articles and letters published in various journals and periodicals, and my position statements (see Appendices) – particularly the potential complications from use of aspartame products by pregnant women, children, and patients with diabetes, hypoglycemia, eye problems, and suspected multiple sclerosis.

These self-named "Roberts' Angels" used every opportunity "to spread the word": the mail; calls to or interviews on radio and television; attendance at professional seminars; meeting strangers at market, airports and various gatherings (especially walk-a-thons for diabetes); and the Internet.

- Without fear or embarrassment, Betty cornered many physicians at meetings – including invited professorial lecturers – to explain aspartame disease when it seemed relevant. Most expressed gratitude for informing them about this subject of which they had been unaware.

- These volunteers literally reached the four corners of the earth by distributing flyers to pilots and flight attendants, and via e-mail.
- Starting from scratch, Betty rapidly became proficient on the Internet, handling an average of 40-50 messages daily!

As a result, scores of persons with aspartame disease submitted their case reports, often utilizing my survey questionnaire (Section 4). The many insights these respondents provided were generally accompanied by expressions of gratitude.

Other Networks

Additional informal networks seeking to inform aspartame reactors came to my attention. (Other types of "victim" consumer groups exist, such as the Audi Victims Network in Plainview, N.Y.) Their ability to find <u>many</u> reactors was impressive in light of the ongoing denials about aspartame disease by physicians and governmental/corporate representatives (Section 7). These individuals in turn repeatedly mentioned other reactors within their immediate circle of acquaintances.

Such encounters proved that astute "laymen" can sense a potentially major public health problem (Section 6) through their own grapevines of communication long before its awareness by the medical profession.

Representative Case Reports

Case I-27

A 37-year-old woman experienced two convulsions and many other symptoms attributable to aspartame products. She wrote

> "I have been giving information to people I know regarding what happened to me, and telling them not to take aspartame. One girl at the office told me she had something similar happen to her – in the sense that she had a strange feeling in her head, like her mind was going away. She went to the doctor. He told her that the symptoms seemed like a temporal lobe seizure. They ran all sorts of tests, EEG, etc., which were normal. So they attributed it to stress."

Case I-28

A 74-year-old woman stated

> "I bought a large carton of powdered aspartame three years ago when I was on a no-sugar diet. Every time I used any part of it in coffee or cereal, I immediately threw up. My doctor told me not to use it any more. I took his advice and threw the balance of the carton in the garbage, where I hope no one ever got it. I did tell all my friends and family how it affected me. They stopped using it, too."

Case I-29

A diabetic woman had been using several aspartame products to avoid sugar. She awakened one morning with "...inability to get my eyes focused. The numbers on the digital clock were all jumbled together. In addition, the room was spinning around. I was very unsteady on my feet, and had headaches every day."

Relating these symptoms to a friend, she was told <u>four</u> other acquaintances had similar problems that subsided after avoiding aspartame. She did so, and "almost immediately my problems cleared up." When she informed her physician about the matter, he volunteered that several of his patients had similar symptoms because "some body chemicals could not tolerate these sweeteners."

OBSERVATIONS BY OTHER PHYSICIANS

As the general press began disseminating information about my research, physicians called to report the remarkable regression of headaches, visual symptoms, and other

complaints noted by their patients after abstaining from aspartame products. Several neurologists and ophthalmologists were especially grateful to hear a candid discussion of aspartame disease from a credentialed physician.

After my first press conference (Overview - F), a few physicians volunteered their heretofore-suppressed suspicions. Some of these communications are incorporated in Sections 2 and 3. A Philadelphia doctor sent this letter.

> "I have had the opportunity to recently have a patient show me an article from Sunday August 3rd issue of the *Philadelphia Inquirer*. In this article, you are quoted as indicating that aspartame may be implicated in certain symptomatology. The article specifically includes headaches, confusion, memory loss, seizures and convulsions. I would appreciate a resume of your experience or references to pertinent articles regarding this as I have had patients myself with seemingly the same complaints that have improved with removal from aspartame. I've enclosed a self-addressed stamped envelope, and would appreciate your reply as soon as convenient."

Several prominent psychiatrists were convinced about the validity of the neuropsychiatric manifestations (Chapters VI and VII) after **personally** experiencing severe reactions to aspartame products. One developed severe fatigue and pain in the right ear every time he ingested an aspartame soda.

Interested clinicians kept finding more cases of aspartame disease in their own practices by (1) routinely questioning patients with unexplained symptoms about aspartame use, (2) noting improvement after its cessation, and (3) and documenting flareups on aspartame rechallenge.

A physician sent this response after receiving information about my publications on aspartame disease.

> "At first I found it hard to believe that aspartame is that dangerous if one consumes it for long periods of time. But I keep meeting more and more people who confirm it is dangerous. One anecdote: Last weekend I met a lady who said she was a food chemist. I said the word 'aspartame.' She instantly pointed at her head and said: 'A neurotoxin. I worked with people who did tests. We can't prove it causes cancer, but many of the lab animals used got brain tumors from prolonged exposure to aspartame.' Her last statement frightened me with how coldly she said it: 'Their behavior changed.' That is, it is truly frightening that 100,000,000 or more people are paying (when they buy these diet products) to be a part of a vast biological human experiment of the kind only someone truly demented could desire doing!"

Table I-1 summarizes the problems reported by colleagues. Such professional feedback reinforced an evolving belief that this enlarged series of aspartame reactors represents a serious public health issue (Section 6).

TABLE I-1

ADVERSE EFFECTS TO ASPARTAME PRODUCTS REPORTED BY OTHER PHYSICIANS

Brain
    Severe headache
    Convulsions (epilepsy)
    Severe depression
    Manic depression
    Insomnia
    Hyperactivity (children; adults)

Eye complaints
    Blurring of vision
    Bright flashes
    Pain
    Tunnel vision
    Blindness (transient; permanent)

Ear complaints
    Tinnitus (ringing in the ears)
    Noise sensitivity

Pain – face; neck; chest; limbs; joints; muscle

Gastrointestinal
    Abdominal pain
    Nausea
    Diarrhea
    Pancreatitis

64

      Skin and Allergies
          Hives
          Itching
          Mouth reactions
          Granulomatous panniculitis (inflammation of fat tissue)

      Menstrual disorders

"SOCIAL HISTORIES"

Discussions with perceptive paramedical personnel, and persons in business or various professions who were not patients strengthened my conviction about the prevalence of aspartame disease. Finding me receptive to their inquiries, nurses and secretaries at my two hospitals gave dramatic stories about headache, depression, changes in vision, menstrual disturbances, or abdominal pain after ingesting diet drinks and other aspartame products. Indeed, once the local media reported on my research, hardly a week passed without some hospital staff member or other acquaintance volunteering a perceived aspartame-related problem. "Casual" questions asked by friends also made it clear that they were probably experiencing aspartame reactions.

> The wife of a prominent elected official queried me during a dinner discussion, "Could aspartame cause palpitations?" I replied in the affirmative. When we parted an hour later, she said, "Thank you so much for telling me about your studies on aspartame... especially the palpitations."

As a corollary, other persons went out of their way to express appreciation for the dramatic improvement of a previously-undiagnosed disorder once they avoided aspartame – in some instances, years later at a social gathering.

Representative Case Report

Case I-30

The wife of a senior executive approached me at the annual meeting of a major organization in Palm Beach County. I had known this woman and her family for three decades. She stated, "I am most grateful for your television interview about aspartame two week ago. I stopped it, and all my symptoms vanished! But my husband is even <u>more</u> grateful. Let him tell you." This down-to-earth, no-nonsense businessman elaborated.

"I didn't know what was happening to me. Come the middle of the afternoon, I felt terribly sleepy and couldn't think straight. It was like my brain was being lifted. I began to wonder about early senility. My wife then told me about her reactions to aspartame. The sleepiness and confusion disappeared right after stopping it, and haven't returned. Thanks, old buddy."

II

CLINICAL DATA ON 1,200 ASPARTAME REACTORS

"Observation is more than seeing; it is knowing what you see
and comprehending its significance. The process is far more
mental than photographic. True observation implies studying
the object and drawing conclusions from what is seen."
Charles Gow

This book focuses on the first 1,200 aspartame reactors in the author's data base. These persons include the following:

- 188 private patients and other individuals who were personally interviewed.
- Complainants who described their aspartame-associated reactions to Aspartame Victims and Their Friends (295), the Community Nutrition Institute (68), and Dr. Woodrow Monte of Arizona State University (28).
- The remainder supplied details of their reactions to the author or to Mission Possible, a volunteer consumer organization (Chapter I). Of this group, 697 (58 percent) completed the 9-page survey questionnaire (Section 4).

Acronym Legend

ACB - aspartame cola beverage
ASD - aspartame soft drink
ATS - aspartame tabletop sweetener

A. GENERAL DATA AND STATISTICS

The general information summarized below will be amplified later. There are minor discrepancies because certain details had been omitted from correspondence or the survey questionnaire. For example, 37 persons failed to give their name or gender for reasons of anonymity.

This chapter references the consumption of aspartame products, the latent period before initial symptoms of aspartame disease, the female preponderance, and seasonally increased intake of aspartame products.

Several important associations became more evident in the enlarged series than the earlier analysis of 551 cases (Roberts 1988, 1989). Accordingly, they were specifically sought among the ensuing 649 reactors.

Gender

There were 838 females (72%) and 325 males (28%) among the 1163 aspartame reactors who indicated their gender.

Age Range

The ages of persons at the onset of their reactions ranged from infancy to 92 years. Most were in their 20s to 50s.

Family History

Two or more close relatives of 211 (17.6%) were known to have had reactions to aspartame products.

Reasons For Consuming Aspartame Products

Approximately half these reactors had used aspartame products because of overweight – real or perceived. Most patients with diabetes mellitus and hypoglycemia consumed them to avoid sugar.

Some examples of other reasons for using aspartame products are cited.

- Patients who had been advised to do so by their dentists because of cavities or related dental problems thereafter developed symptomatic aspartame disease.
- Several reactors ingested aspartame products as part of a perceived "proper nutrition program" for their occupations. For example, a member of the Radio City Rockettes who emphasized this aspect suffered increasingly severe headaches, culminating in an aspartame-induced grand mal convulsion while on tour (Case III-15C).

Interval Between Cessation and Improvement

Nearly two-thirds of these reactors experienced symptomatic improvement <u>within two days</u> after avoiding aspartame. Their complaints usually disappeared with continued abstinence.

Symptoms and Signs

The symptoms and signs of aspartame disease in this series are listed in Table II-1. These reactions, along with less frequent ones noted here, will be amplified in subsequent sections.

TABLE II-1

COMPLAINTS IN 1200 ASPARTAME REACTORS
(ROUNDED PERCENTAGES)
(*indicates data based on the most recent 649 reactors)

Eye

Decreased vision and/or other eye problems (blurred, "bright flashes," tunnel vision)	302	(25%)
Pain (one or both eyes)	87	(7%)
Decreased tears, trouble with contact lens, or both	95	(8%)
Blindness (one or both eyes)	27	(2%)

Ear
Tinnitus ("ringing,""buzzing")	146	(12%)
Severe intolerance for noise	80	(7%)
Marked impairment of hearing	57	(5%)

Neurologic
Headaches	516	(43%)
Dizziness, unsteadiness, or both	376	(31%)
Confusion, memory loss, or both	376	(31%)
Severe drowsiness and sleepiness	150	(13%)
Paresthesias ("pins and needles, "tingling") or numbness of limbs	183	(15%)
Convulsions (grand mal epileptic attacks)	129	(11%)
Petit mal attacks and "absences"	36	(3%)
Nonclassified seizures	21*	(2%)
Severe slurring of speech	124	(10%)
Severe tremors	101	(8%)
Severe "hyperactivity" and "restless legs"	78	(6%)
Atypical facial pain	70	(6%)
Simulation of multiple sclerosis	28*	(4%)

Psychologic/Psychiatric
Severe depression	281	(23%)
Suicidal ideas/attempts	46*	(7.1%)
"Extreme irritability"	194	(16%)
"Severe anxiety attacks"	201	(17%)
"Marked personality changes"	167	(14%)
Recent "severe insomnia"	169	(14%)
"Severe aggravation of phobias"	77	(6%)
"Addiction to aspartame"	32*	(5%)

Chest/Heart
Palpitations, tachycardia, (rapid heart action) or both	193	(16%)
"Shortness of breath"	110	(9%)
Atypical chest pain	85	(7%)
Recent hypertension (high blood pressure)	64	(5%)

Gastrointestinal

Nausea	127	(11%)
Diarrhea	106	(9%)
Associated gross blood in the stools... 16		
Abdominal pain	125	(10%)
Pain on swallowing	61	(5%)

Skin/Allergies

Severe itching without a rash	87	(7%)
Severe lip and mouth reactions	54	(5%)
Urticaria (hives)	47	(4%)
Severe genital itching, rash, or both	25*	(4%)
Lupus erythematosus-type eruption	7*	(1%)
Other rashes	101	(8%)
Marked thinning or loss of hair	71	(6%)
Aggravation of respiratory allergies	17	(1%)
Dual sensitivity to MSG	14*	(2%)

Weight Disorders

Paradoxic marked weight gain	83	(7%)
Marked weight loss	40	(3%)

Rheumatologic/Muscular

Severe joint pains	163	(14%)
"Fibromyalgia""	27*	(4%)
Leg and hand cramps	28*	(4%)
Myasthenia gravis	8	(1%)

Endocrine/Metabolic

Problems with diabetes (loss of control; precipitation of clinical diabetes; aggravation or simulation of diabetic complications)	118	(10%)
Aggravated hypoglycemia ("low blood sugar attacks")	74	(6%)
Menstrual changes	76	(6%)
Severe reduction or cessation of periods ... 42		
Hyperthyroidism (Graves disease)	8*	(1%)

Fluid/Urinary Disturbances

Frequency of voiding (day and night), burning on urination (dysuria), or both	126	(11%)
Intense thirst	116	(10%)
"Bloat"	100	(11%)
Fluid retention and swelling (feet and legs)	43	(11%)
Kidney stones	3*	------

Comparison With FDA Data

As of April 1995, the Food and Drug Administration (FDA) had received complaints from 7,232 consumers who attributed their symptoms and signs to the use of aspartame products (Table II-2). As in the author's series, multiple complaints were common. BUT this agency arbitrarily excluded an additional 649 aspartame reactors reported earlier by the Centers for Disease Control (1984).

These findings are noteworthy.

- Gender - 3271 (76%) of the reactors were female; 1160 (24%) were male
- Age - peak age group 30-39 years, with 847 (25.9%) complaints
- Severity of Reactions - 518 (10.6%) classified as "severe"; 4366 (89.4%) classified as "mild to moderate"
- Recurrent Reactors Following Exposure to a Single Aspartame Product – 1139 (27.6%)

TABLE II-2

SYMPTOMS ATTRIBUTED TO ASPARTAME IN COMPLAINTS SUBMITTED TO FDA

REPORTED SYMPTOMS	NO. OF COMPLAINTS	% OF REPORTS
Headache		
Dizziness/Poor equilibrium	1847	28.1%
Change in Mood	735	11.2%
Vomiting or Nausea	656	10.0%
Abdominal Pain and Cramps	647	9.8%
Change in Vision	453	6.9%
Diarrhea	362	5.5%
Seizures/Convulsions	330	5.0%
Memory Loss	290	4.4%
Fatigue; Weakness	255	3.9%
Other Neurological Symptoms	242	3.7%
Rash	230	3.5%
Sleep Problems	226	3.4%
Hives	201	3.1%
Change in Heart Rate	191	2.9%
Itching	185	2.8%
Grand Mal	175	2.7%
Abnormal Sensation (Numbness; Tingling)	174	2.6%
Local Swelling	172	2.6%
Change in Activity Level	114	1.7%
Difficult Breathing	113	1.7%
Oral Sensory Changes	112	1.7%
Change in Menstrual Pattern	108	1.6%
Symptoms by Less than 100 Complainants	107	1.6%
	1812	—

The types of aspartame products implicated by consumers complaining to the FDA appear in table II-3

TABLE II-3

DISTRIBUTION OF REACTIONS ATTRIBUTED TO ASPARTAME BY PRODUCT TYPE

PRODUCT TYPE	NO. OF COMPLAINTS	% OF RECORDS	% OF COMPLAINTS
Diet Soft Drinks	3021	45.9%	38.3%
Table Top Sweetener	1716	26.1%	21.7%
Pudding/Gelatins	633	9.6%	8.0%
Lemonade	410	6.2%	5.2%
Other	346	5.3%	4.4%
Kool Aid	339	5.1%	4.3%
Iced Tea	319	4.8%	4.0%
Chewing Gum	319	4.8%	4.0%
Hot Chocolate	318	4.8%	4.0%
Frozen Confections	136	2.1%	1.7%
Cereal	119	1.8%	1.5%
Sugar Substitute Tablets	71	1.1%	0.9%
Breath Mints	62	0.9%	0.8%
Punch Mix	45	0.7%	0.6%
Fruit Drinks	24	0.4%	0.3%
Non-Dairy Toppings	8	0.1%	0.1%
Chewable Multivitamins	8	0.1%	0.1%

B. AGE RANGE

The ages of aspartame reactors <u>at the time they or members of their family first experienced complaints</u> ranged from infancy to 92 years, averaging 45 years. The majority were in their 20s to 50s.

The average age <u>when the first aspartame-associated reaction occurred</u> was 43 years. The breakdown by age groups among persons completing the questionnaire appears in Chapter XIX.

<u>Both</u> ends of the age spectrum represent high-risk groups (Chapters XI and XV). For example, an infant developed convulsions as its nursing mother drank an aspartame soda.

Older persons with aspartame disease repeatedly encountered the pernicious attitude of <u>agism</u> as an explanation for their reactions. The implications and consequences of aspartame-induced confusion and memory loss for the elderly are emphasized in Chapter XV.

Representative Case Reports

Case II-1

A mother described multiple reactions to aspartame by her <u>two-year-old</u> daughter. She first developed a "violent rash" after drinking an aspartame soda at school. It recurred after class on the second day, along with the marked facial swelling. Both subsided by the following morning.

Someone then gave her daughter a stick of gum. "She immediately broke out and began swelling. We later found out that the gum had aspartame... but at the time we still hadn't made the connection."

Friends who visited the next weekend brought an aspartame beverage. The rash and swelling recurred as soon as the girl took one drink. The mother observed, "Looking at the bottle, I noticed the aspartame symbol and it clicked!"

Case II-2

I had attended an elderly woman for 21 years when she returned on her 92nd birthday. She was being maintained satisfactorily on a program for heart failure, angina pectoris, obesity and chronic thrombophlebitis of the lower extremities.

The patient recently developed increased thirst, shortness of breath, and a fungal infection under both breasts. Although her fasting blood glucose (FBS) concentrations had been normal (80-115 mg percent) over many years, it now was 161 mg percent. The FBS progressively rose to 185 and 187 mg percent – clearly in the diabetic range. Concomitantly, her blood triglyceride (fat) levels increased to 1,284 and 1,616 mg percent (normal, up to 150 mg percent). The cholesterol concentrations also rose to 354 and 349 mg percent (normal, up to 225 mg percent). When diet alone proved ineffective, a glucose-lowering pill (Glucotrol®) was prescribed.

At the next visit, the patient complained of increasing headache and lightheadedness, a dramatic deterioration of vision, and intense discomfort over the left face, neck and chest areas. Concomitantly, she had become severely depressed. This devout Catholic initiated the visit by saying, "God has forgotten about me because He kept me living so long!"

I then inquired about the use of aspartame. Her daughter indicated that she had been consuming considerable "diet" soft drinks – at least three to four glasses daily over the previous year, but more during the recent hot weather. The patient was advised to continue her basic program but stop all aspartame products. Within one week, most of her symptoms had improved, as did the abnormal tests.

Case II-3

Shortly after seeing Case II-2, I received a letter from another 92-year-old woman who had suffered severe diarrhea and vomiting while taking an aspartame product. These complaints subsided when she avoided it and resumed sugar. She stated, "I have had no problems since. I am 92 years old, and do most of my work from a wheelchair because of a broken leg. I **am** in my right mind."

C. ASPARTAME CONSUMPTION

The prodigious consumption of aspartame was underscored in the Overview. Examples are cited in the representative case reports (as Case III-4), and a review of the survey questionnaire findings (Chapter XIX) which details the amounts of specific aspartame products taken.

- A 29-year-old man (Case III-31) with intensification of prior epilepsy drank 18 12-ounce cans of an aspartame cola daily for one year.

- A 35-year-old woman consumed from 10-15 cups of diet soda, up to 15 glasses of presweetened tea, and considerable amounts of diet cranberry juice <u>daily</u>. In addition to increasing headache, memory problems and anxiety, she complained of "gas" and constipation. (The latter were diagnosed as partial obstruction of the descending colon superimposed upon a "spastic colon.")
- A female aspartame reactor who had suffered headache, vision problems, loss of hair, and a peripheral neuropathy noted marked improvement one week after stopping aspartame products. She had been consuming "almost 350 packets a day, not to mention (a dietary) powder and frozen yogurt."

Several reactors also ascribed their problems to the aspartame present in prepackaged foods they had obtained from weight-loss franchises.

<u>Aspartame addiction</u> contributes to ongoing and increased consumption. This subject is considered in Chapter VII-G.

Representative Case Report

Case II-4

A 34-year-old receptionist with a host of aspartame-related symptoms (see below) listed the following <u>daily</u> intake:

Six 12-ounce cans of several diet cola beverages
One two-liter bottle of an ASD
Five to six packets of an ATS
Several glasses of iced pre-sweetened tea
Eight glasses of aspartame hot chocolate
Eight servings of aspartame pudding
25 to 40 sticks of aspartame gum
12 to 24 packets or teaspoons of other aspartame products

A. Underestimated Intake

Many of my patients did not realize how much aspartame they were consuming until I queried them or their spouses about the <u>specific</u> amounts ingested.

Representative Case Report

Case II-5

A 67-year-old woman had been troubled by increasing confusion, unsteadiness, severe mouth reactions, intense headache, "cracking of the ears," a paradoxic weight gain of eight pounds over 2-1/2 months, and recurrent itching in the afternoon followed by a rash. She brought a list of other recent complaints (the first time she had done so in many years under my care) because of her associated memory impairment. They included increasing pain in both eyes, "thick saliva," atypical pains over the left chest and shoulder area, considerable discomfort in the abdomen, insomnia (waking during the night), difficulty in voiding, and a striking loss of hair. Her physical examination had not changed.

At that point, I inquired about aspartame use. Initially, she admitted to using "only a little" aspartame in her tea at noon. (The addition of saccharin had not been a problem previously.) Her husband then interjected that she also was ingesting considerable aspartame as a diet chocolate pudding. Moreover, he had been adding much aspartame to homemade ice cream in view of the recommendation to avoid sugar because of prior severe hypoglycemic attacks.

In retrospect, this patient's high aspartame intake over a four-month period coincided with the development and progression of her symptoms. They disappeared or markedly regressed within <u>one week</u> after stopping aspartame. Her clinical improvement – both in general appearance and clarity of speech – impressed my staff at the next visit. The scheduled CT scan of the brain, electroencephalogram and neurologic consultation were cancelled. The patient and her husband expressed extreme relief over what <u>really</u> had been bothering them: the possibility of "early Alzheimer's disease."

B. "100 Percent" Aspartame

Several reactors sarcastically mentioned the dramatic exacerbation of their symptoms when using products that had incorporated "100 percent" aspartame.

Representative Case Report

Case II-6

A 31-year-old secretary consumed up to four cans of an ACB daily. She experienced severe drowsiness, irresistible sleep attacks, mental confusion, memory loss, slurred speech, severe depression and irritability, personality changes, rashes, a weight gain of 20 pounds, and the cessation of her periods. She wrote, "When aspartame switched from the blend to full strength, I passed out after dinner three days later."

C. <u>Greater Vulnerability to Certain Aspartame Products</u>

Some aspartame reactors react more severely to some aspartame products than others. A case in point is one popular <u>tabletop sweetener</u>. This may reflect the greater amount of aldehydes therein, which could influence the concentration of its breakdown amino acid stereoisomers.

<u>Aspartame orange soda</u> may contain 333 mg aspartame per 12 fluid ounces, or 930 mg per liter (*Federal Register* February 22, 1984, p. 6677) to preserve the taste, rather than the average of 550 mg per liter for other diet sodas (Section 5).

I repeatedly encountered a history of ingesting considerable aspartame <u>iced tea mixes</u> prior to the clinical onset of aspartame reactions, especially in hot weather.

> A 36-year-old computer programmer experienced many symptoms of aspartame disease after he began using "a line of products containing aspartame." He would ingest as much as three or four quarts of an instant iced tea (in several flavors) on a summer afternoon. His symptoms finally abated after one month of abstinence.

The number of seizures encountered in patients consuming <u>aspartame gum</u> (Chapter II-E) and a popular <u>non-cola lemony diet soft drink</u> was impressive.

D. <u>More On "Aspartame Is Everywhere"</u>

The aspartame-is-everywhere theme (see Overview) repeatedly asserts itself. The labels of EVERY "light" or "lite" product – regardless of the seeming improbability (water; orange juice; beer; non-dairy coffee creamers) – should be <u>specifically</u> inspected by reactors for the presence of aspartame, especially when symptoms persist or recur.

> A couple had considerable difficulty with aspartame products, particularly diet drinks. The husband experienced severe visual difficulty. His wife (a physician) suffered pain in multiple joints, which intensified while making her hospital rounds.

Both improved considerably after avoiding aspartame products. The husband was astonished to read that the first listed ingredient in the "children's vitamin" he used was aspartame. Also finding it in gum, jelly and cough drops, he issued this warning to one and all: "Beware of anything labeled sugar free!"

E. The Sugar Paradox

One might have expected that sugar consumption would decline with the dramatic increase of aspartame use. This has **not** been the case. Indeed, the annual per capita consumption of sugar actually increased according to the United States Department of Agriculture... in part reflecting the craving for calories (both as sugar and fat) by many aspartame consumers (Chapter IX B). A 14 percent rise in the per capita consumption of sugar occurred – specifically, from an average of 113.9 lbs per person in 1965 to 130 lbs in 1985.

A reflection of this paradox is the ingestion of pie, cake and ice cream along with aspartame-sweetened coffee and tea.

D. REACTIONS TO SMALL QUANTITIES

Some reactors evidenced severe symptoms and signs after ingesting or chewing small amounts of aspartame products.

- Mention was made of convulsions occurring in a nursing infant as its mother drank an aspartame soft drink.
- Children developed severe headache, convulsions, or both, within minutes after chewing either acetaminophen (given for fever) or gum containing aspartame (see below under E, and Chapters V and XI).
- A 68-year-old man described his "immediate" reaction to a diet soda. He had no difficulty when previously consuming diet root beer that contained cyclamate. "After drinking one 12-ounce can with the aspartame, I thought I was losing my mind. I had extreme agitation and was too nervous to drive a car."
- A female aspartame reactor experienced severe urinary bladder symptoms simulating infection (Chapter IX-F) after consuming aspartame products. As a diabetic, this created considerable anxiety.

She established the following "strict guidelines": a limit of one 12 oz can of diet soda and one serving of a diet dessert over a week. Any greater consumption of aspartame products caused the bladder problem to recur.

- Case II-15 experienced confusion, memory loss and erratic behavior after drinking <u>one</u> cup of <u>hot</u> coffee sweetened with an aspartame tabletop sweetener just before he played golf. The relationship of <u>heated products</u> to aspartame reactions, noted by other reactors (as Case II-14), will be discussed in Chapter XXV.

- Case III-1, a 31-year-old nurse with an aspartame-induced seizure, subsequently drank "only three sips" of a drink believed to be "regular" soda, but which contained aspartame. She promptly became "very incoherent."

- A chemist who developed migraine from certain foods and additives performed six double-blind studies on himself. He found that as little as 4.0 mg aspartame in a capsule predictably induced headache (Strong 2000).

Several patients with documented aspartame reactions kept retesting themselves with progressively smaller amounts of products containing this chemical... only to suffer the <u>same</u> adverse effects every time.

The precipitation of severe neurological and other reactions within minutes or a few hours after ingesting aspartame (see below) casts doubt on the assertion by the FDA: "The agency does not regard the possible consumption of aspartame in a single large dose as posing any safety problem whatever" (*Federal Register* February 22, 1984, p. 6678).

Representative Case Reports

Case II-7 A

An electronics engineer would feel nauseated and dizzy shortly after she drank an aspartame-containing fruit punch during exercise classes. These symptoms did not occur when she resumed regular colas. She wrote

"I was pleased when, in the summer of 1984, a diet cola came out with a blend of aspartame and saccharin. I thought maybe since it wasn't 100% aspartame, I might not have such a reaction. Wrong! After one week of drinking 1-2 cans per day, all the old symptoms returned."

Case II-7 B

A 28-year-old housewife recalled the "nasty" headaches she experienced since the age of 14 after drinking aspartame sodas. They would recur when unknowingly ingesting aspartame products at the home of friends. Fearing that her children might develop aspartame reactions, she wrote, "I do not allow these products to pass the threshold of my home. I am not a medical professional or a scientist, but I do know what effect aspartame has on my body in very small doses. I can only imagine what it could do in larger doses."

E. ASPARTAME GUM

I have been impressed by the role of aspartame gum in patients suffering severe neurologic aspartame reactions, especially headache and seizures (see below).

- A 24-year-old woman stated that she was "on the very verge of dying" from aspartame disease. Dramatic improvement occurred when she learned about this disorder, and then stopped such products. She emphasized her marked sensitivity to even a single stick of aspartame gum. Symptoms would recur within minutes after chewing it, and lasted one week.
- Aspartame gum was specifically incriminated by Case IX-C-16, a 35-year-old woman with shortness of breath, dizziness, irritability, fatigue, heavy menstrual bleeding, hair loss and weight gain. (She did not drink diet sodas.) These reactions – "within the hour I could not catch my breath"– recurred on multiple retests.

Few realize the enormity of gum consumption. It is estimated that Americans chew $2.5 billion worth of gum annually, the equivalent of 190 sticks per person. Some aspartame reactors chewed 15-20 sticks or more daily, in addition to using other aspartame products (see Case II-4).

Owing to its prolonged sweetness, persons tend to chew aspartame as much as five times longer than regular gum.

Habitual smokers who opt to chew aspartame gum in trying to break their cigarette habit risk aspartame addiction (Chapter VII-G).

Dental/Mouth Considerations

Patients have reported severe aspartame disease while using aspartame gum to have a "sweet breath." Under "Health Facts You Should Know," the *Mayo Clinic Health Letter* stated that sugarless gum "can actually help fight tooth decay."

Additionally, an array of candy-like sugarless gums are alleged to brighten teeth and reduce plaque simultaneously. There is a paradox, however. The recommendation of chewing aspartame gum to help prevent tooth decay by the British Dental Association could actually enhance it by decreasing saliva (Chapter IX-F) and through other mechanisms, such as the aggravation of diabetes (Chapter XIII).

Caffeinated Gum and Other Products

A caffeinated gum containing 50 mg caffeine per stick (the equivalent of one cup of coffee) has been marketed. It is intended for truckers, commuters, college students, and others desiring a "caffeine kick." Unfortunately, the aspartame therein can induce confusion and memory loss (Chapter VI), along with other adverse effects.

The habitual sucking of popular mints containing aspartame may induce seizures and other neuropsychiatric disorders. An aspartame reactor with prior complaints (vision impairment; slurred speech; loss of muscle strength) remained symptom-free after avoiding aspartame. She then experienced "painfully dry eyes" immediately after taking a breath mint containing aspartame.

Absorption

Chewing gum exposes the body to aspartame through its absorption in the upper gastrointestinal tract, and from the lining of the mouth. Additional ingredients could pose added problems. For example, I have repeatedly encountered difficulty with peppermint gum and wafers (Roberts 1983).

The rapidity with which reactions can occur after chewing aspartame gum is not necessarily an "allergy." The prompt absorption of aspartame or its breakdown products (Chapter XXV) from the mouth is akin to placing nitroglycerine under the tongue for the rapid relief of angina pectoris.

Pharmacologists recognize that absorption through the oral mucosa (without swallowing) can be an efficient route of delivery for amino acids and small proteins because the basal lamina under the epithelial layer contains blood vessels. Moreover, the enzymatic activity of the oral cavity is relatively low (principally, an amylase that hydrolyzes only sugars.)

- The blood flow in the buccal mucosa is comparable to that of the sublingual mucosa. Absorbed molecules are collected by the internal jugular veins, thereby directly reaching the circulating blood.
- The buccal route for drug administration is illustrated by its effectiveness in treating childhood seizures with midazolam (Scott 1999). The rich blood supply to the mouth enables absorption directly into the systemic circulation, thereby avoiding the considerable "first-pass" metabolism by the liver. A rapid effect on the central nervous system has been demonstrated electroencephalographically.

Another possible mechanism involves the transport of aspartame from the back of the mouth (oropharynx) <u>directly</u> to the brain. This phenomenon has been documented for small molecules such as glucose, sodium chloride and ethyl alcohol (Editorial, *British Medical Journal* 1:184, 1966; Maller 1967).

Gum-Induced Headache

Aspartame-induced reactions occurred in children who received aspartame gum on Halloween from thoughtful neighbors wishing to avoid giving them sugared gum as presents. Headache was the most frequent reaction; vomiting and severe tremors also occurred.

Blumenthal and Vance (1997) reported three cases of young women with migraine whose headaches could be provoked by chewing aspartame gum.

The promptness with which aspartame gum can precipitate recurrent headache is shown by these encounters.

- A female aspartame reactor developed headache after consuming aspartame in sodas and food. Offered gum in a darkened theater, she experienced severe pain in her face and eyes that radiated to the back of her skull within five minutes of chewing it. She spit it out when her friend confirmed it contained aspartame. The pain subsided over the course of the film.

- A correspondent wrote

  "I decided to lose a few pounds, so I watched my fat and cut out the sugar. I bought diet sodas and other products containing aspartame. Within a week, I started having headaches. My head felt stuffed up, and generally I was not feeling like myself. I happened to see a local news story about the side effects of aspartame and cut out all these products. Within a few days, I started to feel like my old self. About one month later, I accidently had a piece of gum with aspartame; within fifteen minutes, I had a splitting headache."

Gum-Induced Seizures

The precipitation of grand mal seizures after chewing ONE stick of aspartame gum is illustrated below and in Chapter III.

Induced Hunger

Some aspartame reactors described an uncontrollable craving for sweets related to chewing aspartame gum. There are corroborative studies. Tordoff and Alleva (1990) reported greater hunger by oral stimulation when gum base containing aspartame in four concentrations was chewed 15 minutes.

Gum as "Nonexercise Activity"

Levine, Baukol and Pavlidis (1999) recommended continual chewing calorie-free gum as nonexercise activity to achieve weight loss. This novel approach received considerable attention after their letter was published in the *New England Journal of Medicine*. A five-column feature in my local newspaper was titled, "Study of gum suggests you can chew off those excess pounds" (*The Palm Beach Post* 1999; December 30, 1999, p. A-2).

Representative Case Reports

Case II-8

A 19-year-old woman with prior convulsions caused by diet soft drinks remained seizure-free for 11 months after avoiding aspartame products. She then inadvertently chewed
a piece of gum that had been handed to her as presumed "regular" gum while attending a ball game. Multiple grand mal seizures recurred within minutes.

Case II-9

A 52-year-old bank executive in previous good health experienced severe sleepiness, marked depression with suicidal thoughts, intense anxiety, joint pains and a convulsion after consuming six cups of an aspartame hot cocoa mix daily on eight consecutive nights. She also became blind temporarily. Many studies during an ensuing hospitalization proved normal. Her symptoms disappeared within two weeks after avoiding aspartame, enabling her to resume work. When a friend later handed her a stick of aspartame gum in a darkened movie house, she "fell flat on my face in the lobby."

This patient's family history of aspartame disease included a son who developed headache after using aspartame products, and a niece who reacted with tingling of the limbs.

Case II-10

A 32-year-old woman wrote, "I couldn't believe how fast I reacted to the aspartame gum after being given a piece by my boss. I never got dizzy like that before. I had to spit it out." She was pregnant at the time.

Case II-11

A 45-year-old salesman found that even a bit of gum containing aspartame induced extreme drowsiness.

> "Just recently, I discovered as I'm driving my automobile that aspartame gum caused drowsiness after chewing only one-half a stick. It caused me to yawn, and to feel sleepy and weak. Sometimes I had to stop driving and close my eyes for a few minutes."

F. LATENT PERIOD

As a rule, there was a hiatus of from several weeks to months between first using aspartame products and the onset of aspartame reactions. These reactors then felt better by avoiding aspartame. After such "priming," subsequent consumption caused a recurrence within hours or several days. This sequence is reminiscent of allergic reactions to drugs among sensitized patients.

> Studies of hyperactive children (Chapter VI-G) indicate that there is an average interval of 2.3 days from the time some noxious food additive is introduced until abnormal behavior becomes evident.

On the other hand, some persons experienced severe reactions – especially dizziness, itching, swelling of the lips, or a rash – within minutes to an hour after their <u>first</u> known contact with aspartame. Several used the same expression: "I knew almost immediately that it was the cause."

Representative Case Reports

Case II-12

A 38-year-old instructor repeatedly suffered dramatic reactions to diet cola and aspartame hot chocolate. She listed her symptoms as follows:

> "Numbness and heaviness of the hands and feet
> Rubbery legs
> Ringing/roaring in ears
> I feel like my heart is racing
> Pressure over ears
> Tightness in head
> Urgent need to urinate
> Panicky feeling
> A very heavy sleepiness later"

These reactions occurred "immediately" on two retest trials "during which I could not function." There was a history of hay fever, hypoglycemia attacks, and allergy to aspirin and penicillin. She added, "I participated in a 'blind' study by Searle at Duke University. Although I did not have all the listed symptoms, I was feeling very 'shaky' after one test."

Case II-13

A 61-year-old computer operator suffered marked visual disturbances, headache, dizziness, memory loss, facial pains and irritability after consuming aspartame sodas. He stated

> "It seemed to take several weeks to build up the reaction the first time, but when I tested it a month or so after stopping its use, I got the same feelings after just a day or two of use. And one time, someone gave me a glass of a soft drink that I didn't know contained aspartame. I had the same symptoms within one hour or less after ingesting the drink."

Case II-14 A

A woman experienced severe headache, bloat, shaking and general disorientation shortly after drinking her first aspartame soda. These effects lasted one day. They recurred when she drank the beverage a second time.

Case II-14 B

A 42-year-old executive secretary occasionally used an ATS. She then ingested five or six packets in hot tea within less than two hours... the most she had consumed in a day. She wrote

> "I became very ill – nauseated, dizzy, unable to concentrate. I could not make my eyes focus on typewritten material. I was getting worse by the minute. I could not believe that in such a short period of time I had gone from feeling fine to feeling very sick. I had been at work no more than 45 minutes, and decided I had to leave.
>
> "I could not get in to see my boss just then, as he was in a meeting with a client. I called my husband for a ride home... 15 to 20 minutes later, I was amazed that I was beginning to feel better. As it turned out, I did not have to leave for home. I worked the rest of the day and felt better as the day wore on."

88

This woman subsequently read an article about reactions to aspartame, especially after it was heated. She surmised, "The hot tea when I got to work apparently put me 'over the edge'."

G. PERSISTENCE OF SYMPTOMS

Aspartame-induced symptoms may persist months or longer after stopping these products. This problem appears in many of the case reports, especially among aspartame reactors having ongoing visual, neurologic and psychiatric complaints. A number sought "detoxification" (Chapter XXIX).

> A 37-year-old woman with symptoms that began after using considerable aspartame illustrates the problem. She wrote, "I'm quite sure I haven't had any aspartame in three years. Could these ongoing symptoms be related to my past use? Does aspartame cause permanent nerve damage?"

Some of the possible reasons will be discussed in later chapters – including chronic methanol exposure (Chapter XXI). The attending physician, however, must consider a myriad of other diagnostic possibilities. They include complications of previous diseases apparently triggered by aspartame, a superimposed new illness, the side effects of drugs, exposure to other toxic substances, emotional problems, and even the continued use of aspartame (unknowing or intentional). The potential fallacy of making a casual psychogenic diagnosis under these circumstances is discussed in Chapter VII-A.

H. GENDER

Women consistently outnumbered men within every subgroup by a 3:1 ratio. In its monitoring of adverse reactions to aspartame products, the FDA also reported that 77 percent of complainants were female (Tollefson 1987). In this group, 76 percent were between 20 and 59 years, and 10 percent less than 20 years.

Such a gender preponderance can reflect a number of factors. They include the nature of femininity, increased consumption by women, and the reluctance of men to seek medical attention. The NutraSweet Company estimated that low-calorie soft drink consumption by adult women increased from 47 gm/day in 1977 to 105 gm/day in 1985. As more men began using low-calorie products, however, a partial "gender shift" occurred, a five-year trend noted by the Calorie Control Council.

Some of the influences that may contribute to the greater vulnerability of women, especially as they pertain to nervous system disturbances, are relevant.

A. Female Hormones

- Gordan and Elliott (1947) noted that <u>diethylstilbestrol</u> depresses glucose oxidation in brain tissue. Similarly, important energy pathways – for example, those involving some enzymes of the tricarboxylic acid cycle (notably the succinic and malic oxidase systems), and the terminal electron transport pathways within mitochondria – are particularly sensitive to inhibition by diethylstilbestrol (Talalay 1960).
- <u>Pregnant women</u> and those taking <u>oral contraceptives</u> ("the pill") secrete considerably more insulin (see B) and develop a chronic hyperinsulinized state (Spellacy 1966, Javier 1968, Yen 1968). Accordingly, they are likely to experience severe hypoglycemia by simultaneously consuming aspartame and reducing their caloric intake for weight control.
- Neuropsychiatric features are commonly associated with the <u>premenstrual syndrome</u>. (In *Lamentations* [1:17], Jeremiah alludes to the desolate and chaotic melancholy of his era in terms of a "menstruous woman.")

B. Insulin Effects; Diabetes

- Healthy non-obese females evidence <u>greater insulin responses</u> to the oral administration or intravenous infusion of phenylalanine and other amino acids than men (Shah 1986).
- Femininity increases the frequency and magnitude of <u>hypoglycemia</u>. Morton et al (1950, 1953) noted that reactive hypoglycemia tends to be exaggerated before the menstrual periods, especially among young women who experience premenstrual tension.
- <u>Diabetogenic hyperinsulinism</u> (Introduction to Section 2 and Chapter XIV) has been shown to be frequent among relatively young women whose ovaries were removed, and in elderly females (Zeytinoglu 1969).
- Women are more prone to <u>diabetes</u> (Haglund 1986).

C. Pharmacologic Differences

- Pharmacologic studies indicate sex-related differences in the arousal or soporific responses to drugs. Munkelt et al (1962) used seven parameters to investigate the effects of meprobamate (800 mg) and alcohol (0.9 to 1.0%) on the performance of 80 subjects. They noted a greater deterioration in performance among women.

- Tordoff and Alleva (1990) evaluated the increase of hunger by oral stimulation with a gum base containing several concentrations of aspartame. The most effective concentration was 0.3 percent for females, and 0.5 percent for males. Furthermore, the gum base was perceived as sweeter by females in both the 0.3 percent and 0.5 percent concentrations.

- Caballero et al (1991) demonstrated that aging was associated with a significant rise in the plasma concentrations of large neutral amino acids in apparently healthy elderly women, but not men. Specifically, this phenomenon was significant for phenylalanine, valine, leucine, isoleucine and tyrosine.

- Menstruating women with iron deficiency have an impaired ability to convert phenylalanine to tyrosine (Lehmann 1986). Their abnormal response to a phenylalanine load, as evidenced by higher blood phenylalanine levels, normalizes after the repletion of iron stores.

- Women are at increased risk for developing severe depression (Holden 1986). It is estimated that one woman in four is afflicted with a major depression during her lifetime, compared to one in ten for men.

- Gender differences in the concentrations of branched-chain amino acids exist. They are normally higher in men than women, accounting for the low plasma phenylalanine/large neutral amino acids ratio (Caballero 1987).

- Dr. Don McLain (1986), President of the American Association for Clinical Immunology and Allergy, reported that the frequency of allergies – particularly to foods and drugs – is significantly higher among women than men.

- More women manifest disorders of the immune system (Chapter VIII). They include rheumatoid arthritis, lupus erythematosus and myasthenia gravis. (Females also appear to develop fulminant AIDS and succumb more rapidly than men.) Talal (1985) suggested that autoimmune disease is more common among women because of "immunologic imprinting" in an *in utero* hyperestrogen environment. This phenomenon presumably helps protect pregnant women from infectious diseases and other environmental insults.

- The aggravating role of premenstrual and intermenstrual <u>fluid retention</u> on nervous system function (Chapters IX-E and IX-F) was known to Hippocrates.

- A related vicious cycle involves <u>the intracellular retention of water and sodium in the hyperinsulinized state</u> (Roberts 1964b, 1966b; Bloom 1967).

- There are <u>gender differences in brain development</u>. Males have more neurons (averaging 13 percent), whereas the excess of neuropil in females enhances cellular communication.

- The frequency and seriousness of <u>covert alcoholism</u> (Chapter XII) among middle-class women are recognized (Nuckols 1967).

- This gender preponderance may reflect the fact that <u>women tend to outlive men in our society</u>. Accordingly, more women over 50 might visit doctors for aspartame-associated problems -- especially headache, "nerves," severe depression, memory loss, lower urinary tract problems, and aggravated diabetes or hypertension.

I. SEASONALLY INCREASED CONSUMPTION

Many patients in this series volunteered that they increased their consumption of aspartame soft drinks and "presweetened" iced tea during hot weather. It is corroborated by persons living in semitropical and tropical areas.

Some aspartame reactors indicated the extraordinary methods used to accommodate their increased thirst for aspartame beverages during hot weather. One stated, "I drink cans in summer since they are easier to carry in a cooler, and are lighter in weight."

A related clinical issue surfaced. Until the likelihood of aspartame disease was raised, reactors often ascribed recent debilitating symptoms to "the heat." The "aspartame connection" becomes more plausible in light of the body's increased demands for water and energy at elevated temperatures, and the effect of heat on chemical breakdown of aspartame (Chapter XXV). (Physicians in the military ought to be aware of these considerations because recruits can drink up to 10 liters of fluid daily in hot climes.)

This industry's anticipation of increased consumption in hot weather is evidenced by the use of vending machines with a temperature sensor and computer chip that automatically raise prices for cans of soda (*The Palm Beach Post* October 28, 1999, p. A-1).

Representative Case Reports

Case II-15

A 61-year-old executive developed visual problems, confusion and amnesia two hours after drinking <u>one</u> cup of aspartame-sweetened coffee before playing golf. (He usually added saccharin.) Even though he frequently played in similar weather, his golf partners thought he was having "heat stroke" on this occasion.

Case II-16

I had attended a 64-year-old Bahamian executive many years. He presented during July 1986 complaining of recent visual impairment, progressively severe frontal headaches, discomfort and cramps in the lower extremities, and a gain of six pounds.

On direct questioning, he stated that he had been using at least six packets of an ATS in tea daily, and was drinking other beverages containing aspartame. As the weather got hotter, he increased such consumption considerably. All his symptoms disappeared or improved within ten days after discontinuing aspartame products.

Case II-17

A 41-year-old merchandiser experienced a severe convulsion. She neither smoked nor drank alcohol. She explained the circumstances in these terms.

> "We were on vacation at Disney World. It was hot, so I had at least 3 large diet colas for two days only. At the end of the second day, I had a grand mal seizure in my sleep, and was rushed to the hospital. At the hospital, without any real tests, I was told I had a brain tumor. I left the next day on my own because I figured out by then it was the diet cola. Two doctors in Michigan also said it was a brain tumor, but then discovered it was not.

> "I'm glad I never believed them. The side effects from the Dilantin® were almost as bad as the seizure. None of the three doctors wanted to hear about aspartame. My current doctor is much more interested in finding out all he can about it."

Case II-18

A 29-year-old aspartame reactor suffered unexplained loss of appetite and an 80-pound weight loss over six months. She wrote, "We live in Arizona where you have to consume enormous amounts of beverages due to the heat in the summer."

J. FAMILIAL RAMIFICATIONS

The finding of 211 families in which two or more members had aspartame reactions – 17.6 percent of reactors in this series -- was unexpected initially. As many as <u>seven</u> close relatives were so afflicted (see Cases II-19 and 20). This revelation surfaced for Case II-19 at a family reunion.

The survey questionnaire (Section 4) details this familial tendency. Accordingly, *the relatives of aspartame reactors should be considered at higher risk for aspartame disease* (Chapter XVI).

Individual family members may experience different reactions to aspartame products. For example, a boy developed an asthmatic attack after an aspartame drink, while his father would suffer severe migraine shortly after drinking one can.

Bilateral Inheritance

A husband, wife, and one or more children were found to be aspartame reactors in some families. One young woman summarized her family's experience.

> "My four-year-old son has always reacted to aspartame with personality changes, headache and sleep. My husband complains of memory loss with just one bottle of pop containing aspartame. I, myself, react with swelling and headaches. I would like to know more about aspartame and why it affects us like this since we don't have the PKU problem."

Double-Duty Questionnaires

There was an occasional element of humor when two or three members of several families filled out the <u>same</u> questionnaire form. A mother and daughter did so in one instance. Another questionnaire (described below) was completed in different colors – blue for the brother, and red for his sister.

"Anticipation"

I encountered the phenomenon of "anticipation" in families afflicted with aspartame disease. This refers to its occurrence among children and young adults before overtly developing in parents. I previously described this phenomenon in diabetes, hypoglycemia and narcolepsy (Roberts 1964, 1966, 1967, 1971).

Representative Case Reports

Case II-19

A <u>homemaker</u> developed palpitations, depression, recurrent pains in the head, and visual difficulty after drinking considerable aspartame colas. She described her eyes as "getting weaker... as though they had a thumb on them, but when I rubbed them, it didn't help." All her symptoms vanished four days after discontinuing aspartame.

She amplified the reactions of <u>a sister</u> who was described as previously being a "very happy, outgoing person." They consisted of severe depression and unexplained pain in the arms for which no medical problem could be found. She reverted "back to her happy normal self," and without any arm pain, within several days after stopping aspartame beverages.

<u>Another sister</u> also experienced intense depression. "She didn't care if she got up in the morning, and had little interest in anything." On learning of the foregoing reactions by her two sisters, she stopped aspartame... and felt fine within three days.

A non-smoking <u>niece</u> had doctored for unexplained chest pains. They promptly subsided after abstinence from aspartame products.

Her <u>husband</u> also proved to be an aspartame reactor. It was evidenced most noticeably as being "more irritable and edgy." His personality normalized when he avoided all aspartame products.

Case II-20

A 62-year-old <u>female realtor</u> experienced marked decrease of vision in both eyes, ringing in the ears, intense tremors, insomnia, facial pain, slurred speech, depression with suicidal thoughts, severe anxiety, "personality changes," attacks of shortness of breath, palpitations, unexplained chest pains (initially thought to have been a heart attack), diarrhea, severe abdominal bloat, marked itching and severe joint pains.

Her 59-year-old <u>sister</u> developed severe headache, palpitations, depression, and unexplained pains in the chest and joints while drinking five cans of diet cola daily. These symptoms dramatically abated within several days after abstinence from aspartame.

Her <u>two daughters</u> had marked reactions to aspartame products.

A ten-year-old <u>grandson</u> became "very hyper" after ingesting aspartame.

A <u>brother</u> developed "large sores on his face. When I told him how good I felt after stopping aspartame, he stopped and was healed in a few days."

The nervousness and heart symptoms of her <u>husband</u> subsided after avoiding aspartame.

Case II-21

A 38-year-old <u>legal secretary</u> went on a franchised system's program for weight control. She used six packets of an ATS, and drank eight glasses of presweetened iced tea daily. Many symptoms ensued. They included loss of visual acuity, pain in both eyes, recent "dry eyes," difficulty wearing contact lens, severe headache, dizziness, tremors, mental confusion, memory loss, facial pains, extreme irritability, a recent rise in blood pressure, marked bloat, dryness of the mouth and lips, intense thirst, and joint pains. These complaints began to regress within one day after stopping aspartame products, and were gone three days later. The same reactions recurred on two occasions when she ingested aspartame.

The patient indicated in the survey questionnaire that her <u>mother</u> also suffered reactions to aspartame. Responding to "What kind of reactions?", she wrote, "The same as me."

Case II-22

A 62-year-old <u>woman</u> described "immediate difficulty in swallowing" as her most prominent reaction to aspartame. She stated, "I was eating a cereal and did not know that it contained aspartame. My throat became paralyzed and I could not swallow. My daughter asked if I had checked for aspartame. When I did, that's when I realized that I was using it."

Similarly, this <u>daughter</u> had experienced "throat paralysis" as her major reaction to aspartame.

Case II-23

A 64-year-old <u>man</u>, owner of an advertising agency, had been consuming two cans of diet cola daily. His apparent sole reaction was severe insomnia. There was a history of migraine. He indicated, "The lack of sleep created by it made working next to impossible." The insomnia disappeared one day after stopping aspartame. It recurred within a day after retesting himself on <u>three</u> occasions. At that point, he avoided the product.

His <u>wife</u> and <u>a son</u> also experienced aspartame reactions. These consisted of "sleeplessness, chills, and disorientation."

Case II-24

A 53-year-old <u>housewife</u> suffered numerous reactions while consuming two cans of a diet soda and up to six packets of an ATS daily. The symptoms included decreased vision in both eyes, loss of hearing in one ear, severe headache, dizziness, petit mal attacks, tremors, marked insomnia, mental confusion, hyperactivity, tingling and numbness of the limbs, facial pain, slurred speech, intense depression, extreme irritability, a change in personality, the aggravation of phobias, shortness of breath, palpitations, an elevation of blood pressure, abdominal pain, marked bloat, a rash, thinning of the hair, pain on swallowing, intense thirst, cessation of her menses, severe joint pains, swelling of the legs, and a gain of 20 pounds. She saw nine physicians and consultants. Her symptoms began to recede within five days after stopping aspartame. The "esophageal spasms," however, persisted.

She wrote, "This is the very worst experience in my life. It has greatly affected members of my family, physically and mentally."

Her <u>sister</u> and her <u>husband</u> also experienced aspartame-associated headache, nausea, chest discomfort, and aching of the joints. Suspecting that other family members with similar problems were aspartame reactors, she requested that copies of the survey questionnaire be sent to eleven!

Case II-25

A 29-year-old <u>woman</u> would become incapacitated within hours after ingesting any of several aspartame products. She was hospitalized, and then had to stop school. Her reactions consisted of intense headache, dizziness, two convulsions, irresistible drowsiness, insomnia, tremors, mental confusion, depression, slurred speech, marked personality changes, severe anxiety, palpitations, abdominal pain, intense nausea, itching, more frequent periods, joint pains, swelling of the legs, and severe bloat.

Her <u>mother</u> also had multiple aspartame reactions. They included "dizziness, passing out, pain in the stomach, headache, nausea and diarrhea." A diagnosis of "aspartame toxicity" was made by the mother's physician.

Case II-26

Three members of one family had severe reactions from aspartame products.

- The <u>husband</u> developed marked gastrointestinal symptoms. He also was diagnosed as having an "immune deficiency problem" to explain abnormalities of his red blood cells, white blood cells and platelets.
- His <u>wife</u> complained of decreased vision in both eyes, severe headaches, extreme dryness of the mouth, and intense thirst.
- Their 28-year-old <u>daughter</u> suffered multiple grand mal convulsions. Other features included severe headache, marked mental confusion, recurrent depression with suicidal thoughts, a bleeding peptic ulcer, and a 15-pound weight loss.

It was of further interest that this couple's <u>granddaughter</u> had phenylketonuria (Chapter XVII) at birth, and subsequently evidenced marked learning impairment.

Case II-27

A 56-year-old <u>secretary</u> experienced marked decrease of vision, ringing in both ears, severe sensitivity to noise, unexplained head pains, extreme irritability, and atypical chest pain. She had been consuming up to three cans of a diet cola daily.

Her <u>husband</u> became markedly irritable while using "considerable diet colas."

Concerning her <u>sister</u>, she wrote

> "I have sent the other two copies of this form to my two sisters living in Ohio, as they both had much stronger reactions to aspartame than I had – one with pain and depression, and the other with <u>severe</u> depression. Their problems disappeared in a few short days after they quit aspartame drinks."

Case II-28

A 59-year-old <u>secretary</u> suffered severe headaches, marked depression, palpitations, unexplained chest pains, intense discomfort involving the wrist and elbows, and "a weak feeling inside – like I could go down at any time." She had been consuming 4-5 cans of diet cola daily. Her symptoms improved within three days after stopping this beverage, and disappeared by one week.

She indicated that her <u>two daughters</u> also had aspartame reactions. One experienced heaviness in the chest and palpitations. The other had headaches, depression, and a "urinary problem."

She described the reactions of her <u>sister</u> in these terms: "Death wish. Pain from elbow to shoulder. Fatigue. Depression. Looked, walked and acted like she was on her last leg." A remarkable improvement occurred after avoiding aspartame. "The difference in my sister was like a miracle. She even brought me a gift at the end of the no-aspartame week."

Comparable Familial Reactions

Similar reactions to aspartame occurred in multiple family members. This was alluded to earlier (see Cases II-21 and II-22).

- Case IX-D-24 and two close relatives developed <u>diarrhea</u> after drinking variable amounts of aspartame cola.
- Two 40-year-old identical twin sisters experienced <u>severe abdominal pain</u> as their chief reaction to aspartame products.

- Case IV-30 related the <u>visual effects</u> of aspartame disease in a mother and young son.
- A 68-year-old man with severe <u>neuropsychiatric reactions</u> to aspartame volunteered that two grandsons exhibited hyperactivity when they ingested aspartame soft drinks.

The severity of aspartame-induced <u>depression</u> (Chapter VII-B) in the members of families having a tendency to depression was impressive. One patient with extreme depression and other reactions to aspartame related the case of a niece who had been "living on it." She required hospitalization for severe anorexia and bulimia (gorging on food followed by induced vomiting) (Chapter IX-B).

Aspartame-induced <u>seizures</u> occurred among the relatives of aspartame reactors.

- Each of two women with aspartame-related seizures (Cases III-22 and III-23) had several children who also suffered convulsions. They consumed aspartame during pregnancy and while breast feeding.
- A husband and wife (Cases III-26B and III-26C) experienced aspartame-induced seizures and marked motor weakness after consuming a soft drink mix.

Representative Case Reports

Case II-30 and II-31

A 22-year-old <u>Air Force officer</u> and his <u>sister</u> (a 24-year-old landscape foreman) used the <u>same</u> survey questionnaire form to list their aspartame reactions – he with blue ink; she with red ink. Each experienced severe headache and extreme irritability "immediately after usage."

Case II-32 and II-33

<u>Two sisters</u> suffered violent headaches after ingesting small amounts of aspartame. One wrote about the other, "After drinking a cup of hot chocolate sweetened with aspartame, she experienced the worst headache she's ever had."

Case II-34

A 45-year-old <u>interior designer</u> stopped having menstrual periods two weeks after beginning to drink four cans of diet cola daily, along with "diet food meals." There was associated abdominal bloat.

Concomitantly, her <u>two teenage daughters</u> stopped menstruating for three months.

Aspartame was then suspected as the cause. Normal menstrual periods returned <u>in all three</u> within one month after stopping aspartame!

Case II-35

A 31-year-old <u>bookkeeper</u> developed pain in both eyes, ringing in the ears, severe dizziness, attacks of shortness of breath, palpitations, diarrhea, intense itching, a gain of 12 pounds, and marked frequency of urination (both day and night.) She had been consuming up to three glasses of an ASD and ten packets of an ATS daily. There was a longstanding history of hay fever and hypoglycemia attacks. Her symptoms promptly improved after avoiding aspartame products... only to recur within hours on each of <u>three</u> retesting trials.

She concisely described the reactions of her <u>mother</u>: "The same as mine."

Possible Genetic Mechanisms

A clue concerning the familial nature of aspartame reactions emerged from observations by Tobey and Neizer (1987). They suspected congenital deficiency of a major peptidase enzyme in the cytosol of intestinal wall cells (enterocytes) that hydrolyzes much of the aspartylphenylalanine after the cleavage of methanol (Chapter XXV). The subsequent entry of this dipeptide into the system might result in symptoms and immune reactions. Circulating red blood cells could be examined for deficiencies or genetic variants of this hydrolytic enzyme.

Genetic considerations involving methanol metabolism are considered in Chapter XXI.

Congenital deficiency of prolidase, another cytosolic peptidase, also has been reported (Powell 1974).

Presweetened Tea For Two

Mention was made of <u>both</u> spouses being aspartame reactors. The cartoon in Figure II-1, concerning the symptoms of a husband and his wife, illustrates this phenomenon.

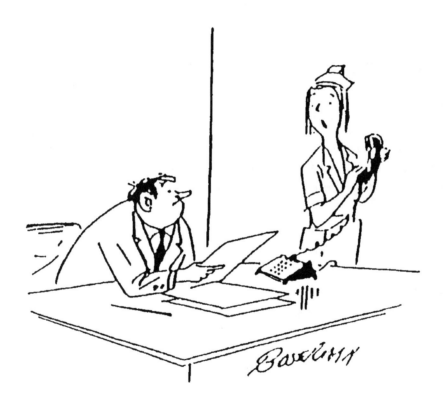

"Dr. Turner has a patient with the same thing his wife had. What did you do for her?"

Reproduced with permission by *Medical Tribune* (September 24, 1986) and William H. Boserman

Figure II-1

K. MULTIPLE REACTIONS TO ASPARTAME PRODUCTS

The multiplicity of complaints <u>specifically</u> attributable to using aspartame products – especially as documented by their marked regression or disappearance after abstinence – is repeatedly evidenced in the preceding case reports. Similar patterns of presenting symptoms appear in ensuing sections.

A number of patients with aspartame disease erroneously believed that their reaction was limited to a single complaint or body system. Inquiry about other symptoms during consultation, or analysis of the details in their completed survey questionnaires, generally indicated additional reactions.

Representative Case Reports

Case II-4 (see above)

A 34-year-old woman consumed large amounts of aspartame products for one and a half years, including eight glasses of a hot chocolate <u>daily</u> (see above). She temporarily lost her job when incapacitated by the following reactions

- A marked decrease of vision and pain in both eyes
- Ringing in the left ear
- Marked sensitivity of noise in both ears
- Severe headaches
- Severe dizziness and light-headedness
- Severe cramping of the toes and legs every day
- Two convulsions
- Marked memory loss ("I couldn't remember something that was said recently")
- Severe tingling, pins and needles, and numbness of the arms and legs
- Severe depression
- Extreme irritability
- Severe anxiety attacks
- Marked "personality changes"
- Fear of crowds and other phobias ("I felt I wanted to ruin someone who ruined me")
- Pain in the abdomen
- Severe nausea and vomiting
- Diarrhea with bloody stools

- Marked abdominal bloat
- Considerable thinning of the hair
- A weight gain of 10 pounds
- Dryness of the mouth
- Intense thirst
- Frequency and burning of urination, with an associated urinary-tract infection

She had seen four physicians and consultants, and was hospitalized once. Multiple studies proved inconclusive. They included x-rays of the head, a CT scan of the brain, an electroencephalogram, two upper gastrointestinal series, two barium enemas, allergy tests, and special examinations of the eyes and ears.

When she concluded that aspartame products had been causing or aggravating her problem, improvement occurred within three days after stopping them. She retested herself more than ten times... with prompt recurrence of the listed symptoms (especially vomiting) on each occasion. At that point, she totally avoided aspartame. ("I now read every label before I take any product.")

Case II-36

A 64-year-old man was seen in August 1986 for his annual checkup. He complained of persistent and increasing headache, especially over the frontal areas. He felt that his vision had deteriorated, but an ophthalmologist could find no significant change. Other recent problems included

- A gain of six pounds
- Marked sensitivity to air conditioning
- Increased stuffiness of the nose and sinuses, with repeated sneezing ("like the beginning of a cold")
- Cramps and numbness of both the legs and feet
- "Getting tired very easily" and a tendency to severe drowsiness

Direct questioning about the use of aspartame products revealed that he had been using at least six packets of an ATS in tea daily since his previous visit. Virtually all the symptoms disappeared within ten days after avoiding aspartame.

104

<u>**Case II-37**</u>

A 38-year-old executive believed that her reaction was "purely intestinal in nature" – namely, severe abdominal bloat (Chapter IX-F). She then admitted to recent "dry eyes," difficulty wearing contact lens, and a gain of 15 pounds.

SECTION 2

ANALYSIS OF ASPARTAME REACTIONS

"To profess what we know, confess what we don't, and interpret from our experience is our duty and privilege as physicians."*
> Dr. Theodore T. Herwig (1986)

"And he (Proteus) will try you by taking the form of all creatures that come forth and move on the earth; he'll be water and magical fire."
> *The Odyssey of Homer*
> (Translated by R. Lattimore
> New York; Harper & Row, 1975)

The chapters in this section describe and amplify major reactions to aspartame products. Some individuals seemingly evidenced a single reaction to aspartame. The vast majority, however, experienced multiple adverse effects (Chapter II-K).

The manifestations of aspartame disease or aspartame syndrome truly can be "protean." This term relates to the ancient God Proteus (see introductory quote) who could assume many forms, thereby eluding his pursuers. One definition of syndrome is the clustering of non-chance associations, which components can be related to a common element (Ferrannini 2000).

While I have limited the representative case reports, every complainant's history was instructive. They encompass my patients' problems, those of individuals interviewed personally or by phone, detailed letters, responses to the Survey Questionnaire (Section 4) containing sufficient information to justify "the aspartame connection," and communications from other physicians.

Similarities in the progression of symptoms and signs often could be detected. Increasingly frequent and severe headaches prior to a grand mal convulsion, and generalized itching preceding hives or other skin eruptions are notable examples of such "syndrome trains." Physicians ought to seek out these sequences. Caleb Hillier Parry (*Preface* Bath, October 1811) wrote

> "In reality, it is not the pomp of language, the 'whistling of a name,' or the simplicity or ingenuity of a pathological theory, that can long give it currency with mankind. The sole point is, whether it is a just arrangement of actual phenomena, of which the operation of remedies form an indispensable part. If it does not include these operations, it is defective; if it is inconsistent with what is known of them it is mischievous. By this test every medical work ought to be tried, and by it the present work must stand or fall."

The pertinent medical details and related clinical/experimental discussions are abbreviated. Some conditions (e.g., narcolepsy) are defined for interested "nonmedical" readers, but familiarity with common conditions such as depression, dizziness and hives is presumed.

COMPARISON WITH FDA STATISTICS

The Food and Drug Administration (FDA) has monitored adverse reactions to aspartame through its Adverse Reaction Monitoring System (ARMS). It subdivided the initial 3,326 complaints into these groups:

- Group A — symptoms recurring each time different products containing the same item were consumed – 13 percent
- Group B — symptoms recurring each time the same product was consumed – 34 percent
- Group C — symptoms associated with the ingestion of a product or products containing the item of interest, but in which there was no rechallenge by the complainant – 17 percent
- Group D — symptoms failing to recur every time the products were consumed, or if a physician stated that a complaint's symptoms were unlikely caused by the substance – 18 percent

Concerning the distribution of consumer reports by products used, 45.9 percent of the total were related to diet soft drinks, and 26.1 percent to tabletop sweeteners (Table II-3).

Table II-2 summarizes the alleged adverse reactions to aspartame products reported to the FDA. The preponderance of neurologic and psychiatric complaints is comparable to my data in Table II-1.

The potential severity of aspartame-associated reactions is indicated by the fact that 10.6 percent of complaints in the FDA's April 1995 analysis of 7,232 complaints were classified as Type I reactions. These were defined as including, but not limited to, "severe respiratory distress or chest pain; cardiac arrhythmia; anaphylactic or hypotensive episodes; severe gastrointestinal distress such as protacted vomiting or diarrhea leading to dehydration; severe neurological distress such as extreme dizziness, fainting, or seizures; or any reaction requiring emergency medical treatment" (Tollefson 1987). Among the first 149 persons reporting aspartame-associated convulsions, however, 129 (87.2 percent) had Type I Reactions.

108

A CLINICIAN'S COMMENTARY

I coined the term **aspartame disease** after much deliberation. In previous texts, I emphasized that the term "disease" can be misleading. The "functional" disturbances evoked by a noxious stimulus – whether chemical, physical or emotional – tend to be in continual flux until irreversible changes occur. Moreover, each tissue or body organ may respond differently at different times, or when there are superimposed stimuli. For example, clinical disorders tend to be provoked by lesser degrees of stress among older persons (Chapter XV).

Another pertinent theme is *the need to understand the adverse effects of foods, drugs and chemicals within the context of our evolving society*. Drastic changes in diet, habits and the ecology can alter physiology. Such a systems analysis approach was emphasized in my books on diagnosis (Roberts 1958), traffic accidents (Roberts 1971b), and the prevention of Alzheimer's disease (Roberts 1995). It also applies to aspartame reactions.

Diabetogenic hyperinsulinism (Chapter XIV) provides a case in point. This condition exists in at least one-third of the general population. It encompasses reactive hypoglycemia ("low blood sugar attacks") and diabetes mellitus. Its clinical spectrum includes recurrent hunger, an intense craving for sweets, pathologic drowsiness (narcolepsy), headache, severe muscle cramps, and a host of other neurologic, psychiatric and metabolic changes that develop after abstinence from food, coupled with the use of aspartame products.

Concomitant caffeinism can potentiate aspartame reactions. Attention is directed to the considerable consumption of aspartame-sweetened colas, coffee, tea and even caffeinated gum (Chapter II-E). The symptoms and signs of caffeinism include severe irritability, tremors, palpitations, insomnia, gastrointestinal distress, the exaggeration of hypoglycemia, and aggravated diabetes (Roberts 1971b).

The adverse professional, business and personal effects of *combined aspartame reactions, caffeinism and hypoglycemia* can be serious, especially for drivers, pilots, persons managing highly competitive industries, and individuals with complex technological skills.

> A 51-year-old woman with multiple severe symptoms chiefly attributable to aspartame disease had increased her intake of both caffeine and aspartame. She experienced dizziness, rapid heart action, an irregular pulse, and extreme "anxiety." Multiple cardiac studies proved normal. She wrote

"My gynecologist told me to quit using sugar in any way, shape or form. She put me on a hypoglycemic diet for menopause and weight control. After two months, I took myself off this diet because I had no energy and felt tired all the time. I tried fooling around to find something that would energize me. I was still drinking lots of coffee (6-8 cups) a day. I needed the caffeine to keep me going... always using aspartame in my coffee."

Awareness of aspartame disease can obviate the many erroneous diagnoses made on patients described in this section. A few examples:

- A man with incapacitating aspartame disease had been misdiagnosed by 21 doctors over eleven years! His dramatic improvement after avoiding aspartame products stimulated him to set up a web site about aspartame disease on the Internet.

- A 43-year-old engineer experienced migraine and marked reduction in vision. He had been a longstanding consumer of aspartame products. Considerable attention was directed to a subarachnoid cyst, which proved to be an incidental benign congenital lesion. Dramatic improvement of vision, headache and dizziness occurred after avoiding aspartame products.

- A woman with previous Lyme disease experienced marked tremors, an upset stomach, and severe headache. She was concerned about the activation of this infection or a delayed complication. The clue to aspartame disease was disappearance of these symptoms on weekends when she did not drink aspartame sodas.

III

EPILEPSY (CONVULSIONS)

"It is of use from time to time to take stock, so to speak,
of our knowledge of a particular disease, to see exactly
where we stand in regard to it, to inquire what conclusions
the accumulated facts seem to point to, and to ascertain in
what direction we may look for fruitful investigations in
the future."

Sir William Osler

GENERAL CONSIDERATIONS

Some of the synonyms for "grand mal" epileptic attacks are convulsions, seizures and "fits." Anyone who has witnessed the severe jerking and loss of consciousness during such an attack can attest to its frightening nature, both for the victim and observer.

At least 1.2 million persons in the United States have epilepsy. Eight percent of the general population is likely to suffer a clinical seizure during his or her lifetime.

Espic (1967) cautioned that epilepsy is neither a single disease or a homogeneous entity. He emphasized that this term should be used only when "intermittent disturbances of consciousness, movement, feeling, or behavior – usually stereotyped – recur as a result of the primary cerebral disorder."

Convulsions may be caused or aggravated by many factors. Aspartame products must be included in the list (Roberts 1988b, e; 1989a; 1992b).

Acronym Legend

          ACB - aspartame cola beverage
          ASD - aspartame soft drink
          ATS - aspartame tabletop sweetener

Classification

The epilepsies are classified in several ways, such as "primary generalized" and "partial."

- Primary generalized seizures are described as tonic, clonic, tonic-clonic (grand mal), myoclonic, atonic and absences.
- Partial seizures originating in various areas of the brain are categorized as sensory, motor, autonomic, hallucinatory, experiential and emotional. (A "simple partial seizure" generally infers that consciousness is spared during the seizure.) These account for between one-half and two-thirds of recurrent seizures. They tend to occur later in life than primary generalized seizures, and may be less responsive to medication.

ASPARTAME-INDUCED GRAND MAL SEIZURES

Most of the 129 persons (11 percent) with grand mal seizures in this series had their first convulsions after using aspartame. Patients who suffered recurrent attacks while taking maintenance anti-epilepsy medication, such as phenytoin (Dilantin®), generally became seizure-free after stopping aspartame products.

The following clinical observations are pertinent.

- Young women with histories of severe migraine, reactive hypoglycemia, and fluid retention (recurrent edema) were more prone to develop convulsions after consuming moderate or large amounts of aspartame.
- Several aspartame reactors with grand mal convulsions emphasized that most of their attacks occurred during sleep. Plausible contributory factors include delayed allergic reactions (Chapter VIII) and nocturnal hypoglycemia (Chapter XIV).
- A normal electroencephalogram in children who ingest these products should alert physicians to the possibility of aspartame-associated convulsions. This finding assumes

further importance because the prognosis tends to be good, medication generally can be limited to a single drug, and anti-epileptic drugs often may be discontinued within one or two years if there are no recurrences.

- Only six of the 50 persons with grand mal seizures who initially completed the survey questionnaire (Chapter XVIII) were on a strict weight-reducing diet when they experienced aspartame-induced convulsions.

- Alcohol intake prior to convulsions was absent or minimum in this group. Two registered nurses who experienced grand mal seizures after drinking considerable aspartame had taken small or moderate amounts of alcohol before their attacks, as did the drug company representative cited below.

- Longstanding changes detected in or adjacent to the brain by computer tomography (CT) scanning proved "red herrings" in several patients with aspartame-associated convulsions. For example, Case III-5 had _five_ CT scans and _four_ magnetic resonance imaging (MRI) studies done because of an abnormal finding. The reviewing radiologist concluded that it represented a congenital vascular malformation.

- Four aspartame reactors with recurrent convulsions continued to use aspartame products, largely because of aspartame addiction (Chapter VII-G).

- Aspartame use can sensitize patients to monosodium glutamate (MSG) (Roberts 1993a) and other neurotoxic additives (Chapter VIII-E). This issue was raised in Case II-1 when a second seizure occurred eight months after avoiding aspartame, but within one day following MSG consumption.

- The frequency of seizures with a brand of non-cola aspartame soda was impressive.

Input From Radio Audiences

My discussion of aspartame reactions on talk shows (Chapter I) predictably evoked calls and letters from listeners who attributed their seizures to aspartame use. The following letter was received after an interview on Philadelphia Station WWDB.

"On November 5, 1985, I suffered a seizure at home. I was rushed to the hospital and stayed for four days. I had blood work, CT scans and EEG. I was discharged and told I had an epileptic condition and low magnesium.. I have been on 300 mg of Dilantin ever since. I also had my driver's license recalled for one year, and as of today it has not been reinstated.

"I was very upset with the epilepsy label that was laid on me. It was very hard to accept...

"I consumed large amounts of aspartame as soda, coffee, and tea. The day I had my seizure my intake of aspartame was quite a lot. I am totally convinced that it triggered my seizure. I have not had a seizure since not using aspartame in any form."

Paramedical Input

The matter of aspartame-induced convulsions surfaced professionally in unexpected ways.

A drug company representative wondered if he could "ask a personal question." The stimulus was my letter in *The Palm Beach Post* (August 21, 1987, pp. E-2) wherein I disagreed with the assertion (based on an animal study), published nationwide, that aspartame does not cause seizures in humans. He had two recent grand mal convulsions while consuming large amounts of aspartame on weekends. Numerous studies failed to reveal any overt cause. When I mentioned that aspartame-related seizures generally occurred during the early morning hours, he replied, "That's exactly when I had my attacks!"

REPRESENTATIVE CASE REPORTS

Many impressive reports were told or submitted by aspartame reactors with convulsions. Others (e.g., Case VIII-22) appear in subsequent chapters.

Case III-1

A 31-year-old registered nurse and health care executive had enjoyed good health her entire adult life. The only aspects of possible significance in her past history were

Sydenham's chorea at the age of three years following several childhood diseases, modest cigarette smoking, intentional but gradual weight loss (from 211 to 135 pounds) years previously, and mild premenstrual fluid retention. No drugs of abuse ever had been taken.

She began drinking one or two glasses daily of an aspartame-sweetened lemon drink for one week. The following Saturday, she consumed 67 ounces (two liters) of the same brand's orange drink. The only other changes in activity or habits were eating more fruit and drinking a small amount of alcohol that day.

The patient was found unconscious and convulsing on Sunday at 4 AM. Her ensuing combative behavior on an emergency floor (which she could not recall) was totally out of character. She also developed itching and a rash over the neck and chest.

Detailed medical and neurologic evaluations during the ensuing hospitalization included a CT scan of the brain, an electroencephalogram, a drug screen, and measurement of blood vitamin B_{12} and folate levels. All were normal. A subsequent hair analysis for toxic minerals proved normal. Phenytoin was prescribed for "idiopathic epilepsy."

This nurse then researched a possible relationship between aspartame intake and seizures in the hospital's medical library. She found several references and case reports comparable to her own. Her neurologist, however, refused to make further inquiry into the matter when she requested him to do so. He suggested, "Stop reading!"

Subsequently researching the aspartame content of diet soft drinks, she found that the orange ones usually had high concentrations – 335 mg aspartame per 12 fluid ounces, or 930 mg per liter – because manufacturers added more to preserve the sweet taste.

The patient became apprehensive over the significance of this seizure, and the impact of an "epilepsy" diagnosis on her professional career and driver insurability. She then saw me in consultation. I concluded that the ingestion of 1,100 mg aspartame within a 10-hour period – about 18.3 mg/kg – had probably caused or contributed to her seizure. Under close observation, she was weaned off phenytoin. There were no further seizures over the ensuing eight months.

Two other factors that probably provoked subsequent seizures thereafter were uncovered: reactive hypoglycemia, and sensitivity to monosodium glutamate (MSG). The role of nocturnal hypoglycemia was raised when she experienced a seizure early one morning after having eaten a popsicle and failed to take the recommended nighttime snack. A subsequent glucose tolerance test (GTT) had to be terminated at 4-1/2 hours because of severe tremors, intense hunger and fatigue. The results (as mg percent, plasma) were as follows; fasting - 112; ½ hour - 185; 1 hour - 131; 2 hours - 95; 3 hours - 96; 3-1/2 hours - 91; 4 hours - 64 (with onset of the reaction); 4-1/2 hours - 67 (severe reaction). The test was concluded at that point to avoid precipitating a seizure.

The patient had another attack after ingesting Chinese food seasoned with MSG two days previously, and eating stuffing that contained MSG the previous day. A repeat EEG and CT scan of the brain were normal. Phenytoin was resumed as a precautionary measure.

The patient subsequently drank "only three sips" of a drink believed to be "regular" soda which contained aspartame. She became "very incoherent" the following morning, but did not develop a seizure.

Case III-2

A 16-year-old student was seen in consultation for recurrent seizures that had not responded to conventional treatment by two neurologists. She was found to have a mitral systolic murmur and click (consistent with mitral valve prolapse), episodic tachycardia by 24-hour monitoring, and a history suggestive of reactive hypoglycemia ("low blood sugar attacks"). Her plasma insulin concentrations (see below) remained elevated two hours after drinking glucose during a glucose tolerance test (GTT). None of the values for seven toxic minerals in a hair analysis reached one standard deviation above the mean.

The patient had no "attacks" for six weeks after being placed on an appropriate diet and digoxin (to prevent or minimize tachycardia). The seizures then recurred on three occasions – either in the late afternoon or three hours after her evening meal. They were characterized by progressive weakness, dizziness, shortness of breath, violent muscular spasms, and altered consciousness. The parents could not detect any change in her pulse during these episodes. She complained of subsequent "extreme exhaustion." Detailed questioning failed to uncover any intercurrent emotional or other contributory influence.

While examining her at 5 PM, she evidenced an incipient attack of generalized muscular contractions, facial grimacing and altered consciousness. Her blood glucose concentration at the time was normal (91 mg per 100 ml). She had taken an aspartame pudding as a snack two hours earlier.

Puzzling over the cause and timing of this seizure, her mother volunteered two crucial clues. First, the paternal grandmother had "a severe allergy to aspartame." Second, the patient was drinking more aspartame sodas in recent weeks after being advised to avoid sugar because of suspected hypoglycemia.

She then remained seizure-free for several weeks after abstaining from aspartame products. With her consent and that of the parents, the patient was rechallenged with <u>one small serving</u> of the same pudding – in the place of glucose – for an "aspartame tolerance test". Her blood glucose concentration fell more rapidly at the second hour than during the prior GTT (see below). Just before the third hour, she evidenced a sweat, confusion, and marked muscular jerking. The test was terminated at that point.

	Conventional GTT		Aspartame GTT	
	Glucose (mg/100ml)	Insulin (μU/ml)	Glucose (mg/100ml)	Insulin (μU/ml)
Fasting	80	8.8	101	9.4
½ hour	123	27.4	130	46.0
1 hour	143	49.5	128	88.3
2 hours	125	136.5	73	13.0
3 hours	104	—	96 (test	—
3-1/2 hours	84	—	stopped)	
4 hours	82	—		
4-1/2 hours	75 (test stopped)	—		

She had no further seizures for nine months after avoiding products containing aspartame.

Case III-3

A 44-year-old sales executive prided himself on "never having been in a hospital a day before in my life." He had consumed two liters of ACBs and three packets of an ATS daily for two years.

He suffered his first grand mal seizure during August 1985. Other symptoms included difficulty wearing contact lenses, ringing and decreasing hearing in both ears, severe insomnia, memory loss, irritability, personality changes, marked loss of hair, frequent urination, and recurrent sores in the nose. The results of a CT scan of the brain, lumbar puncture, an electroencephalogram, and a heart monitoring study were normal. His symptoms improved "immediately" after stopping aspartame. There were no further seizures.

Case III-4

A 35-year-old businessman sought consultation after concluding that his convulsions were likely caused by aspartame.

As the owner of a grocery market, he began using an ATS in 1982 shortly after it came on the market. He consumed other aspartame products when they became available – including ice tea, soft-drinks, gelatins and puddings. His <u>daily</u> consumption as follows:

- 2-4 16 oz. bottles of ACB and ASD
- 1/2-1 large bottle (2 liters) of ACB and ASD
- 2 to 12 packets of an ATS in hot tea
- 4 to 8 regular glasses of presweetened iced tea
- 1 to 2 regular glasses of an aspartame mix
- 2-4 regular glasses of aspartame hot chocolate
- Up to two servings of aspartame-sweetened puddings and gelatins
- Two sticks of aspartame gum

He also ate up to 4 bowls of an aspartame-sweetened cereal a week.

This patient experienced his first grand mal seizure three months after beginning the use of aspartame. The second grand mal convulsion occurred in February 1986. As a pilot who frequently performed in air shows, he was concerned about having a seizure while at the controls. Extensive medical and neurological evaluations (see below) were normal.

Other symptoms included

- Severe headaches with associated visual symptoms "to the point I couldn't even see"
- Attacks of dizziness
- Marked ringing of the ears ("at times I couldn't hear the phone")
- Tingling of the fingers
- Extreme fatigue ("I couldn't even get out of bed in the morning")
- "Terrible depression," irritability and marked phobias
- Severe drowsiness without reason
- Insomnia
- Marked mental confusion and memory loss
- Hyperactivity of the arms and legs
- Slurring of speech
- Abdominal pain and swelling

He was subjected to two CT scans and one MRI study of the brain, two lumbar punctures, four electroencephalograms, and a heart monitor study. The cost of these studies was estimated at $7,000 out of his own pocket, and $6,000 for the insurance carrier.

The patient began to associate his problem with aspartame consumption three months before calling me, and stopped all such products thereafter. He reflected, "It seems that I took a 180 degree turn. I felt like a new person, even when I got up at five in the morning and didn't go to bed until late at night." He had no further convulsions, but lost his pilot's license.

Case III-5

A 29-year-old businessman was seen in consultation for grand mal seizures over a 1-1/2 year period. He began consuming considerable aspartame in soft drinks and other products about six months before the first convulsion. Five major attacks ensued despite relatively large doses of phenytoin (400 mg daily) and six tablets of carbamazepine (Tegretol®) daily. Other symptoms included frequent bowel movements, a weight gain of 30 pounds, severe fatigue (even after a full night's sleep), and pathologic drowsiness. He did not smoke or drink.

By the time this patient was seen in consultation, he had undergone five CT scans of the brain, three MRI studies (each costing approximately $750), and five electroencephalograms. He also had been hospitalized several times at different medical centers. His radiographic studies were interpreted as evidencing "inflammation of either the white or gray matter of the brain."

The physical examination was not remarkable other than for an initial blood pressure of 144/100. His blood and chemistry studies were essentially normal, except for persistent elevation of the blood glucose concentration at 3 and 3-1/2 hours during a glucose tolerance test (while still on phenytoin).

He had no further seizures for six months after stopping all aspartame products. His blood pressure normalized. The writer discussed the case with his neurologist, recommending that he consider a gradual reduction of the anti-epileptic medication while under constant observation. The neurologist promptly told the patient that aspartame "had nothing to do" with his seizures, and insisted that the dosage of both drugs remain the same.

This patient continued to feel well and seizure-free after abstinence from aspartame. A repeat MRI study (performed at my hospital because of the prior dubious finding) was interpreted as representing an incidental congenital vascular malformation.

Case III-6

An 18-year-old man began consuming two liters of aspartame soft drinks daily during the summer of 1984 in an attempt to lose weight. Shortly thereafter, he evidenced memory loss while driving. His mother stated, "He did not know where he was or where to turn for a 5-10 second period while driving in a very familiar area."

This symptom disappeared during the fall. He resumed drinking large amounts of aspartame beverages the following summer, and suffered a grand mal seizure about 5:30 AM. A CT scan of the brain and an electroencephalogram were normal. Anti-epilepsy medication was prescribed.

At that point, a member of his family suspected a link between the seizure disorder and aspartame use. He avoided aspartame products over the ensuing three months; there were no further seizures.

Case III-7

This salesman spent considerable time on the road. He drank at least one quart of an aspartame soft drink daily, and chewed much "sugarless" gum. He experienced a grand mal seizure, followed by residual numbness on the right side of his body and diminished cerebral acuity.

A CT scan of the brain proved normal.

Case III-8

A 26-year-old homemaker consumed up to four liters of an ASD and four packets of an ATS in hot tea daily for one month to control her weight. She then developed frequent severe seizures. She smoked a little, but drank no alcohol.

There were many associated complaints. They included blurred vision, ringing in the ears, severe dizziness, headache, mental confusion, slurred speech, extreme depression (with suicidal thoughts), marked personality changes, unexplained chest pains, swelling of the lips, difficulty in swallowing, a gain of ten pounds, frequent urination, cessation of her periods,

120

and intense joint pain. Describing her emotional problems, she stated, "I went from a fun-loving, carefree person to a monster. My appearance changed, my personality changed, my life changed. At that point I really began to believe I was insane."

Numerous tests were normal. They included two series of head x-rays, two CT scans of the brain, a lumbar puncture, three electroencephalograms, heart monitoring, and special eye tests. She estimated that these medical expenses cost her $3,000 personally, and the insurance carrier $10,000.

The symptoms began to improve <u>within one day</u> after stopping aspartame, and disappeared by ten days. After being seizure-free for months, she suffered a convulsion shortly after unknowingly ingesting aspartame.

Case III-9

A 33-year-old service representative developed convulsions while drinking considerable quantities of aspartame soft drinks. He was seen by four physicians and consultants. The numerous studies performed cost him $12,000.

Concomitant symptoms included visual and ear problems, dizziness, severe drowsiness, impairment of memory, depression with suicidal thoughts, a change in personality, unexplained chest pains, swelling of the tongue, difficult swallowing, and severe joint pains.

The seizures subsided after stopping aspartame. But he had lost his job.

Case III-10

A 43-year-old executive experienced his first grand mal seizure in January 1986. Extensive medical and neurologic evaluation gave no leads. When told of my interview on *A.M. Philadelphia* ten months later, he sent the following letter.

> "All test results were normal. Since I am 43 years of age and in good health with no family history of seizures, the cause of my problem was inconclusive.
>
> "I did point out to my physicians that I had begun a diet some three weeks before the seizure. I believed it to be a sensible one, whereby I simply reduced my caloric intake, eating the

same foods but less. What I did not point out (at the time there was no reason to be suspect) is the fact that I had substituted for my normal beverage of milk an array of diet drinks. Namely, they were two diet colas, and aspartame-sweetened coffee and tea.

While I don't normally consume diet beverages because I find the taste repugnant, I did drink them regularly during the three weeks prior to my seizure. As a matter of fact, I continued to use these products for quite some time later.

"It may or may not be relevant here, but I also continued to experience auras despite the fact that I was taking 500 mg Dilantin daily and my blood Dilantin level was 14."

Case III-11

A 22-year-old emergency-medical-services volunteer experienced a grand mal convulsion while attending a conference on emergency medicine. The attack was witnessed by physicians, nurses and paramedics.

He had been drinking four cans of aspartame soft drinks for three months, and then increased his consumption the preceding day. Working his regular eight-hour shift, he consumed eight cans of "diet pop" just before going to the conference.

Other recent complaints included marked irritability and a change in personality. There was a history of "sinus headaches," hay fever, asthma, and allergy to aspirin.

His symptoms improved within two weeks after stopping aspartame products, and disappeared by one month. There has been no recurrent seizure since abstaining from aspartame.

Case III-12

The 42-year-old vice president of a marketing corporation was in presumed excellent health until suffering two convulsions. He had consumed three or more cans of a diet cola and two or more glasses of other aspartame soft drinks daily for three years.

122

Three consultants saw this patient. A CT scan of the brain, an electroencephalogram, a stress test, and a glucose tolerance test were not revealing. He was placed on phenytoin.

Other complaints included decreased vision in both eyes, insomnia, memory loss, tingling of the extremities, increased irritability and anxiety, severe itching, a nonspecific rash, marked thinning of the hair, and severe joint pains.

During a 24-day trip to the Orient, he consumed no aspartame products or phenytoin. He felt well until returning to the United States. Another seizure recurred after resuming the ACB and other aspartame products. All his symptoms subsequently disappeared after avoiding aspartame.

Case III-13

A 44-year-old "retired" legal secretary began a reducing diet in June 1983. She had enjoyed her work for 13 years, having received repeated compliments as being "one of the best." By December 1983, she was consuming two liters of an ACB every evening. When the 16-ounce bottle became available, she drank four or five during working hours in addition to two liters at home, especially during warm weather.

During the latter part of 1983, she developed extreme changes in personality and mood, actually walking off her job. Severe "sick headaches" ensued, followed by three grand mal seizures one day in January 1985. The convulsions recurred. Numerous tests were normal, including cerebral arteriograms to rule out an arteriovenous malformation.

Other recent symptoms included severe dizziness, marked memory loss, intense depression, anxiety attacks, palpitations, violent nausea, and frequent urination at night.

The revelation that aspartame might be causing her problems occurred after she was released following a nine-day hospitalization.

> "I didn't have one headache all the time I was in there. The only thing I drank during that time was tea, coffee, 2% nonfat milk, and lemon-flavored ginger ale. No diet soda at all. I had never gone for a week before without a severe headache for over a year.
>
> "I came home on the 29th about 11:00 AM, and poured me a diet drink. By 10 AM the following morning, I had one of my sick

123

headaches. I mean a lulu. My husband and I decided the only difference was the diet drink, so we tried doing without it for a while to see just for sure. I found some diet drink that did not have aspartame in it and drank that. It is now April 11th, 1985, and I have yet to have another seizure or sick headache."

In a subsequent letter dated October 24, 1986, she informed me that there had been no further headaches or seizures after ceasing aspartame products. Furthermore, she had discontinued carbamazepine for a considerable period.

Case III-14

A 59-year-old forester experienced his first convulsion in March 1984 after consuming three packets of an ATS and up to eight glasses of an ASD daily. He suffered two convulsions in July 1984 after unknowingly taking aspartame, and seven convulsions in March 1985 within four hours after ingesting aspartame in an unrecognized form.

His seizures and other related problems abated after avoiding aspartame. He then went on a business trip to evaluate timber during July 1985. His wife wrote

"It was a hot day and a tiring trip, so he bought two cans of a soft drink, which he did not realize had been changed to aspartame from saccharin. He drank them, and later on the way home stopped and drank two glasses of punch which we later found out was made with aspartame. When he got home at 7 PM, he wouldn't eat any dinner, was cranky and tired, and went right to bed. At about 5:30 AM, I was awakened again by this roaring sound. He was having another violent convulsion. He dislocated his shoulder and was in lots of physical pain. I asked the doctor if this didn't prove that aspartame causing his convulsions. He said 'maybe.' I said, 'Shouldn't someone write the aspartame company and tell them what had happened?' All he said was 'Yeah, you do it!' We asked to see a neurologist. He was even less interested in aspartame...

"A week later, we went out to dinner at a local restaurant with friends. While we had a cocktail from the bar, he ordered a regular soft drink. They evidently used the nozzle with the

brand's aspartame drink... We came home and went to bed.
About 2:30 AM, he went into the first of seven consecutive
convulsions."

While consuming aspartame products, he also experienced severe headaches, dizziness, unsteadiness, insomnia, marked mental confusion with memory loss, overt hyperactivity, intense depression, irritability, other changes in personality, severe thirst, frequent urination, and a recent rise of blood pressure. These nonconvulsive symptoms improved after three months of abstinence from aspartame. Owing to persistent impairment of his memory and a personality change, however, he was fired.

Case III-15 A

A 31-year-old education consultant developed a seizure after experiencing prior headaches, anxiety attacks, aggravated phobias, and the cessation of her menstrual periods. She also had "epilepsy-like fits without convulsions." This woman had been consuming three cans of an ACB, three packets of an ATS, and six glasses of presweetened iced tea daily. She did not smoke or drink.

In addition to losing her driver's license, this patient described her incapacity in these terms:

"I couldn't drive for three months. I couldn't travel for fear of
a seizure. I delayed the start of a business, and couldn't
complete old business. Anxiety – never knowing when a
seizure might occur, or why medication wasn't working."

A CT scan, an electroencephalogram, cerebral angiograms, and a heart monitor study were not revealing. Her symptoms subsided "immediately" after stopping aspartame products.

Case III-15 B

A 26-year-old special education teacher with prior hypoglycemia suffered four grand mal seizures. Several occurred at school. She had consumed five or six cans of diet cola, four packets of an ATS, and one or two glasses of another ASD daily for several years – including the nine months of her pregnancy.

Other complaints included severe headaches, dizziness, marked drowsiness, tremors, mental confusion, hyperactivity, tingling of the limbs, extreme irritability, anxiety attacks with aggravation of phobias, episodic shortness of breath and rapid heart action, recent hypertension (140/90 on several occasions, compared to previous readings of 102/57), abdominal pain with severe nausea, a loss of 12 pounds, and less frequent periods.

This patient was seen by two consultants, and hospitalized twice. Her symptoms i mproved within five weeks after discontinuing aspartame products. She recalled, "I drank diet sodas all my remembered life, but never had problems until aspartame came about."

Case III-15 C

A member of the Radio City Rockette troupe experienced her first grand mal seizure at the Philadelphia airport in March 1993. A diagnosis of "left frontal lobe epilepsy" was made. She received Tegretol® and subsequent Dilantin®.

The patient attempted to eat properly due to the nature of her occupation and busy schedule. She had been using aspartame products for a decade to avoid sugar. "I sprinkled large amounts of aspartame on all of my cereal, yogurt, fruit and coffee – not to mention drinking diet cola all day long."

Severe headaches began in the early 1990s, and intensified up to her convulsion. Other symptoms included "very strange buzzing sensations in my head," ringing in both ears, confusion and memory loss. ("I lost a day, and had no memory of how I had spent all the hours until 6 PM when a friend came by.")

The patient considered the use of caffeine and alcohol as causes for her seizures, but the symptoms persisted after avoiding them. She began to improve "immediately" after stopping aspartame products, with no recurrence of the headaches, ear ringing or convulsions. She noted, "None of the doctors I spoke with was familiar with a possible aspartame-seizure connection."

Case III-15 D

A 42-year-old woman attended a clinic to lose weight, and began using aspartame products. Her first "simple seizure" occurred several months later. Its cause could not be determined. The seizures continued despite anti-epilepsy medication. Her daughter then read an article about aspartame disease, and suggested discontinuing such products. The patient remained seizure-free thereafter, and was able to discontinue her epilepsy medications.

Case III-15 E

A 32-year-old woman gave the following account of her aspartame-induced convulsions.

> "When the product hit the market in the early 1980s, I was a teenager. Because I was always watching my weight, I drank lots of diet soft drinks. Since aspartame was touted as safe, I, along with everyone else, continued to drink diet soft drinks.

> "Approximately two months after the switchover, I started to have mild seizures. At the time, I was not sure what was happening, and continued to drink diet sodas. As the seizures continued, I was diagnosed as having a mild form of epilepsy. The anti-seizure medicine, Dilantin®, was prescribed at the age of 18.

> "After being on the drug for perhaps six months, my father heard a TV news report that some people were having reactions to the sweetener. I went off anything containing aspartame, as well as my Dilantin, and was completely normal. I am now 32 years old and will not touch aspartame in any form."

Case III-15 F

A previously healthy 33-year-old man consumed considerable diet colas. He developed "horrible headaches, and subsequent unexplained blackouts." His wife indicated that "he would go down like a felled tree." A number of anti-epilepsy drugs caused severe side effects without preventing the seizures.

The patient was subjected to numerous tests – including imaging studies of the brain and "zillions" of blood tests – but to no avail. When hospitalized for transient weakness on one side and slurred speech, studies of the carotid arteries also proved normal.

His wife happened to read about aspartame-induced seizures, and urged him to stop such products. He evidenced dramatic improvement, and gradually reduced the doses of his drugs. They were stopped on Christmas Day 1996. He did not have another seizure over the ensuing nine months.

AGGRAVATION OF SEIZURES

Known epilepsy can be aggravated by aspartame products. Previously-successful maintenance anti-epileptic therapy with phenytoin (Dilantin®), carbamazepine (Tegretol®), and other drugs proved less effective in heavy aspartame consumers.

My observations also suggest that pre-existing brain damage, as from a head injury or severe infection, might predispose to aspartame-association convulsions. The same applies to a congenital vascular malformation (see Case III-5). Although such patients may have had electroencephalographic abnormalities, they were seizure-free prior to using aspartame. Similarly, the importance of a prior head injury should not be exaggerated.

> An Air Force pilot (Case VI-26) experienced a convulsion while consuming one gallon of aspartame beverages daily. Many studies proved normal. His physicians ascribed the seizure to a minor head injury received ten years previously in a car accident. There was no recurrence after abstinence from aspartame.

Dr. Richard J. Wurtman (1987) offered evidence that low doses of aspartame increase the tendency to seizures in animals prone to abnormal brain activity. Transposition of the dosages to humans approximated 12 mg/kg – about three cans of a diet soda. This estimate is within the range of "biological titrations" I determined for aspartame reactors (see Case III-1 and Chapter XXVII).

Abnormal brain function induced by aspartame also might predispose to febrile convulsions in childhood, unprovoked seizures, and perhaps generalized "complex" seizures (Annegers 1987).

Representative Case Reports

Case III-16

An elementary school teacher with epilepsy had been successfully treated with primidone (Mysoline®). She lost 35 pounds weight over a period of 23 months by adhering to a diet. During this time, she added aspartame to coffee and tea, and consumed diet drinks, gum and candy containing aspartame.

Three months after starting aspartame products, she began to suffer increasing lightheadedness. Initially, it was attributed to "too much dieting too fast." She subsequently experienced recurrent moodiness, easy irritability, insomnia (for the first time), and six grand mal seizures. Her physician added phenytoin.

The patient then realized that two of the seizures occurred shortly after ingesting large amounts of aspartame products. When she stopped them and resumed her conventional diet (including sugar), the insomnia and dizziness disappeared "except for a couple of hot days when I had several diet colas." She subsequently remained seizure-free.

Case III-17

A 37-year-old nuclear mechanic with prior temporal lobe seizures consumed up to five glasses of an ASD daily for two weeks. He experienced severe headaches and dizziness, culminating in two grand mal seizures. He lost his driver's license.

The patient was hospitalized and seen by two consultants. He underwent two CT scans of the brain, a lumbar puncture, two electroencephalograms, two heart stress tests, and 24-hour cardiac monitoring.

There was a history of previous migraine and seizures "from a different part of my brain" for which he had been taking phenytoin. He explained:

> "I was having seizures before using aspartame, but they always came from my right temporal lobe. The seizures I had after using aspartame came from my frontal lobe. It lowered my serum Dilantin level to 10; my level needs to be above 15."

Case III-18

A 31-year-old executive had a seizure disorder that was controlled five years with phenytoin and carbamazepine. After consuming four cans of an ACB and three packets of an ATS daily, she experienced dizziness, drowsiness, severe depression, and three convulsions. These symptoms disappeared within two weeks after discontinuing aspartame.

She expressed her frustration to me over the indifference of physicians to the possibility of such an association.

"At this time, I no longer see the neurologist whom I was seeing before. His philosophy is not in tune with my thinking on the subject of aspartame. I would appreciate   it if you could recommend a neurologist in the _____ area. I am desperate to find a doctor since I am aware that with my history I should be under a doctor's care."

CONVULSIONS FROM ASPARTAME IN SMALL AMOUNTS AND UNRECOGNIZED PRODUCTS

Convulsions and other symptoms occurred in aspartame reactors when they consumed small amounts or products not suspected of containing aspartame. This issue was discussed in Chapters I and II, but warrants emphasis in the present context.

The rapidity with which seizures developed in multiple reactors after chewing aspartame gum suggests the prompt entry of aspartame or its metabolites into the brain from the mouth or pharynx (Chapter II-E).

Representative Case Reports

Case III-19 A

A 19-year-old female suffered frequent seizures while ingesting aspartame soft drinks. Once she and her parents appreciated this relationship, she discontinued all aspartame products and remained seizure-free. During this time, she functioned well without anti-epileptic medication which she had refused to take.

Eleven months later, the patient attended a ball game. Someone handed her a piece of gum, which she reflexively began to chew. Within minutes she had several grand mal seizures, followed by violent headaches and depression. The gum contained aspartame.

Case III-19 B

A 27-year-old woman developed recurrent grand mal seizures after chewing ONE stick of aspartame gum. She was hospitalized on each of the three occasions these seizures occurred. Numerous tests proved normal. She experienced severe reactions to Dilantin, and subsequently to Tegretol.

The patient suggested to her neurologist that the seizures might have been triggered by aspartame. "He literally laughed at me and said, 'One stick would not do it.' "

Her chiropractor happened to be interested in aspartame disease. After hearing the details, he concurred. The neurologist's arrogant response to the chiropractor's written opinion was, "I don't see the letters M.D. after his name."

The patient remained seizure-free without medication for several years until flying and inadvertently chewing a stick of gum that was not identified as containing aspartame. She wrote

> "Fortunately, I was buckled in and the flight attendants were well trained. My husband knew what to expect, and there happened to be a doctor sitting behind us. I developed a grand mal seizure on the plane, and the repercussions were great. My speech returned to normal within a few weeks, but my ability to spell and perform mathematical equations took well over a year to recover."

REPORTS BY OTHERS

Several <u>aspartame reactors</u> who experienced convulsions mentioned acquaintances with aspartame-induced seizures in completing the survey questionnaire (Section 4).

<u>Medical colleagues</u> in other communities have reported seizures precipitated by aspartame.

- Dr. Ralph G. Walton (1987) described eight patients in whom seizures appeared to be induced by the ingestion of aspartame.
- One physician informed me of a commercial pilot who lost his license because of unexplained seizures. Deducing they were caused by aspartame, the patient avoided such products and became seizure-free. **Purposefully** challenging himself with an aspartame soda in an attempt to regain his license by demonstrating this specific intolerance, he promptly suffered another seizure.

<u>Dr. David G. Hattan</u>, Chief of the Regulatory Affairs Staff of the FDA Office of Nutrition and Food Sciences, provided a computerized summary of the data submitted to his

agency (as of July 1987) by 149 consumers who attributed their convulsions to aspartame use. This information appears in Tables III-1 and III-2. The FDA classification for determining severities was Type I for severe, and Type II for moderate.

TABLE III-1

ASPARTAME-ASSOCIATED CONVULSIONS
FDA DATA ON 149 CASES

Sex
Females	96	(64.4%)
Males	53	(35.6%)

Race
White	72	(48.3%)
Nonwhite	6	(4.0%)
Unknown	71	(47.7%)

Age Groups (years)
1-19	32	(21.5%)
20-29	28	(18.8%)
30-39	42	(28.2%)
40-49	21	(14.1%)
50-59	5	(3.4%)
60+	6	(4.0%)
Unknown	15	(10.1%)

Time From Ingestion of Aspartame
"Immediate"	24	(16.1%)
1-12 hours	68	(45.6%)
13-24 hours	8	(5.4%)
24 hours	49	(32.9%)

Type of Reaction
I	129	(87.2%)
II	19	(12.8%)
Unspecified	1	

132

Group
A	25	(17.0%)
B	21	(14.3%)
C	29	(19.7%)
D	72	(49.0%)
Unspecified	2	

Aspartame Products Consumed
Soft Drinks	115	(77.2%)
Tabletop Sweeteners	39	(26.2%)
Hot Chocolate	13	(8.7%)
Iced Tea	12	(8.1%)
Gum	11	(7.4%)
Soft Drink Mixes	40	(26.8%)
Puddings/Gelatins	16	(10.7%)

TABLE III-2

ASPARTAME-ASSOCIATED CONVULSIONS
FDA DATA ON 149 CASES

Concomitant Symptoms
Headaches	28	(18.8%)
Depression/Mood Changes	23	(15.4%)
Other	18	(12.1%)
Dizziness	14	(9.4%)
Abdominal Pain/GI Complaints	12	(8.1%)
Memory Loss	9	(6.0%)
Weakness/Fatigue	7	(4.7%)
Visual	6	(4.0%)
Fainting	6	(4.0%)
Hives/Rashes	5	(3.4%)
Sleep Problems	5	(3.4%)
Heart	3	(2.0%)
Bone/Joint Pain	1	(0.7%)
Menstrual	1	(0.7%)

These details are noteworthy.

- The complainants lived in all parts of the United States and Canada.
- The large majority (87.2%) suffered Type I reactions.
- Most had one or more additional aspartame-associated complaints.
- Aspartame soft drinks had been consumed by more than three-fourths, often in conjunction with other aspartame products.

Dr. Richard Wurtman (1986), a Massachusetts Institute of Technology researcher, indicated during a television interview that he knew of more than 100 persons with aspartame-associated seizures. They generally were preceded by headache and nausea. (In my initial survey questionnaire analysis, 30 of 56 persons with grand mal convulsions gave a history of preceding severe headaches.)

- The first three patients reported by Wurtman (1985) ranged in age from 27 to 42 years. They evidenced grand mal seizures after ingesting large amounts of aspartame beverages. Their attacks ceased after avoiding aspartame with the exception of one individual who resumed such diet sodas.
- Another 36-year-old woman, whose case history was submitted by Dr. Wurtman for the public record, abstained from aspartame and other additives during pregnancy. She suffered her first grand mal seizure on resuming aspartame soft drinks and desserts two months after delivery. Extensive medical and neurologic examinations proved normal.

CONVULSIONS IN SELECTED GROUPS

A. **Children** (Chapter XI)

Aspartame may render young persons more vulnerable to epilepsy. In this regard, some health-conscious mothers have fed infants aspartame products in an attempt to prevent tooth decay, obesity, and other problems "caused by sugar."

The onset of seizures in children shortly after consuming aspartame products was occasionally dramatic.

134

- A two-year-old developed a fever for which the mother administered chewable acetaminophen containing aspartame. The child suffered seizures ten minutes later.
- In his testimony to the FDA on April 21, 1986, Dr. Richard Wurtman told of a two-year-old child with seizures whose mother gave him diet soda because her dentist had stressed that "sugar causes cavities."

Representative Case Reports

Case III-20

A 7 1/2-year-old boy experienced a seizure while running to his parent's room "in desperate pain from a headache." There had been no significant prior illnesses. He developed another seizure in the hospital as a lumbar puncture was being performed. A CT scan of his brain was normal. Hives occurred one week after he took medication for epilepsy.

After leaving the hospital, the child complained of "fuzziness" several times daily. Others commented he was irritable, hyperactive, and had difficulty concentrating on his school work.

The parents sought consultation from a "nutritionist." They were advised to eliminate chocolate, wheat and eggs. The mother wrote

> "Since we were going to try the nutrition route, we decided on our own to take him off the aspartame drink he had been consuming for the past four months (ever since I had been on a diet). He was drinking four to six glasses a day (usually one glass was in the form of a frozen popsicle)... He had been a healthy little boy since with absolutely no recurrence of any of the previous problems... It's been five months since the nightmare of the last seizure occurred."

The child's electroencephalograms normalized within two months after aspartame products were stopped.

Case III-21 A

A 2 1/2-year-old boy experienced convulsions within two weeks after beginning to consume aspartame. He was hospitalized when his "blood sugar dropped to 'zero' and IVs were required."

Case III-21 B

A two-year-old boy told his parents prior to sleep that he was thirsty. They gave him a diet cola. About 45 minutes after drinking 12 ounces, the child had a seizure – gasping for air, and turning blue. He received oxygen and resuscitative messages by paramedics, and was rushed to a hospital. (The mother used the name "Sweet Terror" on the Internet in describing this experience.)

B. Convulsions Associated With Aspartame Ingestion During Pregnancy and Breast-Feeding

Two representative families will be described in which each mother with aspartame-associated seizures had the added burden of caring for several epileptic children. They had consumed aspartame both during pregnancy and while breast-feeding.

Representative Case Reports

Case III-22

A 29-year-old credit and collections coordinator had taken aspartame beverages since July 1983. She drank them for nine months during her first pregnancy, for three months during her second pregnancy, and for five weeks while breast-feeding each child.

She experienced severe dizziness, lightheadedness and numbness of the right upper extremity. These symptoms improved within one day after stopping aspartame, only to return within one day on each of the two occasions she rechallenged herself.

Her son (born in September 1983) had two grand mal seizures and petit mal attacks. Her daughter (born in November 1985) had a petit mal attack. Extensive studies were not revealing. She wrote

136

"Right before my daughter was born, my husband had heard (October 1985) on the radio that aspartame may cause seizures in some children. It was then that I quit using aspartame. After she was born, I inadvertently bought diet pop. She was four weeks old and I was breast-feeding. After approximately 4-6 hours of drinking the pop, she went into a petit mal seizure."

Case III-23

A 31-year-old housewife used aspartame early in 1982 when samples of an ATS were received in the mail. Thereafter, she consumed four cans of diet sodas, eight packets of an ATS, up to eight glasses of an ASD, four glasses of aspartame hot chocolate, and three bowls of aspartame-presweetened cereal daily. There was a history of longstanding migraine. She did not smoke or drink alcohol.

The headaches intensified to the point "I couldn't stand them." She subsequently suffered multiple epileptic seizures for which medication was prescribed. Other complaints included severe confusion and memory loss, numbness of the arms and legs, slurred speech, marked depression and irritability, personality changes, aggravated phobias, attacks of shortness of breath, palpitations, abdominal pain, difficulty in swallowing, intense thirst, and the virtual cessation of her menstrual periods.

Her eight-year-old son and three-year-old daughter also became epileptic. She had consumed aspartame during the entire nine months of the second pregnancy, including an aspartame-containing acetaminophen preparation. Both children experienced intense headaches and seizures after taking chewable acetaminophen sweetened with aspartame. (At the time, she did not realize aspartame was an ingredient.) Her son also developed extreme thirst, severe impairment of vision, marked intolerance to noise, and profound depression with suicidal behavior.

C. Diabetics

The diagnostic and therapeutic considerations relating to patients with diabetes mellitus who develop uncontrolled diabetes, severe insulin reactions, or convulsions while consuming aspartame will be considered in Chapter XIII. Insulin-dependent diabetics seem more prone to aspartame-associated seizures, both as grand mal (see Case III-24) and petit mal (see Case III-25).

These problems may be compounded by phenytoin (Dilantin®) treatment. This basic anti-epileptic drug can decrease insulin secretion and aggravate diabetes (Levin 1970). Furthermore, aspartame might interfere with its action (Chapter IX-I), thereby inviting more seizures (see below).

Related medicolegal issues have been raised. One insulin-dependent diabetic with aspartame induced seizures sued the manufacturer on the basis of an alleged violation of a products liability statute (*The Grand Rapids Press* March 6, 1986, p. C-6).

Representative Case Reports

Case III-24

The son of a diabetic woman described her adverse reactions to aspartame on two occasions as follows: "She experienced dizziness and grand mal seizures. She was paralyzed on one side for several hours. Lastly, she had a swollen tongue and mouth." There were no recurrences after stopping aspartame.

Case III-25

A 30-year-old insulin-dependent diabetic developed many petit mal attacks while consuming six cans of ASD and three packets of an ATS daily. Other symptoms included ringing in both ears, severe headaches and dizziness. She stated, "I could not drive on a day when I had more than one soda because a seizure would occur."

The seizures improved within two weeks after stopping aspartame products. They recurred one day after drinking a glass of soda at a friend's home, which she did not realize contained aspartame.

At the time of her communication, there had been no further attacks for over two months. Her initial abnormal electroencephalogram normalized after avoiding aspartame.

D. Familial Aspartame-Associated Convulsions

The family history of reactors to aspartame (Chapters II and XVI) suggests an association between its use and convulsions among members of the same family. The occurrence of seizures in each of two such women and their children was described above.

Although not genetically related, both the husband and wife described in Case III-28 experienced seizures after consuming an aspartame soft drink mix.

Representative Case Reports

Case III-27

A 48-year-old <u>educator</u> developed violent headaches after consuming aspartame beverages. She had a history of mild migraine for two decades. Her 15-year-old <u>daughter</u> developed two seizures shortly after aspartame became available.

Case III-28

A 68-year-old <u>man</u> had consumed considerable aspartame-sweetened cereals, iced tea mixes, and diet soft drinks for "years" because of an overweight problem and hypertension. He neither smoked nor drank alcohol. He was seen by three consultants, for two unexplained convulsions. Concomitant complaints included drowsiness, marked memory loss, various rashes, frequency of urine (both day and night), and intense joint pains. X-rays of the head, a CT scan of the brain, cerebral angiograms, lumbar puncture, gastrointestinal x-rays, and allergy studies failed to reveal a convincing underlying cause. After stopping aspartame on the advice of a personal physician, his symptoms improved... and then disappeared.

A 15-year-old <u>grandson</u> "constantly" drank aspartame beverages, and also suffered seizures.

Case III-29

A <u>housewife</u> suffered a seizure three days after drinking one glass daily of an aspartame beverage. She also had severe tremors, chills, a fever of 101°, impaired ambulation, and transient deterioration of her handwriting. Many studies proved normal.

Her <u>husband</u> experienced a convulsion after drinking three two-liter bottles of the same soft drink weekly. There was concomitant extreme weakness, to the point he could not raise himself from a chair or walk without assistance. He also had difficulty in swallowing. A subsequent unexplained acute intestinal obstruction required surgery and five weeks hospitalization.

In describing her husband's reactions to the FDA, the wife referred to a report in the August 4, 1986 issue of *The Syracuse Herald* that summarized my initial press conference (Overview F). Linking the reactions of both spouses, she wrote, "I <u>certainly</u> agree with him – to my sorrow."

E. <u>Dual Sensitivities to Aspartame and Monosodium Glutamate (MSG)</u>

Convulsions induced by aspartame products also have been precipitated by MSG. My experience in this realm is reviewed in Chapter VIII-E.

Several instances of uncontrollable seizures precipitated by aspartame or MSG were diagnosed as the Lennox-Gestaut syndrome. In two such instances, involving a 2½-year-old boy and a 20-year-old woman, the seizures subsided after avoiding these chemicals, and recurred on rechallenge. The metabolic overlapping of aspartate and glutamate is noteworthy – namely, binding to many of the same receptor sites, common transport mechanisms, and interconversion via aspartate aminotransferase.

NONCONVULSIVE SEIZURES

Nonconvulsive forms of epilepsy – commonly referred to as petit mal and psychomotor attacks (or temporal lobe seizures) – also can be caused or aggravated by aspartame products. They improved in 57 such aspartame reactors (5 percent) after aspartame consumption was stopped.

Patients with these aspartame-induced disorders had a variety of premonitory auras and concomitants features.

- The "bad taste in my mouth" noted by Case III-34 suggested temporal lobe epilepsy.
- The complaint of an odor, "like rubber burning," bothered several aspartame reactors – both with and without seizures. In each instance, this feature disappeared after avoiding aspartame products. For example, a researcher at a neurological institute would awaken "with a feeling of anxiety, and smell a strong order of burning toast." At other times, she smelled "burning rubber" and men's cologne. This person then experienced a complex partial seizure while driving to work. Fortunately, she managed to pull off the road. Her colleagues

mentioned her slurred speech. The postictal "fog" persisted a week. The olfactory hallucinations stopped as soon as she discontinued her large intake of aspartame products. There was no recurrence until she unknowingly ate a popsicle containing aspartame.

Coalfield et al (1992) conducted an independent double-blind controlled study of epileptic children with generalized absence epilepsy using an aspartame product obtained from a grocery store. They reported an increase in the frequency of spiked-wave discharges by electroencephalography.

Representative Case Reports

Case III-31 A

A 29-year-old female had been in good health until developing temporal lobe seizures. Her electroencephalogram evidenced temporal lobe spiking. She consumed from four to six cans of an ACB daily. She described her attacks as "an upset stomach feeling as if it were 'turned inside out,' a tingling sensation, and accompanied by the feeling of what I presume is referred to as déjà vu."

Case III-31 B

A young registered nurse with a history of migraine evidenced a severe reaction to aspartame in the form of multiple "petit mal seizures" that included "feelings of displacement or spacey feelings." This diagnosis was made by a professor of neurology.

Case III-32

A 20-year-old man had consumed up to four liters of aspartame beverages daily for one year. He experienced about 50 petit mal seizures. They were described as "abrupt one-minute-or-so intervals of extreme memory loss, usually noticed while driving." He then suffered his first grand mal convulsion. An electroencephalogram and a CT scan of the brain were normal. He neither smoked nor drank alcohol. Other complaints included slurring of speech, depression, personality changes, marked thirst, and frequent urination. All these features promptly subsided after discontinuing aspartame products.

Case III-33

A 57-year-old secretary had been using large amounts of an ATS when she experienced "spells of split-second power outages in my head – when it seemed as if the lights in the room were suddenly dimmed and then came back on. At the same time, my ears faded as if I'd cupped my hands over them for a split-second." Her neurologist diagnosed "temporal lobe absences." A CT scan of the head was normal. The electroencephalogram revealed a single left temporal sharp wave focus.

Case III-34 A

A 33-year-old nurse had recurrent severe spells five months after beginning to use various aspartame products – including soft drinks, ATS, candy and gum. There was no previous past history or family history of seizures. A consulting neurologist characterized them as consisting of "a disagreeably metallic taste, numbness of the hands, weakness, lightheadedness, and rapid heart beat." The attacks lasted up to 15 seconds, and were occurring two or three times a day. She also suffered frontal headaches several times weekly for which she used Fiorinal® to obtain relief. There was an occasional sensation of quivering or crawling over the left side of the head. An EEG study evidenced right temporal lobe dysfunction. A CT scan of the head was normal. The diagnosis of temporal lobe seizures was made. There were no further spells after the patient discontinued aspartame products.

Case III-34 B

An 8½-year-old girl experienced numerous petit mal seizures. She was studied by more than six physicians in her community, and several consulting neurologists. X-rays of the head, a CT of the brain and an electroencephalogram were not remarkable. Other complaints included pain in both eyes, ringing in the ears, severe headache, slurred speech, a personality change, and intense thirst. In addition, "food didn't taste right."

The patient had been using diet colas, iced tea sweetened with an ATS, and aspartame gum. When her mother learned that a friend's seizures were provoked by aspartame, and made this association, "most of the doctors thought I was crazy."

The complaints subsided over the ensuing months by avoiding aspartame products. The patient then used an instant breakfast containing aspartame while at a soccer camp. The petit mal seizures recurred within several days. The mother became furious on finding that her child had been given an aspartame product. Her recommendation about regulating the use of aspartame was emphatic: "Ban it!"

INTERACTION WITH PHENYTOIN AND OTHER DRUGS

The apparent interaction of aspartame and phenytoin (Dilantin) will be discussed in Chapter IX-I.

A 51-year-old man who drank considerable diet cola daily reported apparent potentiation of valproic acid (Depakene®; Depacote®), another antiepileptic drug. When his physician increased the dose, he became comatose and required hospitalization.

There has been reference to possible epileptogenic potentiation of aspartame by concomitant methyldopa (Aldomet®) and other medications (*Congressional Record-Senate* 1985a, b).

Representative Case Reports

Case III-35

A 29-year-old man had been consuming 18 12-ounce cans of an ACB daily for one year prior to the intensification of service-connected epilepsy. He suffered two grand mal seizures on January 21 and January 29, 1986, during which he broke both ankles. Other symptoms included severe headache, unsteadiness of the legs, and slurred speech. The dose of phenytoin was increased, culminating in clinical phenytoin toxicity three months later. His blood level was 59.6 µg/ml. (The desired therapeutic range is 10-20 µg/ml.)

Case III-36

A 67-year-old retired woman suffered three unexplained seizures. They did not recur when she stopped her daily consumption of aspartame – one can of an ACB, and various brands of cola and puddings. Other complaints included increased sensitivity to noise, palpitations and rapid heart action. She had been taking methyldopa for hypertension.

The possible interaction between aspartame and female hormone replacement therapy is also mentioned in this context.

> A female aspartame reactor who suffered simple partial seizures found that they stopped after she avoided aspartame products. They recurred on three separate occasions when she attempted hormone replacement therapy.

ECONOMIC AND SOCIAL IMPACT

The socioeconomic consequences of aspartame-induced seizures are profound. Some were alluded to in the preceding case reports.

I. <u>Accidents and Deaths</u> (Chapter XXVII)

Convulsions, "fugue states," and "blackouts" are important causes of driving accidents (Roberts 1971b). Accordingly, they pose major considerations relative to driver licensure and insurability. This subject was detailed in *Ignored Health Hazards For Pilots and Drivers* (Roberts 1999a).

- The cited experiences of pilots who lost their licenses because of aspartame-induced seizures underscore this issue.
- A fatal automobile accident involving Case XXVII-7, a young man, was ascribed to a seizure with loss of consciousness while driving his vehicle. He had a number of other complaints while consuming up to four gallons of a diet cola daily. His sister also was an aspartame reactor.

Death following an aspartame-induced seizure has received little attention. For example, Florence Griffith-Joyner, the Olympic gold medalist, suffered an unexpected and fatal epileptic seizure at the age of 38. Witnesses had previously seen her drinking a diet cola while jogging with President Clinton.

II. <u>Medical Costs</u>

The extraordinary costs frequently incurred before making a diagnosis of aspartame-associated seizures appear in the case reports. They are amplified in Chapter XIX. The complications of antiepileptic drugs further compound costs. For example, a woman who had taken Tegretol for an aspartame-induced seizure disorder developed bone marrow depression.

The vulnerabilities of older persons will be discussed in Chapter XV. Stephen and Brodie (2000) reported the increased burden on health care facilities and costs from an increase of seizure disorders in the elderly.

144

Representative Case Reports

Case III-37

A 44-year-old teacher experienced a convulsion while driving. Her longstanding migraine had intensified prior to this attack. Other complaints included severe dizziness, insomnia, memory loss, tingling of the extremities, severe depression, marked "personality changes," and a gain of 15 pounds. She had consumed a variety of products containing aspartame for two years. Her daughter also suffered severe headache and mood swings that were attributed to aspartame.

This patient was seen by multiple consultants, including a psychiatrist. She had three sets of head x-rays, two CT scans, one MRI study of the brain, and three electroencephalograms. All were normal. She estimated these costs at $10,000.

There were no further seizures after stopping aspartame. Her other symptoms also disappeared. The attending neurologist subsequently concluded that the seizures could have been related to aspartame use, and discontinued phenytoin after eight months. She added, "I am lucky that it did not cost me my life. It greatly affected my life, my marriage, and my family relations for over a year."

Case III-38

A 37-year-old administrative assistant suffered two grand mal seizures that were attributed to aspartame use. She had been seen by four consultants, and was hospitalized twice. Her studies included two CT scans, one MRI study of the brain, and four electroencephalograms. She estimated such costs at $8,000 out of her own pocket, and $30,000 for the insurance carrier.

III. Influence On Personal and Business Life

Most aspartame reactors with convulsions suffered severe stress in their personal and business lives. Such incapacitation relative to business and professional careers – especially for medical personnel and nurses (see Case III-1) – will be amplified in Chapter XIX.

- A registered nurse who had experienced aspartame-induced convulsions wrote that "they drastically played havoc with me and my family."

145

- A 48-year-old clerical worker suffered several aspartame-induced convulsions. She succinctly explained the impact on her career: "I lost my driver's license."

PATHOPHYSIOLOGIC CONSIDERATIONS

Aspartame and its metabolites may cause or aggravate convulsions through various mechanisms. The importance of altered neurotransmitter concentrations within the brain (especially serotonin and norepinephrine), the effects of methyl alcohol, and exaggerated hypoglycemia ("low blood sugar attacks") are discussed in Section 5. For example, aspartame and its breakdown products can suppress the synthesis of several neurotransmitters that tend to prevent seizures.

Other mechanisms could contribute to aspartame-induced seizures. They include formaldehyde toxicity (from methanol), altered monoamine receptors in the cerebral cortex, and loss of the protective effect of L-DOPA.

Alterations in brain water, sodium and potassium also may play a role. They were noted in both humans and animals after methanol intake, along with vascular stasis. These assume considerable pertinence in view of the multiple cellular interactions involving calcium, sodium, potassium and chloride that are known to trigger focal epilepsy (Dichter 1987).

Additionally, altered extracellular fluid concentrations of various amino acids, notably glutamate and aspartate, play an important role in the pathogenesis of hypoxemic and epileptic brain injury. Some reference studies are reviewed at the beginning of Chapter VI.

- Tendler et al (1991) found that a noncompetitive antagonist to the MDA subtype of glutamate receptor reduces brain tissue injury for hypoxemia .
- Two toxic amino acids related to alanine can cause convulsions, as well as parkinsonism, dementia and demyelinating disease (Spencer 1987).

Other influences might act as co-epileptogens.

- Aspartame-associated insomnia (Chapter VII) is relevant. Chronic sleep deprivation can induce seizures in animal models, perhaps through norepinephrine depletion.

- The <u>simultaneous administration of caffeine and aspartame</u> lowers the threshold to experimental seizures induced by pentylenetetrazole (Maher 1987).
- Individual case reports of aspartame-associated convulsions by other physicians (Walton 1987) mention the presence of <u>venous malformations</u>, a finding in several of my cases (see Case III-5).

Experimental Observations

Tilson et al (1987) found that aspartame administration to rats significantly reduced the number of cortex stimulations required to induce tonic-clonic seizures. They suggested that "aspartame may facilitate the development of seizures activity" under some circumstances.

Wurtman and Maher (1987) noted that the disproportionate elevation of brain phenylalanine concentrations after aspartame or phenylalanine, compared to tyrosine levels, diminish brain dopamine release. This enhances the susceptibility of rodents to seizures induced by pentylenetetrazole, fluorothyl or electroconvulsive shock. (A problem in interpreting studies involving large doses of phenylalanine given to rodents resides in the fact that tyrosine, the antidote, is also increased owing to their high phenylalanine hydroxylase activity.)

Maher and Pinto (1987) reported that aspartame significantly lowers the threshold to seizures induced by pentylenetetrazole in nonfasted mice. A comparable response occurred with equimolar phenylalanine, but not equimolar aspartic acid or methanol. Conversely, the administration of tyrosine – alone, or with phenylalanine or aspartame – elevated the seizure threshold in this model, as did co-administering valine (another neutral amino acid.)

Wurtman and Maher (1987) attempted to compare the doses of aspartame producing neurochemical effects in rodents and humans. Their data suggest that 15-20 mg/kg diminishes catecholamine release, thereby enhancing susceptibility to seizures.

Hypoglycemia

The hazards of hypoglycemia – or more accurately, cerebral glucopenia (insufficient glucose for proper brain function) – are reviewed in Chapter XIV. I have emphasized the relationship between hypoglycemia and epileptic seizures (Roberts 1964a,b; 1971b). The release of increased insulin following administration of the amino acids contained in aspartame (Floyd 1970, Reitano 1978), coupled with the oft-severe reduction of carbohydrate and calories by weight-conscious persons (see Case III-1) who consume aspartame products, could exaggerate hypoglycemia.

The following observations clarify the epileptogenic potential of severe hypoglycemia.

- Glucose is essential for the aerobic synthesis of the neuromediator acetylcholine, a powerful convulsant, by brain cortex slices (Quastel 1936, Brenner 1942).
- Whereas normal blood glucose concentrations exert a restraining effect on the synthesis and release of acetylcholine within the central nervous system, these processes become markedly stimulated at hypoglycemia levels, even culminating in convulsions (Feldberg 1945).
- Gibbs (1939) noted an increase of 3/second spike-and-wave electroencephalographic activity in patients with petit mal epilepsy when the blood glucose concentrations fell.
- Clinical and experimental data indicate that hypoglycemia can unmask subclinical cerebral lesions." While middle cerebral artery ligation in the cat or monkey generally causes little gross impairment, hemiplegia will ensue if hypoglycemia also is induced (Meyer 1968).
- Tolbutamide-induced hypoglycemia may reveal and magnify a temporal lobe focus causing electroencephalographic abnormalities regardless of whether the clinical attacks were grand mal, psychomotor or syncopal in type (Green 1963).
- Diabetic patients who have epilepsy tend to experience fewer seizures when their blood glucose concentrations remain elevated, and vice versa (Sakel 1958).

Increased Brain Water

The excessive fluid and sodium consumed with aspartame products, especially during hot weather (Chapter II), can contribute to seizures.

- This is even more likely to occur when superimposed upon premenstrual fluid retention. It was noted earlier that women with considerable premenstrual fluid retention and a history of severe migraine seem more vulnerable to aspartame-induced convulsions.

- Wurtman (1987) reported a 35-year-old test pilot who developed a seizure after consuming six liters of an aspartame-sweetened beverage every day following his mid-day jog.

I have reviewed the adverse effects of increased water and sodium on nervous system function (Roberts 1966b,c; 1967b). The intense thirst created by aspartame (Chapter IX-F) also favors increased fluid intake.

The hyperinsulinized state poses another pertinent consideration. Water and sodium migrate into nerve cells following hypoglycemia or the removal of glucose from a perfusing environment (Yanner 1939a,b; Stern 1949; Krebs 1951).

Allergy (Chapter VIII)

The occurrence of seizures during the early morning hours (see Case III-1) might represent a delayed IgE-mediated hypersensitivity reaction to aspartame. This explanation also has been proposed for delayed urticaria or angioedema (Kulczycki 1987).

An allergic background is relevant in such patients. For example, Case III-22, a female with aspartame-induced aggravation of asthma, also suffered two grand mal seizures. She had no prior history of epilepsy.

PROFESSIONAL CONFUSION AND RESISTANCE

The failure to identify aspartame products as a major contributing factor in many patients with "idiopathic" epilepsy because neurologists and other physicians refuse to consider this relationship should be condoned no longer. A recent review of refractory seizures published in the *New England Journal of Medicine* did not mention aspartame. Devinsky (1999) stated, "However, a misdiagnosis of epilepsy can result in social stigma and the loss of self-esteem, employment opportunities or driving privileges or delayed treatment of the real disorder."

Neurologists

Many patients with aspartame-induced convulsions volunteered two major frustrations about their neurologists. First, in the words of one aspartame reactor, these doctors often implied that "the aspartame thing is primarily in my head, and perhaps I should see a shrink." (See Case III-39)

Second, they demanded that patients continue taking high dosages of one or several potent antiepileptic drugs when the seizures no longer had recurred for a considerable period after aspartame abstinence. Most were specifically instructed not to reduce the dosage "under any circumstances without my approval." These individuals understandably expressed concern about taking such medications indefinitely because of their potentially severe side effects – as bone marrow depression (see above).

When seeing these patients in consultation, I attempted to explain both my evaluation and the justification for a cautious reduction in dosage in view of their prolonged seizure-free period after avoiding aspartame. Several neurologists became infuriated. One told Case III-5 that I was "on the wrong track," and insisted she continue taking high dosages of phenytoin and carbamazepine indefinitely.

This attitude among physicians has been influenced by the bold assertion of some organizations that aspartame products do not cause seizures. For example, the chairman of the Professional Advisory Board of The Epilepsy Institute distributed the following letter on March 18, 1986.

> "Recent publicity on aspartame and seizures may have promoted calls from concerned patients. As an organization devoted to people suffering from seizure-related problems, we at The Epilepsy Institute investigated this allegation and found aspartame to be safe for people with epilepsy... As Chairman of The Epilepsy Institute's Professional Advisory Board, I have also reviewed the data and see no cause to link aspartame and seizures."

A representative of The Epilepsy Institute challenged the author's assertion about a link between aspartame and seizures at a national news conference in Washington on October 16, 1986 (Overview F). I pointed out that (a) there already were more than 55 persons in my series who developed grand mal seizures after taking aspartame products, and (b) their attacks predictably recurred or intensified following rechallenge with aspartame. Moreover, I requested any documented position paper or data to the contrary, especially in view of correspondence received from The Epilepsy Foundation stating that it had NOT studied the problem. No response was ever received despite the increasing number of aspartame-induced seizures in my data base and that of the FDA.

Dr. Harold E. Booker, Chairman of the Professional Advisory Board of The Epilepsy Foundation of America, was requested by the United States Senate Committee on Labor and

Human Resources to make a statement concerning any possible risk by epileptic patients taking aspartame products. His correspondence, dated October 31, 1987, read: "As of the last meeting of the Board (April, 1987), the report was that, in their opinion, there was no valid, scientific evidence that aspartame posed any risk for people with epilepsy." Attention is directed to the catch terms, "in their opinion" and "valid."

Representative Case Reports

Case III-39

A 28-year-old hairdresser had been drinking ten cans of an ACB daily in an attempt to lose weight. She developed progressively severe symptoms over the ensuing four months, culminating in two convulsions. She also experienced lightheadedness, unsteadiness of the feet, severe depression (actually contemplating suicide), extreme irritability, anxiety attacks, aggravation of a phobia about crowds, other "marked personality changes," attacks of rapid heart action, diarrhea, ringing in the ears, itching, difficulty in swallowing, recent "dry eyes," intense thirst, and aggravated low blood sugar attacks. Paradoxically, she gained 35 pounds.

This patient was seen by three physicians and consultants. Her studies included a CT scan of the brain, an electroencephalogram, and skin tests. Her mother, an aunt and a sister-in-law also suffered severe reactions to aspartame in the form of headaches, blurred vision, and mouth allergies. On two occasions, her symptoms returned within three days after retesting herself. The patient was told, "It's your nerves," by all physicians except one. She was most upset over the fact that "the doctors still will not admit that it (her medical problem) has anything to do with aspartame."

Case III-40

A 48-year-old woman experienced two grand mal convulsions after drinking up to eight cans of aspartame sodas daily. She neither smoked nor drank alcohol. Two electroencephalograms were normal. She was placed on 400 mg phenytoin daily, and forbidden to drive for six months. The latter rendered her unable to go to work.

The patient's first clue to aspartame disease as an underlying cause for her seizures came while reading a newspaper article. She had no further attacks after stopping aspartame products. Her physician refused to accept the relevance of the newspaper clipping when she showed it to him while stating, "I am afraid of the Dilantin." Her dismay intensified when she received no reply from the FDA after her husband called the agency and offered to submit the pertinent medical records.

A Manufacturer's Position

A statement by the NutraSweet Center titled, "Facts About NutraSweet and Epileptic Seizures," asserted that there is no evidence for an association between aspartame and seizures, even in large doses. It continued to regard reports of aspartame-associated seizures appearing in medical journals and the general press as "anecdotal."

Double-Blind Studies: Some Considerations

Any provocative or double-blind study on aspartame-associated convulsions must take a number of factors into consideration. They include the effects of heat and storage on aspartame products (Chapter XXV) and individual differences.

These topics will be discussed in Chapters XVIII and XXXI. For example, Case III-1 had her first convulsion within 18 hours after beginning to ingest two liters of an aspartame soft drink. On the other hand, most aspartame reactors in this series who experienced convulsions suffered a host of other symptoms (especially headache and personality changes) for days or weeks before their attacks.

It would seem logical to do provocative testing with the **same** product(s) consumed by the patient, as was done in Case III-2. Yet, "negative" corporate-subsidized "double-blind, placebo-controlled, cross-over studies" have been reported on children with seizures who were not given the actual aspartame product that their parents implicated as the cause.

Position of The FDA

Former Congressman Daniel A. Mica forwarded a letter received from the FDA in response to my August 1986 letter, requesting copies of reports submitted to the FDA by aspartame reactors. With reference to seizures, this reply asserted

> "We have reviewed a total of 141 reports of seizures and have found no association between occurrence of seizures and exposure to aspartame-containing products... In addition, clinical studies are being supported by the sponsor of aspartame (G. D. Searle and Company) to assess, under appropriately controlled

conditions, whether it causes or may contribute to the occurrence of seizures in individuals who believe they are sensitive to aspartame. At this time, no evidence has been established for a consistent seizure pattern or dose response relationship."

As noted earlier, the FDA continues to regard this association as anecdotal. The author personally handed the records of Case III-1, a registered nurse with severe convulsions following aspartame ingestion, to an FDA investigator. FDA Commissioner Frank Young told a hearing on November 3, 1987, however, that he had no evidence for such a cause- and -effect relationship. (This patient even came prepared to testify at her own expense, but was not given the opportunity to do so.)

Confusing Clinical Information

In seeking more data concerning aspartame-associated convulsions, I was beset by confusing statements and inferences. For example, one senior FDA physician told me that the Epilepsy Foundation of America had issued a "negative" report on the alleged cause or aggravation of seizures by aspartame. The Director of Research and Professional Education of this Foundation, however, wrote me the following:

"In checking with our information and referral service, I have learned that, since January, we have received an estimated 15 to 20 inquiries on the subject. Our information is not kept in such a way that I am able to tell the substance of the inquiry. However, our director of Information and Referral informs me that these calls were generally for information only and did not involve reports of seizures. I hope this information is helpful."

Confusing Information: Animal Studies

In a letter dated February 3, 1986 to Senator Strom Thurmond, Chairman of the Senate Judiciary Committee, Senator Howard Metzenbaum noted that the key seizure test on aspartame had not been investigated by a grand jury even though all animals given medium or high doses in the company-sponsored monkey study evidenced grand mal seizures. Furthermore, no autopsies had been performed. The Senator stated, "Failure to account for these seizures is of particular significance given current concerns expressed in the scientific community on precisely this issue."

Epileptic seizures occur in Rhesus monkeys fed aspartame in a milk-based formula – presumably because it does not break down as quickly within the stomach owing to the changed acidity, and therefore survives longer within the upper intestinal tract.

By contrast, a Reuters feature titled, "Study Clears Sweetener in Seizures," appeared in *The Palm Beach Post* (August 13, 1987, p.A-5). It stated that scientists at the University of Illinois College of Medicine did not detect seizures in rats given "doses equivalent to what a human would get from drinking 750 12-ounce cans of diet soda all at once." (This study was funded by The NutraSweet Company.)

Even if considerable funding were made available for studies concerning aspartame-induced convulsions in monkeys and other animals, one fact is inescapable: the ultimate "experimental model" remains the vulnerable human aspartame reactor. Dr. Donald L. Schomer (1987) properly stressed that no single animal model involving specific convulsive responses to lowered norepinephrine, dopamine or serotonin concentrations can accurately represent all aspects of human epilepsy.

IV

EYE PROBLEMS

"More is missing by not looking than by not knowing."
Thomas Moore

Eye complaints were prominent in this series of 1,200 aspartame reactors. Decreased vision and related symptoms occurred in 302 (25%), severe pain (one or both eyes) in 87 (7%), and "dry eyes" or trouble wearing contact lens in 95 (8%). Blindness occurred in one or both eyes in 27.

Many of these aspartame sufferees gave further details in the survey questionnaire (Chapter XIX).

VISUAL COMPLAINTS

The constellation of ocular symptoms offered by aspartame reactors was diverse. They included "blurring of vision," "tunnel vision," "visual snow," and clinical blindness in one or both eyes. Others were "bright flashes," "eye pain," intense sensitivity to glare, and "jerking of the eyes." Several had to blink repeatedly in order "to focus my eyes." The diversity of such complaints is illustrated by the following:

Acronym Legend

    ACB - aspartame cola beverage
    ASD - aspartame soft drink
    ATS - aspartame tabletop sweetener

- Case I-29 wrote, "Upon awakening, I could not seem to get my eyes focused. The numbers on the digital clock were all jumbled together, and the room was spinning around."
- A correspondent stated that aspartame "made objects appear to be to one side or the other, and I bumped into them."
- Case VI-2, a 61-year-old executive, described "crossing of my eyes" while playing golf two hours after drinking coffee sweetened with an ATS. He experienced concomitant severe confusion and memory loss.
- A number of persons found that new prescription glasses did not appreciably improve their vision until they stopped using aspartame products.
- Larry R. Taylor, a nurse anesthetist, told the Senate hearing held on November 3, 1987 that he developed visual disturbances while consuming up to six diet colas daily, followed by severe headaches and three grand mal seizures. He stated, "I began having visual disturbances making it difficult to see the monitors in surgery, and to fill out my anesthesia record."
- Aspartame reactors in their 30s had been told they needed bifocals.
- A 52-year-old woman developed "eye seizures" two months after using aspartame. Her description of "the eyes moving back and forth" suggested nystagmus (see below).
- Case VI-4 prided herself on having had "20/15 vision" prior to consuming aspartame. She wrote

> "I suddenly developed dizziness and generally blurred vision. I read an article that stated aspartame could cause blurred vision, and the symptoms should disappear after three weeks. I have not had any aspartame for eight weeks. While the loss of words has disappeared, the blurred vision has not. Incidentally, my eye doctor could not find anything wrong with my eyes."

- A 50-year-old teacher noted a marked decrease of vision in both eyes after drinking diet colas and presweetened iced tea for two years. She commented, "I needed a prescription (for glasses) for the first time in my life!" Other symptoms included tingling of the hands, slurred speech, palpitations, and a symmetric rash. These complaints improved within days after stopping aspartame. She also was being treated for hypothyroidism.

- Several aspartame reactors emphasized awareness of "large floaters" after using aspartame products. There was usually a marked reduction in size, or disappearance, after avoiding aspartame.
- A psychologically-normal female aspartame reactor who experienced complex visual hallucinations was diagnosed as having Bonnet's syndrome.
- A woman experienced "black and white zigzagged vision" on several occasions after cataract surgery. She was able to trace this problem, presumably a migraine equivalent, to aspartame in her cereal and soda – and later in gum. These eye symptoms did not recur when she avoided such products.
- A male aspartame reactor summarized his visual difficulty in these terms:

> "I used to drink diet drinks until they started affecting my vision. The first thing I noticed was a change in the visual acuity of one eye that could not be explained. Also, I noticed glare in bright sun and slight dimming of vision, along with unexplained eye discomfort. All these symptoms went away after I stopped all diet products containing aspartame."

- A female aspartame reactor experienced two attacks of optic neuritis. Each occurred after using aspartame bubble gum. (She could not tolerate the taste of aspartame in diet sodas, yogurt or ice cream.)
- A woman who added considerable aspartame to coffee and cooked with it developed a retinal detachment in the right eye for which laser surgery was performed. She then noticed "an assortment of bright lights in both eyes all over my field of vision that may be silver-white, blue, pink or yellow. Also, I seem to have an exaggerated reaction to looking at bright lights." She stopped aspartame after reading about its ocular effects. "Right away the bright flashes seemed less frequent."

Over-the-counter medications containing aspartame have been incriminated in persistent visual complaints. For example, a woman took a popular aspartame product to alleviate a flu-like episode. She promptly experienced "a bright area in my field of vision" and migraine. The bright spot persisted, however, for which she received extensive consultation. A puzzled ophthalmologist noticed "a breakdown in the matrix of one area of the retina in my right eye." This feature diminished over the ensuing seven years during which she avoided all aspartame products.

Representative Case Reports

Case IV-1

A 66-year-old diabetic had been controlled with diet and an oral hypoglycemic drug. He experienced pain and temporary "loss of vision" in both eyes. Recent "dry eyes" had required the constant application of artificial tears. He also complained of unexplained itching, attacks of "red blotches," severe drowsiness, and a loss of hearing in both ears.

The patient's symptoms abated after abstinence from aspartame products. They had become a preoccupation "because I was afraid I'd go blind."

Case IV-2

A 52-year-old businesswoman consumed six cans of diet colas daily for three months. She experienced impaired vision, "dry eyes," difficulty wearing contact lens, and intense pain in both eyes ascribed to "limbic keratitis."

Other complaints included pain in one ear, lightheadedness, severe depression with suicidal thoughts, extreme irritability, anxiety attacks, a marked change in personality, episodic rapid heart action, a recent rise in blood pressure, diarrhea, and the loss of 20 pounds.

Case IV-3

A 46-year-old director of medical records consumed from six to 12 cans of aspartame beverages daily. She awakened with "pieces of vision missing... I could not always see everything in my path. I ran over wheelchairs and anything in my path. The lower vision was missing." She also suffered severe headaches, dizziness, drowsiness, depression with suicidal thoughts, extreme irritability, marked bloat, thinning of the hair, and intense itching.

Case IV-4

A 40-year-old physician had been consuming about one liter of diet drinks daily for eight years. She developed an optic neuritis of sufficient severity to preclude performing surgery. There were concomitant headaches, menstrual changes (decreased cycles), and memory loss. She also developed Hashimoto thyroiditis with an elevated TSH level of 29 (normal up to 5), and a high antinuclear antibody titer (ANA). All her symptoms improved after stopping aspartame products except the impaired vision. The ANA titer also normalized.

Case IV-5 A

A famous actor consumed 2-4 quarts of an aspartame soda daily because he had been diagnosed as being "pre-diabetic." Although initially dubious about aspartame disease, he became a "true believer" after experiencing visual problems, such as inability to read the labels on medicine bottles. This difficulty disappeared when he discontinued aspartame.

Case IV-5 B

A man drank considerable aspartame soda while on vacation. During and after this trip, he noticed a marked decline of vision. "Four spots of hemorrhaging near my right optic nerve" were found on examination. Happening to hear this discussion with his boss, a coworker mentioned having heard about comparable symptoms caused by aspartame. The patient's vision improved dramatically when he discontinued aspartame products – along with the associated dizziness, confusion, headache and joint pain.

Case IV-5 C

A 72-year-old aspartame reactor previously had enjoyed a saccharin-containing soft drink. When the producer substituted aspartame, he had an "immediate attack" in which "my eyeballs felt as though they would burst and were very painful." He also suffered "a sick stomach and pounding headache." The same reaction recurred several days later when he decided to give this product "a second chance."

Case IV-6

A 36-year-old secretary consumed two 2-liter bottles of an aspartame orange soda, and up to five glasses of presweetened ice tea daily. She experienced recurrent blurring of vision, coupled with pain and "unusual lights and floaters" in both eyes. She neither smoked nor drank alcohol.

Associated symptoms included severe headache, marked memory loss, mental confusion, slurred speech, intense depression and "mood swings," abdominal bloat, itching, and a transient rise in blood pressure. All subsided after avoiding aspartame. She later correctly deduced that her daughter's visual problems and her mother's dizziness were attributable to aspartame reactions.

Case IV-7

A woman who had consumed aspartame soft drinks since their introduction experienced severe visual disturbances over the next two years. They were described as "flashing lights and streaks whenever I moved my eyes back and forth," and "gray shadows and circles." She also suffered severe migrainous headaches during this time. Multiple ophthalmologists and neurologists could find no objective changes. The "gray shadows" became "lighter in color" within six weeks after stopping aspartame.

Case IV-8

A 34-year-old woman described her intolerance to aspartame in these terms:

> "Whenever I drink an aspartame pop, my eyes cloud and I get a mucus covering. I know it is from the pop because I won't have it for a week. Then on the day I have it, my eyes are thick with a mucus covering by night."

Case IV-9

A 45-year-old air traffic control specialist began consuming two 10-ounce bottles of a diet cola daily. He did so to avoid sugar because of hypoglycemic attacks and an overweight problem. Within three days, he experienced intense pain and blurring of vision in one eye, and "dry eyes." He wrote, "The pain was so bad it doubled me up and I could hardly move. I forced the eye open with both hands, and let water spray into the eye. My eye hurt all morning and was red for 24 hours."

Several days later, he awakened to find his vision clouded by a "road map of black blood vessels, which lasted about three seconds after each time I blinked. This condition went away after four or five minutes."

160

He also developed great thirst and an intensification of his "low blood sugar attacks." He retested himself three times before concluding that the aspartame product had caused these problems. The "road map" and eye pain disappeared within two days after stopping aspartame.

Case IV-10 A

A 51-year-old homemaker developed severe blurring of vision in her right eye. A posterior vitreous detachment was found. She had been consuming two cans and two glasses of aspartame soft drinks daily, along with aspartame hot chocolate for one year.

Other symptoms included intense depression with suicidal thoughts, "trouble thinking at times," severe tingling of the limbs, marked irritability, anxiety attacks, a change in personality, aggravation of phobias, diarrhea, severe itching, a rash and joint pain. Although there had been a tendency to slight despondency previously, she volunteered that "the depression while using aspartame was worse than anything before or since." There was a history of allergy to penicillin and sulfa drugs, and intolerance to estrogen replacement therapy. Most of her symptoms began to improve within three days after stopping aspartame except the blurred vision.

Case IV-10 B

A 44-year-old registered nurse in apparent excellent health switched to aspartame sodas, and added aspartame packets to recipes she baked at home. She experienced retinal bleeding in the right eye several weeks later. Several ophthalmologists and her internist were perplexed due to the absence of diabetes, hypertension, or other overt risk factors.

Case IV-11

A 28-year-old electrical engineer consumed two liters of diet cola and up to five glasses of an ASD daily for two years. She described the sequence of ensuing symptoms and signs in a detailed diary. Chronologically, they consisted of hearing loss in both ears, severe ringing in the right ear, daily headaches, pain shooting from the right ear to the back of her neck, a constant pain behind the right eye, blurring of vision in the right eye, and subsequent double vision. A preliminary diagnosis of optic neuritis due to multiple sclerosis was made. A brain tumor also was suspected.

She experienced unsteadiness, severe tingling and numbness over the left head and in the left upper and lower limbs, depression, irritability, a change in personality, and marked thinning of the hair. There was a longstanding history of premenstrual fluid retention.

Six months after these symptoms began, she read an article about reactions to aspartame. The numbness virtually disappeared three weeks after avoiding all aspartame products. As the other symptoms also abated, she resumed her professional career and enjoyed a normal personal life.

Making "The Aspartame Connection"

A number of aspartame reactors consulted me after repeated visits to ophthalmologists for continued and unexplained difficulty with vision. "The aspartame connection" became evident as they responded affirmatively to questions about associated severe headache, memory loss and the other symptoms frequently encountered in aspartame disease. Improvement of vision after abstinence from aspartame, however, was often delayed longer than the dramatic subsidence of other symptoms.

Case IV-12

A 56-year-old engineer had been treated several years for typical reactive hypoglycemia and hypothyroidism, and responded well to appropriate diet and medication.

The patient returned in January 1988 because of unexplained difficulty in vision for several months that his ophthalmologist could not explain. He also had been having severe headache, confusion and memory loss (of particular concern in his professional work), "dry eyes," marked dizziness, tingling or numbness of the limbs, depression, episodic shortness of breath, abdominal pain with diarrhea and blood in the stools, intermittent difficulty in swallowing, intense thirst, and bothersome frequency of urination day and night. Another troubling symptom was severe drowsiness that precluded going out in the evening, and causing him to retire at 9 or 10 PM.

Specific inquiry revealed that he had been taking up to four cans of diet cola, one or two bowls of an aspartame cereal, and other aspartame products daily. Moreover, his daughter had suffered loss of vision from aspartame products.

When seen one week after abstaining from aspartame, the headaches had improved considerably. His clarity of thinking returned two weeks later, along with improvement of vision and other symptoms.

Case IV-13 A

A prominent Philadelphia radio talk-show host interviewed me on the topic of

162

aspartame disease. Two years later, he experienced unexplained double vision. He consulted a cardiologist and a neurosurgeon. Various studies, including an MRI of the brain, were "negative."

Frustrated, he mentioned the problem to his producer. The latter reminded him of my prior interview, and asked if he was still using aspartame sodas. "The light went on." There was no recurrence of the visual problem over the ensuing two years of abstinence from aspartame products.

Case IV-13 B

A physician offered his personal experience with aspartame-induced visual changes.

> "I had been drinking several cans of diet drinks a day for six months. There was a drop in my visual acuity that perplexed me. My eyes were rechecked four weeks later, and the change remained.

> "I accidently came across the problems associated with aspartame on the Internet, and immediately stopped all sugar substitutes. Lo and behold! My vision improved, and the slight haze or blurriness was gone. The colors were more vibrant. I also could tolerate the glare in bright sunlight."

Case IV–13 C

A 48-year-old woman developed severe impairment of vision in both eyes three years previously. It had reached the point she could not read words on her computer screen. An ophthalmologist found "spots on the retina of both eyes that looked like permanent scarring, and still growing." Four retina specialists at a referral medical center in Iowa concurred, stating "they had never seen anything like it, and had no idea what was causing it."

Having finalized plans for a trip to Mexico, she decided to proceed. Using disposable contact lenses, she was able to read a book en route to Denver for the connecting flight. She continued drinking diet colas, and increased her aspartame intake while visiting relatives in Denver. She wrote, "By the next day when we boarded our flight, I could not see some large sign, let alone read a book. It was at that point that I started to suspect the diet pop.

For the next week, I had no diet pop or aspartame in any form. In Mexico, there was only regular pop; no diet sodas were available in most places. By the end of the week, my vision was pretty good again."

On returning, she discussed the matter with her ophthalmologist. He concurred that aspartame might be the problem. Furthermore, he also had been convinced that the headaches <u>his</u> wife experienced were induced by aspartame.

The patient's visual problems stabilized. She emphasized, "If I get any of this by mistake, I can't find my PC for a day or so." She inadvertently ingested some aspartame three years later. "I woke up Monday morning, and had lost depth perception. My left eye burned and was very red, very full of mucus. I could not see for about four days before my vision slowly came back."

There was a strong family history of aspartame disease. One of her daughters experienced severe cramps, diarrhea, a rash and insomnia with aspartame use. Her youngest daughter was affected by severe migraine, mood swings and depression. A nephew vomited and then experienced diarrhea after taking aspartame.

CORROBORATION

After my observations were first published, I received calls from ophthalmologists about patients who had improved dramatically following abstinence from aspartame products. For example, a Pennsylvania ophthalmologist confirmed the regression of eye complaints and associated severe headache in seven of his patients. The doctor's interest initially had been kindled by an aspartame reactor who showed him my survey questionnaire (Section 4) that she had completed.

<u>Dr. Morgan Raiford</u>, an Atlanta ophthalmologist, told me of his experience with 65 aspartame users who had presented with unilateral or bilateral visual deterioration and/or optic nerve atrophy (personal communication, July 10, 1986). These observations reminded him of the ocular complications in methanol poisoning, wherein he had a longstanding interest (Chapter XXI). In this context, "wood alcohol poisoning" was suspected by ophthalmologists in several patients – to their astonishment because little or no alcohol had been consumed (see Case IV-24).

<u>Woodrow C. Monte, Ph.D.</u> (Chairman, Food Sciences Department at Arizona State University) received calls from over 1,000 persons, and letters from more than 300 other individuals (!), after he expressed concern about visual damage in aspartame users (personal

164

communications, July and September 1986). Up to 60 percent of their complaints were ocular in nature – namely., blurred vision, bright flashes, tunnel vision and blindness.

FDA Data

The FDA initially received ocular complaints attributed to aspartame from 177 consumers (Dr. Linda Tollefson, personal communication, August 12, 1987). The data are summarized in Table IV-1. Seventy-five (42.4%) also experienced headaches.

TABLE IV-1
FDA DATA ON 177 CONSUMERS WITH
ASPARTAME-ASSOCIATED VISUAL PROBLEMS

Sex
Female	142	(80.2%)
Male	35	(19.8%)

Race
White	72	(40.7%)
Nonwhite	5	(2.8%)
Unknown	100	(56.5%)

Age Group (years)
1-19	3	(1.7%)
20-29	18	(10.2%)
30-39	33	(18.6%)
40-49	36	(20.3%)
50-59	18	(10.2%)
60+	32	(18.1%)
Unknown	37	(20.9%)

Aspartame Products Consumed
Soft Drinks	119	(67.2%)
Tabletop Sweeteners	83	(46.9%)
Hot Chocolate	17	(9.6%)
Iced Tea	17	(9.6%)
Gum	7	(4.0%)
Soft Drink Mixes	32	(18.1%)
Puddings/Gelatins	32	(18.1%)

Concomitant Symptoms

Headaches	79	(44.6%)
Depression/Mood Changes	30	(16.9%)
Numbness/Tingling/Other Neurologic	29	(16.4%)
Dizziness	64	(36.2%)
Abdominal Pain/GI Complaints	29	(16.4%)
Memory Loss	20	(11.3%)
Weakness/Fatigue	12	(6.8%)
Fainting	4	(2.3%)
Hives/Rashes	8	(4.5%)
Sleep Problems	13	(7.3%)
Heart	4	(2.3%)
Bone/Joint Pain	3	(1.7%)
Menstrual	4	(2.3%)
Breathing Difficulty	3	(1.7%)
Coma	4	(2.3%)

Two patients reported total bilateral blindness to the FDA, which they ascribed to the use of aspartame products.

- A nine-month-old child was "blind due to brain damage since birth." The mother had consumed two aspartame sodas daily during the pregnancy.
- A female aspartame reactor was blinded due to bilateral optic neuritis. She responded to steroid therapy and "fully recovered."

DIAGNOSTIC CONSIDERATIONS AND PREJUDICES

Other ocular diagnoses were convincingly excluded in most of these aspartame reactors – specifically glaucoma, occlusion of a retinal vessel, detachment of the retina, and optic neuritis due to various causes.

The following diagnostic encounters are noteworthy.

- The initial diagnosis of multiple sclerosis (Chapter VI-D) in several young women was retracted after prolonged observation following aspartame avoidance.
- Toxic amblyopia (a type of optic nerve damage) could be ruled out in the majority, especially for patients who did not smoke or drink significant amounts of alcohol (Chapter XIX).

166

- The primary diagnosis of <u>cataract</u> proved erroneous in several older persons (see below).
- The <u>tentative</u> diagnosis of complicating <u>retinopathy</u> was disproved in <u>diabetic</u> patients whose vision <u>promptly</u> improved after stopping aspartame (Chapter XIII).
- The marked decrease of vision in a 52-year-old businessman improved after avoiding aspartame. It had been attributed to "<u>macular degeneration</u>" of unspecified cause. Several other aspartame reactors with marked visual impairment diagnosed as macular degeneration also experienced improvement after stopping aspartame products. When checked by her ophthalmologist 15 months later, the vision of one such woman had normalized. She wrote, "Thank you, Dr. Roberts, for sharing the secret of my 'aging eyes.'"

  The author is not familiar with any study specifically addressing the consumption of aspartame products by patients under the age of 60 diagnosed as having macular degeneration.

- Six aspartame reactors in this series who developed decreased vision, papilledema (swelling of the optic nerve) and headache were diagnosed as having <u>pseudotumor cerebri</u> (Chapter VI-N).
- The diagnosis of <u>Behçet's disease</u> was considered in two patients. Its chief clinical components are eye involvement (uveitis; iritis), ulcers, genital ulcers, recurrent skin lesions, headache, recurrent arthralgia, abnormal neurologic findings and aseptic meningitis.

CT scans and MRI studies of the brain and optic nerves in these patients generally were normal. Minor changes proved nonspecific. For example, Case IV-17 was reported to have "moderate thickening, inhomogeneity, and tortuosity of the optic nerves suggesting either active inflammation (optic neuritis) or cerebrospinal fluid congestion owing to any cause of increased intracranial pressure."

Paradoxically, some aspartame reactors with visual complaints found it difficult to convince ophthalmologists about the reality of their symptoms. Several had been told, "Your eyes are fine. You don't even need new glasses." The "scientific manner" by which these persons subsequently deduced that aspartame was **the** cause for their visual problems is described below and in case histories elsewhere.

Resistance By The Medical Profession

A number of physicians, including ophthalmologists, became interested in aspartame disease when it damaged **their** vision or that of a spouse (see Cases IV-22 and IV-29). One California ophthalmologist noted on the Internet, "There are many ignorant ophthalmologists, such as myself, who have either not heard of potential problems with aspartame, or have not given it much credence. I want to know more."

Some ophthalmologists became incensed at the suggestion aspartame products could cause eye problems. One indicated that he would try to have the America On Line (AOL) account of an aspartame reactor revoked because of such "junk" e-mail... along with presumed "grandstanding" by the author.

The reluctance of physicians to believe that serious eye problems can be due to aspartame effects is detailed in Chapter XIX and Section 7. Furthermore, prominent ophthalmologists (who obviously had not volunteered their time) dogmatically denied on several television programs shown nationally that aspartame has any visual side effects. Others dodged this issue by emphasizing the need for prompt ophthalmologic consultation to rule out retinal detachment, occlusion of a retinal blood vessel, or "brain stem encephalitis."

> During one such program, a neuro-ophthalmologist on the staff at a renowned eye clinic stated that neither he nor three colleagues at that center had ever encountered visual problems attributable to aspartame. He added that this reflected the belief of other eye specialists in a nationwide poll.

BLINDNESS

Twenty-seven persons in this series suffered extreme loss of vision or frank blindness in one or both eyes. Although generally transient, it was permanent in some. Vision is more likely to return if the ocular damage of optic neuritis is in its "wet stage." Comparable case histories have been reported to the FDA (see above).

As noted earlier, no other convincing causes could be found by multiple consultants. Considering the widespread use of aspartame products by young adults, the term "baby boomer blindness" takes on new meaning.

Retinal bleeding and subsequent scarring accompanied aspartame-associated visual loss in Cases IV-12 and IV-13. Neither had diabetes, hypertension, a blood disorder, nor other known disease conducive to hemorrhage.

Retinal detachment occurred in some patients. Its occurrence in the early phase of a double-blind study on depressed patients by Walton (1993) influenced the decision to stop that investigation.

The legal term "willful blindness" assumes greater significance in view of approval of aspartame as a general all-purpose sweetener by the FDA.

Representative Case Reports

Case IV-14

A 37-year-old painter and jewelry artisan consumed considerable aspartame in various beverages over 18 months. She ingested 4 to 5 cups coffee with two packets of an ATS in each cup every morning, one or two cups coffee containing the same amount of ATS in the mid-morning, and up to six glasses of aspartame-sweetened iced tea or diet cola daily during the summer.

The patient experienced constant headache, dizziness, insomnia, fatigue, depression and memory loss. A profound decrease of vision in the left eye on awaking was then noticed. It progressed to complete blindness within four days. Extensive medical, neurologic and ophthalmologic consultations failed to reveal a cause for the presumed optic neuritis. Treatment with prednisone was minimally effective.

On learning that someone had attributed a comparable reaction to aspartame products, she discontinued their use. Her headache, weakness and insomnia subsided within one month. The visual impairment, however, persisted. There was only slight sensitivity to light in the affected eye several years later. She could not resume her previous occupation because of severely impaired depth perception.

Case IV-15

A 41-year-old real estate agent experienced "permanent eye and ear damage" that markedly affected her business career. She had consumed 24 packets of an ATS in tea and coffee daily since 1982 – along with six cans of a diet cola, three glasses of an ASD, two glasses of aspartame hot chocolate, four servings of aspartame puddings or gelatins, and other aspartame-containing products (e.g., diet cheese cake.)

This patient suddenly lost the vision in her <u>left eye</u> during May 1984, and had considerable associated pain. An ophthalmologist diagnosed "optic neuritis of undetermined cause." Light perception began to return in January 1985.

She embarked on a weight reduction program during November 1984, and lost 30 pounds. During this time, she increased her intake of aspartame products. She then lost the vision in her <u>right</u> eye during February 1985 because of an unexplained progressive retinal hemorrhage, complicated by a retinal tear with detachment. Other ocular features included severe pain in both eyes, nystagmus, and "dry eyes."

Concomitant complaints were loss of hearing in one ear, "ringing" and marked sensitivity to noise in the other ear, severe headache, dizziness, memory loss, intense anxiety, palpitations, abdominal pain, marked bloat, swelling of the lips, and atypical mouth and facial pains. "Very little" alcohol aggravated these symptoms. She also had to be hospitalized for recent high blood pressure and a rapid heart rate (146 per minute) for which no underlying cause could be found.

The patient was seen by her personal physician, three ophthalmologists, two neurologists, an internist, a chiropractor, and a temporomandibular joint (TMJ) specialist. She became irate when an ophthalmologist "thought I was hysterical about my loss of vision." One neurologist made the diagnosis of multiple sclerosis, but the other concluded it was not present. Her tests included an MRI study of the brain, an electroencephalogram, heart monitoring, and multiple eye and ear tests. She estimated the costs at $5,000 personally, and $9,000 for her insurance carrier. Summarizing her physician encounters, she wrote, "I visited many doctors trying to find out what was wrong, but never got any answers."

Having been "in perfect health before using aspartame" and not knowing where to turn, this patient decided to analyze the sequence of events herself. By a process of elimination, she concluded that aspartame constituted the only significant "environmental change." Her dizziness, headache and memory loss improved dramatically when she stopped all aspartame products. Three days later, her ophthalmologist (without knowledge of this interim change) expressed surprise on finding that the non-blinded eye had "stabilized."

The patient ingested aspartame one week later "since it was almost impossible to purchase any diet product that did not contain aspartame." Her symptoms <u>promptly</u> returned, with intensification of the eye pain.

The nonocular complaints disappeared totally after avoiding aspartame from May 1985. The right eye vision improved within three months. Fifteen months later, she described her ocular disability in these terms: "I can no longer drive a vehicle because of my eyes. It has greatly decreased my performance in my job because I must depend on my husband to drive me so I can meet my appointments."

Her honor-student sons also suffered severe aspartame reactions. They consisted of dizziness, headaches, visual problems, loss of memory, decreased scholastic achievement, dropping objects, and impaired coordination. These problems disappeared after the entire family strictly avoided aspartame products. She commented, "If aspartame can have such a profound effect on an adult, it is frightening to think of what it may be doing to children."

Case IV-16

A 37-year-old businessman consumed three to four glasses of aspartame beverages daily for one year prior to the onset of severe headaches, impaired vision in the right eye, and intense thirst. His history and commentary are noteworthy.

"My problem started just prior to October 1985. I had been having trouble with my vision and getting headaches. I went to see my ophthalmologist. He was not able to find anything wrong and suggested that I take some time off. I didn't, and just lived with the problem until summer 1986. Toward the end of the summer, the headaches became worse to the point that when I got them I was unable to function, and had to go to sleep for several hours. Also, I started to lose the vision in my right eye. I returned to the ophthalmologist about the beginning of August. He found that I had severe hemorrhaging in my retina, but couldn't explain why. He recommended that I see a retinologist at the _____ Eye Hospital. He too was unable to explain what was causing my problem, and recommended that I see a neuroretinologist at the same hospital. I should mention that I do not drink alcohol very often.

"I went to see the doctor because of the headaches. He put me into the hospital for a full range of tests including a CT scan from head to toe, a full series of blood tests, and spinal taps.

With the exception of seeing some cells in my retinal and spinal fluid, everything came back negative. I continued to see the retinologist who started me on steroids. After the hospital, my vision didn't get any worse nor did it get any better. The headaches stopped and my retina seemed to be healing.

"Coincidentally at about the time I went into the hospital, my wife read an article in the newspaper that cautioned against serving children drinks with aspartame. She stopped making it, and obviously I stopped drinking it because it wasn't around. I didn't make the connection between the aspartame and my medical problems until about two weeks ago when I found a container of an aspartame soft drink and drank two glasses. Within minutes I started to get the headache again. My vision became blurry, and the skin on my skull started to hurt. I discussed the incident with my wife, and we put two and two together.

"Since then I have talked to two other friends who were suffering from severe headaches. Both were users of aspartame drinks. I am convinced that this was the cause of my problems.

"Sadly, there was no reason that my vision should have deteriorated as much as it has. The doctors I saw didn't know the right questions to ask. It would seem that not enough is known about aspartame to allow it to be used without some kind of warning. I hope that your research is well publicized so that other doctors become knowledgeable enough to ask the right questions. Also, I feel that a warning label on products that contain the sweetener is advisable."

Case IV-17

A 38-year-old homemaker experienced bilateral loss of vision. Four physicians and consultants were seen. She stated, "I was suffering with severe headaches when I awoke one day with blurred vision. Within one week, I had lost complete vision in both eyes while in the hospital. Thanks to the Lord, my vision came back in approximately three months."

She had consumed 6-10 packets of an ATS, up to four glasses of aspartame-sweetened iced tea, 4-6 regular glasses of an ASD, and one serving of aspartame pudding daily for four months. There was a weight loss of 15 pounds.

I reviewed the patient's records. The results of a CT scan of the brain, cerebral angiography, and a lumbar puncture were normal. A CT scan of the eyes was interpreted as "moderate thickening, inhomogeneity and tortuosity of the optic nerve suggesting either active inflammation (optic neuritis) or CSF (cerebrospinal fluid) congestion owing to any cause of increased intracranial pressure." The eye consultant concluded that this patient had "marked papillitis bilaterally... with a severe, rapidly advancing case of optic neuritis." Large doses of prednisone were recommended.

The patient retested herself twice before becoming convinced that aspartame was **the** cause of her problem. She felt a return of "the indescribable feeling in my head" within one day.

Three of her friends also had experienced aspartame reactions. These consisted of "blurred vision, halo around eyes, and diarrhea."

Case IV-18

A 63-year-old woman ingested one can of diet cola and 8-10 packets of an ATS daily for four months. She lost most of the vision in her right eye, and noted a marked decrease in the left. Eye pain and recent "dry eyes" also developed. She was seen in consultation by two ophthalmologists who diagnosed "a blind spot and optic nerve damage of unknown cause." At the time of her communication, she could make out only vague shadows on the right; everything else was "hazy and blurred."

This patient also experienced ringing in both ears, severe dizziness, marked insomnia, tingling and numbness of the limbs, episodic shortness of breath, intense itching, hives, severe joint pains, and swelling of the legs. She neither smoked nor drank alcohol.

Case IV-19

A 33-year-old accountant consumed one can of an aspartame soda daily, and one packet of an ATS every two days. She lost her vision in one eye, the condition being diagnosed as "optic neuritis of unknown cause." Two CT scans and an MRI study of the brain, a lumbar puncture, and special eye tests were normal. Her condition improved after treatment with corticosteroids and the cessation of aspartame products.

Case IV-20

A 41-year-old bookkeeper complained primarily of visual problems after consuming aspartame products. She wrote, "If I drink two or three diet colas a day, I lose vision in my right eye for 10-15 minutes each session."

Case IV-21

A 49-year-old personnel assistant consumed up to six packets of an ATS, and eight sticks of aspartame gum daily. She developed total blindness in the right eye, and impaired vision in the left. Other ocular symptoms consisted of pain in both eyes and difficulty wearing contact lens. She neither smoked nor drank alcohol.

The patient also developed severe depression with anxiety, marked memory loss, attacks of rapid heart action, shortness of breath, and bloody stools. Most of these symptoms improved by abstaining from aspartame, but not the blindness in the right eye after ten months.

Case IV-22

A 52-year-old registered nurse had been in apparent excellent health when she lost the central vision in her left eye. Her husband, a professor of surgery at a major teaching medical
center, referred her to an eye institute for extensive study. No cause could be determined. She had been consuming two quarts of an aspartame iced tea mix daily during the preceding summer months.

When rechecked in September, the ophthalmologist found that she still could not see details of the eye chart except by using her residual peripheral vision.

Suspecting the aspartame drink to be a factor, the patient avoided it. She regained considerable peripheral vision in the affected eye over the next year; the central loss, however, was permanent.

An article in the *Philadelphia Inquirer* later asserted that aspartame does not cause eye problems. With this assurance, she drank an aspartame soda at a social function during the Christmas holiday. Her husband reported

"The following morning her remaining vision was so blurred that she could not read the number on the microwave or the headlines in the morning paper. This lasted 24 hours. Her vision then cleared in the good right eye... In February 1990, a second incident occurred. The morning after dinner at a friend's home, she again awoke with blurred vision. On calling our hostess, she learned that the molded salad was made with a gelatin containing aspartame. Her visual blurring again cleared in 24 hours. Our ophthalmologists have not accepted even the remote possibility that my wife's visual loss is related to aspartame. My great concern now is for others!"

Case IV-23

The dramatic deterioration of bilateral vision in a 53-year-old man was described by his wife. Her letter to the FDA supplemented submission of the completed questionnaire (Section 4) to me. His daily intake included six 12-ounce cans of diet cola, one large bottle of diet cola, 8-10 packets of a tabletop sweetener, three regular glasses of an aspartame soft drink mix, two servings of aspartame pudding and gelatins, and a packet of aspartame gum. The details and commentary are relevant.

"My husband suddenly became blind in the left eye (described as a gray cloud covering portions of the eye), which also, a week later, affected the right eye. He was admitted to _____ General Hospital for testing. Upon being admitted, I was answering general questions from his doctor. He asked me if my husband was an alcoholic. I answered that neither one of us drink, not even casually. He then told me that he had symptoms of a person who consumes 'wood alcohol.'

"My husband was told he had high blood sugar (diabetes) on November 20, 1989. I immediately eliminated sugar, and started using aspartame in each large cup of coffee. (Not only coffee, but we used diet drinks, jello, and other products that had no sugar.) Not long afterwards, he started experiencing tingling in the hands, which was later diagnosed as carpal tunnel syndrome. (See Chapter VI-E) This tingling also spread to the legs. A week before he was scheduled to have carpal tunnel surgery, he was admitted to _____ General Hospital for testing (March 5th). He had become blind in the left eye. He was in the hospital for a week, enduring extensive testing. The doctors found NO cause for his blindness other than 'it may be a virus.' During his stay in the hospital, he was still ingesting aspartame.

"After he was dismissed, I heard about the dangers of aspartame, and immediately took him off these products. There has been some improvement in his condition. The tingling in his hands has disappeared, but there is permanent damage to the optic nerve. He still cannot see out of his right eye, and has permanent damage in the left eye. He cannot drive. He cannot read. He lost his job. It has really been a trial.

"I have spoken with a doctor at the FDA. He had a rather 'ho-hum' attitude.

"I DON'T KNOW WHO HAS BEEN 'BOUGHT OFF,' BUT THIS PRODUCT IS A NEUROLOGIC TOXIN!!! POISONING AMERICA FOR THE ALMIGHTY DOLLAR!!!

"I know, without doubt, that aspartame consumption was the cause of my husband's ultimate blindness. Its consumption was the ONLY change in our life-style. We need to get this product OUT of the churches, schools, business places, and OFF the grocery shelves. Sue the socks off the manufacturer who feels people are dispensable for their pursuit of greed. What are a pair of eyes worth?"

Case IV-24

This man developed blindness in the right eye three months after a diagnosis of non-insulin-dependent diabetes was made. Numerous studies at a major eye institution failed to identify a plausible cause for his optic neuritis. He was begun on corticosteroid therapy. His vision then deteriorated in the left eye. Even though the patient did not ingest alcoholic beverages, an attending physician raised the possibility of "wood alcohol poisoning."

His wife "replaced all sugar with sugar-free products" when diabetes was diagnosed. Shortly thereafter, he also complained of insomnia, and severe tingling and numbness of the fingers and hands. The latter complaints were diagnosed as carpal tunnel syndrome by three physicians; surgery was suggested but not performed. Soon after the elimination of aspartame products, the hand neuropathy disappeared. He remained legally blind in both eyes, however, over the ensuing nine years.

CLINICAL CONSIDERATIONS RELATING TO IMPAIRED VISION

A. Vulnerable Groups (see Section 3)

Older persons are more vulnerable to physical and metabolic influences that can damage the eyes (Chapter XV). For example, there is an inverse correlation between recovery from glare and age (Wolf 1960).

Aspartame reactors with coexisting eye disorders are more likely to experience visual complaints. These include cataract, glaucoma, astigmatism, and diabetic or hypertensive retinopathy.

Persons who smoke or drink significantly, and those taking drugs affecting vision may be at increased ocular risk. In my computerized analysis of aspartame reactors with visual impairment, however, there was little to suggest superimposed toxic amblyopia due to tobacco or alcohol.

Patients with diabetes mellitus (Chapter XIII) and severe hypoglycemia (Chapter XIV) are probably more prone to aspartame-induced visual problems owing to the extraordinary metabolic demands of the retina (see below). The simulation or aggravation of diabetic retinopathy deserves reemphasis.

The striking ocular features of multiple sclerosis (or transitional multiple sclerosis) in patients with severe hypoglycemia were discussed in prior publications (Roberts 1966 b, c).

Representative Case Reports

Case IV-25

A 51-year-old insulin-dependent diabetic consumed three cans of diet sodas and eight packets of an ATS daily for three months. He then noted strange visual images. ("I saw things, like a puppy in my kitchen, and we don't have a dog. Also shadows flitting by in my hallway.") Other features included headache, lightheadedness, "pins and needles" in the limbs, palpitations, severe depression (with suicidal thoughts), and marked irritability. These symptoms disappeared within several days after stopping aspartame.

His daughter also experienced headache after taking aspartame products.

Case IV-26

A 40-year-old truck driver presented with poorly controlled diabetes while taking tolbutamide. He complained of progressively blurred vision (attributed to "oozing" in the right eye), and intense neuropathic discomfort of the feet and left hand. The fasting blood glucose (FBS) was 278 mg%. A random blood glucose concentration was 178 mg%.

The patient consumed about four diet sodas daily. He had not drunk alcohol for several years. There was striking improvement of his vision one week after avoiding aspartame – especially the blurring while he drove. His FBS declined to 146-163 mg% within one week.

Case IV-27

A 68-year-old insulin-dependent diabetic man lost an eye due to an injury many years previously. He had done well on a conventional dietary and medical program.

The patient then presented with blurred vision and considerable pain in the remaining eye, more frequent insulin reactions, recurrent intense burning in the feet, and an unexplained rise of glucose concentrations. He was advised to stop aspartame products, but otherwise to remain on the same regimen. When seen ten days later, his vision and eye pain were improved, and the foot discomfort had abated. Concomitantly, his fasting and evening blood glucose concentrations decreased to prior levels.

Case IV-28

A 20-year-old receptionist was an insulin-dependent diabetic. At the age of 18, she began consuming four cans of an ACB, six packets of an ATS, two glasses of presweetened iced tea, one bowl of an aspartame-sweetened cereal, and five sticks of aspartame gum daily. A marked decrease of vision occurred in the left eye when she was 19, with subsequent "permanent damage to the retina." Other symptoms included severe headache, dizziness, marked insomnia, depression, extreme irritability, "severe anxiety attacks," "personality changes," palpitations, swelling of the tongue, abdominal pain and diarrhea.

The patient saw numerous physicians and had been hospitalized <u>five times</u> before aspartame was suspected as a contributory cause. Her studies included a CT scan of the head, cerebral angiograms, an EEG, and multiple eye tests. She experienced marked improvement within two weeks after stopping aspartame products. Her non-ocular symptoms disappeared one week later.

She volunteered that a cousin also reacted to aspartame products with severe headache and "a problem concentrating at work."

Case IV-29 A

A 50-year-old surgeon was diagnosed as having diabetes, and placed on a standard diet and an oral drug (Diabeta®). He began to consume considerable amounts of diet sodas – about two liters daily – in order to avoid sugar. He then experienced marked decrease and blurring of his vision, diagnosed as macular edema. When his vision declined to 20/100, he had to give up both surgery and driving. Laser therapy was administered to one eye.

The patient subsequently obtained information about aspartame, and discovered that it was metabolized to methanol. He discontinued all diet drinks. There was progressive improvement of vision to 20/30 and 20/40, accompanied by near-normal blood glucose concentrations.

Case IV-29 B

A 48-year-old man with recently-diagnosed diabetes experienced marked confusion and memory loss while drinking aspartame beverages. When subsequently seen after stopping these products, he volunteered that he no longer required the special reading glasses purchased. He could now promptly accommodate his vision from one object to another ("just like a photographer attempting to focus the lens"), contrasting with the many seconds to do so recently. He also stated that his confusion and memory loss had subsided.

B. Erroneous Diagnosis of Cataract

Decreased vision was erroneously attributed to cataracts in patients who proved to have aspartame disease. This possibility ought to be considered when the visual problem is relatively recent and rapid in persons with long-standing but asymptomatic lens opacities.

(I have been repeatedly impressed by the paucity of symptoms in some patients with overt cataracts.)

The dramatic improvement of vision within one or several weeks after stopping aspartame products indicated that the presence of a cataract was incidental. The primary role of aspartame was validated in several reactors who had undergone unsuccessful cataract surgery because (1) their visual problems persisted or increased, even with new prescription glasses, before stopping aspartame, (2) other symptoms attributable to aspartame disease existed, and (3) vision improved after avoiding aspartame products.

- Case IX-I-2 continued having visual problems after the removal of a cataract. She also experienced severe headache, lip and tongue reactions, nausea and "nervousness." These features disappeared after avoiding aspartame.

- A 85-year-old man wrote

  > "My health was fair until April 1, 1986 when I started drinking aspartame. I then had a cataract removed from my right eye. I tried three pairs of glasses, but to no avail. I cannot read newsprint. The surgeon now claims this is due to blood pressure which destroyed the eye. I also have trouble with my right ear which started on April 1, 1986."

C. Other Unwarranted Surgery

A young female executive developed visual problems ("my eyes would go out of focus") while consuming three cans of diet soda daily. Before coming under my care, a radial keratotomy had been done on the left eye, and was repeated six months later because her symptoms persisted.

D. Concomitant Systemic Reactions

Most persons with eye complaints had multiple non-ocular symptoms that could be attributed to aspartame disease because they promptly improved after stopping such products. As noted above and in Chapter V, headache was frequent.

180

E. Visual Reactions in Families

The impressive familial ramifications of aspartame disease are described in Chapters II-J and XVI, including the same type of reactions among family members. This applies to vision.

Case IV-30

The mother of a boy in the fourth grade described each of their experiences. They occurred in 1984 when a new aspartame soda became popular. She bought two cannisters that she and her son drank. (No other family members used it.)

Concerning her reaction, she wrote, "All of a sudden, I started going blind. If I looked straight ahead, it was like someone had placed silver dollars over my eyes. I could see out of the corner, but not straight ahead. This lasted about one hour. I was so scared that I drove myself to the hospital, but they could find nothing wrong." She told no one about this incident, presumably a "migraine equivalent." Difficulty with vision persisted thereafter, requiring resort to a magnifying glass. She also developed asthma that had not existed previously.

The following morning, her son jumped up and exclaimed, "Help me, I can't see!" Putting "two and two together," she realized that they were the only ones who had ingested the aspartame drink.

SOCIOECONOMIC AND PUBLIC HEALTH IMPACT

The personal, business and economic toll caused by aspartame-induced visual impairment can be enormous in active adults. Many examples appear above and in other chapters. The relevant responses in the questionnaire (Section 4) are noteworthy.

> A woman experienced her first reaction to aspartame products at the age of 41 when she tried to lose weight. She described her subsequent severe incapacity in these terms: "I had to go on Social Security disability because I had minimal vision in the right eye, and no balance system due to the nerve damage."

The hazards of traffic accidents attributable to visual changes were described in my text on this subject (Roberts 1971b) and *Ignored Health Hazards for Pilots and Drivers* (Roberts 1998). An enlarged "functional blind spot" and increased sensitivity to glare enhance aspartame-associated impairment among drivers.

Representative Case Report

Case IV-31

A 55-year-old priest had difficulty performing his duties due to intermittent double vision and trouble reading. He was drinking three cans of aspartame sodas and used three packets of an ATS daily. Other symptoms included loss of memory, ringing in the ears, slurred speech, severe headache, itching without a rash, and joint pains. All symptoms disappeared within four days after stopping aspartame products, and predictably returned within three days after resuming them.

OTHER PATHOPHYSIOLOGIC CONSIDERATIONS

Aspartame and its components/metabolites (Section 5) can damage the optic nerves, retina and other areas of the eye. Some of the major issues are reviewed here.

A. Methyl Alcohol

Many of the severe visual changes are consistent with methanol toxicity (Chapter XXI). Studies of methanol effects in monkeys emphasized edema of the optic disc (Hayreh 1977), and degeneration of the retinal ganglion cells (Baumbach 1977). There is considerable evidence that methanol is converted from formaldehyde to formate in the eye, even from chronic low-level exposure (Eclos 1996).

In addition to blindness from optic atrophy, patients with methanol intoxication have developed cerebral edema, parkinsonism, dementia, and other neurologic abnormalities (McLean 1980).

The late Dr. Morgan B. Raifford, a prominent Atlanta ophthalmologist, became interested in impaired vision due to methyl alcohol toxicity. He described his findings in a young aspartame reactor who had suffered marked visual damage attributed to aspartame products.

"I observed evidence of effects in her eyes, and the eyes of other patients, that were comparable to the effects observed in patients who had suffered methyl alcohol toxicity in 1952-1953. There was damage to about 225,000 of the central fibers (resulting in optic nerve atrophy), which would be comparable to that observed in patients suffering methyl alcohol toxicity. In this kind of chronic low-dose aspartame exposure, it is likely that patients would experience the impact on the optic nerve differently in each eye."

The profound ocular effects of formaldehyde and formate derived from the <u>free</u> methanol in aspartame are detailed in Chapter XXI. Alcohol dehydrogenase and aldehyde dehydrogenase are the enzymes involved in methanol metabolism. The retina, cornea and liver have high alcohol dehydrogenase activity. The highly reactive formaldehyde molecule, which becomes bound to proteins and nucleic acids, forms adducts that are difficult to eliminate through the usual metabolic pathways. Formate, an inhibitor of adenosine triphosphate (ATP), probably induces retinal damage through energy depletion.

B. <u>Phenylalanine and Aspartic Acid</u>

Aspartame's two amino acids can induce adverse ocular effects.

- Kashida and Naka (1967) reported that certain amino acids play an important role in regulating the general sensitivity of retinal ganglion cells.
- Dolan and Godin (1966) detected ocular cell lesions when rats from one to 21 days of age were given seven percent phenylalanine.
- Other studies demonstrate that aspartame can affect the vision of newborn mice after their mothers had been exposed to it.

Increased intake of the D-aspartic acid isomer in aspartame products, resulting from excessive heat and prolonged storage (Chapter XXII), may influence vision. There is progressive racemization and accumulation of D-aspartic acid in the lens nucleus with aging (Man 1983). By changing their native configuration, altered proteins could impair physiological and biochemical function.

C. Retinal Metabolism

The extraordinary metabolism of the retina renders it vulnerable to impaired nutrition and neurotoxins. To function over a luminous range of about 10,000,000,000 to 1, it requires more energy than any other tissue in the body. Accordingly, interference with basic energy pathways may first become manifest as visual complaints.

D. Hypoglycemia (Chapter XIV)

Hypoglycemia – or more accurately, deprivation of tissue glucose – can adversely influence vision. The breakdown of glucose (glycolysis) plays an important role in photoreception. It is evidenced by certain properties of retinal mitochondria that generate energy. (The mitochondria of photoreceptor cells are concentrated within a small area wherein photoreception occurs.)

Etingof and Skukolyukov (1965) reported the following relevant properties of retinal mitochondria, and observations concerning glycolysis within the retina.

- Mitochondria isolated from retinal photoreceptor cells are endowed with high hexokinase activity that stimulates glycolysis.
- Glycolysis and hexokinase enzymatic activity in the avian retina increases significantly once birds acquire sight.
- Retinal glycolysis can be activated by various substrates of glycolysis, including glucose-6-phosphate and fructose-1,6-diphosphate.

Additionally, certain areas of the brain that influence vision are more vulnerable to hypoglycemia and other metabolic disturbances. For example, there are high enzymatic activities in the lateral geniculate body (Cotlier 1965) – including the succinic, malic, isocitric, glutamic and lactic dehydrogenases, and TPNH and DPNH diaphorases. These enzymatic functions of lateral geniculate body neurons are uniquely dependent upon the intact function of ocular nerves.

E. The Potentiation of Other Drugs and Chemicals

Numerous drugs and environmental chemicals can cause nerve and optic damage. Several astute aspartame reactors were convinced that the side effects of these substances were aggravated by using aspartame products. For example, a 26-year-old female landscaper with severe aspartame disease observed that minimal exposure to cholinergic pesticides became exceedingly toxic for her after ingesting aspartame, most notably evidenced by blurred vision.

"DRY EYES"; DIFFICULTY WITH CONTACT LENS

A prominent businessman accosted me at a social gathering and asked, "Could aspartame cause difficulty in persons wearing contact lens?" Not having been aware of such an effect, I expressed interest in the reason for his question. He stated that he repeatedly noted decreased tears after consuming products containing aspartame, along with irritation of his eyes from contact lens.

This hint led to querying my patients with aspartame disease about such problems. Several promptly confirmed the association. These questions were later incorporated in the survey questionnaire (Section 4).

Ninety-five aspartame reactors (8 percent) reported dry eyes, irritation by contact lens, or both. In most instances, there was prompt improvement after stopping aspartame products.

Patients with dry eyes so induced had resorted to various protective measures for preventing their tear film from evaporating too fast. One involved wearing special moisture-saving glasses from the rim of the glasses back to the forehead, cheeks and each temple.

Several observations are pertinent.

- The use of aspartame products may convert deficient tears (as detected by Schirmer and rose bengal testing) in asymptomatic elderly persons to a clinical problem.
- A medical student who developed "dry eyes" while consuming diet colas was diagnosed as having "giant papillary conjunctivitis."
- Dry eyes served as an indicator to some reactors that they had unknowingly ingested aspartame. For example, a woman with severe aspartame-induced symptoms (vision impairment; slurred speech; loss of muscle strength) became asymptomatic after avoiding these products. Three months later, she experienced "painfully dry eyes immediately after taking a breath mint" containing aspartame.

In attempting to explain this phenomenon, mention is made of aspartame reactors who developed enlargement and tenderness of the parotid (salivary) glands (Chapter IX-D). Similarly, Case II-5 complained of "thick saliva," and Case IV-34 evidenced decreased secretions in other tissues. It therefore seems logical to infer that the lacrimal (tear) glands, having similar secreting structures, might be affected by aspartame.

An association of "dry eyes" and dryness of the mouth with memory loss and psychologic changes (Chapter XIX) was subsequently considered. The prominence of these features in aspartame reactors directed my attention to such complaints in the Sjögren syndrome (see below).

Representative Case Reports

Case IV-32

A 47-year-old woman complained of progressively severe dryness of the eyes. This problem reached the point of requiring one bottle artificial tears a week. Her consumption of aspartame consisted of three cups coffee in the morning to which a tabletop sweetener was added, 10-12 cups of aspartame beverages, and considerable aspartame pudding.

Other symptoms included significant confusion and memory loss, intense headaches (never previously a problem), impaired hearing, lightheadedness, marked "nervousness," muscle cramps, and depression of such severity as to contemplate suicide.

All the patient's symptoms improved or disappeared within several weeks after avoiding aspartame products. Furthermore, she no longer required artificial tears! Her condition improved sufficiently within one month that she was able to join a volunteer church group doing relief work abroad.

Case IV-33

A 36-year-old businesswoman complained of recent difficulty wearing contact lens. She had been consuming considerable aspartame soft drinks and gum. These and other symptoms – including lightheadedness, headaches, and leg cramps – dramatically abated within two weeks after stopping all aspartame products.

186

Case IV-34

A woman over the age of 60 (FDA Project #3659, courtesy of Dr. Linda Tollefson, September 2, 1987) consumed an ATS and other aspartame products from the time they became available until November 1985. Her most severe reactions were extreme dryness of the eyes, mouth and throat, and blurred vision that discouraged her from going anywhere. There also was "constant soreness of the anus for which the doctor could find no cause."

These complaints disappeared within one week after avoiding aspartame products except for the anal difficulty, which also gradually subsided. None of these reactions occurred when she resumed saccharin. She astutely observed, "I think that the membrane of the intestines and anus had simply become dry, as had other membranes of the mouth, etc.... and that caused the trouble."

Case IV-35

A 61-year-old court reporter developed "dry eyes" and bilateral blurring of vision. Other recent complaints included marked memory loss, severe headache, dizziness, atypical facial pain and extreme irritability. As a result, she had been making computer errors.

The patient then "figured out what was causing it" when she felt better "immediately" after running out of aspartame beverages, and resuming regular sodas. She had previously been consuming four cans of aspartame soft drinks, two glasses of aspartame hot chocolate, and six packets of an ATS daily.

Case IV-36

The wife of an aspartame reactor wrote me

"Your writing on the safety of aspartame solved my husband's problem with dry eyes.

"My husband's triglyceride level was very high. On the advice of his doctor, he gave up drinking sugar sodas. Thinking that diet soda was safe, he began drinking up to six 12-oz cans a day of aspartame cola, never giving it a second thought.

"About two years ago, he started having trouble with dry eyes. He had been wearing contact lenses for up to 14 hours a day about 15 years. Now, he had to remove his contact lenses after only wearing them two to three hours. The eye doctor couldn't find anything wrong, so he recommended eye drops to help alleviate the discomfort. This went on for about two years. There were days when he didn't even attempt to put in his lenses. (He hates wearing glasses.)

"I was in the library when I came across your research. My husband was getting headaches, which we just thought were stress related. Having heard that diet soda caused headaches in some people, I thought your work might be enlightening. You mentioned that several people had dry eyes attributed to aspartame. I mentioned this to my husband. We then realized that his dry eyes began about the same time he started drinking diet soda. He stopped using aspartame, and no longer has the problem. And as an unexpected bonus, his headaches diminished!"

Case IV-37

A poignant instance involving aspartame-induced dry eyes pertains to a woman who was unable to produce a tear while mourning the death of her daughter. Once aware of aspartame disease, her severe fatigue, memory loss, anxiety, night sweats and other symptoms – including the dry eyes – abated. She wrote thereafter, "What kind of monsters would poison a planet, and make impossible for a mother to cry for her dead child?"

Case IV-38

An Iowa radio talk-show host interviewed me about aspartame disease. He expressed considerable interest concerning impaired vision, and dryness of the eyes with associated difficulty wearing contact lens.

His reaction to my comments was immediate and unexpected. "I've been consuming large amounts of diet sodas. Since I assumed that I had no problem with them, your concern frankly seemed academic or limited to just a few persons. In recent weeks, however, I have been bothered by unexplained severe dryness of my eyes."

I suggested that he stop aspartame products for at least one week. "You mean that it might improve in only a few days?" My response: "It's happened a number of times."

The Sjögren Syndrome

Aspartame may provoke or aggravate the Sjögren or sicca syndrome. This disorder affects about two percent of the adult population. The patients are predominately women averaging 50 years – as in aspartame disease.

This condition is characterized by reduced or absent secretions from the lacrimal and salivary glands, thereby resulting in "dry eyes" and dryness of the mouth (Chapter IX-F). (Inasmuch as lack of saliva causes lipstick to adhere to the upper front teeth, this can serve as a diagnostic clue.) In addition to the sensations of local discomfort and "sand" in the eyes, the eyelids of such patients tend to become swollen and infected, often with a loss of eyelashes.

> The expression, "There was hardly a dry eye in the audience" is used when referring to reactions over sad movies. In this context, the magnitude of dry eyes has evoked the pun, "There was hardly a moist eye in the audience."

A potential vicious cycle could occur when the associated intense thirst (Chapter IX-F) causes patients with aspartame disease to drink large amounts of diet sodas and iced teas. Weiffenbach et al (1987) demonstrated that taste impairment is not a necessary consequence of salivary gland dysfunction among patients with "dry mouth" caused by the chronic absence of saliva. Accordingly, such individuals may come to prefer the taste of aspartame in satisfying their chronic thirst... with perpetuation of the sicca syndrome.

Dryness of the eyes and mouth associated with aspartame use offers possible insights concerning Sjögren's syndrome. Matsuzawa and O'Hara (1984) detected prompt uptake (within 30 minutes) of isotopically-labeled aspartame in the salivary glands of rats. This association assumes greater importance in view of the finding of cognitive impairment, ranging from forgetfulness to dementia, in as many as one-fourth of these patients (Alexander 1986).

Computerized correlations between aspartame-associated "dry eyes," "marked memory loss," "severe mental confusion," and "severe depression" were done on the first

362 aspartame reactors who completed the nine-page survey questionnaire. (There was a 30.8 percent response to the initial mailing of 1,177 questionnaire.) The correlates were as follows:

- Recent aspartame-associated "dry eyes" and marked memory loss – 20 (5.5%)
- Recent aspartame-associated "dry eyes" and severe mental confusion – 9 (2.4%)
- Recent aspartame-associated "dry eyes" and severe depression – 18 (4.9%)

Various phenomena may contribute to cerebral dysfunction stemming from aspartame use (Chapter VI). They include flooding of the brain with large amounts of phenylalanine (50 percent of the aspartame molecule), the "aging effect" of D-aspartic acid, altered neurotransmitter physiology (especially dopamine and serotonin), the effects of methanol and its breakdown products (formaldehyde and formate), and cerebral glucopenia due to increased insulin release and concomitant decreased food intake in attempting to lose weight.

The Sjögren syndrome is usually regarded as a chronic autoimmune disorder due to lymphocyte-mediated destruction of these glands. The immune effects of aspartame are discussed in Chapter VIII. It is known that other chemicals – including phenylbutazone, busulfan, practolol and epirubicin – can simulate both the primary and secondary types. For example, Oxholm et al (1986) reported a 54-year-old woman who manifested immunological features characteristic of the primary form after receiving treatment with epirubicin for metastatic cancer of the breast. She experienced intense dryness of the mouth and dry eyes following each treatment. The additional finding of antinuclear antibodies, IgM-rheumatoid factor, plasma IgM, and typical histological features in a biopsy of the lower lip were consistent with this diagnosis.

OTHER EYE MANIFESTATIONS IN ASPARTAME DISEASE

A. Nystagmus

Several aspartame reactors described eye symptoms highly suggestive of nystagmus – that is, a rapid jerking of the eyes on lateral or upward gaze (see Case IV-15). My discussion with two female aspartame reactors complaining of "spasm of the eye muscles" revealed that their ophthalmologists had used the term "nystagmus." One patient stated that it finally abated eight months after stopping aspartame products.

190

Representative Case Report

Case IV-39

A 53-year-old office manager wrote, "I still have nystagmus all the time. Sometimes it goes into fast seizures." She had consumed up to three cans of aspartame soft drinks and seven packets of an ATS daily for three months.

Other recent symptoms included the loss of hearing in one ear, severe headache, lightheadedness, memory loss, depression, attacks of rapid heart action, and a 25-pound weight loss. CT scan and MRI studies of the brain, an electroencephalogram, and special studies of the eyes and ears were normal. She had been taking thyroxine for hypothyroidism.

B. Cataracts At An Early Age

The misdiagnosis of cataract as the primary cause of visual symptoms in persons with aspartame disease who happened to have asymptomatic immature cataracts was considered earlier. On the other hand, the development of cataracts in heavy aspartame consumers suggests a possible contributory role of aspartame in cataract formation.

Case IV-40

A 39-year-old clerk became severely incapacitated due to impaired vision, and could not drive. She developed cataracts at the age of 36. The lens of one eye was removed. Other complaints consisted of eye pain, ringing in one ear, headache, dizziness, insomnia, confusion, marked memory loss, numbness of the upper extremities, severe depression, anxiety attacks, phobias, palpitations, unexplained chest pains, a recent rise of blood pressure, marked swelling of the legs, recurrent hypoglycemia attacks, and a gain of 50 (!) pounds.

She had used considerable aspartame sodas and a tabletop sweetener for over a decade. Replacement thyroid was prescribed after the detection of hypothyroidism at the age of 33. Two brothers had probable reactions to aspartame products, especially migraine and depression.

The patient stopped aspartame products after learning that some of her symptoms could be caused by them. She wrote, "Since discontinuing use of aspartame, I have had less water retention, less craving for sweets, no palpitations (I used to have them at least every other day), no hypoglycemia episodes, no lightheadedness, no dizziness, and my memory and thought processes seem sharper. I was a real basket case."

C. Blepharospasm

Several individuals inquired about a connection between aspartame use and "benign essential blepharospasm" – that is, recurrent spasm of the eyelids. This perceived association was based on consuming considerable aspartame before its onset, and improvement of this and other features of aspartame disease following aspartame abstinence.

Several variations are listed.

- A 35-year-old woman with recurrent eyelid spasms and visual difficulty has been diagnosed with having probable Behçet's disease.
- One patient received injections of botulinum toxin to control the spasms.

The occurrence of tremors and spasms in other muscles is discussed in Chapters VI-J and IX-G.

D. Corneal Changes

Several aspartame reactors developed anterior membrane corneal dystrophy.

- A woman who had prior surgery for this disorder was told "to expect more." Learning of eye problems related to aspartame use, she avoided all aspartame products. Her vision then stabilized and corneal tears did not recur. Subsequent eye examination confirmed the considerable improvement.
- A physician-colleague on the staffs of my hospitals developed severe visual changes following the intake of diet sodas. He was found to have a type of dystrophy of the cornea (vortex dystrophy) usually associated with the chronic use of indomethacin and other drugs.

The demonstration of considerable methanol-derived formaldehyde in the cornea, with ensuing cumulative formaldehyde adducts (Chapter XXI), is relevant.

Diminished tears associated with the use of aspartame products probably played a role in otherwise unexplained <u>recurrent corneal ulcers</u>. The dry-eye syndrome was discussed above.

Case IV-41

A 30-year-old media professional was plagued with repeated corneal ulcers over a four-year period. They began in the left eye during June 1983. The right eye became affected in August 1985. Subsequent attacks were more painful and prolonged, requiring artificial tears four to six times daily. His physician could not determine the cause in this otherwise-healthy man.

He had been consuming about 10 packets of an aspartame tabletop sweetener in coffee daily, along with diet soft drinks when they became available.

His wife chanced to see a television program in which aspartame reactors described severe visual problems. The patient's eye complaints subsided dramatically within two weeks after avoiding aspartame products. When served a cola drink containing aspartame two years later, the eye symptoms promptly recurred.

E. **Myasthenia Gravis** (see Chapter VI-M)

V

HEADACHE

"My business is to teach my aspirations to conform
themselves to fact, not to try and make facts harmonize
with my aspirations."
                    Thomas Huxley (1860)

Severe headache was **the** most common complaint among aspartame reactors – being a major symptom in 516 (43 percent). This exceeds by far the conventional estimate of headache in the general population. For example, the overall prevalence of frequent headache in a population sample of 1340 individuals in Baltimore County was 4.1 percent – five percent among women, and 2.8 percent among men (Scher 1999).

The aspartame association was reinforced by improvement of headache when aspartame products were avoided, and recurrence within several minutes to hours after its resumption, often in an unsuspected product (Section 1).

- An aspartame reactor wrote

  "I experienced severe migraine-type headaches after ingesting a little as one sip of diet soda. I am able to differentiate between the taste of regular and diet soda, and without fail, within approximately 90 seconds I have the beginnings of a migraine. If I do not take both antihistamine and headache medication, I will become totally disabled by the headache. I am sending a copy of this letter to the FDA."

Acronym Legend

ACB – aspartame cola beverage
ASD – aspartame soft drink
ATS – aspartame table sweetener

193

- Patients become furious on finding that their recurrent headaches were attributable to the unannounced incorporation of aspartame in products previously lacking it (e.g., frozen yogurt).
- An aspartame reactor who had suffered severe headache was appalled at the approval of an orally-disintegrating tablet containing aspartame for the treatment of migraine. He regarded such action as "the last straw with the FDA... they all are without shame.!"

The FDA data are confirmatory. This agency received 951 (19.3 percent) complaints about headache attributed to aspartame products from 3,326 consumers (Tollefson 1987). A high incidence of headache in persons with aspartame-associated visual problems (Dr. Tollefson, personal communication, August 12, 19987) – 75 (42.4%) of 177 complainants – also exists in my series (Chapter IV).

GENERAL CONSIDERATIONS

Aspartame reactors may suffer the same type of headache they previously experienced – whether classic migraine, other vascular headaches, tension headache, or so-called cluster headache. Many of my patients, however, insisted that their aspartame-induced headaches were "not exactly the same."

The entity of "chemical headache" is well known (see below). Some of the offenders include alcohol, cheese, citrus fruits, tyramine, nitrates, nitrites ("hot dog headache"), monosodium glutamate (MSG), and phenylethylamine ("chocolate headache"). Stress from many other environmental chemicals also can trigger severe headache (Fudenberg 1988).

Recent epidemiologic data are pertinent. Chronic migraine escalated dramatically in the United States following the marketing of aspartame products. The Centers for Disease Control reported that the average prevalence per 1,000 population for both men and women rose from 25.8 per 1,000 population in 1980 to 41.0 per 1,000 population in 1989 (*Morbidity and Mortality Weekly Report* May 24, 1991, pp. 331-338.)

Gender

There is a three-to-one preponderance of females over males having aspartame-associated headache. Such vulnerability of women was noted earlier (Chapter II-H).

Dose Required

The amount of aspartame products required to induce a headache in individual aspartame reactors ranged from minimum (Chapter II-D) to considerable. Examples appear in the Representative Case Reports. The prompt occurrence of headache with small amounts was mentioned above. A chemist who performed six double-blind studies on himself found that as little as 4.0 mg aspartame in a capsule predictably induced headache (Strong 2000).

Continued Aspartame Use

Twenty-four of the aspartame reactors who completed the first questionnaire (Chapter XIX) and continued to suffer headaches were still consuming aspartame. Such reluctance to avoid these products was repeatedly encountered in later submissions, probably reflecting aspartame addiction (Chapter VII-G).

Associated Salicylism

The use of considerable aspirin to relieve aspartame-associated headache spawned or aggravated other problems. Aspirin can irritate the inner ear and upper gastrointestinal tract. Accordingly, it may compound the dizziness (Chapter VI), ringing in the ears or hearing loss (Chapter IX), and esophageal or gastric distress (Chapter IX-D) experienced with aspartame use.

Aspartame reactors who suffer severe headache subject themselves to added problems when they use analgesic drugs that have serious side effects, such as ibuprofen and other nonsteroidal anti-inflammatory agents. Moreover, a vicious cycle occurs when unrecognized aspartame reactors suffering severe headache take over-the-counter analgesics (acetaminophen, ibuprofen, etc.), and become victims of "analgesic rebound headache," a common problem.

Misdiagnosed Aspartame-Associated Pain

Diagnostic errors were the rule among aspartame reactors who complained of persistent severe headache. Some had been jolted by such initial diagnoses as "brain tumor" (Case II-17), "brain aneurysm" (Case V-4), "arteriovenous malformation" (Case III-13), temporomandibular joint (TMJ) dysfunction (Case VI-17), and cervical disc disease. In turn, these patients were subjected to major diagnostic interventions, both noninvasive and invasive. The majority had undergone one or more imaging procedures – that is, CT scans and MRI studies of the brain.

A corollary is evident. *Vague diagnoses should not be accepted as the major cause for recurrent severe headache when the patient is consuming aspartame.* For example, Indo (1987) challenged the concept of "muscle contraction headache" after being unable to find evidence for chronic sustained hypertonicity of muscles in the head and neck.

The severity of concomitant facial and neck pain will be discussed in Chapter VI-H.

A recent change in the concern of children having aspartame-induced headache is shared by their parents: the possibly of an existing brain tumor (Chapter XXVII-F).

The Cumulative Chemical Effect

Persons with prior migraine must add aspartame to the list of chemicals capable of triggering their attacks. A 48-year-old teacher wrote

> "I developed classic migraine (flashes of light, numbness on one side of my head, impairment of my power to use words, nausea, vomiting, etc.) immediately after drinking beverages sweetened with aspartame. I have discovered over the years that the same thing happens when I ingest phenyl-propanolamine in some cold pills and diet pills. Wine flavored with woodruff also gives me migraine headaches. Obviously, I have learned to completely avoid aspartame, phenylpropanolamine and woodruff!"

Aspartame also exacerbates the headache induced by certain foods and additives. They include chocolate, cheese, nuts, alcohol, and monosodium glutamate (MSG) (Roberts 1993a). A similar response can occur with other substances in the diet (e.g., nitrites, phenylethylamine; tyramine) known to provoke migraine (Dalessio 1972, Raskin 1980, Johns 1987).

Aspartame As a Co-Epileptogen in Migraineurs

The greater likelihood of convulsions occurring among aspartame reactors with migraine who continue to consume aspartame products (Chapter III) is noteworthy. Among the 397 respondents to the initial survey questionnaire, 30 (7.5 percent) with aspartame-associated headaches and convulsions gave a history of prior migraine or other severe headache. Case III-3 described the symptoms preceding his first grand mal convulsion as "of gradual onset, like having a migraine headache all the time to the point of affecting my vision."

This "train" or "march" of events culminating in a seizure seems more frequent among women taking oral contraceptives ("the pill"), and those with considerable premenstrual fluid retention and nervous tension prone to severe hypoglycemia ("low blood sugar attacks"). The combined effects of aspartame and "the pill" even might be conducive to subsequent stroke in younger women (Chapter VI), particularly when the blood pressure becomes increased (Chapter IX-C).

Representative Case Reports

Case V-1

A 48-year-old university educator had intermittent mild migraine for two decades. After consuming six or more cans of diet colas over a three-year period, her headaches "often were so violent I thought I would have a stroke." Propranolol (Inderal®) (40 mg twice daily) and considerable Fiorinal® failed to reduce their frequency. While taking aspartame, the headaches intensified whenever she drank wine or liquor.

Other features included severe insomnia, slurred speech, palpitations, and a gain of 50 pounds. She was seen by four physicians and consultants; none suspected aspartame as a contributing cause. The patient had hypothyroidism and was allergic to penicillin.

A friend with aspartame-induced convulsions mentioned the possible relationship of her headaches to aspartame use. After discontinuing these products, she experienced only two headaches in a two-month period, compared to two or three attacks a week previously.

Her 15-year-old daughter developed two seizures shortly after aspartame came on the market.

Case V-2

A 61-year-old therapist had increasing headaches, an unexpected gain in weight, and visual problems for five months. The latter consisted of difficulty in reading conventional newspaper print, and severe sensitivity to headlight glare.

On direct questioning, he began consuming large amounts of aspartame three months before the onset of these symptoms. He drank 10-15 servings of aspartame daily as soft drinks, and put two packets of an ATS into each cup of coffee. Within three days after abstinence, the headaches receded. They were gone by one week, coupled with dramatic improvement of his vision.

Case V-3

A 27-year-old retail manager was incapacitated for more than one year because of intense headaches. She had been a "regular user of a diet cola since the spring of 1984, averaging two cans daily." Other complaints included severe sensitivity to noise in both ears, marked depression, "puffiness of my face," and "hypersensitivity to smells." She underwent two CT scans and two MRI studies of the brain, and cerebral angiography. Four consultants and three clinics had not considered the possible contributory role of aspartame.

The patient's fiancé had been with her "every day during this ordeal." He offered the following account.

> "Before she stopped using aspartame, F__ Was in chronic pain, 24 hours a day. She took about 8-12 Fiorinal per day, along with Percodan® (up to two daily). She lay in bed and squeezed her head as if to squeeze the pain away, describing her intense pounding pressure. She couldn't do anything. She was very depressed. This was every day from July 1984 to April 1985.

> "During this period, she went to see many doctors in New York City, New Jersey, and the _____ Clinic (Boston), in addition to local physicians. These were the finest and best in their field. Not a single one suggested that she stop using aspartame, or even suggested it as a cause. (Although each recommended a migraine diet, none specified the hazards of aspartame...

> "I have to say at this point that F__ hoped it was a brain tumor so she could rid herself of it and those dreadful headaches. After these many consultations, F__ now was at square one, still suffering from horrible headaches. During this time, F__ did not work. She left her job with Macy's in July, knowing the pain was too much to handle, and too excruciating to tolerate.

> "It was not until April, 1985 that aspartame was blamed. F__ ordered diet cola, and I a regular cola. When our glasses got mixed up, I had a sip of diet cola for the first time. The difference was easily recognizable. Not only was the taste

different, but I felt lousy after drinking it. That is when I suggested F_____ stop drinking it completely. She was apprehensive. After a few days her severe pain turned to moderate, almost nonexistent pain. We thought then that perhaps it was the combination of the aspartame and her medications. She slowly went off Inderal, and did not even need the Percodan or Fiorinal. Now completely aspartame-free and medication-free, F__ was HEADACHE-FREE !!!!

"While we were experimenting, the newspapers had an article on the questionable effects of aspartame. F_____ was now convinced after reading about the symptoms that she was not alone in such suffering."

Case V-4

A 27-year-old ophthalmic assistant had consumed up to eight cans of diet cola and eight one-liter bottles of diet cola daily. She began to suffer increasing pain on one side of her head along with numbness, dizziness and nausea. When seen in an emergency room, a neurologist stated that she was either "having an aneurysm, or your problem may be related to stress." She refused to accept the diagnosis of "tension headache."

"From that point on, I started making checklists to see if anything else could be causing the pain. Dentists, sinus and ophthalmic examinations all checked out okay. Then I took a look back two months to see if anything had changed in my diet. That's when I realized I had started drinking the new diet cola with aspartame in it. I stopped drinking the pop, and the pain began to diminish day by day. In one week, I was not experiencing any dizziness or nausea, and I didn't feel like I was in a fog anymore... It is now three weeks since I ceased drinking these diet colas. I am today experiencing almost no symptoms except an occasional burning sensation on my scalp. I know now that it was definitely the aspartame."

There was a history of mild hay fever. Her grandmother and husband also had severe aspartame reactions. Their symptoms included headache, dizziness, mood swings and depression.

To add insult to injury, the patient's insurance company would not pay for the emergency room visit because "it was not a matter of life or death since I did <u>not</u> die!" She added, "Can you believe that? And here the E.R. doctor tells me I probably have an aneurysm!"

Case V-5

A 24-year-old housewife suffered increasingly severe headaches while consuming up to three liters of an ACB daily. She commented on her first awareness of its relationship to this product.

> "If it wasn't for the *Consumer's Report* Special, I might have never associated my severe headache (everyday) with the aspartame. Only God knows what would be wrong with me now. The night I saw the show, I immediately stopped drinking diet drinks. The next night the headaches were gone."

Case V-6

An active 72-year-old female had been in good health. She ate a large bowl of aspartame chocolate pudding daily and drank diet cola.

The patient then experienced headaches, dizziness and diminished vision for two months. (She denied prior headaches.) There also had been three episodes of palpitations and "blacking out" around breakfast. A CT scan of the brain, an electroencephalogram and other studies were normal.

I happened to discuss aspartame reactions in the context of her husband's condition. She thereupon also stopped using aspartame products. The headaches and episodes of "blacking out" disappeared, and did not recur. She further volunteered that her nephew (a dentist) had severe headaches caused by diet colas.

OTHER REPORTS

The <u>FDA data</u> were mentioned earlier in this chapter.

<u>Johns</u> (1986) reported a 31-year-old female who had "throbbing vascular headaches with associated gastrointestinal symptoms" within one or two hours after ingesting two or

three cans of diet cola. They were reproduced within one and one-half hours after rechallenge with pure aspartame (500 mg in 14 fluid ounces), but not with comparable amounts of saccharin or sucrose.

Ferguson (1985) described a 22-year-old woman who had severe headaches when she used about ten packets of an aspartame sweetener. In <u>five</u> separate trials, her headache abated within several hours after avoiding aspartame beverages, and predictably recurred (along with a flush and sweat) when she resumed them.

<u>Koehler et al</u> (1987) performed a controlled nine-week, double-blind, randomized crossover study to determine the frequency and intensity of aspartame-induced migraine. The capsules of aspartame and a matched placebo were taken at meals and at bedtime for four weeks, separated by an interim "wash-out" period of one week. The frequency of migraine headaches increased significantly with aspartame intake.

A randomized crossover trial by <u>Van Den Eeden et al</u> (1994) validated headache as being <u>specifically</u> attributable to the ingestion of aspartame.

<u>Blumenthal and Vance</u> (1997) reported three young women whose migraine could be provoked by aspartame chewing gum.

<u>Lipton et al</u> (1988) found aspartame to be the precipitating cause of headache in 8.2 percent of 171 patients consecutively evaluated at the Montefiore Headache Unit. They commented that double-blind trials tend to be an insensitive method for identifying dietary factors as a cause of headache, in part because of the heightened expectation by subjects that a headache may develop.

PATHOPHYSIOLOGIC MECHANISMS

There are multiple possible mechanisms for aspartame headache. They include altered concentration of brain amino acids, neurotransmitter dysfunction, reactions to the diketopiperazine metabolite (Chapter XXV), aggravated hypoglycemia (Chapter XIV), the ingestion of large amounts of fluid in response to increased thirst (Chapter IX), and allergy (Chapter VIII). Methanol-induced cerebral edema, alterations in brain water, sodium and potassium, vascular stasis (Menne 1938, Bennet 1953, Erlanson 1965, Rao 1977), and the neurotoxic effects of formaldehyde and formate also may be operative (Chapter XXI).

Neurotransmitters

The effects of aspartame and phenylalanine and neurotransmitters are described in Chapter XXIII. They have considerable relevance to the headaches and atypical facial/neck pain experienced by aspartame reactors.

The apparent benefit of a tyramine-restricted diet in treating migraine suggests adverse effects by other amino acids. Such a diet afforded relief from severe headache and petit mal episodes in an elderly aspartame reactor.

Hypoglycemia

The aggravation of severe hypoglycemia – or decreased glucose availability to the brain (cerebral glucopenia) – was mentioned as a mechanism whereby aspartame can trigger migraine and related headaches. This is likely in the case of women having "functional" hyperinsulinism (Chapter XIV) who attempt to lose weight by decreasing food intake drastically and concomitantly engage in strenuous exercise.

I have reviewed the interrelationships between migraine and hypoglycemia (Roberts 1967d, 1971b). Only a few of the evidences are cited here.

- Attacks of vascular headache are <u>predictably</u> precipitated by prolonged delay in eating, increased activity, ingesting sugar or alcohol, and increased insulin release from oral contraceptive use.
- The patient's <u>exact</u> headache often can be reproduced by fasting, or triggered when reactive hypoglycemia develops during a glucose tolerance test.

Allergy

Nocturnal aspartame-induced headache could reflect delayed IgE-mediated hypersensitivity (Chapter VIII). This may be comparable to aspartame-induced delayed urticaria (hives) or angioedema (Kulczycki 1987).

Other instances have been dramatically rapid.

> A woman wrote: "I am allergic to aspartame. If I break open a packet containing it, and inhale the powder, I instantly develop a headache. I was fortunate enough to have had an anatomy teacher in college who knew about how aspartame was approved by the FDA."

RELATED CONSIDERATIONS

Diagnostic Costs

Physicians who are not aware of the relationship between severe headache and aspartame use are likely to order electroencephalograms (EEGs), and CT scans or MRI imaging studies. Concomitant complaints by aspartame reactors – confusion; memory loss; visual disturbances; personality changes – also reflexively generate these studies and neurologic consultation. The high medical costs (Chapters II and XIX) so incurred may surpass the limits set by insurance carriers.

Position of the FDA

The attitude of the FDA concerning aspartame reactions is reviewed in Sections 6 and 7. Its data on 951 consumers who complained about aspartame-associated headache, noted above, did not evoke recommendations relative to regulation or labeling.

> In reply to my request for copies of reports sent to this agency by aspartame reactors under the Freedom of Information Act, a staff member wrote Congressman Dan Mica on September 8, 1986: "G.D. Searle and Company have funded a study focusing on the possibility that consumption of aspartame induces headaches solely because of the frequency with which headaches have been reported. There has been no consistent pattern or type of headache syndrome associated with aspartame consumption." (My analysis of the report suggested that its basic design was flawed for reasons detailed in this and subsequent chapters.)

Shortcomings of Double-Blind Studies

The reservations concerning "double-blind" studies involving the use of aspartame capsules or freshly-prepared cold aspartame solutions are discussed in Sections 6 and 7. For example, a double-blind study by Schiffman et al (1987) concluded "aspartame is no more likely to produce headache than placebo." But the investigators did not replicate the reality of adding aspartame to hot water, tea, coffee or chocolate, or giving subjects the same incriminated products obtained from market shelves.

Two other vexing issues involving presumed double-blind studies have been raised by other critics. One relates to the nature and amount of the "aspartame" supplied. The other entails the possible inclusion of monosodium glutamate or other excitotoxins in the "placebo" administered.

VI

OTHER NEUROLOGIC COMPLICATIONS

"Finally, we should learn a lesson from the NutraSweet®
experience. If a food additive has potential neurological or
behavioral effects, it should undergo human clinical testing,
similar to the process a drug must undergo, before it is put on
the market."

> Senator Howard M. Metzenbaum (1987)

Aspartame reactors frequently experience disorders of the brain and peripheral nerves
in addition to convulsions (Chapter III) and headache (Chapter V). These include severe
dizziness, unsteadiness, confusion, memory loss, motor and sensory disturbances affecting
the limbs, atypical pain, slurred speech, tremors, pathologic sleepiness (narcolepsy), sleep
apnea and intellectual deterioration. I summarized the neurologic, psychiatric and behavioral
reactions in the initial 505 aspartame reactors for the First International Conference on
Dietary Phenylalanine and Brain Function (Washington, D.C., May 8-10, 1987).

Pro-aspartame advocates repeatedly deny these reactions, and raise the issue of "only
anecdotes." On the other hand, the National Research Council (1991) perceptively stated,
"Anecdotal reports of neurotoxicity in humans need to be pursued vigorously with clinical
surveillance and followup."

Input From Neurologists

Neurologists have contacted me about a variety of aspartame-related neurologic
complaints. On finding that problems of their patients improved or disappeared within

---

Acronym Legend

        ABC - aspartame cola beverage
        ASD - aspartame soft drink
        ATS - aspartame tabletop sweetener

206

several days or weeks after stopping aspartame products, they wished to validate my observations. Most neurologists, however, adamantly denied any connection. One preferred to diagnose a female aspartame reactor with bilateral eye symptoms and multiple neurologic features as having "multiple migrating ailments and the restaurant syndrome."

Input From Aspartame Reactors

The public expressed its concern over aspartame-induced neurologic complications to the Congress, the FDA, and many organizations (Chapter XXX). Case VI-1 illustrates the matter. Its resentment of neurologists who adamantly refused to consider the possible contributory role of aspartame products will be discussed in Chapters XIX and XXIX.

> A male nurse anesthetist told a November 3, 1987 Senate hearing that he had experienced visual complaints, headaches, memory gaps, hives and then a convulsion while consuming 4-6 diet colas daily. When he suggested aspartame as a factor, his neurologist replied, "Wouldn't it be a shame if all that's wrong with you is aspartame?"

Representative Case Report

Case VI-1

A 61-year-old woman suffered severe dizziness, convulsions, insomnia, memory loss, irritability, and a fear of crowds after consuming multiple aspartame products. I received copies of her correspondence to the manufacturer and the FDA. She asserted, "Frankly, I think in deference to we few, you should place a warning on aspartame products reading: 'If a neurological problem is present, do not use this.' "

A. GENERAL CONSIDERATIONS

An abbreviated overview of diagnostic considerations and pathophysiologic mechanisms relating to aspartame-associated neurologic disorders is appropriate. The relevant changes in body chemistry (including neurotransmitters) are amplified in Section 5.

Young children are highly vulnerable. The density of synapses reaches its maximum at the age of three years, concomitant with peaking of the cerebral metabolic rate between 3 and 4 years (Huttenlocher 1990).

The financial arrangements and corporate affiliations of physician-lecturers who emphasize the use of drugs for treating neurological disorders herein discussed are often impressive (Section 7). Few make any reference to the contributory role of aspartame and other neurotoxins in their presentations.

Diagnostic Reservations

Aspartame disease should be considered when a "mysterious-whatever" neurologic problem affects weight-conscious persons.

The diagnosis of multiple sclerosis ought to be made with considerable reservation in aspartame consumers. This warning is essential when based primarily on the occurrence of unexplained optic neuritis (Chapter IV). In such instances, a definitive diagnosis of multiple sclerosis ought to be deferred at least several months in order to observe the patient's response to abstinence from aspartame products (see below).

Similar concern applies to aspartame consumers who present with other of the neurologic features described in this chapter. Two examples are cited.

- Pseudotumor cerebri (Chapter VI-N) occurred in 12 persons with aspartame disease. This condition is characterized by headache, convulsions, confusion, a high cerebrospinal fluid pressure, and an enlarged blind spot with visual changes due to optic nerve pressure and swelling. Its frequency in children and overweight young women is noteworthy.
- Several aspartame reactors were diagnosed initially as having Behçet's disease. This disorder consists of headache, abnormal neurologic findings, aseptic meningitis, oral and genital ulcers, joint pains, and eye involvement (uveitis; iritis).

The Plasticity of Nerve Tissue

Another important perspective involves the considerable plasticity of the central nervous system in recovering from exposure to neurotoxic injury. This contrasts with the fatalistic view expressed by Ramon y Cajal in 1928 in which "the nerve paths are something fixed, ended immutable. Everything may die, nothing may regenerate."

Admittedly, neurons cannot be replaced once they are lost as a result of trauma, disease or toxic exposure. The remaining neurons, however, retain the capacity for a remarkable array of responses through mechanisms such as immediate activation of proto-oncogenes c-fos and c-jun within neurons (Jenkins 1991), a number of growth related proteins, interleukin-1, and various cytokines. Indeed, reactive gliosis may constitute an attempt to contain and combat potentially harmful neurotoxins.

Amino Acid Influences

The ingestion of neurotoxic amino acids can cause or exacerbate pathologic conditions associated with endogenous neurotoxic amino acids (Samuels 1994). The following observations concerning amino acid effects (Section 5) are germane.

- Phenylalanine has a higher affinity for transport across the blood-brain barrier than other circulating neutral amino acids (Partridge 1981).
- Brain scanning and positron emission tomography (PET) studies verify the reduced brain uptake of other amino acids (such as methionine) in the presence of elevated phenylalanine concentrations.
- Excitotoxic amino acids initiate the release of considerable free radicals that can oxidize cell membranes, as well as other consequences of lipid peroxidation. Toxic substances generated by the latter (as 4-hydroxynonenal) occur in high concentrations in the brains of patients with Alzheimer's disease and Parkinson's disease.
- The inhibition of specific ATP-sulfurylase activity in the central nervous system by high concentrations of phenylalanine decreases the synthesis of sulfatides (Chapter XXII), followed by changes within the brain and myelin sheath.
- Dr. Woodrow Monte (personal communication, July 1986) detected selective brain and nerve injury in aspartame-treated rats, especially cells having high concentrations of corticosteroid receptors.
- Aspartic acid is importantly involved in brain metabolism (Chapter XXII), but excessive amounts can adversely affect its function.
- Further damage to the brain and peripheral nerves may be superimposed by caloric reduction due to suppression of the desire for food by aspartame (Chapter IX), and amino acid-induced release of insulin with hypoglycemia (Chapter XXIV).
- Yamatsui et al (1996) demonstrated the replacement of valine by phenylalanine at position 642 in amyloid precursor protein (APP) among families with inherited Alzheimer's disease.

- A demyelinating neurologic disorder resembling amyotrophic lateral sclerosis has been attributed to an alanine-related plant neurotoxin (see below).

The Blood-Brain Barrier

The blood-brain barrier has been variously described as a "chemical filter" and "biogenic wall." It appears to be altered by aspartame, its breakdown products, and monosodium glutamate (MSG).

The "tight junctions" of capillaries in the brain are the chief anatomic basis for the blood-brain barrier. The importance of such protection is suggested by the development of these junctions toward the end of the first trimester of pregnancy.

Major carrier-mediated transport systems to the brain involve the delivery of glucose and large neutral amino acids. These substances must be delivered from the blood stream since they are not manufactured by brain cells. Recent studies have identified a receptor in the brain regulating the blood-brain barrier, with emphasis on two proteins (zonulin and zot) that are also involved in absorption from the intestine.

The efficacy of the blood-brain barrier, however, is limited. Dr. Adrienne Samuels (1994) pointed out that it may not exclude neurotoxic amino acids – notably glutamic acid, aspartic acid, and L-cysteine (a dough conditioner and color preservative for fresh fruit). She
emphasized that ingested neurotoxic amino acids can cause and exacerbate pathologic conditions associated with endogenous neurotoxic amino acids.

Aspartate and Glutamate as Excitotoxins

Entry of excitotoxic breakdown products of aspartame into the brain are probably greater than heretofore realized. Studies on the neurotoxicity of aspartate and glutamate demonstrate that several small regions of the brain lack a blood-brain barrier, thereby enabling these blood-borne substances to penetrate freely. Dr. John W. Olney (Professor of Neuropathology at Washington University School of Medicine) wrote the following explanation to Senator Howard Metzenbaum on December 8, 1987:

> "If glutamate and aspartate are released from cells and not
> rapidly taken back up, they flood the excitatory receptors on the
> external surface of nerve cells and excite nerve cells to death.

It has recently been shown that certain drugs which block the action of Glu and Asp at these excitatory receptors can protect the animal brain against damage associated with stroke, cardiac arrest or perinatal asphyxia. Thus, *it is an ironic fact that today knowledgeable neuroscientists in many parts of the world are working fervently to develop methods for preventing endogenous excitotoxins from damaging the human brain, while other elements of society, including the FDA, are promoting and sanctioning the adulteration of foods with unlimited amounts of exogenous excitotoxins which are known to destroy nerve cells in the mammalian brain following oral intake.*"

The interest of scientists at G. D. Searle & Company concerning memory loss and related realms appeared as full-page ads in the *Journal of the American Medical Association* (December 16, 1986) and other journals. Specifically, their attention focused on the search for antagonists capable of blocking amino acid receptor systems that might prevent "neuronal dysfunction and disruption." The advertisement addressed the possibility that increased excitatory amino acids could damage nerve cells in a mammal comparable to the findings in "Alzheimer's, Huntington's chorea, and other degenerative diseases."

Overstimulation of receptors for excitatory amino acids, including aspartate and glutamate, is believed to represent a "final common pathway" for both many acute neurologic disorders and chronic neurodegenerative states (Lipton 1994). Glutamate, the principal excitatory neurotransmitter in the brain, has interactions with specific membrane receptors that affect cognition, memory, movement and sensation. Activation of glutamate receptors results in an excessive influx of calcium into neurons, and subsequent neuronal injury.

Roelofs et al (1991) reported a significant negative association between dietary intake of glutamate and aspartate, and the serum levels of these excitatory amino acids, in patients with amyotrophic lateral sclerosis. These findings also suggest altered metabolism of ingested glutamate and aspartate.

Neurotoxicity

The methanol component of aspartame contributes to the neurologic and psychiatric manifestations of aspartame reactors (Chapter XXI). Dr. Herbert S. Posner (1975), the National Institute of Environmental Health Sciences, emphasized methanol's "delayed and irreversible effects on the nervous system... at small widely varying levels of exposure and at rather low levels." Brain edema, altered cerebral sodium and potassium concentrations, and vascular stasis have been noted after methanol intake by both humans and animals (Menne 1983, Bennet 1953, Erlanson 1965, Rao 1977).

The neuropsychiatric features of chronic toxicity from methyl alcohol and other organic solvents were reviewed by the National Institute for Occupational Safety and Health (NIOSH) in *Organic Solvent Neurotoxicity* (*Current Intelligence Bulletin* 48, March 31, 1987). They range in severity from a mild "organic affective syndrome" characterized by fatigue, impaired memory, irritability, mild mood disturbances and difficulty in concentrating, to severe toxic encephalopathy with irreversible dementia.

The cumulative deposition of formaldehyde and formate, its breakdown products following chronic intake of methanol (Chapter XXI), is highly relevant. The effects of chronic methanol poisoning in man, rabbits and monkeys (Rao 1977) include multiple sclerosis-like features. They may compound the altered water metabolism noted in multiple sclerosis patients thorough the further ingress of fluid into nerve tissue (Roberts 1966b,c).

Cumulative Influences

Severe brain damage can be caused by the summation of aspartame-induced reactions and other influences. Examples of the latter are excessive caffeine, nicotine and alcohol, exposure to cholinergic pesticides, "the pill," and drugs exerting a depressant effect on the neuromuscular junction. The latter include beta adrenergic blocking agents (Herishanu 1975).

Representative Case Report

Case VI-2

A 31-year-old woman had been taking an oral contraceptive, and was consuming 12 cans of an aspartame soda daily. She developed intense migraine, hypoglycemia, hypertension and a subsequent stroke with left-side paralysis. Although the contributory role of the oral contraceptive seemed most likely to her attending physician, he suspected aspartame disease after becoming aware of its complications. Her severe headaches disappeared following avoidance of aspartame.

The important contributory role of hypoglycemia – or more accurately, reduced glucose concentrations at the tissue level – in nerve injury will be discussed in Chapters XIII and XIV. Numerous pertinent studies have been cited in my previous publications.

Yasaki and Dyck (1991) demonstrated that the induction of severe and prolonged hypoglycemia induces damage within both the central and peripheral nervous systems of young rats as nerve glucose and ATP levels become significantly decreased. A significantly greater decrease was found in the distal sciatic and proximal tibial-peroneal nerves.

Epidemiologic Evidences For Environmental Factors in Neurologic Disorders

Aspartame has been on the market since 1981. Accordingly, changes in the incidence of major neurologic disorders possibly associated with its consumption require consideration and careful monitoring – particularly epilepsy (Chapter III), headaches (Chapter IV), brain tumors, and the conditions discussed in this chapter.

- The alleged increase of multiple sclerosis during 1985 and 1986 is noted below.
- Any disproportionate increase of brain tumors among aspartame consumers demands scrutiny in view of the brain tumors in documented experimental animals (Chapter XXVII).

The data inferring an influence of aspartame on the ecogenetics of neurologic disorders, such as parkinsonism and Alzheimer's disease, obviously require careful analysis to avoid overlooking trends existing prior to the general availability of aspartame. For example, deaths due to primary brain tumors increased from a rate of 4.9 per 100,000 in the 1953-1957 period to 5.9 per 100,000 for the 1967-1973 period, and to 9.2 per 100,000 in 1981 according to the National Institutes of Health. (This trend has been most apparent in communities and countries having higher medical capabilities.)

Calne et al (1986) hypothesized that several major degenerative diseases reflect the adverse effects of environmental factors on specific regions of the central nervous system. They include the substantia nigra (parkinsonism), the medial basal forebrain (Alzheimer's disease), and the motor neurones (motor neurone disease). It is my opinion that aspartame products qualify as an "environmental factor" (Roberts 1995b). In the present context, Joseph Foley (1987), Chairman of a National Institutes of Health consensus panel on "Differential Diagnosis of Dementing Disease," wisely asserted that "our first obligation is not to allow the remediable to get out of hand."

The damage by ecologic pathogens may remain "subclinical" or "transitional" for one or several decades. During this time, compensatory reactions within the brain take place.

They are evidenced as sprouting of extensive synapses with other nerve cells, increased synthesis of neurotransmitters, a rise in the number of receptors, and greater sensitivity of post-synaptic structures.

A number of observations strengthen these suspected environmental relationships. They include the onset of parkinsonism after use of methylphenyltetrahydropyridine (MPTP), the delayed post-poliomyelitis syndrome following prior poliovirus infection, and the amyotrophic lateral sclerosis-parkinsonism complex in Guam caused by some unidentified agent. Calne and his colleagues also stressed possible prevention by removing or minimizing those environmental factors known to be capable of causing "abiotrophy" (the premature and selective destruction of functionally related neurones.) It is in this sphere that aspartame consumption by patients at risk warrants study.

> The postpoliomyelitis syndrome surfaced in recent years among persons who had clinical poliomyelitis as long as four decades earlier. Their complaints – including new weakness, fatigue, pain, loss of function, and intolerance to cold – might reflect the superimposed effect of toxic substances on remaining nerve cells that innervate muscles and other organs.

The "environmental hypothesis" for major neurological diseases has been strengthened by the data of Spencer et al (1987). These investigators linked a high incidence of the amyotrophic lateral sclerosis-parkinsonism-dementia syndrome among the indigenous (Chamorro) population of the Marianas Island of Guam and Rota to the large intake of highly toxic seed of the false sago palm (*Cycas circinalis*). The following findings favor an etiologic relationship to this "slow toxin."

- The prevalence of this disorder declined significantly after 1955 when use of this plant as a traditional source of food and medicine decreased.
- No inherited or viral factors could be demonstrated in affected patients.
- The feeding of the *Cycas* amino acid (B-N-methylaminolalanine) to monkeys resulted in corticomotorneuronal dysfunction, parkinsonian features, behavioral abnormalities, and severe degenerative changes of motor neurons in the cerebral cortex and spinal cord.

The foregoing observations are relevant to the neurological complications associated with aspartame use because of the presence of an unusual nonprotein amino acid derived from alanine-namely, B-N-methylamino-L-alanine (L-BAMA). It bears a chemical and neuropharmacologic relationship to B-N-oxalylamino-L-alanine (L-BOAA). The latter induces severe corticomotorneuronal deficits in primates after repeated oral administration. (These amino acids also cause convulsions in rodents.)

Several correspondents raised the issue of aspartame-induced stroke. There is some experimental evidence to support a contributory role for aspartic acid (and glutamate). Butcher et al (1990) analyzed amino acid release and neuropathologic outcome in the rat brain following occlusion of the middle cerebral artery. Proximal occlusion of the vessel resulted in large increases of aspartate and glutamate, and increased phenylalanine. A comparable massive release of these amino acids has been reported during global ischemic insults in adults.

B. DIZZINESS AND UNSTEADINESS

In this series of 1,200 aspartame reactors, 376 (31 percent) complained of dizziness, unsteadiness or both. Recurrent dizziness is also referred to as "benign positional vertigo," vestibular neuronitis, "central vestibulopathy" and "peripheral vestibulopathy," but all require clarification as to cause. Related ear problems will be discussed in Chapter IX-A.

Among 397 reactors who initially completed the survey questionnaire (Section 4), 174 (44.3 percent) reported "severe dizziness or feeling lightheaded," and 61 (15.3 percent) "severe unsteadiness of the legs."

FDA data (Tollefson 1987) corroborate the results. These symptoms were attributed to aspartame use by 419 persons who complained to this agency.

There have been isolated case reports. Gulya et al (1992) described a patient whose symptoms of episodic vertigo and continuous unsteadiness resolved after avoiding aspartame products.

Related Clinical Considerations

Several aspects of patient complaints warrant mention.

- Reactors often volunteered related descriptive terms such as "giddiness" and "vertigo."
- Some emphasized that they felt dizzy primarily on flexing the head or looking down – as while washing their hair or bending over to reach a low shelf.

- Aspartame-associated dizziness could persist for a considerable period. A 51-year-old woman wrote, "After not using aspartame for 17 months, I still have trouble with lightheadedness, dizziness and memory recall."

- Another contributory factor was the use of considerable aspirin to relieve aspartame-induced headache (Chapter V) or joint pains (Chapter IX-G).

Unexplained recurrent dizziness requires extensive medical and neurologic evaluation of the patient for possible underlying causes. They include episodic rapid or irregular heart action, high blood pressure, anemia, hypoglycemia, carotid artery disease, and tumors or other disorders in or near the inner ear and brain. Concomitant hearing and visual changes, confusion, headache, and convulsions underscore the importance of proper diagnosis. Accordingly, many of these aspartame reactors had been subjected to radioimaging studies of the brain, Holter monitoring for abnormal heart rhythms, and cardiac stress testing (Chapter XIX) before aspartame disease was considered.

The primary or aggravating role of aspartame products was demonstrated by improvement or cessation of symptoms when they were stopped, and their prompt recurrence after being resumed. This twofold diagnostic sequence convincingly relieved the anxiety of many who worried about having a brain tumor, "small strokes," a "silent heart attack," and atypical insulin reactions. Aspartame-associated unsteadiness among older individuals also had been erroneously attributed to "normal aging."

An aspartame reaction should be considered when entertaining the diagnosis of "benign paroxysmal vertigo of childhood" in which there is no loss of consciousness.

Mechanisms similar to those by which aspartame contributes to convulsions (Chapter III), visual disturbances (Chapter IV), and headache (Chapter V) are relevant. The high metabolic requirements of the vestibular system within the inner ear that maintains balance are germane. Additionally, other amino acids and peptides are known to cause severe unsteadiness – for example, so-called gluten ataxia among susceptible individuals who ingest gluten (Hadjidassiliou 1998).

Representative Case Reports

Case VI-B-1

A 30-year-old computer programmer ingested an average of two cans diet cola daily for weight control. He concluded that this beverage was the cause of his recurrent lightheadedness and abdominal pain.

> "Within minutes of drinking one diet cola, I feel lightheaded. In 15-30 minutes, I am better. I have switched back to regular cola. Every now and then, I'll accidently buy a diet soft drink, and become dizzy within minutes. Then I remember that I shouldn't be drinking drinks containing aspartame."

Case VI-B-2

A 59-year-old fashion coordinator <u>immediately</u> suffered a violent reaction after ingesting <u>one</u> cup of aspartame-containing gelatin. She described her reaction in these terms: "I felt as if adrenalin was shooting through my head. My head was swimming with dizziness, along with slight nausea and head pounding."

Case VI-B-3

A 63-year-old woman developed intense dizziness after consuming four packets of an ATS and one glass of ASD daily. Other symptoms included marked drowsiness and rapid heart action. She wrote, "The dizziness was so severe that I could not lift my head off the pillow without passing out. This went on for months. I could only stay up short periods of time."

Her symptoms markedly improved after stopping aspartame, but required six months to disappear. They recurred within three days on the one occasion she retested herself.

Case VI-B-4

A chemist suffered episodes of severe dizziness and manic episodes with visual delusions while consuming considerable aspartame. These symptoms continued six years, during which he estimated experiencing "over 1000 Meniere attacks." In desperation to survive, he decided in 1996 "to stop eating all man-made foods, including aspartame." Such action was influenced by his professional knowledge about multiple chemical sensitivity. He described the results in these terms: "I have not had even one manic episode since 1996, nor one Meniere's attack since 4-19-97."

C. CONFUSION AND MEMORY LOSS

Severe confusion, impairment of memory, or both, were prominent complaints in 376 (31 percent) of 1,200 aspartame reactors. In the present context, "memory loss" means gross impairment of memory... not a brief inability ("senior moment") to recall some name or number which most active adults experience when their attention is diverted.

"Severe memory loss" was reported by 102 (25.6 percent) of the initial 397 persons answering the questionnaire (Chapter XIX), and "severe mental confusion" by 75 (18.8 percent). The breakdown by age groups of the 102 respondents with "severe memory loss" was as follows:

10 - 19 years ...	4
20 - 29 years ...	14
30 - 39 years ...	26
40 - 49 years ...	23
50 - 59 years ...	18
60 and older ...	17

Patients with aspartame disease who repeatedly experienced confusion and memory loss after inadvertently ingesting aspartame products could identify with the term "dementia roulette."

Even relatively small amounts of aspartame products induced confusion and memory loss in some individuals, as Case III-1. The prompt subsidence of these features after stopping aspartame not only afforded improvement, but also emotional reassurance that clinical Alzheimer's disease was not present

- A high school teacher began drinking considerable diet cola after being advised to avoid fruit juices because of fructose intolerance. His memory loss became so severe – including inability to remember the names of students – that they referred to him as "Mr. Alzheimer."
- A 51-year-old woman who described her severe confusion and memory loss as "the old age syndrome," thought she was "a candidate for Alzheimer's disease." There was dramatic improvement after avoiding aspartame products. She made the analogy to "finding the lost piece of a puzzle."

Aspartame disease should be suspected when diabetic patients who consume aspartame are diagnosed as having "diabetic dementia" or "diabetic encephalopathy."

Attempts to define and quantitate aspartame-induced memory problems may frustrate researchers. This is due to vague terminology ("long-term," "short-term," "remote"), and the limitations of brief screens (such as recall of a name or address, and digit repetition) in the clinical setting.

Manifestations

Confusion and memory loss associated with aspartame use became manifest in many ways, both overt and subtle. The following examples of "forgettings" are supplemented by more detailed descriptions in the representative case reports.

- A 30-year-old female sales consultant noted, "I could not consciously remember what I had done or said before."
- An engineer had trouble remembering "names and descriptive adjectives."
- A building inspector volunteered, "I could not think straight."
- An 18-year-old male experienced severe confusion while driving in his neighborhood because he kept forgetting where he was or where to turn. At the time, he was drinking two liters of aspartame sodas daily.
- A 47-year-old woman expressed extreme concern over impairment of her prized "photographic memory."
- Several confided that they occasionally couldn't remember their own names while consuming aspartame.
- Aspartame reactors repeatedly stressed "difficulty in concentrating."
- Experienced secretaries (as Case II-21 and Case VI-13) were troubled because they made many typing and computer errors.
- A 34-year-old instructor in English and Spanish had "trouble sequencing assignments" after consuming two cans of diet cola daily.
- A 66-year-old man summed his most troublesome reactions to drinking three or four cans of aspartame soft drinks as "inability to read, and inability to remember."
- The executive director of a major organization repeatedly could not remember whom he was calling after dialing the number. Being in his early 50s, he raised the possibility of "early Alzheimer's disease." His wife urged him to cease the considerable intake of aspartame sodas after hearing about such an association. The memory problem disappeared within several weeks, and did not recur.

- Case III-1, a 31-year-old nurse with an aspartame-induced seizure, became "very incoherent" the morning after drinking "only three sips" of an aspartame beverage.

- A 48-year-old administrator noted as his only significant reaction to aspartame in the survey questionnaire: "BECAME VERY FORGETFUL." He had consumed 4-5 packets of an ATS daily for six months. His memory improved within four weeks after stopping this product. The problem recurred within several days during two subsequent rechallenges.

- A highly qualified school teacher described her confusion while drinking aspartame sodas as feeling she was "in a small room with all these names swirling around me, but I could never quite grab the right one for the person I was trying to remember."

- A woman with other manifestations of aspartame disease (depression; visual changes) described her confusion in these terms: "I have problems with short-term memory. Sometime I feel like a computer hard drive which needs to be defragmented. I know that data are there, but I'm just not sure where it went!"

- A businessman experienced a "short-term memory deficit" while consuming aspartame products. He gave this description: "My symptoms included (1) the feeling like something is taking over my thoughts, like a big, slow wave would engulf a swimmer on the beach, and (2) an inability to remember just about anything, including my whereabouts and what it is I'm saying or doing."

- The 45-year-old superintendent of a large school system began drinking one can of a diet cola daily at 2 PM for weight control. Within two hours, he would experience "inability to concentrate fully, lightheadedness, and headache feelings." This sequence occurred on eight rechallenges, the symptoms disappearing within two days after then avoiding the beverage.

- A 43-year-old man had consumed diet colas for 15 years. He experienced numerous manifestations of aspartame disease, on the basis of which multiple sclerosis was suspected. He described his memory impairment: "Forget where I put things. Forget appointments, clients information, details of work, tasks that need to be done, etc. Lose everyday objects like keys, medications, shoes, etc., and can't remember where I put them."

- A woman had complained that her husband "was on my case for years because of the large number of diet colas I drank each day." She ignored his concern until having "the biggest scare of my life when I just went blank while talking to a friend on the phone. I could not recall the names of people, places or things." She added, "By the way, my mother has Alzheimer's, and also was a big diet cola drinker."

There were some bittersweet anecdotes about the memory loss of aspartame reactors. In an attempt to comfort a young mother of three boys who had debilitating confusion and memory loss, her husband said, "Look on the bright side. You can hide your own Easter eggs and you'll never see reruns on TV."

Corroboration By FDA Data

Dr. Linda Tollefson provided information on 129 consumers who complained to the FDA about memory loss while using aspartame products. The data are summarized in Table VI-1.

TABLE VI-1

FDA DATA ON 129 CONSUMERS WITH
ASPARTAME-ASSOCIATED MEMORY LOSS

Sex
Female	109	(84.5%)
Male	20	(15.5%)

Race
White	43	(33.3%)
Nonwhite	0	
Unknown	86	(66.7%)

Age Groups (years)
1-19	6	(4.7%)
20-29	11	(8.5%)

30-39	28	(21.7%)
40-49	21	(16.3%)
50-59	13	(10.1%)
60+	12	(9.3%)
Unknown	38	(29.4%)

Aspartame Products Consumed

Soft Drinks	81	(62.8%)
Tabletop Sweetners	57	(44.2%)
Hot Chocolate	14	(10.9%)
Iced Tea	16	(12.4%)
Gum	6	(4.7%)
Soft Drink Mixes	23	(17.8%)
Puddings/Gelatins	25	(19.4%)

Concomitant Symptoms

Headaches	58	(45.0%)
Depression/Mood Changes	46	(35.7%)
Numbness/Tingling/Other Neurologic	24	(18.6%)
Dizziness	43	(33.3%)
Abdominal Pain/GI Complaints	14	(10.9%)
Weakness/Fatigue	13	(10.1%)
Visual	20	(15.5%)
Fainting	4	(3.1%)
Hives/Rashes	6	(4.7%)
Sleep Problems	8	(6.2%)
Heart	4	(3.1%)
Bone/Joint Pain	1	(0.8%)
Menstrual	2	(1.6%)
Breathing Difficulty	1	(0.8%)
Coma	2	(1.6%)

Input From Radio Interviews

Relatively young adults repeatedly mentioned their confusion and memory loss during my interviews on talk shows. The gratitude of persons who had gone through this ordeal can be summed in the title of a familiar song, *Thanks For The Memory*.

- One caller to an Iowa station had been troubled by inability to remember "even simple things." Her husband constantly teased this young housewife about it. She had been consuming considerable amounts of diet soda. Her sister, an aspartame user, was also experiencing unexplained confusion and memory loss. Both had anguished over the prospect of having familial Alzheimer's disease.

- A woman in her early 30s began by listing a number of symptoms experienced after consuming aspartame products. They included severe memory impairment, tremors, headache, dizziness, "stomach spasms" and intestinal bleeding. These problems persisted despite many consultations. She chanced to hear my discussion about aspartame disease on radio, and quit using these products. The relief was gratifying, especially improvement of memory. On the one occasion she rechallenged herself, the first symptom to recur was memory loss.

Representative Case Reports

Case VI-C-1

A 61-year-old advertising executive related his experience with aspartame products. In retrospect, he had a similar reaction several times after drinking coffee to which an ATS had been added. He felt "dizzy and very uptight," followed by severe insomnia. At the time, he did not relate these symptoms to the use of aspartame.

Several months later, he stopped at a fast-food outlet for a snack and coffee prior to playing golf. He requested a saccharin sweetener. Since it was not stocked, he received a packet of aspartame sweetener.

During the game, his "eyes crossed." Realizing that he was confused and behaving erratically, his golf partners suspected "possible heat stroke," and took him home. The next thing he remembered, about two hours later, was having his pulse and blood pressure taken. It was the first time he ever "lost my memory."

Chancing to read the details of my recent press conference, he immediately suspected having had an aspartame reaction. None of the foregoing mental or visual problems recurred after avoiding these products.

Case VI-C-2

A registered nurse and successful businesswoman suffered progressive memory loss, lethargy, dizziness, irritability and depression shortly after she began using an ATS. An endocrinologist could find no underlying cause. Her symptoms intensified on a recommended vacation, during which she continued using this product.

She happened to hear a reference to aspartame reactions on television. Her response to stopping the product was described in these terms: "The results were dramatic! Within days, I was feeling better, and soon back to all my activities I had given up. I often wonder what would have happened if I hadn't seen that news spot." She reported these adverse effects to the Food and Drug Administration on November 11, 1983.

Case VI-C-3

A housewife described herself as a "diet soda fiend" because of her heavy consumption of aspartame soft drinks. She developed "trouble thinking of ordinary words while in mid-sentence." Its relationship to using these beverages crystallized when her husband **also** began evidencing similar difficulty while drinking diet sodas. In addition, she experienced visual difficulty, a source of considerable concern for one who had always prided herself on "20/15 vision." She wrote

> "I suddenly developed dizziness and blurred vision. I then read an article that stated aspartame could cause blurred vision, and the symptoms should disappear after 3 weeks. While the loss of words has disappeared, the blurred vision has not. Incidentally, the eye doctor could not find anything wrong with my eyes."

Case VI-C-4

A 36-year-old registered nurse suffered severe reactions to aspartame products. They consisted of confusion, decreased vision in one eye, marked sensitivity to noise, severe headache, dizziness, unsteadiness, insomnia, shortness of breath, abdominal pain and intense thirst. All these symptoms subsided within 15 days after stopping aspartame products. Her son became "hyperactive" when he drank aspartame beverages.

Case VI-C-5

A 50-year-old diabetic social worker was treated with diet and chlorpropamide (Diabinese®). She began consuming two cans of aspartame sodas and two packets of an ATS daily. Severe mental confusion and memory loss developed. She wrote, "In social situations, I was unable to communicate. The confusion and memory loss made conversation impossible."

Other complaints attributed to aspartame disease included slurring of speech, extreme irritability, altered personality ("the total personality change was frightening"), and intense itching. She neither smoked nor drank alcohol. Most of these symptoms disappeared within two weeks after avoiding aspartame. They predictably recurred within one or two days during three retesting trials.

Case VI-C-6

A 43-year-old attorney/nurse called about her recurrent problems with diet drinks and other aspartame products over six years. The symptoms of greatest concern were confusion, memory loss, blurred vision, and nocturnal anxiety attacks.

These symptoms occurred while in law school. ("I couldn't finish my thoughts.") With her medical background, she arrived at the conclusion that aspartame products were the probable culprit. Her mind cleared totally after discontinuing them.

Four years later, she decided to try diet beverages again to lose weight... rationalizing that the previous difficulty had been related to "stress." She became confused during her first trial. (Fortunately, the presiding judge helped her through the procedure.) The visual difficulty and nocturnal anxiety attacks also recurred. Her confusion and memory loss increased to the point that "it's the closest I ever want to be to having Alzheimer's disease." She then experienced a "total blackout" while driving, and made an erroneous left turn that demolished her car. At that point, the importance of total abstinence from aspartame products became evident. She perceptively stated in retrospect, "The thing that is so disturbing to me is that the symptoms are so subtle it would be difficult to convince the jury of their causation by these products."

Case VI-C-7

A 58-year-old patient requested an earlier appointment because of profound memory loss and intermittent confusion since his last checkup. His memory had become "so bad that if I am cooking something in the kitchen, I'm likely to forget about it." He also suffered headaches, dizziness, decreased vision, and depression over the previous month. These symptoms virtually vanished within one week after stopping his considerable intake of aspartame sodas, and did not recur over the next five years.

Case VI-C-8

A 61-year-old court reporter developed marked memory loss, blurred vision in both eyes, "dry eyes," severe headache, dizziness, facial pains, extreme irritability, episodic shortness of breath, and unexplained chest pains. She was particularly concerned over making many computer errors and becoming "very nonproductive." She consumed four cans of an ASD, six packets of an ATS, and two glasses of aspartame hot chocolate daily. She wrote

> "I am usually a very sharp quick person. Suddenly I had a general feeling of malaise, dull-witted, couldn't concentrate, began to forget things, felt fuzzy-headed and very unstable. I had been drinking a lot of aspartame. I then ran out of it, drank some regular soda, and began feeling better immediately."

Case VI-C-9

This prominent businessman, an insulin-dependent diabetic, had felt well until consuming beverages and gelatin sweetened with aspartame. He presented with dramatic memory loss and severe confusion – as evidenced by having lost his wallet, and misplacing his keys several times. He also forgot to take several doses of insulin, resulting in markedly elevated blood glucose levels. There was striking improvement within three days after discontinuing aspartame products.

Case VI-C-10

A 44-year-old educator was increasingly concerned about developing Alzheimer's disease over the previous two years. Her uncle suffered from this disease. She had been a heavy consumer of aspartame products for over a decade.

Her concern stemmed from the following behavior:

- Inability to recall writing checks, and to recognize her signature on them

- Finding notes she had written, but having no recollection of doing so
- Inability to remember the location of common objects, such as the knob on her car radio or the brake pedal
- Getting lost while driving
- Reaching for the wrong object, such as a perfume bottle instead of a deodorant, or shampoo instead of toothpaste
- Giving her class tests that she already had given and graded

Other manifestations of probable aspartame disease included depression, a change in personality, anxiety attacks, and a craving for diet soft drinks. Within two weeks after stopping aspartame products, this craving disappeared.

Case VI-C-11

A 29-year-old molecular biologist and trained toxicologist (pesticides) had studied the saccharin controversy three years previously. As a result, he avoided saccharin, and drank three cans of diet cola daily because aspartame contains "naturally occurring chemicals." He subsequently suffered a number of neurologic problems that were described in this correspondence.

> "I lost much feeling in my body. When I sat down, I did not feel the chair; when I lied down, I did not feel the bed. I then felt pins-and-needles sensations whenever my body came in contact with anything.

> "There was also marked memory loss. It had been so good that I memorized almost every entry of the Oxford English Dictionary in order to qualify for a scholarship in the U.S. It was really strange when I forgot things I had done just recently, and asked people the same question I asked a few days previously. I now spent minutes or hours laboring to remember something.

> "During a long meeting with a colleague, I asked whether he cared for a drink because I always have diet cola in the refrigerator. He then stated that aspartame is no good. I suddenly woke up to the fact that my symptoms were linked to the use of diet cola, and rapidly improved after stopping it. I feel very lucky that some persons with a burning desire to

spread information about reactions to aspartame are out there. You have done so far what no hero in the history of modern toxicology can parallel."

Case VI-C-12

A 50-year-old woman experienced severe confusion, memory loss, headache, fatigue, "anxiety attacks," aggravation of phobias and personality changes while consuming aspartame sodas and "diet" ice cream. Other features included decreased vision, ringing in the ears, a recent rise of blood pressure (previously always low or normal), severe nausea, diarrhea, a facial eruption., the loss of 30 pounds, marked frequency of urination, "low blood sugar attacks," and severe bloat. Three physicians and consultants had been seen. Two MRI studies of the brain excluded a brain tumor.

The patient herself suspected aspartame products as the cause after learning about aspartame disease from the media. She had never smoked or consumed alcohol. Her symptoms virtually disappeared within several weeks after avoiding aspartame. They recurred the one time she rechallenged herself.

The family history was impressive. Her daughter had become markedly confused and depressed while "drinking cases of the 12 oz cans because it was on sale." An aunt and uncle had histories suggestive of Alzheimer's disease; indeed, the patient had feared that she "might be in the first stage."

Occupational and Safety Implications

Aspartame-induced confusion and memory problems can have serious professional, business, educational and personal ramifications. Their occurrence in drivers and commercial pilots may endanger public safety (Chapter VII and XXVII) (Roberts 1998d).

- Aspartame reactors repeatedly mentioned loss of confidence in continuing or resuming their professions and occupations. Case VII-33, a registered nurse, illustrates this issue.
- A number of teachers stated that aspartame-induced confusion and memory loss affected their ability to teach (see Case VI-C-10).
- Business managers and professionals were reluctant to joke about their "pseudosenility" attributable to aspartame-associated confusion and diminished memory because of the possible stigma of being considered a "nemesis on the premises."

The extreme interest in this realm by members of the print and electronics media was noted in Chapter I. After my initial press conference, they sought appearances on talk shows and television programs. The reason soon became apparent: these hosts were concerned over <u>their</u> intermittent confusion, memory gaps, and wide swings of mood that posed career threats. Most were health-conscious individuals who had been drinking considerable amounts of diet sodas or coffee sweetened with aspartame. After reading about my studies, the dramatic clearing of these symptoms following abstinence from aspartame generated the best reward they could offer – coveted interviews for their audiences.

Pathophysiologic Mechanisms

The mechanisms by which confusion and memory loss might be caused are discussed in Section 5 and in my book dealing with the prevention of Alzheimer's disease (Roberts 1995b).

The essential memory circuits in the mammalian brain continue to be investigated, along with clarification of the neurochemical, molecular and biophysical substrates of memory. Reviewing the neurobiology of learning and memory, Professor Richard F. Thompson (1986) (Department of Psychology, Stanford University) stated, "A wide range of chemicals can influence memory performance, and learning involves many alterations in neurotransmitter systems and other chemical processes."

A committee of the American Academy of Neurology assessed the neuropsychological features from neurotoxic exposure (*Neurology* 1996; 47:595). It emphasized that the first complaints following such exposure are often poor concentration, impaired attention, and abnormal memory.

Several reports are pertinent.

- In studies on early-treated phenylketonuria (PKU) subjects whose intake of dietary phenylalanine was increased for one week, Krause et al (1987) found prolongation of performance time on a choice reaction test, decreased concentrations of neurotransmitters in the plasma and urine, and decreased EEG mean power frequency (a reflection of brain dopamine).
- Aspartate and glutamate are critically involved in learning and remembering new information, based on the identification of binding sites for these excitatory amino acids (excitotoxins).

- Cholecystokinin is involved in the modulation of memory. Accordingly, changes in its metabolism by aspartame or phenylalanine (Gibbs 1976) might contribute to impaired memory.
- Brain edema and vascular stasis due to methanol (Rao 1977) may be contributory.
- Dementia from a related plant neurotoxin (Spencer 1987) was discussed above.

Misdiagnoses

Confusion and memory loss are nonspecific symptoms that occur in many disorders. Accordingly, numerous tests were performed on symptomatic aspartame reactors. The present discussion focuses on drugs, Alzheimer's disease and the Sjögren syndrome.

I. Drugs

Several patients initially refused to concede that aspartame products could be the primary cause of their confusion and poor memory, preferring to attribute them to prescribed drugs. They frequently incriminated beta-blockers, such as propranolol (Inderal®), commonly used in treating hypertension and angina pectoris.

Representative Case Report

Case VI-C-12

A 62-year-old businessman with angina pectoris had been taking the same dose of propranolol for a considerable period. He presented with increasing confusion, memory loss, and visual difficulty after using three packets of an ATS daily. He agreed to stop it, albeit reluctantly. Two weeks later, his mental clarity had normalized without any change in the dosage of this or other medications.

II. Alzheimer's Disease

As emphasized earlier, many younger aspartame reactors expressed the identical worry, "Could I be developing early Alzheimer's disease?" Most were reassured when their memory loss and confusion promptly improved after abstaining from aspartame products. This subject is further considered in Chapter XV.

The association of "memory loss" and "Alzheimer's disease" is not surprising because of increasing focus on this disorder by the media. Well-meaning support groups and organizations reinforce such an association.

> An ad in *The Miami Herald* (September 29, 1986, p. A-14) carried the caption ALZHEIMER'S in bold capital letters. Its message began: "If you or a loved one are experiencing memory loss, then you are invited to contact us. Our programs are conducted by board-certified neurologists with extensive experience in the treatment of Alzheimer's disease, stroke and general aging."

An equally disturbing issue must be raised – the possibility that Alzheimer's disease CAN be triggered or aggravated by chronic aspartame use (Chapter XV). In describing researches on memory loss and related areas by its scientists, G. D. Searle & Company published full-page ads in the *Journal of the American Association* and other medical journals stating "excessive activity of the excitatory amino acids might cause nerve cell destruction resembling the changes noted in Alzheimer's disease, Huntington's chorea, and other degenerative diseases."

In view of the confusion and memory loss also experienced by aspartame reactors when they took phenylalanine, and the considerable phenylalanine present in bee pollen, it is of interest that President Reagan had been taking bee pollen since 1961 as an "energy restorative" (*Parade Magazine* December 13, 1987, p. E-9) prior to developing overt Alzheimer's disease.

III. Sjögren's Syndrome

The association of "dry eyes," dryness of the mouth, and memory loss in aspartame reactors may be a clue to the presence of Sjögren's syndrome (Chapter IV), or a greater predisposition to it. The primary form of this disorder, currently presumed to be an autoimmune state, affects about two percent of the adult population. Up to one-fourth of such patients have severe cognitive dysfunction ranging from forgetfulness to dementia (Alexander 1986).

D. SUSPECTED MULTIPLE SCLEROSIS

My observations justify the conviction that *no patient suspected of having multiple sclerosis (MS) who consumes aspartame products should have this diagnosis finalized until being observed many months after abstaining from them.*

More than 50 aspartame reactors in this series anguished over having presumed multiple sclerosis. The dozens of representative case reports cited in this and other chapters validate the foregoing assertion. It is underscored in the case of persons with aspartame disease whose neurologic features are accompanied by visual symptoms (Chapter IV).

The author's emphasis upon this issue assumes even greater significance in view of recent consensus statements recommending vigorous drug intervention therapy for early MS, including patients with "clinically isolated syndromes" such as an attack of optic neuritis. These agents – including interferon beta 1b, interferon beta 1, and glatiramer acetate – can have serious side effects.

Several diagnostic pitfalls will be emphasized. For example, *the finding of minor abnormalities in a few small areas by a CT scan or MRI studies is NOT necessarily diagnostic of multiple sclerosis* (see Case IV-10.)

Concerned individuals have provided pertinent insights. For example, the engineer-father of a young female aspartame reactor who had been misdiagnosed as having MS carefully scrutinized the available medical and biochemical literature, including the alteration of myelin after injection of synthetic peptides. He wrote

> "I am identifying aspartame as a possible causal factor of central nervous system problems because of the inexplicable outbreak of MS-like symptoms across the nation.

> "Can aspartame be initiating a chemical process in the body that could subsequently produce some of the same symptoms that would otherwise be attributed to MS?

> "Can aspartame cause the body to attack its own myelin, thereby generating CNS lesions and MS-like effects in people that could be mistakenly diagnosed as MS? Perhaps the molecular mimicry premise provides the key to understanding MS."

Representative Case Reports

Case VI-D-1

The following detailed letter from a young aspartame reactor suspected of having MS is reproduced because it illustrates the foregoing issues.

* * * * *

"I experienced a strong adverse reaction to aspartame products. Being a moderate to heavy consumer of its many available forms – be it diet soda, diet milkshakes, gelatins, puddings, fruit drinks, cocoa and the like – I had no qualms about my own consumption. I also purchased and prepared these foods for my family. Because I had been "assured" of its safety, I continued my use of aspartame during pregnancy.

"In the spring of 1986, following the birth of my daughter, I became determined to lose weight. I didn't eat much, but instead drank large quantities of sodas, milkshakes and other aspartame products. The foods I did eat included aspartame sweetened puddings, gelatins, etc.

"On June 7 of the same year, I noticed an increased sensitivity to light and blurring in my right eye. Within three days I could not read a book or newspaper, was unable to see the reflection of my own face in the mirror, and was unable to properly care for my infant. Because of the visual loss, I could not work for nearly nine weeks.

"I sought professional care immediately. I first consulted an ophthalmologist. The doctor performed a comprehensive exam, but was unable to offer a clinical explanation. He then referred me to my personal physician who performed a neurological exam and followup. This entailed two neurological workups, a complete blood chemistry profile, and skull x-rays; none revealed any problem. I was told I probably suffered from an inflammation of the optic nerve (retrobulbar neuritis).

"On August 12, 1986 I was examined by a neuro-ophthalmologist at Michigan State University. One of the first questions he asked was if I had been working with or exposed to any chemicals. At the time, I was totally unaware that I had indeed been ingesting a neurotoxin (aspartame), so I replied no to his question.

"I then underwent a battery of tests. They involved more blood work, an evoked visual response, fundus photos, and finally a Magnetic Resonance Imaging scan of the brain.

These tests showed some demyelination of the optic nerve and some plaque formation. The physician believed I "maybe...possibly" had multiple sclerosis. The doctor went on to say I would never see any better than I did on that day, and that no further testing was necessary. I was still very confused and horrified.

"Going back to my own physician with these findings, I had another neurological exam, and again passed it with the proverbial flying colors. At this time, my doctor told me to put the notion of MS out of my mind because until I could "prove" I had this disease, I didn't have it. Even though I had this visual loss and the chronic aching sensation, especially in my legs, these were not regarded as true symptoms of MS. So after a battery of medical tests, doctor bills, and lost time from work, I decided to just get on with my normal routine, even though I continued to be concerned why all of this was happening. Was it something that I brought on myself?

"As time went on, I began to read and hear bits and pieces of information about people all over the country who had experienced assorted medical problems from aspartame products. I decided I had nothing to lose at this point, so I immediately ceased my consumption of aspartame in its many forms. Within a month or so, I became increasingly aware that I no longer "ached" as I had before, and that vision in my right eye was much clearer than it had been in many months!

"Since that time, I have been in touch with Shannon Roth and Aspartame Victims and Their Friends. When I initially discussed the problems with Ms. Roth, she knew exactly what I was talking about – having experienced many of the same problems. This was incredible because I had never imagined there would be someone who could match me word for word, and for symptoms, of what I had been going through.

"I have since gathered a hefty collection of information and recently presented it to my physician who had doubted the diagnosis of MS. He feels I did indeed suffer from methyl alcohol poisoning, and this is what caused the damage to my optic nerve. As the doctor said, 'I'd rather be fat than blind.'

"Now that some time has passed, other problems I experienced while using aspartame have ceased since discontinuing its use. These were headaches, loud ringing sensations in my right ear, dizziness, lightheadedness, and even short term memory loss."

Case VI-D-2

A 29-year-old sales assistant for a major company was diagnosed as having multiple sclerosis in 1988. She had been consuming 6-8 cans of diet cola and other aspartame products for five years. Her symptoms included marked decrease of vision in both eyes, ringing in the ears with marked sensitivity to noise, severe unsteadiness of the legs, impaired memory, tingling and numbness of the limbs, depression with suicidal thoughts, severe itching, intense thirst, marked frequency of urination, joint pains, and swelling of the limbs. She had been treated with a corticosteroid for two years. A fusion of the right ankle was performed in 1997 due to local injuries resulting from falls because of her marked weakness. She summed her problem in these terms: "I could not work, walk, or drive. I lost my job, and was facing a possible divorce because of this stress."

Her husband found an article about aspartame disease "as a fluke" in December 1998. Improvement was both prompt and dramatic within three days! Most of her symptoms disappeared within one week. During a personal interview five months later, the patient indicated that the remission persisted. Her main problem at that point was difficulty in walking because of the fusion.

Case VI-D-3

A 28-year-old woman began consuming diet colas and numerous aspartame products (including yogurt and chewing gum) shortly after matriculating in medical school. She developed a number of health problems that culminated in her dismissal. They included severe headache, insomnia, forgetfulness, extreme fatigue, visual difficulty, nausea, bloat, constipation, a gain of 24 pounds, loss of hair, irregular menses, intense thirst, "asthma," and voiding at least four times at night. She then experienced numbness and tingling in her hands and feet, as well as repeated tripping and falling. A consultant neurologist made the diagnosis of "probable multiple sclerosis" on the basis of her symptoms and hyperreflexia.

In desperation, the patient called a biochemistry teacher who had been her mentor. He sent an article about aspartame disease mimicking MS. She promptly accessed the Internet, and then stopped all aspartame products. Dramatic improvement ensued. After 19 months, she wrote, "I sleep regularly, am employed, swim over one-half mile, no longer have imbalance problems, am ovulating again, walk distances, can wear heels again, and no longer have the frequent urgency to use the bathroom."

Related Considerations

The familial ramifications of aspartame disease (Chapter II-J) were evident in this context. For example, two sisters in their 30s had been diagnosed as having MS. They experienced prompt and dramatic improvement of neurologic and other symptoms within several weeks after avoiding aspartame.

The occurrence of multiple sclerosis and amyotrophic lateral sclerosis in members of the same family who consumed considerable aspartame further evidences its potential extensive neurotoxicity among different individuals at risk (see under Chapter VI-F).

I have received dozens of <u>letters expressing gratitude</u> from persons with aspartame disease who had been misdiagnosed as having multiple sclerosis. All experienced gratifying remissions after abstaining from these products.

- A secretary stated, "I had all the symptoms of MS for 10 years. I kept getting worse, but no one knew why. My migraine headaches (at least three a week), cramps, muscle spasms, joint pains, and skin lesions also are now gone."
- A 31-year-old woman had been diagnosed as having multiple sclerosis for ten years. She suffered "debilitating headaches, severe muscle spasms, anxiety attacks, and loss of sensation, memory, and nearly half the vision in my right eye before quitting my 15-year addiction to diet cola. I was confined to a wheelchair for 8 months. My doctor was amazed at the difference in my health when I stopped aspartame."
- A 34-year-old woman consumed considerable amounts of aspartame products because of diabetes. She often drank a gallon of diet ice tea daily, along with several cans of diet cola. Her symptoms included visual difficulty, headache, vertigo and "task perversion". Several physicians attributed her neurologic and metabolic problems to the diabetes. Another physician diagnosed multiple sclerosis. Within days after discontinuing aspartame, she felt "100,000,000 times better, and have continued to feel pretty good since."

There may be <u>medicolegal problems</u> for physicians who incorrectly diagnose multiple sclerosis due to unawareness of aspartame disease, especially neurologists.

- The Supreme Court of Israel upheld a lower district court conviction of malpractice that had resulted from ignorance of the current medical literature (Fishman 1998). Its judicial opinion in this matter asserted that doctors have "personal responsibility" in their "professional duties to remain updated with medical literature" to be aware of alternative diagnoses, opinions and recommended treatments.

- A patient who had been diagnosed in 1994 as having multiple sclerosis was shocked to learn of its simulation by aspartame disease. She wrote,

  "I drank diet drinks for years. I would start drinking at 6 AM, and would continue until after 10 PM each day – always on an empty stomach."

Mechanisms

The selective localization of lesions in multiple sclerosis requires comment. I have attributed them in large measure to energy (glucose) deprivation and fluid retention within the central nervous system (Roberts 1966b, c). Aspartame disease involves both, as well as direct neurotoxicity. Indeed, aspartame-induced dysfunction of nerve cells and their axons may have greater importance than myelin changes.

Significant biochemical differences are known to exist in various central tracts, even though they may appear identical histologically. The concentration of glucose-6-phosphate dehydrogenase activity, for example, is three to four times greater in the heavily myelinated central tracts than the lightly myelinated ones, whereas the reverse applies for glutamic aspartic transaminase (McDougal 1961, 1964).

This orientation is germane because fluid retention is enhanced by the hyperinsulinized state (Chapter XIV) and impaired water metabolism (Chapter IX-F). The ingress of water into myelin can disrupt its intermolecular cohesion and functional integrity (Vanderheuvel 1964).

An autoimmune response may be triggered by aspartame (Chapter VIII). The possible mechanisms include formaldehyde-induced protein changes (Chapter XXI), and increased leukotrienes, 15-hydroxyeicosatetraenoic acid, and other arachidonic acid metabolites after the exposure of macrophages to aspartame (Hardcastle 1997).

E. ATYPICAL PERIPHERAL NEUROPATHY ("NEURALGIA")

In this series of aspartame reactors, 183 (15 percent) presented with sensory or motor symptoms diagnosed as unexplained peripheral neuropathies. They complained of "pins and needles," "tingling," "crawling," "numbness," and "burning" sensations. These featuers also characterized many of the cases reported in other chapters

Representative Case Report

Case VI-E-1

A male reactor experienced "the loss of feeling in my feet, and legs so painful that I could hardly stand my pants touching them." He was consuming two liters of an aspartame soda daily. Other symptoms included memory loss and severe dizziness. After avoiding all aspartame products, these complaints disappeared or were markedly improved within two weeks. He later experimented by drinking a small glass of aspartame soda, and suffered a recurrence of leg pain within an hour.

General Considerations

The causes of peripheral neuropathy are numerous. Physicians and medical students resort to the mnemonic scheme of "DANG THERAPIST" – standing for diabetes, alcoholism, nutrition, Guillain-Barré, toxic metals, heredity, etc. Aspartame disease should be added to the list. (The 24-page booklet published by The Neuropathy Association [April 1999] titled, *A Guide to Peripheral Neuropathies*, did not mention the causative or contributory role of aspartame products.)

Several misdiagnoses are noteworthy.

- The aggravation or simulation of diabetic neuropathy by aspartame products is discussed in Chapter XIII.
- The "stocking-glove" distribution of sensory alterations in heavy aspartame consumers led to the inference of hysteria in several instances.
- Three patients had received a provisional diagnosis of the Guillain-Barré syndrome – also referred to as acute polyneuritis and ascending paralysis.

The amount of medication currently being prescribed for "idiopathic neuropathy" is impressive. Indeed, interest in this subject by nonprofessionals led to creation of the publication *Neuropathy News*.

Representative Case Report

Case VI-E-2

A 49-year-old insulin-dependent diabetic patient with diabetic retinopathy used considerable aspartame soft drinks. He developed neuropathic symptoms that were diagnosed as a "chronic inflammatory demyelinating polyradiculoneuropathy, which is a peripheral version of multiple sclerosis or a slow version of Guillain-Barré."

The Carpal Tunnel Syndrome

The carpal tunnel syndrome (CTS) refers to irritation or compression of the median nerve at the wrist. Surgical "decompression" is usually recommended when other measures prove ineffective.

The carpal tunnel syndrome, both unilateral and bilateral, occurred in eight patients who consumed considerable aspartame products, especially diet sodas. They also experienced other features of aspartame disease. The hand neuropathy improved dramatically or disappeared after avoiding these products, even obviating surgery (Roberts 2000b).

Representative Case Reports (also see Case IV-23)

Case VI-E-3

A 39-year-old sales representative with reactive hypoglycemia began using an ATS when it became available. She also drank three to four cans of an ACB daily for two years. During the previous year, she developed numbness of the upper limbs "like 50 pounds of dead meat." This was followed eight months later by "scalding and burning in my legs," with associated marked loss of muscle tone. Several physicians diagnosed carpal tunnel syndrome combined with neuropathy of the lower extremities. She did not smoke or drink alcohol. Electromyography (EMG) or the right upper limb evidenced muscle and nerve damage.

Other complaints included a marked decrease of vision in both eyes, severe sensitivity to noise, unsteadiness, recurrent migraine, intense insomnia, depression with suicidal thoughts, anxiety attacks, less frequent periods, swelling of the legs, and intensified hypoglycemia reactions. She also awakened during the night to drink diet cola because of intense thirst.

Within 2½ weeks after discontinuing aspartame, the neuropathic and other symptoms improved.

Case VI-E-4

A man had been suffering severe tingling in the fingers and arms, and marked impairment of vision. Two days before scheduled surgery for carpal tunnel syndrome, he became acutely ill with "symptoms of wood alcohol poisoning" (the diagnosis of an emergency floor physician) requiring hospitalization. At that point, he stopped his large intake of diet sodas. The neurologic symptoms promptly disappeared <u>without</u> surgery, but his impaired vision persisted.

Case VI-E-5

A 53-year-old man was diagnosed as having diabetes. He eliminated sugar, and began using considerable amounts of aspartame products. He then experienced tingling of the hands (diagnosed as "carpal tunnel syndrome"), which spread to his legs. Blindness ensued – first in the left eye, and then in the right. The neuropathic symptoms disappeared after stopping aspartame, but the eye damage remained.

Case VI-E-6

A 35-year-old woman was consuming two liters of an aspartame cola daily when she developed carpal tunnel syndrome in <u>both</u> upper extremities. Other features included confusion, memory loss, marked irritability, depression, loss of menses, and rapid graying and thinning of her hair. Many of these features improved after avoiding aspartame products.

Case VI-E-7

A 35-year-old diabetic man had been using aspartame products "in mass quantities," including one gallon of sugar-free ice cream weekly. He developed severe neuropathic and arthritic symptoms two years previously, requiring surgery for carpal tunnel syndrome on one hand... and later on the other. These persistent symptoms were not attributed to diabetic neuropathy by his physicians. Concomitant shoulder and hip pain precluded working. Dramatic improvement of his neuropathic and other symptoms occurred within two weeks after avoiding aspartame products at his fiancee's suggestion when she read about aspartame disease.

Case VI-E-8

A man recently diagnosed as having non-insulin-dependent diabetes developed severe tingling and numbness of the fingers and hands after using sugar-free products. Three physicians made the diagnosis of carpal tunnel syndrome; and suggested surgery. These symptoms disappeared shortly after stopping aspartame products... without surgery. Unfortunately, his blindness in both eyes persisted.

Commentary

More than 200,000 carpal tunnel release surgical procedures are performed annually in the United States, costing in excess of $1 billion (Franzblau 1999). Aspartame-associated CTS provides insights relative to this disorder and the neurotoxicity of aspartame products.

CTS probably represents the cumulative effect of many contributory factors. They include anatomic, occupational, metabolic, neurologic and toxicologic influences causing nerve swelling or degeneration, and increased intracarpal canal pressure that reduces median nerve perfusion.

- Median nerve movement tends to be reduced in the carpal tunnel with wrist flexion (Greening 1999).
- Atroshi et al (1999) found CTS among 14.4 percent of 170,000 persons in a South Sweden population.
- The observations that there is a strong association between obesity and CTS, and that CTS is almost four times more prevalent among women (Chapter II-H), are relevant.

Accordingly, superimposed exposure to the aspartame, a neurotoxin, could precipitate clinical CTS.

Aggravation of Other Neuropathies

Several persons with unexplained exacerbation of other types of peripheral neuropathy were heavy aspartame users.

- A patient with progressively severe neuropathy affecting the lower extremities was presumed to have narrowing of the spinal canal (spinal stenosis). The dosage of corticosteroid therapy, prescribed for symptomatic relief, could be reduced shortly after stopping aspartame.

- The adverse neurologic effects of aspartame are illustrated by the responses of many patients with Charcot-Marie-Tooth disease in a survey questionnaire by CMT International (kindly supplied by Mrs. Linda Crabtree). Under "diet," a number of respondents indicated aspartame products had caused severe reactions, particularly headache.
- An aspartame reactor suffered recurrent Bell's palsy. There were no further problems after avoiding aspartame.

Mechanisms of Aspartame Toxicity

Each of the three components of aspartame – phenylalanine, aspartic acid, and a methyl ester (10%) that promptly becomes free methyl alcohol (methanol) after ingestion – and their multiple breakdown products following exposure to heat or during storage are potentially neurotoxic. The mechanisms may involve dopamine (derived from phenylalanine), cerebral cholecystokinin (CCK), serotonin, endorphins and other important neurotransmitters, insulin, the unique permeability of the blood-brain barrier to phenylalanine, and the "aging" effect of the stereoisomer D-aspartic acid (Section 5).

The chronic intake of free methanol is highly pertinent to the peripheral neuropathies herein reported. This subject is reviewed in Chapter XXI. Six years before FDA approval of aspartame, Dr. Herbert S. Posner (1975), the National Institute of Environmental Health Sciences, wrote a review titled, "Biohazards of Methanol in Proposed New Uses." He stressed the failure to recognize the "delayed and irreversible effects on the nervous system" of methanol... at widely varying levels of exposure and at rather low levels."

The marked improvement of carpal tunnel syndrome in patients with aspartame disease without surgery after abstaining from aspartame products not only may reflect the chemical's neuropathic effects, but also changes within surrounding soft tissues from chronic formaldehyde toxicity (Chapter XXI).

F. SEVERE MUSCLE WEAKNESS; SUSPECT MOTOR NEURONE DISEASE

Several muscle weakness was the most disabling symptom for several aspartame reactors. One neurologist-patient (Case VI-F-4) expressed concern about developing motor neurone disease. A diagnosis of various myopathies had been made in some instances.

Wokke (1996) appropriately warned physicians about making an erroneous diagnosis of motor neurone disease or amyotrophic lateral sclerosis.

Other rheumatologic and muscular aspects of aspartame disease are discussed in Chapter IX-G.

Representative Case Reports

Case VI-F-1

A housewife indicated her intense muscle weakness in these terms:

> "I was unable to open a jar, or lift a roasting pan from the oven, or stand at the sink to wash dishes – so many things I once took for granted. After stopping aspartame, I am grateful for now being able to do some of the everyday things that I could not do for so long, that is, cook, wash dishes, laundry, vacuuming, wash a window occasionally, and take a walk by myself on a good day."

Case VI-F-2

A 59-year-old man developed polyneuropathy with severe muscle weakness and "restless limbs" when he consumed three liters of aspartame beverages daily. He was diagnosed as having "kinesthetic dystonia" after being subjected to numerous neurologic studies.

Case VI-F-3

A 62-year-old woman with aspartame disease described her condition as "a living hell." She had become virtually immobilized at the age of 53 with severe weakness and aching of the muscles, presumably due to polymyalgia rheumatica. Prednisone was prescribed. She saw two cardiologists, three ophthalmologists, an ear specialist, two neurologists and other physicians. This retired school teacher chanced upon my first book on aspartame disease. Her improvement after avoiding aspartame products was dramatic and sustained – including the subsidence of muscle pain and weakness. (She used "AspRac 657" as her e-mail address, a reference to the fact that I listed her as Case 657 in my data base.)

Case VI-F-4

A 30-year-old female neurologist was suspected of developing motor neurone disease until her recognition of aspartame disease. This explanatory letter is reproduced because of the clinical and scientific insights provided.

*　　*　　*　　*　　*

"I was very interested to read your book about the possible dangers of the artificial sweetener aspartame. I am writing to you now with yet another 'anecdotal' report concerning symptoms that I developed over the course of prolonged intake of aspartame foods and drinks.

"Aspartame was introduced into foods and drinks in the UK around 1983. I consumed large amounts of yogurt, soft cheeses and drinks containing aspartame. On many days my entire intake consisted of aspartame-containing substances.

"I had a baby in April 1990. Four months later (around August 1990), I began to have problems using my hands and arms. I have always been physically strong, having swam competitively, so I was surprised at the difficulties I was experiencing with simple things like
picking up my son, undoing tight jars, etc. Initially, I put the problem down to overuse of my arms, and didn't think much of it. However, I also noticed that my shoulder and forearm muscles had decreased in bulk.

"Around Christmas 1990, I began to notice a cramp in my right leg while walking, especially in the cold. In January 1991, I noticed fasciculations in the small muscles of my hands occurring many times a day. I began to notice them also in my shoulder muscles, forearms, calf muscles and thighs. At this stage, rightly or wrongly, I began to associate the problems using my arms (which had not improved) with the wasting in my shoulder and forearms, and finally with the fasciculations. I initially panicked, thinking that I might have motor neurone disease. Of course, knowing how rare this was in someone my age, I began to think of alternative explanations.

"As my research involves producing animal models of neurodegenerative diseases in seeking novel treatments for Parkinson's disease, I was aware of the toxicity of aspartame and glutamate to motor neurones. Early one morning, it occurred to me that my problem might be due to the huge amounts of aspartame I'd been consuming. It was then that I began to look through the literature for problems attributable to aspartame, and came across

244

your book. Of my own accord, I immediately cut out all aspartate- and monosodium glutamate-containing substances from my diet. Within a month, my symptoms and the frequency of fasciculations improved markedly.

"I did, with great embarrassment, approach a very sympathetic colleague (a professor of neurology at a London teaching hospital) who examined me and could find no pathological signs. He also arranged for EMG and nerve conduction studies to be performed; but by the time the appointment for these came through, my symptoms had almost completely resolved. (I had been off aspartame for nearly three months). The studies were normal.

"I adhere firmly to aspartame being responsible. Benign fasciculations would not explain either the difficulties I was having using my arms, or the disappearance of the fasciculations. In further support of my suspicion is the fact that elevated aspartate levels have been found in the cerebrospinal fluid of patients with motor neurone disease. Some patients with motor neurone disease have also been found to have abnormal metabolism of aspartate and other excitatory amino acids. It is therefore possible that some people (like myself) may have an unusually slow metabolism of aspartate, so that accumulation occurs – and subsequent neuronal damage if large amounts of aspartate-containing foods are consumed. This would explain why the symptoms I had have not been more widely observed, or at least not attributed to aspartame.

"Incidentally, I also suffered increasingly from insomnia and migraine over the past few years. These have almost disappeared since eliminating aspartame from my diet."

Commentary

The probable pathophysiologic basis for these neuromuscular features was reviewed earlier in this chapter.

Intriguing observations about the suspected role of aspartame disease in other muscle disorders are germane. For example, a non-diabetic man in his mid-50s and daily consumer of aspartame products, experienced marked weakness of both arms with an associated elevation of the serum creatine phosphokinase (CPK) to 420.

Amyotrophic Lateral Sclerosis (ALS). ALS is the most common form of progressive motor neuron disease. Initially, it selectively involves neurons primarily in the spinal cord (as spinal muscular atrophy) or the brain stem (as pseudobulbar palsy and primary lateral sclerosis)... with devastating progressive nerve and muscular effects.

The contributory role of aspartame to ALS was suspected in several instances. This association became more impressive when close relatives developed related neurologic disorders.

> A man with adult-onset diabetes used considerable aspartame, especially as a tabletop sweetener in his oatmeal and coffee. He developed severe and ultimately fatal ALS. Two daughters suffered severe aspartame disease, one having been initially diagnosed as multiple sclerosis.

Patients afflicted with <u>mitochondrial myopathy</u> have an inherited inborn error of metabolism causing deficient synthesis of adenosine triphosphate (ATP). Such persons should avoid aspartame and other products that contain methanol or break down to formic acid and lactic acid owing to difficulty in handling these metabolic wastes.

> A woman and two children with mitochondrial myopathy indicated that aspartame use could result in acidosis and aggravation of the degenerative process. (Her husband was a director of the International Mitochondrial Disease Network.)

G. ATTENTION-DEFICIT/HYPERACTIVITY; "RESTLESS LEGS;" THE TOURETTE SYNDROME

Seventy-eight (6%) of aspartame reactors in this series evidenced hyperactivity, "restless legs," or both. Their restlessness often was expressed as "the need to keep moving."

I. Attention-Deficit/Hyperactivity

Magnitude of the Problem

The attention-deficit/hyperactivity disorder (ADHD) has become a common neurobehaviorial disorder of childhood.

- An estimated 10-15 percent of all school children in the United States – 1.8 million to 2.7 million – manifest ADHD.
- The annual number of outpatient visits for ADHD increased dramatically by a factor of 2.48 (from 1,687,000 to 4,195,000) from 1990 to 1993 (Swanson 1995).

- This disorder appears to doubling every three to four years among children, concomitant with the quadrupling of methylphenidate (Ritalin®) use between 1990 and 1997. (An estimated 4 million children currently take methylphenidate.) More than ten tons were produced in 1997.

The Aspartame Connection

Generalized hyperactivity associated with aspartame use has been striking among children (Chapter XI). Others have noted this association.

- The Centers for Disease Control (1984) cited a child in whom hyperactivity was aggravated after his physician administered aspartame in a double-blind study.
- A Boston physician notified the FDA in April 1984 of "personal experience with toddler children ingesting this substance (aspartame) in whom it has produced hyperactive behavior."

Sally Bunday, Director of the Hyperactive Children's Support Group, wrote the author (October 21, 1999) because of increased concern over these effects of aspartame. She stated, "We have grave concerns for the children. Almost every new parent-caller gives them aspartame drinks, believing the avoidance/reduction of sugar is 'better for the children.' "

Adult aspartame reactors are similarly affected. For example, a 26-year-old landscaper experienced "muscle twitches all over my body" immediately after taking aspartame. He stated, "My thumbs were jumping around, my eyelids were twitching, and the muscles in my thighs were rolling".

Commentary

The combination of aspartame intake, calorie-deficient diets, and aggravated hypoglycemia (Chapter XIV), and sleep deprivation deserves careful consideration when dealing with both children and adults having ADHD. The reflexive prescription of psychotropic drugs for children manifesting behavioral and neurological problems caused primarily by these disorders has contributed to the "generation Rx."

- I reported on the importance of hypoglycemia and poor nutrition among hyperactive children three decades ago (Roberts 1969b).

- Zametkin et al (1990) found that global cerebral glucose metabolism was 8.1 percent lower among adults with hyperactivity than in normal controls. Moreover, glucose metabolism was significantly reduced in 30 of 60 specific regions of the brain, compared with the values in controls.
- The failure of children to obtain adequate sleep resulting from late-night television viewing – termed "bedtime resistance" – can summate upon the effects of aspartame to intensify daytime drowsiness and attention deficit.

As noted, my interest in the problem of attention deficit and hyperactivity began decades before the availability of aspartame. The major component of narcolepsy suggested the limited use of Ritalin as *part* of the therapeutic program... the chief focus being proper diet. Failure to recognize the aggravating role of widespread aspartame use and other undesirable habits in recent years fueled allegations about "the Ritalin conspiracy" – with accusations that children having ADHD are being "drugged" by "doctor-pushers."

Representative Case Report

Case VI-G-1

A registered nurse deduced that aspartame was the cause of her hyperactivity.

> "I become exceedingly restless when I drink a beverage containing aspartame. I have to keep moving for no apparent reason. If I consume anything having this sweetener, no longer can I sit still and read. I have to get up and wander around. The first time this happened to me, I was frankly amazed, and never considered that it was due to this low-cal drink.

II. Restless Legs

So-called restless legs is characterized by continual involuntary movements of the lower extremities. Patients with this disorder frequently complain of numbness, "crawling," "pins and needles," weakness, discomfort on contact with the other extremity or bedding, and spontaneous leg cramps.

Representative Case Reports

Case VI-G-2

A 55-year-old secretary had enjoyed excellent health aside from mild nasal allergies. She watched her diet closely, and even attended a "diet workshop."

She began ingesting aspartame as an ice tea mix during August 1983. Within one week, she experienced "restless legs" and associated aching at night. These complaints subsided in the fall. She resumed this mix during the summer of 1984. "Almost immediately I noticed the same symptoms. When I stopped using the product, the aching of the legs ceased."

She drank and ate other products sweetened with aspartame the following year. Her subsequent course was described in this correspondence.

> "For about three weeks this summer, in July and August, I began again to drink and eat products sweetened with aspartame. They included gelatin, instant puddings, diet colas and an iced tea mix. I began to have the same symptoms but simply dismissed them as 'all in the mind.' The week of August 11, I began to experience slight memory loss – nothing substantial, but disturbing. For example, I put a chunk of hard cheese in the freezer instead of the refrigerator, and only found it by searching the whole kitchen, pulling out drawers, finally looking in the freezer out of desperation! There were several other small 'forgettings.'

> "On August 8, I realized some dizziness, and my whole body ached from my toes to my neck. I felt as though I had arthritis. It hurt badly even to move an arm or my hand. I also felt severely depressed. At 10 PM, I took two acetaminophen tablets and went to bed; slept soundly, and arose in the morning feeling much better. I also began to drink considerable water to get the substance out of my system quickly.

> "Since that time, I have not touched anything sweetened with aspartame, and have experienced no unusual aches, memory loss or dizziness."

Case VI-G-3

A female aspartame reactor was delighted because of the dramatic improvement of her joint and muscle pain, confusion and impaired concentration after avoiding aspartame products for seven weeks. She had previously consumed diet colas daily. She added, "Another thing that has 100% disappeared is this awful restless and fidgeting feeling in my legs, especially during rest. For the past several months, I regularly felt like I wanted to crawl out of my own skin. That has vanished!"

III. The Tourette Syndrome

The Tourette syndrome is a chronic disorder characterized by motor and vocal tics generally beginning in childhood. (The condition and its comorbid psychiatric features is more appropriately termed "tic-related disorder.") These quick and involuntary movements occur repeatedly and nonrhythmically in the same way. The disorder probably represents neurotransmitter malfunction within the brain, current research focusing on postsynaptic dopamine hypersensitivity involving the basal ganglia.

These patients may suffer additional neuropsychiatric disorders – including hyperactivity, attention deficit disorder, learning disabilities, obsessive-compulsive behavior, sleep problems and inappropriate sexual activity. An impressive aspect being encountered at present is racial cursing.

I have urged the avoidance of aspartame products in this disorder (Roberts 1973c). Sheila Rogers, Director of the Alternative Therapy Network for Tourette Syndrome, informed me that some patients afflicted with the Tourette syndrome develop tics after ingesting aspartame products (personal communication, 1993). (Also see Chapter XVI)

In view of the possible genetic component, other family members also ought to avoid aspartame products.

Representative Case Report

Case VI-G-4

A 13-year-old boy was diagnosed as having a "motor tic disorder." His symptoms included twitching and jerking of the head and arms, coupled with anxiety attacks. Suspecting aspartame sodas as a responsible factor, his mother discontinued them. There

250

was steady improvement over the ensuing months. Shortly after he resumed drinking diet sodas four months later, the boy evidenced repetition of his "twitching and jerking."

IV. <u>Dopa-Responsive Dystonia</u>

Hereditary progressive dystonia is another neurologic disorder that usually affects children. It is exquisitely responsive to levodopa. Patients with this condition (at times misdiagnosed as cerebral palsy) can be adversely affected by ingesting phenylalanine because of decreased hepatic phenylalanine hydroxylase activity (Hyland 1997).

H. ATYPICAL AND UNEXPLAINED PAIN

A number of aspartame reactors complained of atypical pain in the face, neck, chest or abdomen. The nature of such peripheral nerve and spinal cord dysfunction proved baffling until improvement after the avoidance of aspartame products. It is probably a form of "visceral hyperalgesia" (*The Lancet* 2000; Volume 356:1127-1128).

There is repeated reference to "aches and pains" in other sections. For example, a 52-year-old antique dealer suffered severe pain in the face, at the base of her neck (for which she wore a neck brace), across both shoulders, and in the right hip area.

The subject of aspartame-induced joint pain will be discussed in Chapter IX-G.

Physicians have submitted case reports of atypical pain experienced both personally and by their patients while consuming aspartame products. The *Cortlandt Forum* published several.

- The April 1991 edition (p. 70) described a patient presenting with unexplained flank pain of several months duration that resolved when he stopped drinking iced tea containing aspartame. Another patient suffering low back pain became asymptomatic when switching to plain water or iced tea containing sweetened with sugar. The editor commented: "We have received several reports incriminating aspartame as a cause of muscle pain."
- A Miami physician reported that he had been playing tennis for 30 years without experiencing cramping of the muscles. When this problem occurred one year previously, the only change was the addition of aspartame to coffee and diet drinks. The cramping ceased when he avoided aspartame (October 1990, p. 44).

- Dr. William Duerfeldt asked the editor, "Are there any studies linking the artificial sweetener aspartame with musculoskeletal pain and weakness?" (February 19, 1990, p. 79). This query stemmed from several patients who insisted that aspartame caused muscle pain, weakness, tender points, fatigue and morning stiffness. Their symptoms disappeared after eliminating aspartame products.

I. Facial Pain

Atypical facial pain occurred in 70 (6 percent) of 1200 aspartame reactors.

Dentists are more likely to encounter this problem. In fact, my initial awareness of its severity occurred while interviewing a dental surgeon who had unrecognized aspartame disease. His severe facial pain disappeared shortly after discontinuing aspartame products. Owing to this personal interest, he promptly found two of his patients with unexplained facial pain who used considerable aspartame.

Correspondents who had suffered intense facial pain expressed frustration and anger over the failure of doctors to inquire about their high aspartame intake. A Pennsylvania patient wrote

> "I have been under a neurosurgeon's care for a number of years for the treatment of trigeminal neuralgia and severe daily headaches. Recently I had an MRI, and CT scans prior to that. Since many of the resulting problems from consuming aspartame also seem to be mine, and having been an almost daily user of diet sodas, we of course are wondering whether this could be a contributing factor to my problem."

Representative Case Reports

Case VI-H-1

A 42-year-old man developed severe pain and loss of feeling over the left face. He had been consuming two cans of diet cola and six packets of an ATS daily. Numerous studies for these and concomitant symptoms during two hospitalizations proved normal. They subsided shortly after stopping these aspartame products.

Case VI-H-2

A young woman spoke to me during a Cleveland radio talk show about her prior severe symptoms caused by aspartame products. The most distressing had been unilateral facial pain for three years. She also experienced severe headaches. She consulted many physicians, and had both CT scans and MRI studies. These complaints ceased when she stopped aspartame as a result of her own intuition.

II. Misdiagnosed "Headache"

Various erroneous diagnoses had been made for the atypical severe "headache" in patients with unrecognized aspartame disease. They included cranial and cervical neuropathies and temporomandibular joint (TMJ) dysfunction. None responded satisfactorily until stopping aspartame.

Representative Case Report

Case VI-H-3

The 44-year-old president of a large insurance firm had been troubled with headache for six months. It was sufficiently severe to "cause me to be short with my staff and clients." His pain had been attributed to the TMJ syndrome, but persisted after extensive dental work for this alleged condition.

Other problems developed. Blurred vision of both eyes began to affect his performance. An elevation of blood pressure was found for the first time notwithstanding his ideal body weight.

I then questioned him about the use of aspartame products. He had been consuming three 12-ounce cans of diet sodas and five sticks of an aspartame gum daily. His symptoms improved shortly after discontinuing them. He retested himself ten times – with predictable recurrence of his complaints – before becoming convinced that aspartame triggered them.

III. Chest Pain

Eighty-five aspartame reactors (7 percent) experienced unexplained chest pain. This subject will be considered in detail in Chapter IX-G.

Physicians must consider a number of diagnostic possibilities in patients who present with atypical chest pain. They include disorders of the heart; chest wall tenderness, pleurisy from various causes, vertebral collapse associated with osteoporosis, tumors, and esophageal problems. A trial of abstinence from aspartame is indicated in persons who consume considerable amounts, especially when all studies prove normal.

I. SLURRING OF SPEECH

Overt slurring of speech – that is, when noticed by others – occurred in 124 (10 percent) aspartame reactors. It was <u>not</u> related to medication, a prior stroke, or drinking alcohol. This problem **promptly** subsided after abstinence from aspartame in most instances, and predictably recurred following rechallenge.

Slurred speech was particularly disturbing for professionals and persons in business whose jobs entailed personal interviews and frequent phone calls.

- A physician consuming large amounts of aspartame beverages told a nutritional consultant that he "looked wasted all the time, and eventually my speech became slurred" (cited by Reschersky 1986).
- One heavy user of aspartame sodas stated, "I've been having slurred speech with depression, and it scared me to death!" Both symptoms disappeared shortly after stopping aspartame.
- A 59-year-old man experienced attacks of slurred speech lasting two to eight hours, in conjunction with "crackling" and diminished hearing in both ears, while consuming three liters of aspartame beverages daily.
- A 55-year-old woman complained primarily of slurred speech and vision problems. Out of desperation, she typed "slurred speech" in a search engine on the Internet, and found a reference to aspartame disease. Her symptoms promptly improved after avoiding these products.

Aspartame-induced slurred speech initially had been attributed to a prior head injury in several instances (see Case VI-I-3), thereby compounding the diagnostic confusion.

<u>**Representative Case Reports**</u>

Case VI-I-1

A 53-year-old woman consumed considerable aspartame in cereal, coffee, tea and various soft drinks. She placed two envelopes of an aspartame packet into each cup of coffee. Speech became increasingly slurred. Her employer assumed it was due to a recent set of false teeth. Intense headaches, dizziness on sudden motion, and extreme depression also were experienced.

She then read an article about reactions to aspartame that mentioned her symptoms. All disappeared within three weeks after stopping aspartame products.

Case VI-I-2

A housewife expressed concern over "a bad problem with slurring of my words." Her family joked about it and the concomitant "lack of memory." She also experienced considerable visual difficulty, but an ophthalmologist could detect no problem.

While reading about comparable symptoms in aspartame disease, this association crystallized. She had been using an ATS and diet soda. Improvement promptly occurred when she avoided these products.

Case VI-I-3

A 22-year-old student sustained a head injury during an automobile accident in January 1986. He manifested slurred speech shortly after leaving the hospital. ("I could not effectively communicate verbally.") Concomitantly, there was extreme irritability and a striking change in personality.

To avoid gaining weight, he had been consuming 8-16 cans of diet cola and soft drinks, along with three packets of an ATS and one glass of presweetened iced tea daily.

Speech retraining was instituted. It seemed successful at first, but he regressed. At that point, "A friend of my father indicated that some of the speech problems I had been experiencing could be caused by aspartame. My mother sent for more information. Then I quit." His speech and other problems improved within two weeks, and disappeared by six weeks. The symptoms returned within two days after one rechallenge. He summarized his ordeal in these terms:

"Aspartame really had a devastating effect on my speech. Perhaps the depression or irritability was caused because I felt bad concerning the effect it had on my verbal communication. Quitting my consumption also has had a very favorable effect on my speech and demeanor."

J. TREMORS: POSSIBLE INSIGHTS CONCERNING PARKINSON'S DISEASE

One hundred and one (8 %) aspartame reactors in this series developed severe tremor. The condition usually represented exaggeration of the slight tremor demonstrable in most persons. A number of correspondents referred to this feature as "the twitch."

The subjects of hyperactivity and "restless legs" were considered in Chapter VI-G.

Essential Tremor

Aspartame-induced accentuation of "benign tremor" ("essential tremor") can spawn serious occupational and social problems. For example, a senior engineer found it difficult to control his handwriting when he consumed aspartame products.

Under these circumstances, patients with severe tremor are likely to seek medical consultation because they fear Parkinson's disease ("the shaking palsy"). The absence of muscle rigidity and other parkinsonian features, along with added clinical findings, generally indicate that this disease is not present. In the present context, prompt improvement after avoiding aspartame usually resolved the matter.

Aspartame users frequently inquired about their severe tremors during my talk-show interviews. This is illustrated by a woman who expressed concern over the recent intensification of her tremor on the Irv Homer program (Station WWDB in Philadelphia). Propranolol (Inderal®) had controlled it for several years. The tremor intensified, however, when she ingested considerable aspartame, notwithstanding a considerable increase in the dosage of propranolol.

Other Tremors

Other types of aspartame-associated "shaking" were encountered. For example, the "thumb twitches" in Case I-4 that developed shortly after consuming aspartame were subsequently diagnosed as "focal seizures."

Representative Case Reports

Case VI-J-1

The sister of a 59-year-old mentally retarded woman described the patient's "horror story" with aspartame. She started drinking 4-5 glasses of aspartame iced tea and diet sodas in July 1986. Shortly thereafter, she began "turning her head from side to side constantly, and was diagnosed as having Parkinson's disease." Progressively increased doses of Sinemet® afforded little improvement. A neurologist suspected a slight stroke.

After hearing me on a radio interview, the sister wrote

> "Since March 11, 1987, my sister has had nothing with aspartame, and her head no longer twists and turns. Before, she could not control the movement at all. It was constant and very annoying to her. While her consumption was not excessive – no more than four or five glasses of the drinks combined – it was enough to trigger her problem, which disappeared when aspartame was withdrawn."

Case VI-J-2

A 75-year-old homemaker consumed diet cola, ASDs, an ATS, aspartame chocolate mixes, presweetened iced tea mixes, and "sugar free" chewing gum. She feared having

> "... contracted a nervous condition since I had no control of my hands, feet and legs. I also had a slobbering condition. It was very discouraging and embarrassing, whether awake or asleep. The saliva poured out of my mouth, ran down my chin, and dripped onto my clothes. My clothing was always so soaked you could wring it out."

In addition to the tremors, she experienced severe headache, a marked decrease of vision in both eyes, unsteadiness of the legs, intense drowsiness, restless legs, and discomfort on swallowing. She pinpointed aspartame products as the cause when her symptoms improved several weeks after discontinuing them.

> "I was in and out of the hospital three times from May to July. During this time I was so ill I could not keep food or liquids down. Thereafter nothing with aspartame. I was home for a while after the third visit when I realized these conditions had left me. Since then, I will take nothing that might have aspartame in it. It was a <u>very frightening</u> time for me. I will <u>never</u> chance going through that experience again!"

Case VI-J-3

An Air Force fighter pilot told the U.S. Senate hearing held on November 3, 1987 that he developed uncontrollable tremors of the left arm while drinking "close to one gallon" of an aspartame soft drink mix daily. They were preceded by an aura of "butterflies in the stomach." In view of his marked sweating and thirst while stationed in hot climates, he would bring along a supply of the beverage on flights.

The tremors disappeared for six months when he was assigned to a remote area in Korea where he could not obtain this aspartame product. They recurred <u>one day</u> after ingesting it during October 1984 when he received a package from home. His considerable intake of aspartame resumed during January 1985 on returning to the United States, as did the tremors. He subsequently suffered a grand mal seizure which his physicians tried to relate to a minor head injury in a car accident ten years previously.

There was no recurrence of the tremor or seizure for two years after avoiding aspartame. Unfortunately, he was permanently grounded (with reduced pay) for an "idiopathic partial seizure disorder."

Case VI-J-4

The wife of a diabetic husband reported aspartame-induced tremors in this correspondence.

> "My husband started having shaking of the arms and legs, and would become very ill – requiring his being in bed for days at a time. The doctor ordered an MRI, but could not

give us a reason for these symptoms. We then noticed that he would have these symptoms, sometimes severe, whenever he took anything with aspartame. We finally decided to no longer use anything with aspartame. He has not had an attack since."

Case VI-J-5

A 62-year-old woman experienced violent and disabling reactions to aspartame products, from which she recovered after avoiding them. A major complaint was severe tremor.

The patient subsequently wrote about <u>her sister</u> who had been experiencing "terrible tremors." She was given information about aspartame-induced tremors. I received this message one month later: "My sister immediately stopped aspartame, and the tremors have decreased by 95 percent!"

Case VI-J-6

A 42-year-old woman described her "living hell for five months" because of "unbelievable tremors... sometimes light, but most often violent." She had been a heavy consumer of diet colas and an aspartame tabletop sweetener. After having been seen by four family physicians, three neurologists, and two emergency room doctors, "I decided to take a break from doctors, and started doing my own research." Improvement promptly followed aspartame abstinence.

Case VI-J-7

A female aspartame reactor stated, "I had muscle tremors while trying to go to sleep. They made it feel like we were having an earthquake. I completely stopped consuming any aspartame products the last five years, and have had no shaking sensations. But when I ate desserts not known to be sweetened with aspartame, the tremors returned."

Cases VI-J-8 and J-9

A home health aide described aspartame-aggravated tremors in herself <u>and</u> a patient.

Her previous "familial" tremor intensified to the point she could not drink a cup of coffee or play solitaire with the right hand. This proved highly embarrassing when she "shook worse than the people I am caring for." Her sister happened to visit, and suggested that she obtain information about aspartame disease. Within two weeks after avoiding aspartame products, "I could hold a cup in my right hand and play solitaire again." She subsequently helped care for a 43-year-old woman who was recovering from surgery. Commenting on the aide's slight tremor, the patient said that she also had it while drinking two liters of diet cola daily, with considerable improvement following aspartame abstinence.

Pathophysiologic Considerations

The "pacemaker" for essential tremor has been localized among serotonin-activated neurons in the inferior olivary nucleus (Longo 1985). The bilaterally increased glucose metabolism therein, demonstrated by position-emission topographic (PET) studies in patients with essential tremor (Boecker 1998), probably renders these areas more vulnerable to the metabolic effects of aspartame.

The alteration of serotonin and dopamine concentrations in the brain by phenylalanine and aspartame will be reviewed in Chapter XXIII. The following observations are germane.

- The enzyme phenylalanine hydroxylase converts phenylalanine to tyrosine. Tyrosine is first transformed into dihydroxyphenylalanine (levodopa), and then to dopamine.
- The two dopamine receptor subtypes (D1 and D2) exert synergistic effects on the firing rates of basal ganglia neurons (Walter 1987).
- The importance of dopaminergic pathways in severe tremor is further suggested by the effectiveness of levodopa in treating both parkinsonism and "restless legs" (von Scheele 1986).
- There is a reduction of brain dopamine in the presence of high concentrations of phenylalanine (*Congressional Record-Senate* 1985b, p. S 10846).
- Chronic exposure to excess phenylalanine and aspartic acid can decrease the levels of serotonin and other neurotransmitters within several regions of the brain. These changes, presumably compensatory adaptive mechanisms, may disturb important diurnal variations associated with feeding and the light/dark cycle.
- An ad by G. D. Searle & Company in the *Journal of the American Medical Association* (December 16, 1986) implied that excess activity of these excitatory amino acids could cause nerve cell destruction resembling the changes in degenerative disorders of the nervous system.

An Aspartame-Parkinsonism Connection?

These observations raise the question, "Can aspartame products initiate or aggravate changes in the brain that contribute to parkinsonism – specifically, within the substantia nigra which produces and stores dopamine?"

As many as one million persons in the United States are afflicted with parkinsonism, most over the age of 60. (The "idiopathic" form accounts for 85 percent of cases.) Its prevalence among persons older than 40 years approximates 357 per 100,000 population. It occurs less frequently in underdeveloped countries – e.g., 57 cases per 100,000 in China.

There is considerable evidence for a reduction of brain dopamine in parkinsonism. Conversely, levodopa and anticholinergic drugs have therapeutic benefit. The latter decrease the concentration of acetylcholine, a neurotransmitter that may cause a parkinsonism tremor when dopamine levels are reduced.

Repeated references to clinical deterioration and erratic therapeutic responses were encountered when patients with parkinsonism ingested aspartame products.

- Betty Martini, founder of Mission Possible (Chapter XXX), wrote

> "A friend was diagnosed with Parkinson's disease, and he appeared to be dying. His arms and legs would kick out and he had a hard time forming words. He was like a toy soldier out of control. He was an outstanding speaker, full of vim and vigor. It was shocking to see him being almost carried to a podium to speak, and have to read a prayer because he couldn't remember. It was at that time I called Dr. H.J. Roberts. He told me that aspartame changes the dopamine level of the brain, and to get him off aspartame right away because it was interacting with the L-Dopa he was taking. As soon as he abstained from aspartame he returned to normal; the kicking stopped, and he began to remember again. Five years later, when he celebrated his 50th wedding anniversary, I wept because I knew he would not have been alive had we not gotten him off aspartame."

- One patient who had done well on levodopa suffered intensification of his symptoms when the drug was "washed down with artificially sweetened black current." His symptoms dramatically improved after switching to the sugar-sweetened variety.
- Yale researchers reported considerable improvement of the crippling fluctuations of motor performance among patients with Parkinson's disease treated with levodopa by eliminating protein from breakfast and lunch (Pincus 1986). The antagonism of levodopa by protein – and presumably phenylalanine and other amino acids – probably reflects interference with its transport by neutral amino acids across the blood-brain barrier.
- Pincus et al (1987) demonstrated that elevated levels of the large neutral amino acids correlate with aggravated parkinsonian symptoms despite elevated plasma levodopa concentrations. These motor fluctuations decreased when the amino acid levels declined.

Additional information concerning the prevalence, clinical features, and deranged neurochemistry of parkinsonism suggest other possible adverse effects by aspartame. They may involve presynaptic dopamine deficiency, and alteration of the fine balance between dopaminergic and cholinergic systems within the brain. (An overbalance by the cholinergic system exists in parkinsonism.)

- The incidence of parkinsonism among younger persons has increased in recent years.
- There is greater awareness that patients with Parkinson's disease and dementia may manifest some of the "specific" symptoms (such as aphasia and visuospacial disturbances) present in Alzheimer's disease (Chui 1986, Roberts 1995b).
- Several authorities believe parkinsonism can be caused by environmental toxins that damage the substantia nigra, leading to "abiotrophy" (the premature and selective destruction) of functionally related neurones (Calne 1986). As a case in point, this disorder has occurred in young drug users exposed to illicit neurotoxic drugs, especially 1-methyl-4-phenyl-1,2,3,6-tetrahydropyridine (MPTP) and its metabolic product 1-methyl-4-phenylpyridine (MPP).
- A comparable interrelationship is the amyotrophic lateral sclerosis-parkinsonism complex in Guam caused by ingesting one or several alanine-derived amino acids (Spencer 1987). Such damage may remain "subclinical" for several years or decades.

Other biochemical observations are relevant.

- Aspartame can interfere with dopamine release in the brain (Chapter XXIII).
- Whereas the intraperitoneal administration of phenylalanine to rats in doses from 200-500 mg/kg increases basal dopamine release, the administration of 100 mg/kg reduces dopamine release (During 1987).
- The methyl alcohol derived from aspartame (Chapter XXI) probably plays a role. McLean et al (1980) reported parkinsonism and other neurologic abnormalities in two patients with methanol intoxication. Methyl alcohol appears to cause parkinsonism through postsynaptic dysfunction, perhaps by interfering with dopamine reuptake at nerve terminals.
- Symmetrical necrosis and hemorrhage of the putamen have been found in a number of patients with methanol intoxication.

Returning to the question introducing this section, Elble (2000) editorialized on the pathophysiology of essential tremor, parkinsonism and cerebellar intention tremor. Although they involve different parts of the motor system, he noted that "the collective rhythmicity of widely distributed neuronal networks seems to be necessary for the clinical expression of tremor."

K. NARCOLEPSY; SLEEP APNEA

Severe sleepiness and related "extreme fatigue" not attributable to other causes was a prominent complaint by 150 aspartame reactors (13 percent).

- Some developed pathologic drowsiness after chewing only single stick of aspartame gum (see Case VI-K-1).
- Case VI-K-2 suffered these symptoms and aspartame-associated intellectual deterioration.

Clinical Considerations

Narcolepsy is a <u>common</u> condition characterized by inappropriate and oft-uncontrollable drowsiness and sleep. Its subtleties and medical ramifications are legion. Three decades ago, I estimated that it afflicts at least 10 million persons in the United States (Roberts 1964b,c; 1971b).

The prevalence of narcolepsy can be inferred from entrenchment of "the coffee break" and "the cola break," as well as our society's enormous consumption of caffeine and other stimulants. I have personally observed and documented more than 1,100 patients with the syndrome of narcolepsy and hypoglycemia (Roberts 1964, 1971).

The four components of the narcolepsy complex are referred to as "the narcoleptic tetrad." Whenever narcolepsy was encountered in aspartame reactors, one or more concomitant features often could be recalled.

- Narcolepsy. *Narcolepsy is diagnosed largely on the basis of an adequate history.* Its hallmarks are irresistible drowsiness and inappropriate sleep. An important criterion is intrusive somnolence after a conventional night's rest, the absence of physical fatigue, and under conditions ordinarily conducive to enhanced alertness (e.g., driving a vehicle).
- Cataplexy. Cataplexy describes brief attacks of decreased muscular tone or flaccid paralysis, especially in the lower limbs while standing. It is commonly precipitated by some sudden emotional episode such as laughter, surprise or anger. During an attack, the person feels limp; at times the legs may buckle.
- Hypnagogic hallucinations. These hallucinations – or vivid dream-like experiences – have a more nightmarish impact than conventional dreams. They may be visual or auditory.
- Sleep paralysis. Such "night palsy" describes a brief inability to move the extremities. The frightening attack may occur either on awakening (postdormital) or before falling asleep.

Many physicians are reluctant to make a diagnosis of narcolepsy because of its social, economic or psychologic threat, and the need to monitor prescribed alertness-inducing (analeptic) drugs. As a result, substitute diagnoses are made, such as "chronic psychosomatic fatigue."

The symptomatic benefit of methylphenidate (Ritalin®) in narcolepsy (Roberts 1964; 1971b) and attention-deficit disorder/hyperactivity (Roberts 1969b) also reflects its action as dopamine reuptake inhibitor – that is, enabling more circulating dopamine.

Aspartame and Narcolepsy

Aspartame can precipitate or aggravate severe sleepiness (see representative case reports). Some of my patients in their 30s and 40s developed aspartame-induced narcolepsy of such magnitude that they infrequently went out in the evening, and would have to retire as early as 8 PM. While the caffeine present in coffee, tea and cola drinks can partially ameliorate their drowsiness, any aspartame therein is likely to counteract the analeptic effect.

Alterations of neurotransmitter activity affecting wakefulness, especially norepinephrine (Chapter XXIII), are likely mechanisms. A brief commentary on the phenomenon of alertness appears in Chapter VI-L.

The initiation or aggravation of narcolepsy by aspartame and its metabolites poses another major health issue: safety (Chapters VII and XXVII) (see Case VI-K-3). I reviewed this subject in *Ignored Health Hazards for Pilots and Drivers* (Roberts 1998d).

- The National Highway Transportation Safety Administration found that driving when drowsy accounted for 100,000 motor-vehicle crashes a year between 1990 and 1995.
- Irresistible sleep in commercial airline pilots ("navigator snooze") has become a major problem in aviation safety (*The Miami Herald* December 23, 1986, p. A-11). The same applies to air traffic control personnel.
- The potential hazards of dozing by on-duty operators and supervisors at the control room of nuclear power stations is regarded by the Nuclear Regulatory Commission as "an immediate threat to the public health and safety" (*Sun-Sentinel* Fort Lauderdale, April 1, 1987, p. A-3).

The localized neurotoxic effects of aspartame and its breakdown products are inferred from the narcoleptic dog model. Siegel and colleagues (1999) demonstrated a degeneration of axons in the forebrains of these dogs peaking just before or at the onset of narcolepsy. (These observations also extend to the neurotoxic effects of MSG and other excitotoxins.) The absence of cells in the hypothalamus that secrete a hormone called hypocretin (orexin), noted independently by several observers (*Nature Medicine* August 30, 1000), is consistent with their destruction by a neurotoxin such as aspartame. The classic features of narcolepsy occur in genetically engineered mice that do not produce this hormone.

Representative Case Reports

Case VI-K-1

A 45-year-old salesman listed severe drowsiness as his foremost reaction to consuming aspartame. This sequence was repeated on at least four occasions. He stated, "Just recently I discovered as I'm driving my automobile that chewing aspartame gum caused drowsiness, even after chewing only half a stick. It caused me to yawn, and to feel sleepy and weak. Sometimes I had to stop driving and close my eyes for a few minutes."

Other aspartame-induced complaints included dizziness, unsteadiness, marked hyperactivity of the limbs, abdominal pain, weight gain, frequency of urination (both day and night), and poor control of diabetes notwithstanding strict adherence to diet and taking his oral medications.

Case VI-K-2

A 48-year-old word-processing coordinator experienced intense drowsiness within one day after ingesting aspartame soft drinks. This sequence recurred on two retesting trials. She then had to discontinue such products because the sleepiness was undermining her performance at work.

Case VI-K-3

A 51-year-old letter carrier developed "drowsiness, sleep apnea and narcolepsy while consuming aspartame, both as diet colas and a tabletop sweetener." He had increased their intake greatly over the previous six months. Other complaints included severe dizziness, marked memory loss, "personality changes," shortness of breath, nausea, intense thirst,, frequent urination at night, a marked decrease of vision in one eye, and ringing in one ear. The cost of consultations and tests – including a CT scan of the brain, lumbar puncture, electroencephalogram, a cardiac stress test, and special eye and ear studies – was estimated at $3,500.

He rechallenged himself with aspartame products two times before becoming convinced they induced these symptoms – that is, his complaints predictably recurred within three days. Although most disappeared within four weeks after abstaining from aspartame, the tendency to severe drowsiness persisted.

Case VI-K-4

An 80-year-old homemaker developed many symptoms after drinking aspartame in soft drinks and hot chocolate. The most disturbing was severe sleepiness. She stated, "I fell asleep suddenly at such places as hockey games, baseball games, church, etc."

Other complaints included blurred vision, ringing in both ears, severe headache, dizziness, marked unsteadiness of the legs, "inside shaking," mental confusion, memory loss, slurred speech, extreme irritability, "anxiety attacks," palpitations and abdominal bloat. Her daughter also experienced headache, ringing in the ears, and visual difficulty after using aspartame products.

Sleep Apnea

Sleep apnea is increasingly recognized as a serious problem. Patients with this disorder generally complain of intense fatigue, drowsiness and "insomnia." They may not breathe for a minute or longer during sleep. (The severe "snoring" that ends apneic episodes serves as a diagnostic clue.) A concomitant decrease of oxygen to the brain and heart could be disastrous.

Several callers to talk-show hosts interviewing me about reactions to aspartame products spontaneously raised the associated problem of sleep apnea. Moreover, they volunteered this information in the absence of any reference to breathing problems (Chapter IX-C).

The significant cognitive impairment that may develop in patients with sleep apnea can improve dramatically with appropriate treatment (Scheltens 1991b). It consists of weight reduction, the avoidance of alcohol, smoking and sedatives, mechanical or surgical procedures that insure an adequate airway, and some drugs. Avoidance of aspartame products must be added to this list.

Relatives of several heavy aspartame consumers who had "stopped breathing" while asleep suspected an aspartame reaction. They were told that the cause of death was "not getting enough oxygen because of inefficient lungs" and "something was wrong with the communication center of the brain." Indeed, one explanation for sleep apnea is neurotransmitter dysfunction (Chapter XXIII) involving an area in the brain stem that controls respiration.

Representative Case Reports

Case VI-K-5

A 75-year-old patient had been treated for hypertension and a myocardial infarction (heart attack). His wife subsequently analyzed the recent deterioration of his memory, coupled with severe daytime drowsiness. She volunteered concern over the lapse of a minute or longer before he resumed breathing while asleep. As a result, she had been staying up most of the night to monitor him.

In view of his consumption of aspartame, I recommended a trial of abstinence from these products. The sleep apnea, drowsiness and confusion improved dramatically, and did not recur over the next eight months of observation. Accordingly, the planned referral to a sleep apnea center was cancelled.

Case VI-K-6

A 44-year-old nonobese woman was seen by several internists and neurologists for severe sleep apnea. Two sleep studies had failed to clarify the cause. This patient also had "gasping attacks" and severe headache during the day. When she discontinued her considerable intake of diet sodas, these complaints ceased.

L. INTELLECTUAL DETERIORATION

My personal consultations, considerable correspondence, many telephone calls, and the detailed notes accompanying completed survey questionnaire provide poignant evidence that profound intellectual deterioration can be attributed to aspartame disease. The implications are profound.

Associated confusion and memory loss (Chapter VI-C) also posed great problems for students, professionals and persons in business. In some instances, they persisted months or longer after the cessation of aspartame products.

These problems become compounded when other treatable medical disorders remain unrecognized. Case VI-L-2 illustrates the importance of undetected hypothyroidism and hypoglycemia in persons manifesting aspartame-associated intellectual and behavioral changes.

Individuals involved with the care of mentally handicapped persons anguished over their consumption of aspartame products. A Philadelphia woman wrote, "I work at a residential facility for multi-handicapped young adults. I am concerned about the amount of aspartame consumed there."

Representative Case Reports

Case VI-L-1

A 29-year-old public relations executive consumed up to three packets of an ATS and one glass of aspartame hot chocolate daily for two years. Her ability to read became severely impaired. She described "letters transposing themselves. I thought I was losing my mind." Other problems included "floating spots" in both eyes, severe headache, marked irritability, a change in personality, palpitations, a nonspecific rash, and marked thinning of the hair.

These symptoms improved within one week after stopping aspartame products when she read an article about aspartame disease. They recurred within several days during retesting trials.

Case VI-L-2

An 18-year-old college student used diet colas and an ATS in an attempt to control her weight. She also chewed several sticks of aspartame gum daily.

This outstanding student previously had been in good health. She also was a skilled typist and pianist. The director of an honors program at a major university even congratulated her for proficiency in the introductory economics course during the previous semester. He wrote, "On the basis of your performance, you appear to be an excellent candidate for the honors program."

Dramatic intellectual deterioration coincided with her continued consumption of aspartame. Her I.Q. dropped 20 points, and she became incapacitated academically. Other features included severe headache, a marked decrease of vision in one eye, dizziness, unsteadiness, intense drowsiness, tremors, insomnia, depression with suicidal thoughts, extreme irritability, a change in personality, abdominal pain, recurrent nausea, cessation of her menstrual periods, and a weight gain of 15 pounds.

She was seen by many physicians and consultants, and underwent numerous tests – including two CT scans and one MRI study of the brain. An electroencephalogram suggested petit mal. Multiple medications for a presumed primary depression and possible organic brain syndrome proved ineffective.

I saw this patient in consultation during December 1986. Other important aspects of her history that had not been previously ascertained included the following:

- She predictably experienced drowsiness after using aspartame, such as falling asleep in class about 9 AM and during the early afternoon. Furthermore, she began to doze while driving on several occasions. Suspecting inebriation, a policeman stopped her one morning.
- She felt recurrent severe weakness, "draining of my energy" and intense hunger, particularly after exercising.
- Marked "twitching" and tremor of the hands made typing and playing the piano increasingly difficult.
- Overt restless legs was noted during the initial interview.
- Other features included intermittent severe itching, burning on urination, and the absence of menses for six months while on aspartame. (Her periods normalized after discontinuing it.)
- Her skin became markedly dry, and she was highly intolerant to cold.
- There was a history of both diabetes and goiter in close relatives.

Many of the patient's symptoms already had improved within one month after stopping aspartame products on the advice of friends. Her headache, dizziness and inability to concentrate, however, persisted at the time of my consultation.

Dry skin and a café-au-lait spot were noted on physical examination. Supplementary studies revealed the presence of hypothyroidism, the thyroid stimulating hormone (TSH) level being 13.2 (normal 1-5). She also evidenced reactive hypoglycemia during a morning glucose tolerance test. The study was terminated prematurely (at 3-1/2 hours) because of a clinically-severe hypoglycemic reaction. The results were as follows:

	GLUCOSE (mg percent)	INSULIN (μU/ml)
Fasting	115	6.6
½ hour	230	73.8
1-hour	127	54.3
2-hours	120	89.2
3-hours	81	-----
3-1/2 hours	70* (test stopped)	

The patient was advised to continue aspartame abstinence, and given an appropriate diet and a prescription for thyroxine (Synthroid). Gratifying clinical and academic improvement ensued.

Case VI-L-3

A 23-year-old student had been consuming aspartame cola beverages. She developed severe drowsiness, marked memory loss, confusion, petit mal seizures, tremors, tingling and numbness of the limbs, intense depression with suicidal thoughts, extreme irritability, anxiety, and other personality changes. She also complained of decreased vision in both eyes, marked sensitivity to noise, attacks of rapid heart action, abdominal pain and nausea, bloody diarrhea, joint pains, and the loss of menstrual periods.

Her mother also suffered severe reactions to aspartame, especially the precipitation of migraine attacks. She conveyed the magnitude of her daughter's mental and intellectual deterioration in this letter.

"My daughter's reactions to products containing aspartame has been far more serious than mine for several reasons. For nearly two years, she was unaware of the possible connection between her medical problems and aspartame. Her father and I were not aware of the nature of her problems. We were therefore unable to suggest a possible connection between the two. She continued to consume aspartame, and her condition worsened.

"J___ was living in another state, completing her graduate studies, so we did not have the opportunity to see her very often. However, her behavior became more and more bewildering. My mother's intuition told me that something was amiss. I hammered at her relentlessly by phone. She was reluctant to discuss her health with me by telephone or letter, so I tried to visit her. I was unable to find her in her apartment. Finally, and nearly too late, she announced (April 1986) that she was experiencing bizarre symptoms with increasing frequency. She said that she thought she was losing her mind, so she had consulted a neurologist (late 1985). He diagnosed her as having temporal lobe epilepsy. At the time, she decided to learn to live with 'epilepsy' and not even tell her family about it. Much later (May or June of 1986), when I spoke to him, he said that his diagnosis 'was not etched in granite.'

"After my daughter told me of her symptoms, I pondered for several days. It suddenly occurred to me that aspartame could have triggered her seizures, etc., since I knew that beverages sweetened with aspartame caused me to experience migraine attacks. I explained my theory to J＿ over the telephone and in letters.

"However, her personality had changed so much that she was totally uncooperative, and simply would not listen to me. Her behavior was most peculiar and uncharacteristic. It took me five months to track down her friends, and convince them to beg J＿ to stop drinking aspartame sodas. Only after she stopped consuming them did she realize that aspartame had ruined her physical and mental health.

"J＿ began an excellent job as a financial analyst for a large corporation in April 1986. At the time, she was still drinking products sweetened with aspartame because I had not yet convinced her to stop. After 5 weeks, she was too 'disabled' to continue. I wasn't the least bit surprised! She was having headaches, hallucinations, déjà vu, abdominal cramps, acid stomach, menstrual irregularities, unbelievable mood swings, paranoid states, depression, sleep problems, diarrhea, etc. She was vomiting often, especially after eating meat or dairy products. She also noticed blood with her bowel movements. From then on, her physical and mental health continued to deteriorate at a rapid rate until September 1986, when she finally was convinced to stop consuming aspartame in any form.

"J＿ is an uncommonly brilliant girl with the possibilities of a magnificent future. (When in high school, she won a Telluride Association Scholarship. She competed with more than one million students from the entire United States for this honor.

She was two years younger than all the other students. As an example, she scored in the 98th percentile nationally in all areas on her GMATs.) I sincerely believe that her life and her future have been jeopardized by aspartame.

"In addition to her other problems I mentioned, J__ divorced a wonderful husband. She eventually lost the ability to remember, all before she was finally convinced to discontinue the ingestion of aspartame it was an unbelievably frightening, frustrating time for J__, her ex-husband, her friends, and her family. It is thanks to you and Shannon Roth, and the information you have provided, that my daughter is feeling better each day. She is trying to pick up the pieces of a life shattered by aspartame. Everyone is praying that the situation will be completely reversible, but only time will tell."

In a subsequent telephone discussion, the mother stated that her daughter had continued to abstain from aspartame since our initial correspondence, and was feeling better everyday. In fact, she had since applied for a Ph.D. program. Unfortunately, she relapsed several years later and suffered aspartame addiction (see Chapter VII-G.)

Case VI-L-4

This correspondent joined the Air Force at the age of 18. Obtaining a perfect score on the Armed Forces Qualifications Test for general intelligence, he was sent to a university for training in the Russian language. A classmate accused him of having a "photographic memory." After leaving the military, he received an appointment as press secretary to the governor of his state. He subsequently wrote speeches for four governors.

"The Dark Ages" occurred after September 1982 when he began using aspartame products in an attempt to avoid sugar. There was a "constant downward spiraling" in his personal and professional life, during which "my ability to be creative ceased to exist." He also suffered severe headaches, numbness in the fingers and toes, extreme fatigue, knee pain, outbursts and poor judgment. His difficulty in both memory and language fluency (including German) proved frustrating, and caused him to lose one job after another.

He wrote, "I concluded in July 1991 that something serious was wrong with my brain, and intuitively felt the problem had to be chemical. The only 'foreign' substance in my diet was caffeine-free aspartame cola."

His "renaissance" came within three days after avoiding all aspartame products – most notably with a return of mental clarity. He now could meet people and remember their names. His remarkable memory and creativity returned as evidenced by the writing of poetry, songs and a self-help book, and the enjoyment of reading complex material. "I am convinced beyond a reasonable doubt that aspartame, used even in modest quantities, negatively affects the central nervous system of virtually all, if not all, human users of it."

Case VI-L-5

A teacher with aspartame disease suffered fibromyalgia and neuropathic symptoms. It also triggered Graves disease (Chapter IX-E).

Another manifestation involved difficulty in speaking languages. "Brain fog" while consuming aspartame products not only impaired her ability to speak Italian and Spanish, but also English. These and the other symptoms disappeared after aspartame avoidance. An exacerbation lasting one week occurred when she later inadvertently drank an aspartame soda.

Case VI-L-6

A 21-year-old student had been "highly functional" until developing depression, severe irritability and a dramatic personality change for which she was hospitalized four months. She had become "almost non-verbal" prior to hospitalization. Other features included marked unsteadiness, "silent seizures," severe insomnia, confusion, memory loss, and hyperactivity. She had been consuming various aspartame products – including sodas, puddings and gum.

A professor of psychiatry and pediatrics made the diagnosis of "mental retardation." The patient's grandmother, however, was concerned about aspartame disease. Although she presented considerable information about aspartame reactions to her granddaughter's attending physicians at the hospital, they would not consider this possibility! Within one week after stopping aspartame products, the patient "improved immensely".

Case VI-L-7

The following communication was received from the husband of a 31-year-old professional who suffered severe confusion, memory loss, and an impressive decline of her IQ.

*   *   *   *   *

Dear Dr. Roberts,

My wife was diagnosed in 1991 as being hypoglycemic. When advised to cut down on her use of sugar, she switched to aspartame products. She used a lot as she had always had a sweet tooth. Even so, she maintained her body weight at around 100 pounds. Her height is 5'6".

She is a Certified Public Accountant and was the controller for an electronics manufacturing company at the time. She began having difficulty at work, and worked longer and longer to keep up. Eventually, she was working seven days a week for 10 to 14 hours a day. Her health began to deteriorate. Finally, I convinced her to resign, thinking the company was making unreasonable demands on her.

I helped her get a job as office manager for a real estate company through contacts I had, thinking this would give her a change of pace and let her recover from near burnout. She was laid off from this job in less than six months. She then took a position as a parttime bookkeeper, but was laid off from that job as well. I told her to just quit as we didn't really need her income, and take some time off. We were now approaching the end of 1992.

She started helping me in my business (mortgage loans). I discovered she had difficulty following simple directions. It also was incredibly hard to teach her new software programs. It became clear to me she was having difficulty with short-term memory. We went to our medical provider to discuss this. She was referred to a neurologist, received a CT scan, and had complete neuropsychological testing in 1993. No problem could be discovered other than suffering severe short-term memory loss and confusion. I think they suspected physical abuse, but later ruled that out as I have never struck or threatened to strike my wife. (We were married in 1967. Neither of us had been married previously.)

In early 1995, we repeated the neurologic review and neuropsychological testing. She showed a decline in IQ from the 93 scored in 1993 to 72 in 1995! Again, we were given no probable cause for the difficulty.

We visited a naturopathic doctor in mid-1995 and were referred to Dr. _____. He had a complete blood chemistry examination done, but could find no abnormality. While visiting him, I discovered your letter on page 99 of the August/September 1995 issue of the *Townsend Letter*. Dr. _____ confirmed that my wife's condition could be caused by aspartame if your studies were correct. My wife immediately quit using aspartame, and has not used it now for over a year. She still suffers from some short-term memory loss and confusion. Another MRI showed no overlooked cause.

Comments on Perception and Attention

Some of the biophysiologic derangements in aspartame disease that can influence alertness, perception and attention were mentioned in Chapter VI-C. Others are considered in Section 5. These functions influence a dynamic state of cerebral activity that affects intellectual performance.

Only a few references to the vast research and literature involving this realm are presented. They are fundamental to understanding "intelligence" and impaired alertness (See Chapter VI-K).

- Audley (1964) asserted that perception conveyed by the senses encompasses all the processes involved in an organic transaction with the environment, including a virtual reconstruction of the world based on numerous fragmentary clues.
- Lindsley (1960) closely allied attention to arousal and wakefulness, being a graded phenomenon that extends from general alerting to specific alerting.
- Arousal involves a heightening of attentiveness that helps individuals to act and learn (Berlyne 1966). The term "collective stimulus properties" designates certain aspects of behavior influenced by novel, complex, surprising, puzzling or ambiguous stimuli.
- The reticular activating system of the brain is crucial to such arousal by sharpening sensory, musculoskeletal, and reflex preparedness (Franch 1957). Metabolic and neurotoxin-induced dysfunction therein may be manifested as severe sleepiness.
- Ittleson and Kilpatrick (1951) described perception as a functional phenomenon based on action, experience and probability – the thing perceiving being "an inseparable part of the function of perceiving, which in turn includes all aspects of the total process of living."

M. MYASTHENIA GRAVIS

Myasthenia gravis is a form of generalized muscular weakness in which one or both upper eyelids characteristically droop (ptosis). It is usually diagnosed by demonstrating prompt but transient improvement after the intravenous administration of edrophonium chloride (Tensilon®). Treatment consists of pyridostigmine bromide (Mestinon®) and other measures.

I attended three female patients in whom overt drooping of the eyelids and marked muscle weakness **first** developed after consuming aspartame products (Roberts 1991c). The diagnosis of myasthenia gravis had not been raised in any examination during at least a decade of doctoring. All experienced improvement of other aspartame-related complaints when they avoided aspartame, but not of the ptosis or severe fatigue. Each patient evidenced a diagnostic response to intravenous edrophonium, and subsequent improvement on pyridostigmine. Two were able to stop this drug after avoiding aspartame, but not Case VI-M-1.

These observations and others (see below) suggest that aspartame can precipitate or aggravate latent myasthenia gravis.

Representative Case Report

Case VI-M-1

An 82-year-old insulin-dependent diabetic presented with drooping of the right eyelid, a finding not noted during many years of personal observation. At times, she had to manually elevate the lid. Her ophthalmologist recommended an operation to "pull up the skin."

The contributory role of aspartame was suggested by the large amounts she had been consuming prior to the onset of generalized muscle weakness. Associated symptoms included memory loss, confusion, dizziness, insomnia, and loss of diabetic control despite careful home glucose monitoring and appropriate adjustments of insulin dosage. Within one week after stopping aspartame products, these problems improved except for the eyelid drooping.

Three observers witnessed a dramatic response to edrophonium testing. Pyridostigmine afforded gratifying improvement. The ptosis promptly returned two months later after a brief attempt to discontinue it, however, necessitating resumption of the medication.

Input From the Questionnaire (Section 4)

Six other aspartame reactors who completed the survey questionnaire reinforced this association. Two with both ptosis and virtual inability to lift themselves out of bed had been diagnosed and treated for myasthenia.

The drooping of one or both eyelids, and the generalized muscle weakness in two other aspartame reactors had been attributed to "aging" by their physicians.

A 31-year-old woman indicated that she had been taking pyridostigmine two years for myasthenia gravis. She previously consumed three cans of diet soda daily to lose weight. On retesting herself three times, she predictably experienced severe headache, dizziness, tremors, insomnia, nausea, diarrhea and vomiting within one day.

The additional case of a man with aspartame-related "ocular myasthenia" was submitted by his wife.

Pertinent Shortcomings of the Questionnaire

Inasmuch as an aspartame-myasthenia connection had not been considered when devising the initial survey questionnaire, it did not inquire about drooping of the eyelids.

Another problem was the inability to document details of other persons with aspartame disease and suspected myasthenia because they wished to remain anonymous, and failed to provide their addresses.

Commentary

Mention was made in Chapter IV of the inability by ophthalmologists to detect intrinsic eye problems in most aspartame reactors who complained of trouble focusing their eyes. In retrospect, some may have had weakness of their extrocular muscles due to myasthenia gravis.

278

The precipitation or aggravation of latent myasthenia gravis by aspartame reflects pathophysiologic changes induced by this chemical and its three components (phenylalanine; aspartic acid; methanol). The likely mechanisms include metabolic effects on muscle or the neuromuscular junction, and altered neurotransmitter function, especially cholinergic transmission (Section 5).

One of these patients previously developed anemia from methyldopa (Aldomet®) that had been prescribed for her hypertension. Since myasthenia is currently regarded as an autoimmune phenomenon, this autoimmune response is consistent with other immunologic observations (Chapter VIII).

N. PSEUDOTUMOR CEREBRI

Six patients in this series were formally diagnosed by neurologists as having pseudotumor cerebri (benign intracranial hypertension) before aspartame disease was considered -- generally by the patient, relatives or friends after reading about aspartame reactions.

All were women in their 20s and 30s. Concerned about weight, they consumed considerable aspartame, chiefly as diet sodas. Their extensive studies and treatments are illustrated in the case reports. These ranged from repeated lumbar puncture for reducing cerebrospinal pressure to ventricular shunt procedures.

Diagnostic Considerations

The diagnosis of pseudotumor cerebri is generally based on evidence for increased intracranial pressure, and the absence of a mass lesion (brain tumor), infection, obstruction of the brain's ventricular system, or focal neurologic signs. The most prominent features are headache and eye abnormalities (decreased vision; papilledema; visual field loss; extraocular palsies).

- None of the patients had taken corticosteroids, excessive vitamin A, or other drugs incriminated in this disorder (e.g., tetracycline; nalidixic acid).
- One patient developed concomitant diabetes insipidus. It also improved dramatically after aspartame avoidance.

Representative Case Reports

Case VI-N-1

The mother of two young children stated, "I used to drink aspartame by the hour." She was diagnosed by <u>five</u> neurologists as having pseudotumor cerebri.

This patient suddenly developed "floaters" and a large blind spot in the left eye. She also suffered severe nausea and fatigue. A neuro-ophthalmologist told her that she would be blind unless a ventricular shunt was performed to drain the excess cerebrospinal fluid causing pressure on the optic nerve. The surgery was done in March 1998. Most of her symptoms persisted, however, especially severe headache, nausea, and numbness of the feet and fingers.

Several persons, including her father-in-law, had given her information about aspartame disease. She initially ignored it, but finally decided to stop aspartame products. "I saw major results. The headaches were not as bad, and the other symptoms did not bother me as much. My children didn't believe I was actually with them!"

Case VI-N-2

A registered nurse with an extensive professional background in neurology and psychiatry was diagnosed as having pseudotumor cerebri in February 1997. Intent upon losing weight, she had consumed considerable amounts of aspartame products beginning in January 1997. She then experienced "fullness in my head, dizziness that wouldn't go away, panic attacks, and a squishy feeling in my head." Severe headache ensued, leading to multiple neurologic consultations and studies.

This nurse then realized that the only significant change in her habits had been use of aspartame products. She stopped them in April 1997. Her symptoms virtually disappeared. The "headache and strange feelings" would recur, however, if she drank any aspartame soda. In the meantime, the numerous lumbar punctures to lower cerebrospinal fluid pressure were discontinued.

Case VI-N-3

A 31-year-old woman with diagnosed pseudotumor cerebri wrote

280

"I used aspartame in my tea in the morning, diet cola during the day, and aspartame sodas all evening. Nothing touched my lips unless it was aspartame. When someone told me about reactions, I stopped using aspartame, and am doing much better!! They may not even do the brain surgery now to relieve the increased pressure."

Commentary

In a previous medical textbook (Roberts 1958, p. 336), I noted that "the greatest frequency of this disease is among women under the age of thirty." Similarly, Wilson and Gardner (1966) emphasized the association of obesity and pseudotumor cerebri. Forty-eight of their 61 consecutive cases were characterized as "fat young women."

The importance of considering aspartame disease under these circumstances is obvious. Such patients usually have a good prognosis, and can be spared much anxiety and formidable medical or surgical interventions if aspartame disease is recognized.

Several attending physicians confirmed the striking improvement after aspartame abstinence. For example, the decreased vision and headaches markedly improved in a patient (not cited above) after avoiding aspartame several weeks. Her physician was impressed that there were only three or four blind spots in her visual fields, whereas "the whole outer circle had been grayish for almost halfway in."

Additional patients with aspartame disease probably fell in this category, but were excluded because other diagnoses had not been definitively ruled out.

A third-year medical student was not included because "a membrane blockage between the third and fourth ventricle" had not yet been analyzed. She refused to quit aspartame products despite pleas from her parents (each a nationally known author). They stated that "she gives the typical medical arguments to refute what you (the author) says."

This patient had developed blurred vision, severe headaches, and problems with speech while consuming considerable diet sodas and coffee sweetened with an ATS prior to her final exams. An MRI study suggested enlargement of the lateral and third ventricles "but they are not sure." At the time, a "natural shunt" was being considered.

In addition to the <u>pathophysiologic mechanisms</u> reviewed earlier, aspartame-induced fluid disturbances (Chapter IX-F) and cerebral edema caused by methanol poisoning (Chapter XXI) may contribute to pseudotumor cerebri.

O. UNEXPLAINED "BLACKOUTS"

Individual patients with unexplained "blackouts" were encountered in whom the only common denominator was use of considerable aspartame. They had been extensively studied for abnormal heart action, transient cerebral ischemic attacks caused by small clots from the heart or neck (carotid) arteries, and atypical seizure disorders, but these could not be documented. (For example, a 37-year-old woman experienced déjà vu feelings followed by a "blackout" while consuming 1-2 liters of diet cola daily.) These persons had complete or significant relief after abstinence from aspartame products.

<u>**Representative Case Report**</u>

<u>**Case VI-O-1**</u>

A 78-year-old man was seen before his next scheduled appointment because of recent "blackouts". He was considering the cancellation of a long-planned cruise to Alaska because of this development. A detailed physical examination, coupled with pertinent laboratory tests and imaging studies of the brain, failed to reveal a cause.

At this point, he was questioned about dietary changes. The **only** significant deviation had been the use of diet sodas for several weeks. When seen two weeks later after avoiding all aspartame products, there had been no recurrences.

The "happy ending" occurred five weeks later when I received a postcard titled, "Alaska's Arctic." My patient wrote, "This is a fantastically beautiful country, and has to be seen to be fully appreciated. No more blackouts. (No more aspartame)."

P. DIFFICULTY IN EXPRESSION

"Difficulty in expressing myself" represents another aspect of impaired brain function attributable to aspartame products. It could fall in the category of "progressive aphasia."

The related problem of dyslexia or reading disability deserves mention. It is commonly associated with hyperactivity and attention-deficit disorder (Roberts 1969b) (Chapter VI-G). An aspartame reactor with dyslexia wrote, "In addition to nasty headaches, aspartame increases my dyslexia problem. I tend to transpose letters (sometimes entire words are written backwards), and I have problems speaking quickly."

These individuals understandably feared having "early Alzheimer's disease" (Chapter VI-C), but were reassured by the gratifying improvement after aspartame avoidance.

Representative Case Reports

Case VI-P-1

A 65-year-old woman had been using an aspartame tabletop sweetener 15 years when she read a reference to my work in the *Saturday Evening Post*. She wrote about the intermittent difficulty in expressing herself.

> "It seemed like the word was hard to come up with, so I'd have to explain myself in detail rather than using that word I knew would tell people what I wanted. My husband later noted that I'd say words which didn't make sense.

> "I also found that I would have to say one word at a time when reading the newspaper. As a result, I hardly got the meaning. But if I looked away from the printing a few seconds, and then went back to it, I could read it without any problems.

> "After reading these articles about problems from the effects of aspartame, I avoided all such products. I am now much improved."

A 49-year-old diabetic woman had to retire because, as described by her daughter, she can no longer communicate with us in full sentences that make sense." She had previously been "a funny lively person, but now seems trapped within herself." The patient also suffered from longstanding severe migraine headaches.

Her garage was found to be "lined up on the shelves with tons and tons of diet sodas."

VII

PSYCHOLOGIC, PSYCHIATRIC AND BEHAVIORAL PROBLEMS

"Some strange commotion is in (your) brain."
Shakespeare (*Henry VIII*)

"There is no doubt in my mind that most of the common
diseases depend upon food for cause and cure save those from
wounds, injuries, contagion and infection... Patients, cooks
and almost all the laity are not willing to deny their appetites,
and had rather eat and die than eat to live."
Dr. Ephraim Cutter (1893)

The following psychiatric and behavioral problems occurred among 1200 aspartame reactors.

Severe depression	-	281	(23%)
"Extreme irritability"	-	194	(16%)
"Severe anxiety"	-	201	(17%)
"Marked personality changes"	-	167	(14%)
"Recent severe insomnia"	-	169	(14%)
"Severe aggravation of phobias"	-	77	(6%)

The frequency in persons who completed the survey questionnaire (Section 4) was higher because some related questions had not been routinely asked early in this study or were not volunteered by correspondents. Furthermore, many described their mental reactions in vague terms such as "feeling spaced out" and "much more intense stress."

Additionally, emotional disorders were exacerbated or rekindled by aspartame consumption.

Acronym Legend
ACB - aspartame cola beverage
ASD - aspartame soft drink
ATS - aspartame tabletop sweetener

- A scientist with prior minor emotional problems, who had been under my care several years, commented, "Aspartame adds badness to an already bad emotional problem."
- A 51-year-old homemaker with a previous tendency to depression emphasized that "the depression while using aspartame was worse than anything before or since."
- A 50-year-old woman characterized the severity of her reaction to aspartame products in these terms: "During the last two weeks of my illness, I was sure that I was going to end up in a mental ward."

In the context of the foregoing mental and behavioral reactions, excessive aspartame consumption could qualify as "substance abuse." This will be amplified below under "aspartame addiction."

A. GENERAL COMMENTS AND CAVEATS

The existing magnitude of mental illness underscores the public health dangers of continued use of neurotoxic chemicals if they can be reasonably linked to its causation or aggravation. A federally funded study indicated that one in five Americans has some form of mental illness (*Newsweek* May 20, 1996, p. 20). It found that 12.6 percent of the population suffers anxiety in the form of phobias, panic disorders or obsessive-compulsive disorder, and 9.5 percent experiences depression.

Every patient presenting with unexplained "emotional problems" should be queried SPECIFICALLY about aspartame use. I emphasized this theme at the First International Conference on Dietary Phenylalanine and Brain Function (Roberts 1987b).

The following observations and caveats deserve emphasis.

- Unexplained mental deterioration while on a regimen that had been effective previously ought to prompt such inquiry.
- The difficulties facing aspartame reactors often were increased by physicians, psychiatrists and psychologists who (a) dogmatically asserted that their symptoms primarily reflected "the somatization of a deep-seated emotional disturbance" or some equivalent statement, and (b) the averred association with aspartame use reflected a hypochondriacal obsession ("cyberchondria").

- Aspartame-related "executive stress" was manifest as marked irritability with employees, inability to concentrate, decreased interest in one's work, and difficulty in coping with the pressures of entrepreneurship.
- The unrecognized aggravation of schizoid behavior by aspartame can become compounded when psychiatrists prescribe potent psychotropic medication.
- A female aspartame reactor had been diagnosed as having Bonnet's syndrome reference to psychologically normal persons who experience complex hallucinations.
- The problem of intellectual deterioration suffered by aspartame reactors (Chapter VI-L) has been exacerbated by psychiatric misdiagnoses.
- Profound mental disturbances can accompany the considerable weight loss due to "anorexia" and "pernicious vomiting" (Chapter IX-B) in aspartame disease. Moreover, patients with prior depression who develop aspartame-associated anorexia or bulimia seem prone to exacerbation of depression and suicidal thoughts.

The impact of aspartame disease in children cannot be ignored (Chapter XI). A dramatic increase in the prescription of psychotropic medications for preschoolers (ages 2 to 4 years) occurred between 1991 and 1995, based on analysis of the ambulatory care records from two state Medicaid programs and a salaried group-model health maintenance organization (Zito 2000). The majority of these prescriptions were for stimulants, 90 percent for methylphenidate (Ritalin). The other major ones were clonidine and neuroleptics.

Resistance By Psychiatrists and Psychologists

A number of my patients and correspondents with aspartame disease had been categorized as "the worried well" when their studies proved normal. They took double delight when the correct diagnosis of aspartame disease was made. First, their complaints improved or disappeared after avoiding these products. Second, they were vindicated of the "phantom disease" or the "it's-all-in-your-head" stigma.

It was noted above that some psychiatrists and psychologists reject the possibility that these problems can be related to aspartame use. This theme repeatedly surfaced as patients with severe aspartame disease described their predicament when inflexible mental health professionals labeled them as hypochondriacs on the basis of allegedly having been victimized by information on the Internet and "chat rooms."

> A young woman discovered the problem of aspartame disease on the Internet. She wrote, "I suffered with panic disorder for over 15 years, and attribute its severity to aspartame use. Since removing it from my diet over a year ago, I have suffered only one panic attack." (See VII-C)

This reflexive attitude of physician-colleagues is understandable. It has become ingrained by the denial from self-serving corporate interests. On the other hand, the multiple criteria for invoking aspartame disease are the same as for "medical" problems described throughout this book... particularly the prompt exacerbation on rechallenge.

The Issue of "Functional Somatic Syndromes"

Seasoned clinicians are aware of the many "functional somatic syndromes" (Wessely 1999) frequently encountered in practice, especially among women with current or previous anxiety and depression. They include the irritable bowel syndrome, the hyperventilation syndrome, the chronic fatigue syndrome, atypical facial pain, and so-called fibromyalgia.

Such patients ought not be regarded as merely "the worried well," particularly if disabled by their symptoms. Special care must be taken to avoid lumping aspartame sufferees in this category for two reasons. First, their complaints subside or improve after avoiding aspartame products. Second, they are exactly reproducible on rechallenge. Some of these patients admittedly may be experiencing functional somatic complaints while under great stress, but must not be denied a specific recommendation: the avoidance of aspartame products.

Dr. Thomas Szasz (1991) aptly warned about the shortcomings of psychiatric diagnoses. He asserted: "If mental diseases are diseases of the central nervous system, they are diseases of the brain, not the mind." The importance of this attitude is reinforced by the dramatic response to drug therapy of some disorders previously regarded as solely "psychiatric" (e.g., Tourette's disease).

The Input of Correspondents

Some brilliant descriptions of the psychological afflictions suffered by aspartame reactors appear in this chapter and elsewhere.

Dozens of grateful correspondents wrote letters of appreciation to the author, as Cases VII-A-3 and VII-A-8. The dramatic emotional improvement of an aspartame reactor after avoiding aspartame products was expressed in these terms: "My energy levels have increased fivefold, and my sunny disposition has awakened from hibernation. My stomach is happier too."

Drug–aspartame interactions (Chapter IX-I) pose an added problem, as in Case VII-A-3. A noted physician observed that many of his patients using fluoxetine (Prozac®) consumed at least a gallon of aspartame diet sodas daily. Similarly, nurses and other workers at mental health institutions have been impressed by the adverse reactions to aspartame products among patients under their care.

> A male nurse at a residential facility for the mentally disabled was responsible for 134 patients. Many had behavioral disorders and seizures. Once aware that **he** was an aspartame reactor (depression and "mental fog"), he recognized the "monumental task" of attempting to convince other members of the staff <u>and</u> patients about the need to avoid aspartame products.

Representative Case Reports

Case VII-A-1

A female aspartame reactor sent a detailed letter with her completed questionnaire. It began: "My epic journey starts in 1986 with this 'new and wonderful' aspartame product. When the diet cola came out, I thought I had died and gone to heaven." She held a fine job and had a happy marriage. After using aspartame, she experienced progressive impatience, paranoia, insomnia, a "dark bottomless depression," diminished hearing, and impaired vision.

Case VII-A-2

A 28-year-old woman had been afflicted with severe depression, marked lethargy, an extensive eruption, arthritic symptoms, a 30-pound gain in weight, insomnia, and "mental fog." Dramatic improvement occurred when she abstained from aspartame products. She wrote, "In a sentence, I could say that aspartame effectively ruined my physical and emotional health for the better part of ten years."

The Input of Relatives

The spouses and relatives of aspartame reactors often supplemented the survey questionnaire with independent corroboration of their psychiatric affliction and behavioral aberrations.

Representative Case Reports

Case VII-A-3

A 42-year-old homemaker experienced marked depression with suicidal thoughts, convulsions, tremors, severe mental confusion, and frequency of urination (both day and night). She drank up to four two-liter bottles of diet cola daily. These symptoms disappeared within two weeks after discontinuing the beverage. Her husband offered this addendum.

> "My wife has been under the care of a psychiatrist all her adult life. For the past 5-10 years, her medicine has been primarily Librium® and Stelazine®.

> "She has always been a big cola drinker and, being overweight, she opted for diet cola. In 1984, she began to deteriorate physically and mentally. It was gradual. The doctors could not come up with any answers as to the cause. During 1985, she became very bad. In December, she suffered a total collapse. She was hospitalized, and immediately put into the ICU.

> "When I got her home, I was determined not to let her become re-addicted to the cola, so I would not allow her to have any. She started to show improvement once again. It was about that time I saw an article in a news magazine that called attention to the fact that aspartame was detrimental to health, particularly to those with nervous conditions.

> "I am out of town frequently. Several times during the following months, she was able to secure the diet cola; each time it made her sick."

Case VII-A-4

The sister of an "aspartame junkie" chanced to find a copy of my first book on aspartame disease. She insisted that the patient read it after being told by a psychiatrist that her "symptoms were a hodgepodge." They included severe anxiety, panic attacks, intense depression, marked weakness, itching of the skin, dizziness and clumsiness.

The patient heeded her sister and stopped all aspartame products. She first noticed an ability to think more clearly. Her sobering addendum is noteworthy: "I told my psychiatrist about your book, and left it with her for a couple months, but she didn't read it. I was not taken seriously when I told other doctors what was happening to me. As a result, I have been without medical attention for several years."

Case VII-A-5

A 31-year-old insurance administrator suffered severe depression, three convulsions, intense drowsiness and dizziness while consuming four cans of an ACB and three packets of an ATS daily. X-rays of the head, a CT scan of the brain, two electroencephalograms, and other studies were normal. Her symptoms disappeared within two months after avoiding aspartame. She resented having been told that "it was all in my mind."

Case VII-A-6

A 32-year-old woman developed intense depression, dizziness, insomnia and headaches while using considerable aspartame in various products for weight control. These symptoms vanished <u>within one week</u> after avoiding aspartame, coupled with improvement of her "anxiety level." Describing these experiences, she wrote, "I did discuss this with my medical doctor. He felt that the symptoms and controversy over aspartame were too subjective to be able to say my symptoms were from aspartame."

Case VII-A-7

A "former diet soda drinker" provided this summary of her devastating reactions to aspartame products.

> "Approximately six months ago, I discovered on my own – with NO help from the three family physicians, two psychiatrists, or three psychologists – that aspartame was responsible for my five years of anxiety/panic attacks, insomnia, heart palpitations, and the list goes on and on."

Case VII-A-8

A female reactor provided this "horror story about aspartame," "I am a 21-year-old who felt as though I was 95. I had a list of symptoms as long as my arm, and was convinced that my entire life was on a downward spiral to destruction.

"Once I learned about reactions to aspartame, and stopped these products, I felt like a new person. The panic/anxiety, depression and nastiness just faded away. My sleeping patterns returned to normal. I can move like I used to without pains and aches. It was a good thing that my boyfriend loved me enough to stay with me through all the horrible mood swings and things I put him through. I am 21 again, and just so happy I could scream!!"

Long-Term Implications

The potential for behavioral abnormalities and impaired intelligence in the offspring of mothers who consumed aspartame during pregnancy will be discussed in Chapters X and XI.

There is considerable evidence that subsequent behavior and intelligence can be influenced by exposure of a fetus to neurotoxic chemicals which cross the placenta. This is well known in the case of ethyl alcohol, and also may apply to methyl alcohol (Chapter XXI).

One large longitudinal study by the Department of Psychiatry and Behavioral Sciences at the University of Washington addressed the status of children born to mothers who drank alcohol during pregnancy. They were found to have shorter attention spans and slower reaction times (*The Palm Beach Post* January 17, 1987, p. A-1).

Biophysiologic Perspectives

Anxiety, depression, headache (Chapter VI), attention-deficit disorder (Chapter VI-G), and narcolepsy (Chapter VI-K) ought to be considered symptoms of underlying brain dysfunction rather than specific diseases. They may be caused or aggravated by multiple physiologic and biochemical aberrations. For example, the severe premenstrual syndrome is often associated with fluid retention, aggravated hypoglycemia, and unrecognized hypothyroidism.

Considerable information exists concerning marked neuropsychologic changes when dopamine-serotonin balance is altered. These neurotransmitters will be discussed further in Chapter XXIII.

I. Serotonin

Decreased brain serotonin has been associated with insomnia, depression, anxiety, panic attacks, hallucinations, suicidal attempts, hostility and psychopathic states.

Experimental reduction of serotonin in humans confirms the ensuing tendency to aggressive behavior. Several studies have utilized the technic of feeding subjects a diet low in tryptophan (from which it is derived) for a day, followed by milk shakes (containing multiple amino acids) to further deplete tryptophan (Maugh 1995).

Aspartame and its components can lower brain serotonin levels through several mechanisms.

- Dr. Richard Wurtman demonstrated that aspartame inhibits the carbohydrate-induced synthesis of serotonin (*Congressional Record-Senate* 1985a, p. S 5511). Serotonin is an important component of the feedback system that helps limit one's consumption of carbohydrate to appropriate levels by blunting the carbohydrate craving.
- The amino acid tyrosine, derived from phenylalanine, reduces the amount of tryptophan that can cross the blood-brain barrier for utilization in serotonin production.

II. Dopamine

The mounting scientific evidence for altered brain dopamine concentrations (Chapter XXIII) in mental illness is relevant.

- The injection of dopamine (a metabolite of phenylalanine) into the brain ventricles of humans can precipitate psychotic episodes, including hallucinations.

- Wong et al (1986) studied the D_2 dopamine receptor density in the caudate nucleus of normal volunteers and patients with schizophrenia by positron emission tomography (PET). Higher densities were noted in the schizophrenic group, even without prior neuroleptic drug treatment.
- Several aspartame reactors with severe neuropsychiatric features evidenced brain changes by SPECT imaging studies.
- The dopaminergic influences in aspartame and other addictions are considered in VII-G.
- More numerous D_2 dopamine receptors have been found in the basal ganglia of schizophrenic patients obtained at postmortem examination, compared to persons having no history of neurologic or psychiatric disease.

III. Other Changes

Dr. Ralph G. Walton (1986) urged physicians to bear in mind "the possible impact of aspartame on catecholamine and indolamine metabolism, and inquire about use of this artificial sweetener when assessing patients with affective disorders."

The brain edema and vascular stasis due to chronic methanol intake (Chapter XXI) could contribute to the neuropsychiatric manifestations of aspartame reactors.

The observation that tryptophan depletion in nonalcoholic young men can induce behavioral changes is pertinent in view of the depletion of tryptophan by aspartame consumption.

B. DEPRESSION

Severe depression afflicted 281 (23 percent) of 1200 aspartame reactors. Of the 397 aspartame reactors who completed the initial survey questionnaire, 144 (28.7 percent) suffered depression; 39 (9.8 percent) had suicidal thoughts. (Twenty-two were on a "strict diet.") Ten continued using aspartame despite its apparent contribution to their depression.

Suicide has become a public health crisis. One occurs every 17 minutes in the United States, ranking it third among causes of death for young people, and second for college students. Accordingly, any substance that may contribute to suicide cannot be ignored, particularly when consumed in large amounts.

General Considerations

The onset or recurrence of severe depression may be triggered by multiple interrelated social, economic, interpersonal and medical events. In view of the significant incidence of "endogenous" depression in the general population, commonly used chemicals that might aggravate it – as aspartame products – deserve close scrutiny.

The National Institute of Mental Health (NIMH) emphasized the epidemic nature of depression in the United States (Holden 1986). Its analysis revealed

- About six percent of the population experience clinical depression within a given six-month period.
- The average age of onset has declined from 40 years to the mid-20s.
- Women are more likely to be afflicted with a major depression – namely, one in four within their lifetime, compared to one in ten for males. The preponderance of female aspartame reactors (Chapter II-H) is germane.
- Depressed persons requiring hospitalization suffered a relapse rate of about 85 percent.

Depression often interferes with one's occupation, schooling and personal life. Its many manifestations include loss of interest in pleasurable activities, sleep disturbances, impaired appetite, unexplained fatigue, difficult concentration, the feeling of worthlessness, and suicidal thoughts.

Observations Concerning Aspartame-Associated Depression

A. Older persons (Chapter XV) tend to be affected severely. They often interpret inability to concentrate and mental blocking as evidences of "old age" or even early Alzheimer's disease. A comparable diagnostic error by professionals compounds the "irony of the psychiatric megatrends" for the elderly (Glass 1987). Dr. Robert H. Willis (1987) reported that suicide is successful in only one of 100 attempts by adolescents, but in nearly all first-time attempts among persons over 60.

B. Young individuals are highly vulnerable. An estimated ten percent of teenagers suffer significant depression. Furthermore, the suicide rate for the 15- to 19-year-old age group has more than tripled. The contributory role of aspartame products is inherent in mounting concern over "junk food" taken by weight-conscious teenagers.

The young friend of an aspartame reactor required psychiatric admission shortly after beginning to use a popular aspartame reducing "formula." Once she discontinued this formula and aspartame diet sodas, she improved dramatically and could omit the prescribed lithium.

Whereas depressed adults often express unremitting sadness and a sense of foreboding, depressed teenagers tend to withdraw socially. They lose interest in school achievement and sports, as well as food. A vicious cycle then may be generated by considerable aspartame consumption and decreased caloric intake.

C. Depression may be a response to the aspartame molecule or its three components. One patient convincingly found that L-phenylalanine alone caused it. This prominent writer initially suffered extreme depression while using aspartame sodas. When she tried L-phenylalanine one year later, hopefully to abort recurrence of her depression, it intensified.

D. De novo depression occurred in persons with no prior history of this disorder after they used aspartame products.

- A successful business executive experienced severe depression, headache and lethargy while drinking aspartame beverages. She stated, "I didn't even want to go out into the sun and enjoy the summer. I even looked forward to the rain. (I love summer and hate rain.)" Her symptoms disappeared shortly after stopping aspartame products.
- A 33-year-old office manager with multiple reactions to aspartame wrote, "I was extremely depressed, and it was hard to work. I didn't lose my job because we're self-employed.

E. Suicidal Thoughts. Among the more recent 649 aspartame reactors in this series, 46 (7.1%) admitted to contemplating suicide! (See Case VII-B-6).

Physicians, psychologists and social workers recognize that depressed individuals with suicidal thought require prompt treatment and counseling, especially young persons. In this context, the March 1986 *Morbidity and Mortality Weekly Report* emphasized an age shift to younger individuals, especially white males less than 40.

Special emphasis ought to be directed to aspartame reactors with suicidal thoughts after losing considerable weight. A patient who attempted suicide twice asserted, "All my problems began with drinking diet cola."

Representative Case Reports

Case VII-B-1

A prominent radio announcer in his mid-30s called one week after my initial press conference on aspartame disease to volunteer a personal report. His joyful attitude and perceived brilliance had been appreciated throughout the community. A consultant therapist was unable to explain his feeling of "something dragging me down." A news colleague who had taped my remarks insisted that he listen to the recording. While doing so, he analyzed his own "terrible mood swings and inappropriate depression" over the previous four months. One week after stopping aspartame, he gratefully acknowledged that his symptoms had abated.

Case VII-B-2

A 43-year-old attorney and trust officer quit several positions because of presumed "job-related depression" and suicidal thoughts. He had been drinking three or four cans of diet cola daily. Other complaints included extreme irritability, "anxiety attacks," a change in personality, and the fear of crowds.

He deduced that aspartame beverages were the cause after retesting himself on four occasions. His symptoms improved "immediately" each time he stopped them. A niece also suffered severe depression and menstrual changes from aspartame disease.

This lawyer was emphatic in his perceptive recommendations about the regulation of aspartame products. "Please research as many suicides as you can regarding quantity consumed prior to the act. Also child abuse. Watch in particular the teen suicide situation!"

Case VII-B-3

A 29-year-old homemaker drank "enormous amounts" of diet cola. She developed many symptoms – including "mood swings," "personality changes," "crying for no reason," and "severe suicidal thoughts." She stated, "I never was depressed before, so why now? I have two beautiful kids and a husband with a good job."

Case VII-B-4

A 43-year-old nutritionist and health educator suffered intense depression within one week after consuming ten or more glasses daily of an aspartame soft drink. It recurred after one retest trial.

"I was depressed (sad, crying etc.) for no reason. I was on vacation at the time and having a good time. I started drinking aspartame on vacation because of thirst. I do professional counseling. My clients also have experienced depression and vision problems with aspartame."

Case VII-B-5

A 26-year-old woman experienced severe depression, suicidal thoughts, and marked personality changes after consuming aspartame sodas. All began to improve within one day after stopping them, and disappeared in ten days.

"I went from a fun-loving, carefree person to – as I would like to refer – a monster. My appearance changed, my personality changed, my life changed. At that point I really began to believe I was truly insane."

Case VII-B-6

This woman had consumed saccharin-containing soft drinks until they were no longer available. She then drank two to three cans of diet cola daily. Within a week, she experienced severe depression that had not been experienced previously. She wrote, "One day, I was so distraught and crying continuously that I decided to get in my car and find a bridge to drive off. Fortunately, I passed a doctor's office before I found one, and just walked in – crying and carrying on. The doctor agreed to see me on the spot." He prescribed an antidepressant, which only sedated her.

While in bed praying for help, "A voice told me to stop drinking those sodas. (No, I don't normally hear voices.) Within 24 hours of stopping, I felt much better. Within 48 hours I felt like a brand new human being."

This patient's conclusion was bolstered on meeting another woman who described a comparable mental reaction after consuming aspartame soda.

Case VII-B-7

A college student suffered "major depression" while drinking 6-8 diet colas daily. On learning about aspartame disease, she stopped these products. She reported

"After a couple of months off the soda, I was at a speaking competition, doing very well, and in a good mood. Within minutes after drinking a diet soda, I felt teary and was shaking. Since that time, I have not had so much as a stick of aspartame gum. There have been no more depressive episodes."

Familial Predisposition to Aspartame-Associated Depression

A large body of information confirms the familial tendency to depression. Debate continues as whether the chief provocative influence is genetic or environmental. A single genetic abnormality has been found among one large Amish family with many depressed members.

Aspartame products appear to have initiated or aggravated depression in members of afflicted families. Examples are cited in Chapters II and XVI. The following letter from a woman who had read about aspartame reactions illustrates this issue.

"Yes. I definitely experience side effects when I use aspartame regularly – especially depression! I am a happy, up-beat person and never feel "down" unless I've been using aspartame.

"I have a 28-year-old daughter who suffers from heart palpitations and depression when she uses aspartame.

"I also have a 22-year-old daughter who feels depressed if she uses aspartame."

Aspartame-induced depression in relatives offers leads about future research. For example, neurotransmitter and metabolic alterations could be studied by position emission tomography (PET) (see VII-A) in members of depression-prone families following aspartame challenge.

Representative Case Report

Case VII-B-6

A 62-year-old woman suffered severe depression with suicidal thoughts. She felt "just miserable, hating every day." Other complaints included marked visual changes in both eyes, ringing in the ears, personality changes, severe insomnia, tremors, facial pain, slurred speech, shortness of breath, palpitations, diarrhea, abdominal bloat, itching and joint pains. Striking improvement occurred within six days after discontinuing an aspartame beverage.

Her sister, her husband, a grandson, a brother, and a sister experienced comparable severe reactions that promptly improved or disappeared when they avoided such products.

Mania and "Bipolar" Depression

Several aspartame reactors in this series had "bipolar" depression wherein the depression would alternate with periods of manic behavior characterized by intense excitement and overactivity. As many as two million Americans suffer manic-depression.

The ability of phenylalanine to stimulate the central nervous system, directly or through its conversion to other neurotransmitters (Chapter XXII), is germane.

Some studies suggest that bipolar and unipolar affective disorders are distinct entities – that is, in terms of familial prevalence, genetics (including twin studies), prognosis, and response to treatment (Schwartz 1987). Several observations are pertinent

- Women outnumber men with unipolar depression by about two to one.
- Differences in unipolar and bipolar depression are reinforced by positron emission tomography studies (Schwartz 1987). Patients with unipolar depression have significantly higher local cerebral metabolic rates for glucose, but these are reduced in bipolar depression. Accordingly, a further reduction of the cerebral metabolic rate caused by aspartame or its byproducts might precipitate clinical depression in predisposed individuals.
- A subset of manic-depression appears linked to a dominant gene on the tip of the short arm of chromosome 11. The tyrosine hydroxylase gene (Section 5), which cascades the synthesis of dopamine, exists in this region.
- Whereas the cyclic antidepressants are more effective than lithium in unipolar depression, they tend to cause more behavioral disturbances in bipolar depression.

Representative Case Report

300

Case VII-B-7

A 67-year-old man had been treated for bipolar depression, essential tremor, and a labyrinthine syndrome. He fared well for several years on small doses of propranolol and lithium.

One month prior to his June 1986 visit, the tremor and vertigo intensified, coupled with "increased mood elevation." On direct questioning, he admitted to recent consumption of aspartame products. His symptoms promptly subsided when he avoided them and did not recur over the ensuing year, notwithstanding enormous stress because of his wife's serious illness during that period.

The Studies of Walton et al

Walton, Hudock and Green-Waite (1993) dramatically demonstrated the adverse effect of aspartame intake in patients with a history of depression. They administered aspartame (30 mg/kg) daily or a placebo for seven days in a double-blind challenge to 40 patients with unipolar depression, and a similar number of persons without a history of psychiatric problems. The NutraSweet Company apparently refused to supply these researchers with aspartame, so analytically certified USP grade aspartame was purchased from a chemical distributor.

The frequency and severity of depression, headache, nervousness, difficulty in remembering, insomnia, fatigue and malaise were striking among patients with a history of depression after ingesting aspartame, compared to the placebo, both in these patients and nondepressed volunteers. Persons without a history of depression did not manifest frequent or severe symptoms when given aspartame. The severity of reactions among patients with a history of depression proved sufficiently alarming that the Institutional Review Board had to halt this project prematurely.

- Three participants spontaneously volunteered that they felt "poisoned" after taking the product later determined to be aspartame.
- A 42-year-old Ph.D.-psychologist with a history of recurrent severe depression experienced pain in one eye, followed by retinal detachment (Chapter IV) requiring emergency surgery.
- Another depressed patient evidenced conjunctival bleeding for the first time during the week she ingested aspartame.
- Individual patients with a history of depression experienced swollen lips, a bad taste in the mouth, facial numbness, weight gain and irritability – complaints not reported by nondepressed volunteers.

This experience also has raised questions about the nature of the aspartame supplied for published "negative" double-blind studies (Section 7).

Some Pathophysiologic and Pharmacologic Considerations

My experience underscores two important factors that should be considered when persons present with "endogenous" depression: severe hypoglycemia (Roberts 1964, 1971b) and aspartame disease. They also ought to be sought when depressed patients unexpectedly suffer severe relapse while on conventional anti-depressant treatment. In this regard, aspartame may interfere with the action of imipramine (a tricyclic antidepressant) and other drugs influencing neurotransmitters that are used in managing depressed patients (Chapter IX-I).

The decrease of serotonin by aspartame administration (see VII-A) has considerable relevance to depression and other psychological problems, particularly among weight-conscious women who severely restrict their carbohydrate intake. Smith et al (1997) reported that the rapid lowering of brain serotonin can precipitate clinical depressive symptoms in untreated individuals vulnerable to major depression.

The subject of neurotransmitter alteration in depression and other mood disturbances was mentioned in VII-A, and will be amplified in Chapter XXIII. It has been hypothesized that depression results from decreased brain serotonin. Conversely, drugs such as imipramine tend to increase serotonin, and sensitize the brain to norepinephrine.

- There is considerable evidence for the diminished turnover of brain serotonin in depression and behavioral disturbances, including suicide (*The Lancet* 1987; 2:949-950).
- Aspartame decreases the availability of L-tryptophan (a precursor of serotonin) and alters its balance with norepinephrine, another important neurotransmitter. Some have likened its effects to that of a lesion in the lateral hypothalamus causing depression, other psychiatric problems, and eating disorders.
- Impairment of serotonin metabolism appears to summate upon the high insulin levels and reactive hypoglycemia found in violent offenders and arsonists (Virkkunen 1982, 1983, 1984, 1987).

The reduction or absence of carbohydrate in aspartame products also can contribute to depression. Dr. Harris R. Lieberman (1987) asserted that carbohydrates exert an

302

antidepressant effect in a subgroup of obese individuals who use them as snacks for combating mood changes without risking altered alterness. This phenomenon may reflect changes in serotonin synthesis and release.

C. ANXIETY ATTACKS AND PHOBIAS

In this series of 1200 persons with aspartame disease, 201(17 percent) used the term "severe anxiety attacks" to describe their emotional reaction.

Anxiety can assume one of several forms – panic attacks, generalized anxiety, marked irritability, phobias, and obsessive-compulsive behavior.

- <u>Panic attacks</u> refer to sudden episodes involving the feeling of intense terror or impending doom. Associated sweats, rapid heart action, feelings of smothering and faint, dizziness, trembling, and the sense of alienation are common.

  A female aspartame reactor could precisely date the onset of her panic attacks to use of diet sodas. They occurred after a new fountain was installed in her corporate break room. This led to binging on aspartame beverages. "When I went back to drinking water, the panic attacks stopped!"

  Drake (1986) also reported panic attacks in a 33-year-old woman who consumed considerable aspartame cola drinks.

- <u>Generalized anxiety</u> describes a persistent sensation of tension. It is commonly coupled with sleep problems and the inability to concentrate. Palpitations, sweating, jitteriness and mild depression also may be present.
- <u>"Extreme irritability"</u> was mentioned by 194 (16 percent) aspartame reactors.
- <u>Phobias</u> intensified in 77 (6 percent) of the aspartame reactors. They described extreme fear of a particular situation, object or activity. It may be evoked by exposure to heights, enclosed spaces or crowds (agoraphobia). One aspartame reactor developed a marked phobia for dogs.

- Obsessive-compulsive behavior refers to recurrent and persistent ideas or repetitive behavior, at times assuming the nature of a ritual.

The unexplained recurrence of severe anxiety after previously successful medication, counseling, and behavior modification therapy should prompt therapists to inquire about aspartame use. This issue assumes added pertinence when these patients are known to be dieters subject to hypoglycemia (Chapter XIV).

> A psychiatrist interested in morbid agoraphobia described the reaction of some patients en route to work as "an attack in which they become dizzy and unstable, sweaty and warm all over, shaky on the outside and inside, heart pounding and beating rapidly, mouth dry, lump in throat, weak legs, stiff ness, and crawling guts" (*Medical Tribune* October 2, 1969, p. 2). These symptoms often characterize "low blood sugar attacks" as well as aspartame reactions.

There is a consensus that agoraphobia, including its broader definition as the fear of panic attacks, stems from "stress" and negative thoughts or perceptions. In the present context, however, panic episodes (or "passive aggressive behavior") that had been triggered by aspartame consumption were often obviated by avoiding this chemical.

A number of observations concerning the neurobiology of panic attacks involve abnormal cerebral glucose metabolism, disturbances of various neurotransmitters (including cholecystokinin and serotonin), dysfunction of the locus ceruleus, and altered aspartate receptors (Roy-Byrne 1998). These were cited in VII-A, and will be amplified in Section 5.

Representative Case Reports

Case VII-C-1

A 34-year-old registered nurse developed severe "anxiety attacks" after consuming up to eight cans of a diet cola and ten sticks of aspartame gum daily. Other complaints included headache, lightheadedness, "epilepsy-like fits," marked memory loss, slurred speech, sensitivity to noise in both ears, difficulty with contact lens, diarrhea, severe joint pains, and less frequent periods. Her symptoms disappeared within six weeks after avoiding all aspartame products. She wrote

"My doctor told me I was having anxiety attacks. However, I have not had that feeling since I quit using aspartame. I had to convince my physician that aspartame, and not neurosis, was my problem. Luckily for me, my friend developed seizures and linked it to aspartame. I got off it before this happened to me."

Case VII-C-2

A 32-year-old man with severe reactive hypoglycemia responded well to a conventional diet and supportive measures. He subsequently evidenced increasing irritability and anxiety for which a psychiatrist was seen.

The patient returned because of persistence of these features, along with "feeling woozy" and having memory problems. The physical examination and routine studies were normal. On direct questioning, he stated that he drank four liters of a diet cola daily. He thereupon volunteered that his sister also experienced marked confusion and dizziness after using aspartame.

When seen three weeks after stopping aspartame products, the foregoing symptoms had virtually disappeared.

Case VII-C-3

A 52-year-old bank executive developed convulsions after drinking an aspartame hot chocolate mix for eight consecutive nights. She also experienced severe anxiety, marked aggravation of phobias, and intense depression with suicidal thoughts. She recalled, "I wanted to jump off the top of a parking garage."

Case VII-C-4

The following correspondence from a registered nurse described her reactions to aspartame products.

"The onset of symptoms is very subtle so it is difficult to put your finger on the source of trouble. At first, I noticed that I became not only very depressed but also developed a feeling of irritability. I had extreme mood swings between these two. My temper developed, and was instant and very sharp. I would get very angry over nothing, and yell and throw temper tantrums. I felt as though I not only could get extremely violent and probably kill, but also that I had no feelings of remorse. I knew I was acting bad. I also knew when I was being too angry, but I didn't try to stop and didn't care. That was the scary part. It was all very overwhelming, and finally scared me because I knew something was very strong.

"I was about to go seek help when I realized that it might be the aspartame. After discontinuing the product, it took about two to three weeks for the worst of the symptoms to disappear.

"I lost total control of myself during the time I was using the aspartame. It seems so strange because I used it to help me diet, but I couldn't stop eating. Because of this lack of control, I gained more weight than I had ever done before in my life. I had extreme anxiety attacks over nothing, especially when I went out any place."

She elaborated upon some of the other "little things that happened" while taking aspartame.

- "My eyes went from OK to not even being able to focus."
- "My loss of memory is strange because I forgot things I did yesterday, which is like a senile person. Also things I knew in the past, as vocabulary words, were totally foreign to me. I've been scared to go back to work as an RN because of this memory loss."
- "My hair had been falling out since then."
- "I've practically lost self-respect and feel bad about myself, which is something new for me."

With reference to the depression, she wrote

"I've been diagnosed as having severe depression, yet every antidepressant I have taken caused severe reactions (seizures; an extrapyramidal syndrome; disorientation; blurred vision). I believed I was crazy. I signed myself into a mental institution, but was told after three days that I was not crazy."

It was her mother who finally made the diagnosis: "aspartame poisoning."

Case VII-C-5

A 36-year-old janitor was urged by his dentist to drink diet sodas when he developed several cavities. Shortly thereafter, he experienced "panic attacks," considerable facial pain, a tremor, and increasing nervousness. He also had abdominal discomfort, diarrhea, insomnia, confusion and memory loss. ("I found my mailbox stuffed full, with postmarks nearly two weeks old.") A psychiatrist told him that he had "a fixation with the number 6." Another diagnosis was "male menopause." His neighbors became concerned about "my possibly using drugs and going crazy."

After reading an article on aspartame disease, his mother asked about the use of aspartame products. His symptoms promptly subsided after avoiding aspartame. He wrote, "Thank you again, and please don't give up on your research. If I had my way, they'd un-invent aspartame!"

An impressive family history of aspartame disease unfolded. His sister had severe anxiety attacks when taking aspartame. A younger brother and his mother developed gastrointestinal complaints from diet sodas. The mother also recently developed "borderline diabetes."

Case VII-C-6

A 46-year-old woman had been diagnosed as having a "panic disorder" six years previously. Other prominent symptoms included headache, chronic fatigue, lightheadedness, and "dazed feelings." She rejected the assertion that "stress" was a major factor. Her symptoms "vanished" after avoiding aspartame products. She stated, "For the first time in years, I feel I am in charge of my life again."

Case VII-C-7

A female aspartame reactor described her aspartame-induced panic attacks in these terms:

> "I would get a very uncomfortable tight feeling in my chest, and
> sometimes my heart would race or beat irregularly. The doctors
> thought I was crazy or that it was linked to some sort of mental

illness. I went through extensive testing. They found me perfectly healthy, with no heart problems or other physical problems that would be causing this pain. I also would frequently feel dizzy while just walking for no apparent reason. I had extreme mood swings and anxiety. A week after I stopped ingesting aspartame, all my symptoms disappeared and I have not had any of these problems since. It makes me extremely angry how this information is hidden from the public."

D. "PERSONALITY CHANGES" AND ABNORMAL BEHAVIOR

I. Personality Changes

"Marked personality changes" occurred in 167 (14%) of the 1200 aspartame reactors in this series. Their vivid descriptions appear below and in other chapters.

- The wife of a patient with aspartame disease described how this "very outgoing and vibrant-on-action man" had become transformed into an "in-spirit-nothing" person. He also experienced dizziness shortly after ingesting an aspartame beverage on several retrials.
- A 39-year-old homemaker evidenced a marked change in personality, irritability, memory loss and insomnia while consuming aspartame. She stated, "I was amazed by the total personality change. Doctors think I'm 'nuts' to think a sweetener would be the problem."
- A 34-year-old teacher exhibited personality changes whenever she drank a diet cola. They consisted of "trouble with co-workers, mood flare-ups, and two arguments with the principal of the school even though we previously got along OK."

II. Abnormal Behavior

Evidences of abnormal behavior by aspartame reactors, with or without confusion (Chapter VI-C), are cited in other chapters.

- Several victims described in Chapter VI-L suffered grossly abnormal behavior, personality changes, and severe intellectual impairment.
- The wife of a businessman volunteered that leaving an untidy desk and failure to turn off the lights were uncharacteristic of him.

- Mothers anguished over their irritability, erratic behavior, and potential for child abuse while ingesting aspartame products. For example, a 38-year-old accounting clerk "lost my temper and found myself screaming at my son" after drinking a diet cola the previous day. Such behavior promptly recurred on three retesting challenges with two other brands of aspartame cola.

- An experienced coordinator of special programs for Minnesota high school students with disability from emotional/behavioral disorders (E/BD) became increasingly convinced about a relationship between the phenomenal rise of such disability over the last decade and consumption of aspartame products.

Health care professionals who had personally experienced aspartame reactions of this nature repeatedly conjectured about the potential for psychopathic behavior. They linked newspaper accounts of strange behavior with the presumed intake of aspartame products.

> The *Orlando Sentinel* (August 18, 1986, p. B-1) reported that a 39-year-old nude burglary suspect was apprehended after the sound of glass breaking had been heard. A communications supervisor at the Sheriff's office stated, "They did not find his clothes. He does not know anything about how his clothes were taken off him, and the last thing he remembers is having a drink of (a diet beverage), and lying on the couch."

The dramatic increase of highway violence (Section 6) (*The Wall Street Journal* August 3, 1987, p. 1) has coincided with heightened aspartame consumption. Previously responsible persons engaged in fights, shootings and other mayhem after some minor stimulus – e.g., the flashing of high beams by an oncoming car, or failure of a driver to yield.

Aspartame disease may contribute to "road rage." The American Automobile Association reported a 51 percent increase of overtly hostile manner by motorists since 1990 (*The New York Times* September 20, 1997).

The recent emphasis upon unexplained "air rage" among passengers in planes is relevant, especially by persons chewing aspartame gum (Chapter II-E). Their bizarre and unexpected behavior after being served diet drinks has raised the possibility of an aspartame reaction. These individuals tended to have an "anxious look" and "glassy" eyes, but no memory of such behavior thereafter.

Courts have denied the so-called Twinkie defense in cases wherein depression and other psychiatric aberrations were attributed to "junk food." In the case of persons consuming considerable aspartame, however, this possibility does exist.

The dramatic increase of <u>criminal activities by children</u> below the age of ten in recent years – ranging from armed robbery to sadistic murder – has alarmed police, judges and criminologists (*The Miami Herald* December 29, 1986, p. A-16). Others have stressed the need to rethink the roots of violent behavior. While many socioeconomic factors influence adolescent violence, the possible contributory role of aspartame-induced aberrant behavior has hardly been addressed.

In an attempt to understand violence better, Alice Miller (1983) suggested discarding theories that have proved of little value. Dr. John R. Hamilton (1987), Section on Forensic Psychiatry at the Institute of Psychiatry in London, emphasized an interlinking of the physical, psychologic and social effects of violence.

The <u>abnormal behavior of young children</u> consuming aspartame will be described in Case VII-D-4 and Chapter XI. The <u>Tourette syndrome</u> (Chapter VI-G), an extreme form, was reported by one mother. This disorder, possibly familial, is also characterized by chronic intermittent motor and speech tics.

The following scientific observations are germane.

- Behavioral changes may occur early in life after the experimental administration of aspartame. Dosing mice with it during late pregnancy delayed achievement age for visual placing in the offspring (Mahalik 1984).
- The choice reaction time in adults decreases as much as ten percent with a 250 µmol/L increase in the plasma phenylalanine concentration (Krause 1985).

Reports suggesting that aspartame does not affect the behavior of children require close analysis, especially when the studies were corporate-sponsored. Kreusi et al (1986) concluded that neither sugar nor aspartame significantly disrupted behavior in 30 preschool boys. However, they kept the sweeteners in a refrigerator and on crushed ice, and the drinks were served cold. The significance of these details is discussed in Section 5.

Representative Case Reports

Case VII-D-1

This housewife experienced many difficulties three months after beginning to consume aspartame products. They included crying, headache, extreme fatigue, diarrhea, rashes, weakness, loss of appetite and weight, "flashes of darkness like I was going to pass out, and jerking in my insides."

She also expressed great concern over "fussing at my husband every minute he was home after we had always had a beautiful relationship." She added, "I think my husband thought I was psychotic – and frankly, so did I." These problems increased despite the prescription of an antidepressant drug.

A cousin then informed the patient about an article discussing aspartame disease. She described her response to abstinence in these terms:

> "About 24 hours after I took my last diet drink, I suddenly felt better than I had in months. I have been fine ever since. I have continued to stay away from aspartame, and nobody will ever convince me that it was not the cause of all my problems. I credit my cousin for saving my life because if she hadn't told me about that article, I believe it would have killed me."

Case VII-D-2

A 42-year-old registered nurse developed extreme irritability and anxiety, severe depression with suicidal thoughts, a change in personality, and aggravated phobias while consuming two glasses of aspartame-sweetened iced tea and two packets of an ATS daily. She had switched to these products because of the alleged cancer risk of saccharin, even though the latter had not caused her any obvious difficulty.

Other complaints included decreased vision in both eyes, dizziness, tremors, mental confusion and memory loss, numbness of the arms, slurred speech, palpitations, unexplained chest pains, abdominal distress (for which she began taking ulcer medication), nausea, marked abdominal bloat, thinning of the hair, and a 20-pound weight gain. She had hay fever for 20 years.

Her mental changes became so severe that she quit her work and supplementary courses. She added

> "I could have killed if provoked. That's why I was going to seek help. I also noticed I lost my inhibitions and any guilt feelings for acting bad. I still don't feel I can work as a nurse because I've forgotten so much, and things are all confused in my head.

> "I continually make a fool of myself because of being so stupid now. I've lost all self-confidence and self-esteem. I continue to be depressed because of this. How long will I feel bad? I spoke to three doctors about my symptoms being caused by aspartame, and they all just about laughed in my face. How do you work with this?"

As this nurse was arranging to see a psychologist, she deduced that her symptoms could be related to using aspartame. There was decided relief within two weeks after stopping such products... especially her anxiety attacks. The depression and memory loss, however, persisted at the time of her communications.

She offered this thought about abnormal behavior by other aspartame reactors: "Can anybody know if these bizarre killings aren't aspartame induced? I know I could have done so."

Case VII-D-3

A 41-year-old legal secretary took great pride in her work over a period of 13 years. She described her changed mood and personality during the several months she consumed aspartame.

> "I would come home from work and the least thing that happened would bring on a crying fit. I was so sensitive that if someone even said 'good morning' to me, I would go off on a tangent. My husband felt it was the pressure of my job, and told me several times he was going to make me quit. I then began to believe it was the job because I couldn't seem to cope with the simplest things; co-workers and bosses alike seemed to get on my nerves. These were people I had known and loved all those

years. In July of 1984, I walked off my job. (I had been in the work arena for 28 years and never did such a thing.) The moodiness didn't quit, it just got worse."

Case VII-D-4

The concerned father of a 12-year-old boy observed his son's aspartame-induced behavioral changes. He had become highly irritable, emotional and seclusive, coupled with plummeting grades. The lad "started sneaking it (aspartame) behind my back." An endocrinologist found low blood sugar levels (in the 40's). When the boy was then allowed to have sugar products, he evidenced marked improvement. After drinking a diet soda while eating with his family, he promptly "felt tired and sick."

The boy's symptoms left with aspartame abstinence. He received all A's and B's grades in several months.

E. SEVERE FATIGUE

Many aspartame reactors complained of severe "fatigue." It improved or disappeared after aspartame was avoided, thereby confirming the causal relationship.

I did not include this term in the initial survey questionnaire because of its vagueness and limitations. Fatigue may variously refer to a decline in performance during prolonged or repeated tasks, decreased attention or concentration, somnolence, or a symptom accompanying depression and viral syndromes.

Many aspartame reactors were initially reluctant to attribute their severe fatigue to the use of aspartame. This relationship crystallized, however, when they stopped these products as part of a "two-week test" or "four-week test." The concomitant regression of other complaints reinforced the validity of such causation.

Representative Case Report

Case VII-E-1

A male aspartame reactor wrote

"It has been 34 days without any aspartame, and I feel great. Looking back, it amazes me that I was just going along when I <u>really</u> realized that I was less fatigued and not in as much pain. I wasn't twisting all over the sofa trying to get comfortable. I am now doing my gardening and general house work without much pain. Before, I would have to lay down, and nap or at least rest. I feel like I am getting my life back. My friends have noticed that I am much nicer to be around, and am not always spending my energies on fighting pain."

Commentary

A. <u>Awareness</u>. The issue of aspartame disease as a basis for chronic fatigue surfaced during my interviews. One young man wondered if his prior "half diagnosis" of "chronic fatigue syndrome" could be related to the large consumption of aspartame sodas ("a gallon or more daily").

The awareness by persons who had suffered severe aspartame disease led to some striking interpretations of problems encountered by others. Several experienced vivid déjà vu recollections on seeing a film titled, *The Wedding Gift*.

The plot was based on the true story about a woman in her late 30s who had developed progressively severe fatigue, blackouts, convulsions, extreme muscle weakness, and joint pain over a three-year period during the mid-1980s. When her devoted husband asked about the diagnosis, she replied, "No idea. No cure. No hope." Three hospitalizations, visits with numerous consultants, and a muscle biopsy were summarized as "hysteria." This woman, who subsequently died, wanted a wife for her husband so that he would not be alone after she died. The account of this tragedy brought world attention to the "chronic fatigue syndrome."

B. <u>The "Unnamed Disease."</u> Syndicated health columnists receive requests for advice concerning young persons with unexplained severe fatigue and other features that probably often represent aspartame disease. For example, a concerned mother wrote about her son, who had been active in sports but recently felt weak without obvious cause (*The Palm Beach Post* April 2, 1999, p. F-2). He also experienced marked dryness of the mouth and intense thirst (see Chapter IX-F).

C. "The Yuppie Plague." Doctors have dubbed a severe affliction affecting highly educated adults between 20 and 40 years, particularly single women, as "the yuppie plague." It is characterized by extreme weakness, depression, inability to concentrate, headache, dizziness and lightheadedness. Although commonly attributed to a preceding viral infection, particularly the Epstein-Barr virus (see below), aspartame disease must be considered when such persons consume these products in large amounts.

D. "Chronic Infectious Mononucleosis." This term usually represents a "fad" diagnosis. In my experience, the large amounts spent for Epstein-Barr virus antibody tests and related studies in persons having chronic nonspecific fatigue, headache, joint aching and depression were generally wasted.

> Neither the Epstein-Barr virus nor another infectious organism could be detected among 178 persons in close contact with each other who suffered from "an outbreak of chronic fatigue." Dr. Dedra Buchwald (1987) studied this Nevada cohort. The majority were women averaging 38.5 years, who experienced symptoms comparable to those in aspartame disease – namely, headaches, nonspecific aching, and difficulty with concentration. Furthermore, 26 of the 78 patients evidenced neurologic features such as seizures, unsteadiness, and cognitive impairment suggesting an organic brain syndrome. Buchwald aptly asserted that a "common-source exposure to some environmental toxin might also be responsible."

E. The Chronic Fatigue Industry. An entire industry aimed at persons with "the chronic fatigue syndrome" has evolved in recent years. For example, a physician placed a full-page ad in *The Palm Beach Post* (March 18, 1997, p. A-15) for patients with this diagnosis – as well as the Epstein-Barr virus syndrome, fibromyalgia, Gulf War illness, depression, etc. They allegedly had been "successfully treated with our breakthrough methodology without the use of antidepressants." The "mini test" included in this ad could also serve to describe the complaints of many patients with aspartame disease.

F. <u>Proneness to Accidents</u>. The importance of aspartame-associated fatigue is underscored by the major role of "driver fatigue" and "pilot fatigue" in accidents (Roberts 1971; 1998d). Further details appear in Chapter XXVII.

Many drivers and pilots attempt to combat fatigue by drinking considerable caffeine as an "upper." Unfortunately, <u>caffeinism</u> (see introduction to Section 5) can compound aspartame disease.

G. <u>Frequent Concomitant and Overlooked Causes</u>. Numerous medical and psychologic problems can contribute to "chronic refractory fatigue." In my reviews of this subject (Roberts 1964c, e; 1995b), I emphasized the frequency of unrecognized narcolepsy (Chapter VI-5) and severe hypoglycemia (Chapter XIV), each of which also may be aggravated by aspartame. A factor that frequently summates upon the effects of aspartame is failure to obtain adequate sleep as a result of late-night television viewing.

F. INSOMNIA

"Recent severe insomnia" was a major complaint by 169 (14 percent) aspartame reactors. Most gave impressive histories of improvement after stopping aspartame, and prompt recurrence when they ingested it again... at times inadvertently.

<u>Representative Case Reports</u>

<u>Case VII-F-1</u>

A husband wrote this account about his 36-year-old wife who had suffered recent severe insomnia.

> "My wife used to drink diet cola religiously. We live in South Texas, a hot and humid climate. She then couldn't sleep, and had heart palpitations and flutterings. She is a nonsmoker and nondrinker, and exercises regularly. She weighs approximately 107 pounds. I hate doctors, but after two nights of no sleep, I did what doctors do: ask questions. And the only unhealthy thing I could fathom was diet cola. She has been in the pink ever since stopping, with one exception – the day she drank four ounces of the stuff, and her symptoms reappeared. Glad to have my wife back."

316

Case VII-F-2

A 32-year-old legal assistant greatly increased her consumption of various aspartame products in an attempt to lose weight. Shortly thereafter, she began experiencing severe dizziness. ("I would have to hold on to furniture to walk.") She also suffered severe headaches that repeatedly caused her to borrow aspirin. The diagnosis of "a major depression" was made, and antidepressant medication prescribed.

Her most severe complaint, however, was insomnia ("I stopped sleeping") which the antidepressant drugs failed to alleviate.

The patient subsequently read an article about aspartame disease. After stopping all such products for one week, she stated, "I felt profoundly better. My anxiety level and insomnia improved, and I have continually improved since then."

Case VII-F-3

A 64-year-old advertising executive with longstanding migraine began consuming two cans of diet cola daily. Severe insomnia ensued. ("The lack of sleep created by it made working next to impossible.") This problem disappeared <u>one</u> day after stopping the aspartame drink, but predictably occurred on each of three occasions he retested himself.

His wife and a son also suffered aspartame reactions consisting of "sleeplessness, chills, and disorientation."

Case VII-F-4

A young mother heard me discuss aspartame disease on a talk show. She described her aspartame-associated insomnia in this letter.

> "I've found aspartame to cause insomnia and pain in my eyes. I used to live on such products, but when I became pregnant, I stopped them for fear of what it would do to the baby. <u>All of a sudden, I could sleep at night</u>!! After three months, I started back on some diet sodas, just one a day, and could no longer sleep. I also noticed a sharp pain in my eyes. It was during this time I heard you on the radio program."

Commentary

Aspartame-induced insomnia should not be equated with a primary depression. This could pose a dual diagnostic dilemma when depression is also caused by aspartame products (VII-B).

The problem becomes compounded when long-acting hypnotic or tranquilizing drugs are prescribed, particularly for older individuals. The ensuing disturbance of rapid-eye-movement (REM) activity during sleep may initiate a vicious cycle of insomnia and inverted sleep rhythms – that is, the person may sleep during the day, but remain awake at night.

Insomnia constitutes a major public health hazard because of associated fatigue, poor performance at work, and driver/pilot error. About one-third of Americans have 6 ½ hours sleep or less a night during the work week. (It has been punned that adequate sleep has become a perk of the refreshed and successful executive in our high-tech and information-driven economy.)

Sleep deprivation among high school students becomes a serious problem when it reflects the combination of early morning classes, "night owl" habits ("bedtime resistance"), and aspartame-induced insomnia.

I have detailed my clinical and experimental researches in narcolepsy and other sleep disorders (Roberts 1964, 1965c, 1967b, 1970, 1971). They afflict millions in the United States at enormous annual cost from lost productivity, and accidents on the road and in the work place.

Related aspartame effects may have other serious consequences.

- Sleep debt has a detrimental impact on carbohydrate metabolism and endocrine function. It includes decreased glucose tolerance, and altered thyrotropin and cortisol concentrations (Spiegel 1999).
- The possible contribution to sleep apnea was discussed in Chapter VI-K.
- Chronic sleep deprivation enhances susceptibility to seizures, perhaps through norepinephrine depletion.
- The occurrence of early morning insomnia attributable to aspartame might represent a delayed IgE-mediated "brain allergy," perhaps comparable to delayed aspartame-associated urticaria (Kulczycki 1987).

318

Aspartame-associated insomnia in part reflects an influence on the thalamus involving specific protein receptors or enzymes. Certain thalamic areas (notably its anterior and dorsomedial aspects) not only integrate and express sleep, but also influence neuroendocrine circadian rhythms and autonomic nervous system functions.

G. ASPARTAME ADDICTION

The habitual consumption of "diet" products containing this chemical not only risks aspartame disease but also clinical addiction (Roberts 2000). Prior aspartame addicts repeated volunteered, "I could hardly go anywhere without a diet cola in my hand." An aspartame reactor in Scotland joked that there is only a "c" difference between "additive" and "addictive."

Thirty-five (5.4 percent) of 649 aspartame reactors in my most recent data base found it difficult or impossible to discontinue these products because of severe withdrawal effects. They or their reporting relatives (especially parents of afflicted children) **specifically** used the terms "addict" and "addiction," notwithstanding the absence of these words in my 9-page Questionnaire Survey form (Chapter XVIII). Others who used comparable terms were excluded even though they experienced similar withdrawal symptoms. (Case VII-A-4 was an "aspartame junkie.")

Violent prolonged withdrawal reactions and "losing control" are hallmarks of addiction. Recovered alcoholic patients repeatedly stated that they felt worse after stopping aspartame than alcohol. Some asserted that they had traded one addiction for another in becoming "chain drinkers" of diet sodas. They adopted the Alcoholics Anonymous principle of "one day at a time" to get themselves through aspartame withdrawal. These victims invented expressions such as "recovering aspartolic," and "diet croak."

The addictive potential of caffeine (present in two-thirds of soft drinks sold nationwide) can summate upon that of aspartame. It has been quipped that businessmen desire products that are habit-forming. Examples are coffee and cola drinks as "delivery systems" for caffeine. Adding aspartame to these elixirs clearly invites dual addiction. A female aspartame reactor who suffered blurred vision, confusion, mood swings, depression, panic attacks, hunger and weight gain wrote the FDA that diet colas were "like a drug I can't resist... I stay thirsty and drink more."

The rapidity of addiction of aspartame colas impressed many, especially college students. (This phenomenon is comparable to observations by various researchers on nicotine dependency, who were impressed by evidence of addiction among teenagers within <u>days</u> or <u>weeks</u> of smoking their first cigarettes.) For example, an undergraduate chemistry major emphasized her escalating consumption within several months, even after switching to caffeine-free diet colas (up to two liters daily). She experienced aspartame disease – most notably as severe headache, ringing of the ears, intense thirst, "dimming of my vision," dizziness, marked fatigue, loss of hair, and problems with equilibrium. She volunteered that her initial symptom of anxiety was the first to abate after four days abstinence.

Persons who had recovered from aspartame addiction, and then unsuccessfully attempted to warn friends about this affliction, were amazed at the <u>resistance</u> they encountered. One such individual commented, "What does it take for a seemingly reasonable and intelligent human being (in this instance, a friend of 12 years) to be able to process information from another seemingly reasonable and intelligent human being who has experienced aspartame disease? What is it that makes them think we are lying to them?"

At a time when public health officials and politicians espouse a "drug-free America," aspartame has become "Satan's sweetener." There have been dramatic instances involving <u>famous personalities</u>. The addiction of Christina Onassis to diet cola (Roberts 1992, page 110) has been repeatedly confirmed – as the statement by Prince Dimitri of Yugoslavia: "She'd carry a magnum (of diet cola), literally, and drink and drink all day" (*The Miami Herald* May 16, 1999, p. I-2)

Victim Data

Gender and Age. There were 24 females and 11 males. Most were between 25 and 50 at the time of consultation or correspondence. They also include four children – ages 2-1/2, 3, 6 and 9-1/2.

Consumption. The amounts of aspartame products consumed daily ranged up to, or exceeded, six liters or 12 cans of sodas, 20 or more packets, and considerable gum.

- A 54-year-old woman was phoned by her daughter who had just learned about aspartame disease. "When I called her with the information, she had already taken 15 aspartame packets. Mother told me this was usual for her since the product had come on the market."

- One "huge consumer of aspartame" conjectured that such sodas are ideal for addiction because "they first quench thirst, and then cause thirst." His side effects of dry mouth and dry eyes are experienced by many aspartame reactors (Chapters IV and IX-F), even in the absence of marked sweating or hot weather.

- A correspondent consumed at least a 12-pack of diet cola daily "for many years." She previously felt "devastated" when saccharin-containing diet sodas were withdrawn, but then "quickly got the taste" for their aspartame counterparts.

- A male aspartame reactor had consumed two to three two-liter bottles of diet soda daily, along with 20 aspartame tablets in cups of coffee. When he stopped using these products, he vomited for 12 days and required hospitalization.

- A woman with aspartame disease used up to 44 (!) aspartame-containing popsicles daily.

- A correspondent indicated her addiction to diet colas was so severe that she would bring a can when visiting friends in the event they didn't have any. Similarly, dental technicians encountered aspartame addiction in patients who brought diet sodas with them.

- A woman with aspartame disease described the severe addiction of her brother, a college graduate who repeatedly suffered withdrawal symptoms. In an attempt to lessen his family's concern, he would buy multiple cartons at a country store, and then hide them in the trunk of his car or the laundry room.

Familial Aspects. Several instances of multiple family members being addicted to aspartame products are cited in Chapter XVI.

Addiction and Withdrawal

The pathos of aspartame addiction appears in the representative case reports and elsewhere (see Case VII-A-3). Withdrawal symptoms – notably, severe irritability, tension, depression, tremors, nausea and sweating – usually abated promptly on resuming aspartame, as did the intense craving for these products.

- One woman noted, "This was as bad as when I quit smoking 13 years ago."

- Many relatives and friends urged "aspartame junkies" to stop aspartame products, but to no avail. One frustrated mother commented, "The problem with some people is that they either are addicts or just plain stubborn."

- A 49-year-old woman with severe rheumatologic complaints reported

  > "For the first two weeks after removing aspartame, I was listless, tired, craved sweet foods, and found my legs were restless. I felt incredibly ill; but, after about seven days, I found I no longer had the drug, insomnia, mental confusion, and bouts of feverishness."

- A 34-year-old man who drank at least two liters of a diet cola daily described himself as a "slave" to this product. He was able to tolerate a week of severe withdrawal symptoms with the help of a support group of friends. He stated, "I never would have thought that the one drink I enjoyed could be doing so much harm to me and to those around me."

Some <u>pertinent clinical aspects</u> are noteworthy.

- As with other addictions, denial and distortion were encountered. The mother of two young children stated, "I didn't want to believe aspartame was the cause of my problems. Even though anything with it made me crave carbohydrates, I dismissed this as my imagination."
- Aspartame addiction can recur, even after abstinence for years. This phenomenon is well known among "former" alcoholics. The mother of Case VI-L-3 provided this poignant 12-year followup.

  > "About eight months ago, unknown to me, she began drinking considerable diet soda. I learned a few days ago that she started drinking alcohol, plans to leave her fiancé, and bought a motorcycle – exactly as she had done 12 years previously when drinking diet soda. Her aspartame addiction makes her totally irrational. She crusaded against aspartame for 12 years, and is now drinking it. I don't know where to go for help, especially because most doctors I know think aspartame is just wonderful!"

322

- Diabetics addicted to aspartame depended on it for their "sugar fix."
- Several pregnant women resumed aspartame products, notwithstanding their great misgivings in doing so, after experiencing severe withdrawal symptoms.
- A young mother was told by her allergist that her withdrawal reaction was "as similar to heroin withdrawal as one could get."
- There were dramatic stories of patients with aspartame disease who experienced severe withdrawal symptoms when they traveled abroad, and were unable to purchase aspartame sodas. Considering the possibility these features represented caffeine withdrawal, they tried drinking more caffeine, but to no avail.
- Addiction has occurred to specific types of aspartame products. One victim wrote, "I don't drink diet sodas, but I have noticed that I crave aspartame chewing gums to the point that I have to go and buy it. I get quite put out if I can't get to buy it. It's like an addiction. I simply crave it, and don't feel OK until I'm chewing it."

Representative Case Reports

Case VII-G-1

The anguished friend of an aspartame addict stated, "She could hardly walk. She could hardly see. She was already going to a neurologist because they thought she had multiple sclerosis. But she told me not to talk about it even though her physician already told her that aspartame was the problem, especially after he started researching its role in brain tumors – because two persons in her family died from brain tumors! When told aspartame would kill her, she said, 'I'm addicted to it and can't live without it. If they try to take it off the market, I'll get it on the black market!' "

Case VII-G-2

The wife of an addicted aspartame reactor wrote, "I've told my husband over and over again, as have several physicians, that his problems would probably go away if he got off aspartame. But he says he is addicted and can't." Provoked by her continued purchase of aspartame sodas, the daughter-in-law asked whether she would hand him a gun if he wanted to commit suicide. She responded, "Please don't say anything else. It's hard enough to watch him lose his memory, fall, and hardly be able to walk. I just want to make him happy."

Case VII-G-3

A patient with previous alcoholism expressed concern that he traded it for aspartame addiction. He observed, "There are MANY just like me. You will rarely see a recovered alcoholic without a drink in hand, day or night, whether it be coffee or soda... usually DIET. We can hardly keep sweeteners on hand at our meetings. MANY of us suffer from tremendous mood bouts. If aspartame has contributed to the difficulties I have had with depression and mood swings, I WANT TO KNOW!"

Case VII-G-4

A woman with aspartame disease misdiagnosed as multiple sclerosis stated

> " I am convinced that aspartame was at the root of my problem. It is hard to convey just how much of this stuff I was using. I used at least one large box of aspartame a week... for myself! After my husband heard on a radio broadcast that it was bad, he told me not to use it, and refused to buy it for me any longer. I then literally bought it weekly, hid it in the kitchen, and used it when he was out of the room. And people still don't believe it is addictive???"

Case VII-G-5

A young man with longstanding symptoms ascribed to aspartame sodas wrote

> "I drank a lot of pop with aspartame when I was a kid in the 1980s, and felt bad. After reading a page on the net about insomnia, lightheadedness, ringing in the ears, and feeling unreal 'like I was on something,' I stopped. But it's hard to make yourself stop. It took about two months before I felt better. I think most people who drink diet pop get addicted to it, like me. At first you don't seem to like the taste; then you crave it."

Case VII-G-6

This statement was made by a hospital pharmacist with considerable knowledge about addictive substances and drug abuse.

"I have been a chronic user of diet drinks for years, and always joked that I was 'addicted' to aspartame. Recently, I decided to stop them, but I couldn't do it no matter how hard I tried. When I'm not drinking these drinks, the people I work with and my family have all commented that I act as if I'm going through heroin withdrawal. I also experienced many problems while drinking them, the most profound being joint pain."

Case VII-G-7

A woman became a "heavy diet cola drinker" at 20, but had consumed aspartame sodas since the age of 13. Her intake increased at 16 because she could obtain them at no charge when she began to waitress. By 22, her "addiction" amounted to a 12-pack daily. She experienced many symptoms attributable to aspartame disease – including joint/neck/back pains, a constant throbbing headache, recurrent yeast infections, intense leg cramps, anxiety attacks, marked palpitations, constant intense thirst, insomnia, a facial rash, and heartburn. Within one day of avoiding aspartame, and drinking water "by the gallons," her headache was gone and the other symptoms began to improve.

Case VII-G-8

A 14-year-old girl read about aspartame disease, and sought advice after having experienced intense withdrawal symptoms when she tried to stop diet colas. ("They sky-rocketed into absolute agony.") She had consumed considerable amounts over the previous two years. In a remarkable letter, she wrote, "I have been in doubt and denial. I am only 14, and don't like having what feels like a death sentence hanging over me."

Case VII-G-9

A nurse with depression, fibromyalgia, chronic headache, joint pains, and unexplained rapid heart rate drank three 2-liter bottles of diet cola daily. She attempted to quit when informed by her sister about aspartame disease. The ensuing hallucinations and suicidal thoughts necessitated hospitalization with suicidal precautions.

Case VII-G-10

A 28-year-old woman stated, "I was an addict. I could drink 10 to12 20-ounce diet colas a day... hot or cold!! I was so addicted that I would even drink a diet cola that had been in my car all day in 100 degree weather." Her symptoms included extreme fatigue, sleepiness, loss of hair, depression, severe neck pain, and reduced sexuality. ("I was a walking time bomb waiting to happen... and it did happen.")

She avoided aspartame sodas when her marriage became threatened. She felt "recovered" one year later.

Commentary

I. Exclusion of Related Terminology

By excluding aspartame reactors who continued to consume large amounts of aspartame, despite debilitating symptoms, because they failed to use the terms "addict" or "addiction," the prevalence of aspartame addiction in this series was underestimated.

- Many aspartame reactors described their "unnatural craving" for aspartame products. It was not limited to diet sodas – e.g., persons with a severe "craving" for aspartame gum. The threat posed by the habitual chewing of such gum is considered below and in Chapter II-E.
- An aspartame reactor referred to herself as "a 10-year-plus aspartame junkie." Another stated she had been "a dietcolaholic" for 12 years.
- Three women indicated that they had been "hooked" on diet sodas for a decade.

This correspondence from a 29-year-old woman with severe aspartame disease, who was referred to me by her physician to confirm the diagnosis, bridges the terminology of "addiction" and "craving."

> "As I do not use any sugar, I have used aspartame and saccharin. The disturbing phenomenon is that I now have intense and abnormal cravings for aspartame, and find myself using more and more of it... like an addictive cycle. Without it, food seems flat. I have tried eliminating it altogether, and find that this actually intensifies the cravings even a week later! I would like to know if you have ever heard of anything like this before, or have advice as to dealing with it. Besides the aspartame cravings, I have also continued to have inexplicable bouts of itchy skin, hives, and quite a bit of swelling in the face and legs. The legs are often numb, and I am extremely fatigued most of the time."

II. Children

The apparent addiction of four children to aspartame poses a serious problem. Their case histories are summarized.

- A 9-1/2-year old boy exhibited "extreme hyperactivity." Every time he opened the refrigerator and found only regular cola sodas, he would exclaim, "I can't believe they didn't get even one diet cola!"

- A 2-1/2-year-old girl had been weaned off baby fruit juices, and was begun on aspartame drinks on the premise of preventing sugar-induced dental problems. She developed an extensive rash that subsided after stopping aspartame. Her mother wrote, "For the first five days, she was like someone in withdrawal – aggressive and craving the substance."

- A 6-year-old girl was diagnosed by a pediatric neurologist as having attention-deficit disorder and a "mild encephalopathy of unknown origin." Her mother drank an aspartame beverage during the pregnancy because of marked morning sickness and a severe yeast infection. She wrote

  > "Little did I realize what I was doing to myself, let alone my fetus who also developed the yeast infection. By the time she was three years old, we were both using sugar-free products – including yogurt, popsicles, gum, soda pop, candy, ice cream, pies, puddings, and hot chocolate. (She also sneaked them in.) I developed a brain tumor (oligodendroglioma), and underwent surgery and radiation. Fortunately, my mom came across two articles on aspartame a year ago, after which we quit these products."

- A 3-year-old girl repeatedly developed a rash and behavior problems after taking aspartame products. Her mother stated, "For at least five days after stopping them, she craved the former drink, and was extremely hyperactive and aggressive."

Other indications of aspartame addiction among children appear in the media. For example, a syndicated health column carried the headline-title, "Can a young child become addicted to a cold remedy?" (*The Palm Beach Post* April 9, 2000, p. D-3). This inquiry had been received from concerned sister-in-law of a mother who had been giving her 17-month-old daughter a popular antihistamine-decongestant, presumably in palatable syrup form, since the age of three months "to help her sleep better."

III. **Comments on Addiction**

The continued heavy consumption of aspartame products by persons with aspartame disease qualifies as "substance abuse" relative to causing, aggravating or prolonging their physical, mental and behavioral problems. As with other forms of chemical dependency, aspartame abusers are likely to deny or distort symptoms. The erroneous assertion that this addiction solely represents caffeinism was noted previously.

In his classic description of "addictive eating and drinking," Randolph (1956) emphasized that small quantities of a specific excitant can perpetuate an addiction response owing to the extreme specific sensitivity commonly involved. He included various sugars, alcoholic beverages and monosodium glutamate (MSG).

Each of the three components of aspartame (phenylalanine; aspartic acid; the methyl ester that promptly becomes free methyl alcohol after ingestion), and their multiple breakdown products following exposure to heat or during storage, are potentially neurotoxic and addictive (Section 5). The mechanisms may involve dopamine, serotonin, cerebral cholecystokinin (CCK), endorphins, other important neurotransmitters, insulin, and the unique permeability of the blood-brain barrier to phenylalanine. Only several aspects will be discussed here.

The transformation of phenylalanine to dopamine and dopamine metabolites is highly relevant. Addictive drugs flood synapses with dopamine, which carries a "pleasure message" from one nerve cell to another in the "reward pathway"... thereby creating a "high." For instance, cocaine blocks the reuptake of dopamine, and acts as an indirect dopamine agonist. Such repeated rushes can result in desensitization of the brain to dopamine, and perhaps a reduction of dopamine receptors.

- During et al (1987) demonstrated that changes in brain phenylalanine may selectively affect production of the dopamine molecule that becomes preferentially released into synapses.

- Aspartame-altered dopamine metabolism includes blocking of dopamine D_2 receptors in the mesolimbic circuitry of the brain (Wang 2000). Persons with low numbers of D_2 receptors may be more vulnerable to addictive behaviors, apparently representing a "reward deficiency syndrome."

- Persons with few dopamine D_2 receptors appear to be at greater risk for abusing psychostimulants. Volkow et al (1999), Brookhaven National Laboratory, consistently found this among all persons addicted to cocaine, alcohol and heroin who were tested.

- Myers and Melchior (1977) reported that a dopamine-dopaldehyde condensation product (tetrahydropapaveroline) caused rats to drink increasingly large amounts of alcohol solutions which normally would have been rejected.

- Researches have advanced the concept that increased dopamine influences the addictive effects of cocaine, and dopamine-receptor agonists themselves might be addictive in cocaine users (Koob 1998).

- Aspartame has been shown to increase morphine analgesia (Nikfar 1997).

Suggestions about minimizing the severe effects of withdrawal offered by addicted individuals who had diet sodas by their side "24/7," based on personal experiences and research, appear in Chapter XXXIV. Noni juice has been used with apparent success by some patients with aspartame addiction, presumably due to its ability to increase serotonin (Chapter XXIX).

The habitual chewing of aspartame gum poses a unique threat, as evidenced by dramatic precipitation of systemic reactions (Chapter II-E). Its flavor and sweetness can last 30 minutes, compared to five minutes for sugar-sweetened gum. The chemical may be absorbed through the mucosa of the mouth (as used therapeutically with nitroglycerin), and via simple diffusion from the oropharynx directly into the brain. The latter phenomenon has been demonstrated with small molecules such as glucose, sodium chloride and ethyl alcohol (Maller 1967).

As noted earlier, some persons who opted to chew diet gum containing aspartame in an attempt to break the smoking habit actually transformed their nicotine addiction into an aspartame addiction.

IV. <u>Chronic Methanol Toxicity and Addiction</u>

The chronic intake of free methanol is germane to aspartame disease and addiction, particularly for alcoholics. Several aspartame reactors demonstrated their gratitude in having been informed about this problem by joining anti-aspartame consumer groups. As a recovered alcoholic and a member of Alcoholics Anonymous for 25 years, one stated that she could probably appreciate "the addictive nature of wood alcohol."

The daily intake of methyl alcohol from natural sources is less than 10 mg. Aspartame beverages average 55 mg methanol per liter, and nearly double as much in some carbonated orange sodas. Persons ingesting five liters a day can therefore consume over 400 mg methanol. The subjects of methyl alcohol metabolism reviewed in Chapter XXI.

Two commentaries deserve restatement.

- Six years <u>before</u> FDA approval of aspartame, Dr. Herbert S. Posner (1975), National Institute of Environmental Health Sciences, wrote a review titled, "Biohazards of Methanol in Proposed News Uses." He stressed that failure to recognize the "delayed and irreversible effects on the nervous system" of methanol... at widely varying levels of exposure and at rather low levels." Furthermore, he suggested that "when a safer compound is available, methanol should not be utilized."
- Huge C. Cannon, Associate Commissioner for Legislative Affairs of the FDA, commented about the methyl alcohol component of aspartame in a letter dated September 8, 1986: "The Agency has recently become aware, however, of clinical data that indicate that the toxic effects of methanol are due to formate accumulation and not to formaldehyde which is itself formed from the metabolism of methanol."

Another possible complication of chronic methanol intake from aspartame addiction is an increasingly frequent form of chronic liver disease known as nonalcoholic steatohepatitis (Chapter IX-K).

VIII

ALLERGIES AND SKIN REACTIONS; IMMUNOLOGIC PERSPECTIVES

"It is hard to estimate how many people who already have
allergies are suffering from food additives."
Dr. William C. Grater (1969)

"With the frequent introduction of new foods and beverages
into our diets, it is becoming more difficult to establish
etiological factors responsible for hypersensitivity reactions."
Dr. Stephen D. Lockey, Sr. (1973)

Patients in this series attributed the following allergies and skin reactions to use of aspartame products.

Severe itching without a rash	-	87 (7%)
Severe lip and mouth reactions	-	54 (5%)
Hives (urticaria)	-	47 (4%)
Severe genital itching, rash, or both	-	25* (4%)
Other skin eruptions, including lupus erythematosus	-	108 (9%)
Aggravation of asthma and other allergies	-	17 (1%)
Marked thinning of hair	-	71 (6%)
Dual sensitivity to monosodium glutamate (MSG)	-	14 (2%)

* -- data based on most recent 649 reactors

Acronym Legend

ACB - aspartame cola beverage
ASD - aspartame soft drink
ATS - aspartame tabletop sweetener

A. GENERAL CONSIDERATIONS

The broad implications of introducing a chemical currently being used by over half the population that can affect the immune system are considered in this chapter.

The term "allergy" indicates an abnormal reaction to some substance. The offending agents (allergens) may be dust, pollen, molds, foods, drugs and other food additives. Such persons tend to be allergic to other substances. They also often have close relatives afflicted with allergies.

Manifestations

Allergic reactions can manifest themselves in various ways. They consist of severe itching, a localized or diffuse rash, swelling of the nose and sinuses, joint pains, and the destruction of blood components (autoimmune anemia; aplastic anemia). One patient with aspartame disease asserted, "It was almost as if I was allergic to myself."

Anaphylactic shock occurred in four aspartame reactors. It entails severe obstruction of the larynx and upper airways, spasm and swelling of the bronchial tubes, and a drop in blood pressure from marked dilation of the blood vessels. I pointed out this omission in commenting on a review of anaphylaxis that failed to mention aspartame products (Roberts 1996).

Representative Case Reports

Case VIII-A-1

A health professional gave this account of his severe allergic reaction to aspartame:

> "I experienced an anaphylactic reaction following a drink presweetened with aspartame. Within 15 minutes of drinking an 8 oz. glass, I found myself gasping for air, and having hives the size of a baseball mitt and at least one inch raised off the skin. Lucky for me, I worked in a department adjacent to the emergency room of a community hospital. The ER doc in charge knew me, and immediately recognized the severity of the situation. From the time I walked to the ER, I could barely

stand, and then collapsed. I was intubated (which I don't recall). Being a pharmacist, I realized that I had just experienced a near-fatal reaction when I regained my wits and whereabouts."

"I notified the manufacturer of the sweetener at the time."

"For months after that, and months on prednisone and topical creams and ointments for the pruritus and hives that continually reappeared, I finally did return to a normal state. Since then, even someone opening a packet of aspartame in a restaurant, and flicking the packet to assure it was empty, has been sufficient to generate an allergic response."

Aspartame may aggravate <u>respiratory allergies</u> (VIII-C). This assumes considerable significance in the case of asthmatic children. The incidence and severity of asthma among younger persons have increased steadily over the past two decades, notwithstanding improved therapies.

Several <u>dermatologic "idiosyncrasies"</u> are discussed in this chapter. They indicate the need for considering an aspartame reaction in patients presenting with unexplained persistent or recurrent eruptions, especially when extensive testing and skin biopsies have shed little light.

A related consideration involves persons with documented or suspect <u>lupus erythematosus</u> (VIII-E). Such patients should be queried about aspartame consumption.

Female Preponderance

The preponderance of women having aspartame disease was noted in Chapter II. Dr. Don McLain (1986), President of the American Association for Clinical Immunology, indicated that women have significantly more allergies to food and drugs than men.

Women are also more vulnerable to autoimmune diseases, such as rheumatoid arthritis (3:1 ratio) and lupus erythematosus (10:1 ratio).

- One possible explanation is the greater orientation of the female immune system to autologous antigens with aging (*Science* Volume 238: 159, 1987).

- Talal (1985) suggested that autoimmune diseases are more common in women because of "immunologic imprinting" in a hyperestrogen environment *in utero*. This phenomenon presumably serves to protect pregnant women from infectious diseases and other environmental insults.

Prior History of Allergies

Analysis of the survey questionnaire (Section 4) revealed known allergies to dust, pollen, molds, foods, drugs and other additives in nearly one-third of aspartame reactors. They included hay fever, asthma, and allergies to one or more medications. The following patient illustrates such an allergic background.

Representative Case Report

Case VIII-A-2

A 60-year-old housewife attributed recent headache, tingling of the limbs, extreme irritability, palpitations, abdominal pain, nausea and diarrhea to the consumption of aspartame products. She promptly became "very ill with flu-like symptoms." There was a history of previous asthma and severe sensitivity to penicillin. A grandson also became "extremely nervous when he takes anything with aspartame."

On the other hand, an allergic history may be absent, especially in persons experiencing an allergic-type reaction for the first time. One young Iowa woman stated, "As soon as I drank a diet soda for the first time, my lips and mouth became swollen, and I developed terrible pain shooting to my head and chest!"

Other presumed allergic responses are cited elsewhere. Some examples:

- Case IV-M-1 evidenced myasthenia gravis while consuming aspartame. (This condition is regarded as an autoimmune phenomenon.) She had previously developed anemia from alpha methyldopa (Aldomet®) prescribed for hypertension.

334

- Case IX-D-7 described <u>swelling of her salivary glands</u> "as large as golf balls" 15 minutes after drinking a diet cola.

Familial Aspects

The familial ramifications of aspartame disease were discussed in Chapter II-I. They are evidenced in several of the case reports to be cited (VIII-A-2, VIII-B-16, VIII-B-19, VIII-C-3).

Other family members may experience acute reactions to aspartame products that are not typically "allergic" (see Case VIII-A-3). For example, a man suffered severe migraine after drinking one can of aspartame soda. His son, however, would begin wheezing when he consumed an aspartame drink.

Representative Case Report

Case VIII-A-3

A 36-year-old architectural designer experienced intense and prolonged headache ("as though my brain was swollen and trying to crawl out of my ears"), and pain in both eyes "immediately" after drinking an aspartame soft drink. This sequence recurred on three retesting trials. She gave a history of hypoglycemia. Her daughter evidenced hyperactive behavior (Chapter VI-G) after consuming aspartame.

Aspartame in Drug Products

The incorporation of aspartame in drug products is widespread, particularly pediatric and antihistamine formulations (Chapter II and XI).

Persons with severe allergic reactions to aspartame have expressed their concern to pharmaceutical companies selling products that contain aspartame, especially in chewable form.

Aggravated or Enhanced Allergies

Aspartame reactors seem to exhibit more frequent and severe reactions to drugs. For example, aspirin and nonsteroidal anti-inflammatory analgesic drugs (such as ibuprofen) induced violent dizziness and other symptoms in several patients with prior aspartame-associated headaches or impaired vision. Reactions attributed to pharmacologic interactions with aspartame intake are discussed in Chapter IX-I.

<u>Subsequent allergies to other substances and food additives were encountered among aspartame reactors</u> (see Cases VIII-B-1 and VIII-B-2). Dual sensitivity to aspartame and monosodium glutamate (MSG), and the multiple chemical sensitivity syndrome are discussed below.

- Cases VIII-B-1 and VIII-B-4 later developed milk intolerance.
- "Universal allergy" to numerous natural and man-made substances (see Cases VIII-B-1 and B-2) is an extreme form. Unfortunate individuals with this condition, also referred to as "environmental disease," obtain relative relief only by living in allergy-free rooms ("cocoons") covered with aluminum foil.

The Need for Testing "Real World" Products

The need to use commercially-available products when testing subjects/patients for aspartame reactions is again emphasized. The reasons focus on sensitivity and toxicity to aspartame breakdown products (Section 5), especially after exposure to heat and prolonged storage. Unsuccessful attempts to replicate documented adverse reactions to aspartame products after administering "non real" substances are underscored.

- Downham (1992) was able to reproduce a variety of allergic-type skin reactions (see below) by having patients drink a diet soda – rather than swallowing aspartame in capsule form – in his series of 23 such cases.
- Kulczycki (1995) challenged the presumed infrequency of aspartame-induced hives based on the foregoing deficiencies involving a corporate-sponsored study.

Costly Diagnostic Studies

Many aspartame reactors emphasized the considerable – and in retrospect needless – expense of extensive allergy tests to which they had been subjected. Case VIII-B-1, a physician, illustrates this issue and the numerous erroneous diagnoses. Moreover, most of these costly studies proved of little value. An exception was the markedly positive RAST test to aspartame in Case VIII-B-13.

Possible Mechanisms

Allergic reactions may be due to the aspartame molecule, its three components, or the approximate ten breakdown substances (including stereoisomers and the diketopiperazine derivative) associated with heating and prolonged storage (Chapter XX). As noted, they might not be reproduced by administering a capsule or freshly prepared cool solution containing aspartame.

The diketopiperazine metabolite may initiate an allergic response through haptene-protein conjugates. (This is analogous to penicillin allergy wherein a derivative of penicillin binds to endogenous proteins.) An IgE-mediated reaction generally occurs after exposure for several weeks.

Aspartame-induced inflammatory, allergic and anaphylactic reactions may result from the production of leukotrienes. This group of biologically active compounds is derived from arachidonic acid via lipoxygenase enzyme pathways. They are released from a variety of human cells – including macrophages, polymorphonuclear leukocytes, mast cells and monocytes. The ensuing inflammatory responses could contribute to many of the problems encountered in aspartame disease such as skin reactions, allergic manifestations, gastrointestinal symptoms, and joint complaints.

> Hardcastle and Bruch (1997) treated macrophage cells with aspartame. They found the production of leukotrienes and other arachidonic acid metabolites, most notably leukotriene C_4, leukotriene B_4, and 15-hydroxyeicosatetraenoic acid. The aspartame-treated macrophage cell cultures produced three times as much arachidonic acid metabolites as did untreated control cell cultures.

The rise of cytokine concentrations, notably interferon and tumor necrosis factor, provoked by food intolerance (*Lancet* 2000; Volume 356: 400-401) could account for the allergic and other symptoms these patients experience, such as joint/muscular pain, headache, and respiratory/abdominal complaints.

The occurrence of aspartame-induced hives or seizures during the early morning hours could be explained in part by a <u>delayed hypersensitivity reaction</u>.

Tobey and Heizer (1986) suggested another mechanism for aspartame-induced systemic symptoms and immune reactions. It involves <u>deficiency of a major peptidase enzyme within the cytosol of intestinal-wall cells</u> that hydrolyses the aspartylphenylalanine dipeptide. Circulating red blood cells might be used to screen for such an enzymic deficiency, or genetic variants thereof. Congenital deficiency of prolidase, another cytosolic peptidase, is a recognized disturbance might involve <u>mast cell dysfunction</u>. Mast cells cultured in aspartame evidence enhanced rates of proliferation (Sczuc 1986).

Grateful Patients

Paradoxically, some patients expressed gratitude because these associations were detected. A woman who developed an extensive rash from using aspartame products wrote, "I think I'm lucky that I am sensitive. I believe that the cumulative effects for those who are not so sensitive will later become evident, but the person may not draw the connection until it is too late."

B. ITCHING AND HIVES

In this series of 1,200 aspartame reactors, 87 (7 percent) developed severe itching without a rash, 47 (4 percent) hives (urticaria), and 108 (9 percent) other eruptions. The latter – including acne rosacea, eruptions resembling lupus erythematosus, and photosensitivity – are discussed in VIII-F.

The sequence of regression after abstinence, and predictable recurrence following rechallenge was diagnostic. As with other foods and additives, hives due to ingesting aspartame products generally occurred within 6-12 hours. Analyzing their episodes of "stray hives" provided aspartame reactors with insights about the causation.

This frequency of skin reactions exceeds the overall reaction rate of 2.2 percent for drug-induced skin reactions reported in a large study of consecutive medical inpatients monitored by the Boston Collaborative Drug Surveillance Program (Bigby 1986). The high incidence of such reactions among females (see above) is also noteworthy.

Importance of Careful History Taking

It was necessary to query patients with unexplained rashes **repeatedly** and **specifically** about the use of aspartame-containing products. For example, the issue of a delayed reaction to an antibiotic arose in a patient who developed itching and hives several weeks after taking it. She initially denied taking aspartame, but then admitted to its use when several diet beverages were named.

The complex problem of chronic and recurrent urticaria warrants specific inquiry about aspartame use (Roberts 1996). Dr. Kenneth P. Mathews (Professor of Medicine, University of Michigan Medical School) asserted, "When it comes to chronic urticaria, 95% of cases, except for the physical urticarias, are never solved" *(Internal Medicine News* November 1, 1986, p. 53).

Dose Responses: "Biological Experiments of Nature"

Aspartame reactors who <u>predictably</u> develop an itch or rash on challenge constitute pertinent "biological experiments of nature." They also provide insights relative to THEIR <u>maximum "safe" daily intake</u> (Chapter XXVII). The occurrence of an overt allergy in some patients (as Case B-14) seemed an "all or none" phenomenon – that is, reactions developed only after a threshold quantity had been taken.

It was mentioned earlier that these individuals regard themselves as fortunate, compared to aspartame reactors with more subtle changes (especially of vision and brain function) who continued using aspartame products.

Inadvertent Rechallenge

Several patients – as Cases VIII-B-6, B-7, B-11 and B-12 – illustrate the prompt recurrence of symptoms after ingesting products they did not suspect contained aspartame.

Representative Case Reports

Case VII-B-1

A physician and former industrial research chemist had suffered severe itching and a rash for four years. Several prominent physicians and a professor of dermatology had variously diagnosed his disorder as "nerves, allergies, and vasculitis." At the time of his correspondence, he had remained symptom-free for four months after discontinuing aspartame products.

Case VIII-B-2

A 50-year-old woman suffered severe symptoms after drinking one 12-ounce can of an aspartame soft drink or chewing up to four sticks of aspartame gum daily. She used these products to avoid sugar (because of reactive hypoglycemia) and to control weight.

Her reactions consisted of a rash, headache, dizziness, mental confusion, memory loss, hyperactivity, tingling or numbness of the limbs, profound depression (with suicidal thoughts), severe anxiety, unexplained chest pains, nausea, a metallic taste in the mouth, and exaggerated "low blood sugar attacks." On the occasions she retested herself, these symptoms were experienced "the moment I swallowed it." She qualified her subsequent disability in these terms.

"About one or two months after I stopped using aspartame, I started reacting to other foods, and then chemicals. Eventually, just about everything provoked symptoms identical to those provoked initially by aspartame. The condition continues with nervous system distress, vision problems, breathing problems, headaches and memory problems. I now react to most foods, molds, chemicals. My doctor feels the use of aspartame may have triggered this condition.

"Since my experience with aspartame and the general spread of hypersensitivity to all chemicals and most foods, my life has become a nightmare. My doctor says that this condition is usually precipitated by exposure to some toxic substance. Since aspartame was the only thing that was changed in my routine, and because it was the first thing to which I reacted, I feel strongly that there is a connection between aspartame and my current health problems."

Case VIII-B-3

A 52-year-old homemaker developed itching and hives. She had been consuming six packets of an ATS, three glasses of presweetened iced tea, two glasses of aspartame hot chocolate, and two servings of aspartame puddings or gelatins daily in an attempt to lose weight. "Anything that has aspartame, I bought."

She became virtually incapacitated by these and other complaints. They included headache, dizziness, drowsiness, memory loss, decreased vision and pain in both eyes, facial pains, slurred speech, severe depression and a marked change in personality. Additional problems were abdominal bloat, recent "dry eyes," and sensitivity to noise. Her symptoms improved within six weeks after stopping all aspartame products, but recurred within eight hours on the two occasions she retested herself.

Additional intolerances ensued even though there had been no prior allergic history. She wrote, "Today, after two years of being off aspartame, I notice sensitivity to all food additives and other environmental toxins."

Case VIII-B-4

A 29-year-old chemist experienced swelling of her lips, eyes, hands and feet within less than an hour after ingesting aspartame soft drinks. This sequence, often with concomitant swelling of the tongue, recurred on rechallenging herself more than 20 times! She abstained from aspartame products thereafter. Her only relevant history was an episode of hives (attributed to chocolate) at the age of eleven.

Other allergies developed. She stated, "Then suddenly, milk products started causing the same reaction. I was never allergic to milk before."

Case VIII-B-5

A 59-year-old housewife developed an extensive rash and difficulty in swallowing within one day after consuming aspartame. This sequence was repeated on each of the three occasions she tested herself. Other symptoms included "dry eyes," ringing in both ears, insomnia, marked thirst, frequent urination, joint pains, and a gain of 15 pounds. She gave a history of allergy to penicillin and sulfa drugs.

Case VIII-B-6

A young woman discontinued aspartame because she developed a severe rash whenever using products containing it. She successfully substituted saccharin-containing beverages. The producer of one such cola drink subsequently substituted aspartame without indicating this on the label. She promptly suffered intense itch after drinking the new formulation.

Case VIII-B-7

A 54-year-old woman developed a rash extending from the neck to knees. After deducing that it was due to the aspartame in her soft drink and chewing gum, she shifted to soft drinks containing saccharin. The eruption gradually subsided.

An inadvertent rechallenge occurred when the manufacturer of a diet cola incorporated aspartame without her awareness of this shift. Severe itching recurred after she drank several bottles.

Case VIII-B-8

This aspartame reactor **precisely** timed her one, and only, encounter with aspartame. She wrote

> "On April 16, 1984, I had my first glass of diet cola sweetened with aspartame. Approximately one-half hour later, I experienced generalized itching with giant hives on my back, chest and arms. There were approximately 100. I never had such an experience. In approximately 3 hours, the eruption was alleviated with an antihistamine and cortisone."

Case VIII-B-9

A 49-year-old tennis professional had been "miserable and discouraged by the continual outbreaks of hives for one year." She also experienced swelling of the lips and eyes. Treatment with a corticosteroid and antihistamines was required. Concomitantly, she had heavy menstrual bleeding.

Three physicians and consultants could not identify the cause despite extensive allergy testing. She tried eliminating "all chemicals, certain foods... you name it" – but in vain. "I seemed allergic to everything."

She then chanced to view a television program on the subject of aspartame reactions. After stopping such products, the hives did not recur. In retrospect, she recalled that they developed several weeks after she began consuming a "sugar-free" gelatin. "I really feel that aspartame use triggered the hives."

342

Case VIII-B-10

A diabetic female developed "large sores over my head, face and back" shortly after she began drinking two cans of an aspartame soft drink daily.

Case VIII-B-11

A female reactor provided the following chronology of recent skin reactions to aspartame.

"Sat. 9/14   I had <u>hives over much of my body</u>: under arms, legs from crotch to knees, chest and neck Went to Baptist Hospital Emergency. Doctor J__ gave me shots of adrenalin and Benadryl. He said the cause might never be known and perhaps it would clear up by the next day. <u>I had sweetened coffee served by a friend with aspartame</u> Friday and Saturday.

"Sun. 9/15   Hives had not improved. Called Doctor C__ who prescribed Decadron and Lidex Creme.

"Mon. 9/16   No improvement. Went to Dr. C__'s office. He prescribed Trilafon, Celestone and Lidex Creme (3 tubes were used). Hives continued to come and go all week, and by Friday and Saturday was quite improved.

"Mon. or Sat.   I ate a serving of a cereal sweetened with aspartame. The following day the hives were back, spreading to new areas not itching before. I began to suspect aspartame. Dr. C__ agreed that it was likely a reaction to the artificial sweetener.

"Mon. 9/30   The hives had cleared enough that I could go to water exercise class. Small itchy spots appeared from time to time. It had been more than 2 weeks.

"Thurs. 10/10   A friend served hot tea mixed with a tea mix sweetened with aspartame. The following morning I broke out with a rash. I rook 50 mg Benadryl and it subsided.

"I have never had this problem before. The last three times I used aspartame I had a reaction. There is now no question in my mind that this artificial sweetener is the cause."

Case VIII-B-12

A 43-year-old man suffered recurrent hives over most of his body for two months. The "blotches" measured about the size of a quarter, and lasted from 20 minutes to eight hours. Numerous studies failed to unravel the cause. His only known prior allergy was a sulfa drug reaction during childhood.

He and his wife then began a process of "one-by-one elimination." The attacks cleared when he stopped aspartame beverages. He stated, "My doctor is fairly convinced our own detective work did the job." An unsuspected challenge offered further proof.

"While on vacation in British Columbia several weeks ago, I bought what I thought were two regular soft drinks out of the machine. Within twenty minutes of drinking them, I began to break out and itch. Within eight hours, I was completely covered with wheals all over my upper torso and neck."

Case VIII-B-13

A 31-year-old dentist had been in excellent health until November 1985. He developed itching within two weeks after ingesting aspartame beverages. Antihistamine therapy provided no relief. Numerous studies were not revealing. Subsequent severe extensive hives and dermographia (wheals at the site of stroking) forced him to stop practicing!

He was seen by several allergists. One found that the RAST test to aspartame was positive in a 1:1,486 dilution (greater than 1:750 being a positive reaction). Positive RAST tests to cinnamon and vanilla, but of lesser degree, also were noted. He was able to resume his practice after avoiding aspartame.

Case VIII-B-14

34-year-old woman suffered recurrent severe itching of the limbs and a subsequent rash. A cortisone-type injection afforded only transient relief.

She kept a diary, which was analyzed with a nurse. Both implicated the diet cola she consumed (two liters daily) as the likely cause. The following additional correlations were made.

- The rash generally occurred within two hours if she ingested enough of these beverages.
- The itching and eruption did not occur when she limited her intake to four glasses a <u>week</u>. Both developed within two hours, however, after drinking four or more glasses a day.
- Aspartame-associated itching and rash tended to occur sooner when she exercised and became overheated.
- Aspartame also provoked lightheadedness and "low blood sugar attacks."

Case VIII-B-15

A 21-year-old student noted that "my cheeks would swell up, my eyes would close, and my sinuses would fill up" after drinking up to four 12-ounce cans and a one-liter bottle of an ACB daily. There were associated headaches and irritability. She had hay fever for 11 years, and asthma for five years.

This patient's symptoms improved within a week after avoiding aspartame products, and disappeared the following week The reaction recurred within several hours when she once retested herself.

Case VIII-B-16

A 63-year-old writer had consumed one glass of an aspartame beverage and one packet of an ATS daily for three weeks prior to developing an "unexplained red rash on my leg." Other complaints included severe headache, dizziness, tingling of the limbs, irritability, a rise of blood pressure, abdominal cramps, debilitating nausea and diarrhea, joint pains, and swelling of the legs. Her symptoms disappeared within one week after stopping aspartame.

She stated, "I am allergic to medications and many foods with MSG, sulfites, additives, chocolate, many oils, oranges, milk." There was a history of prior asthma and an underactive thyroid. Her daughter also experienced abdominal distress from aspartame products.

Case VII-B-17

A 25-year-old male dietitian suffered unexplained severe itching, recurrent hives, a rash of both eyelids, dramatic thinning of the hair (despite conditioners), and swelling of the lips. Other complaints included decreased vision, dry eyes, ringing in both ears, intense thirst, severe sensitivity to noise, unsteadiness, drowsiness, insomnia, memory impairment, slurred speech, severe depression with suicidal thoughts, irritability, anxiety attacks, personality changes, marked bloat, and unexplained pain in the right hip. He had been consuming aspartame sodas since the age of thirteen.

The patient experienced dramatic improvement when he avoided aspartame products – especially of the skin rashes and slurred speech. The eyelid reaction recurred shortly after he unknowingly ingested an aspartame product. He wrote

"The changes that have occurred for the better since my elimination of aspartame are nothing short of a miracle. It's scary to think that half the population is consuming some form of aspartame. I am doing as much as I can to have my friends and family eliminate these products. I am glad that at age 25 I was able to save myself from further toxic effects. I hope that the American Dietetic Association will someday accept the fact that aspartame is harmful. I can't thank you enough for your information."

Case VIII-B-18

A teacher described her severe aspartame-associated itching and rash in a letter written shortly after learning of my studies.

"Fortunately, my reactions to aspartame have been relatively mild compared to many people, if one considers the maddening itch a mild reaction. I have been seeing dermatologists, allergists and our family doctor for at least three years only to be told that it either wasn't their problem, or that the rash was parapsoriasis or of no known cause. I couldn't accept their conclusions as I feel that there has to be a cause. I might add that I refuse to believe that I am a hypochondriac, and rarely lose a day of work in my teaching profession.

"If the rash appears on the top of one leg, it will show up at the exact same place on the other. Likewise, on the inside of both forearms, and the tops of both ankles.

"Several weeks ago, I decided to eliminate aspartame from my diet. This meant making adjustments since I had just completed losing forty pounds on a weight-watching program. Within several days, the rash lost most of its redness. I am now able to sleep at night without scratching myself to the point of bleeding in my sleep. The areas involved have subsided to a dull discoloration and somewhat dry feeling. I suppose that it might take some time for all of this to leave my system permanently."

Case VIII-B-19

A young woman had severe urticaria for seven months despite referral to two allergists. Many allergy tests "came up negative." Her mother captured the pathos of the situation. "This poor girl had to exchange her wedding gown for one with long sleeves because the hives were so bad. Her eyes and lips would swell until it looked like her lips would burst." Her rash and other symptoms were gone after one day of abstinence from the diet cola she drank!

Reports by Others

In its initial monitoring of adverse reactions to aspartame, the FDA received reports of 111 rashes and 80 cases of hives among 3,326 aspartame complainants (Tollefson 1987).

Kulczycki (1986) initially described two patients with aspartame-induced hives and angioedema.

- Hives of the eyelids, lips hands, face and trunk, along with shortness of breath and joint swelling, were precipitated by diet colas and an ATS in a 23-year-old female. The causative role of aspartame was confirmed by open challenge and by two double-blind challenges using opaque capsules of aspartame or a placebo. Itching and hives occurred within one and a half to two hours after swallowing the aspartame. Their severity tended to correlate with the challenge dose (25 or 50 mg).
- A 42-year-old woman developed hives and angioedema within one hour after swallowing aspartame drinks. They recurred within 90 minutes after challenge with 75 mg aspartame in a double-blind study.

Kulczycki (1987) subsequently reported an additional 224 patients who contacted him for possible aspartame sensitivity; 154 had chronic hives, angioedema or both. Fifty of the first 75 refrained from ingesting aspartame for two weeks, and noted complete resolution of their hives. Of these 50 patients, 22 reacted positively when rechallenged with aspartame.

Downham (1992) reported 23 patients with hypersensitivity skin reactions attributable to drinking 12-72 ounces of aspartame sodas daily. Twenty were women. Their reactions included urticaria (19), angioedema (2), macular purpura (2), panniculitis (2) (see below), and eczematous dermatitis (1). In each instance, the reaction recurred after rechallenge with a diet soda, or coffee/tea sweetened with an aspartame product.

C. OTHER ASPARTAME-ASSOCIATED ALLERGIES

I. Respiratory Tract Allergies

The precipitation or aggravation of bronchial asthma, and allergic reactions involving the nose and sinuses were prominent complaints in 17 aspartame reactors. This relationship became evident in some when aspartame products were discontinued because of other aspartame reactions.

- A female aspartame reactor with longstanding upper respiratory symptoms and "a constant buzzing" decided to avoid aspartame products. She stated "I can breathe through my nose for the first time in years, and my sinus infections have stopped."
- A correspondent from Finland wrote that she began having asthmatic symptoms after ingesting a juice containing aspartame. The problem promptly disappeared after discontinuing this product.

- An asthmatic man related the induction or aggravation of his asthma to aspartame cola beverages. He stated, "When I drink more than one diet cola, I have to reach for my inhaler within a couple of hours."

A striking increase in mortality from asthma occurred after 1981, the year aspartame became available. This is relevant because of questions repeatedly raised concerning the role of environmental agents in asthma, including food additives *(The Wall Street Journal* February 18, 1987, p. 29.) The prescription of chewable tablets containing aspartame, especially intended for asthmatic children, requires reflection in this context.

Representative Case Reports

Case VIII-C-1

The mother of a five-year-old boy described his severe choking and cough 30 minutes after drinking an aspartame soda. "It progressed to where he could hardly breathe. His trachea swelled, and only croaking noises were emitted when he tried to talk." An emergency room physician treated this reaction with injections of epinephrine and an antihistamine. There were no recurrences after abstinence from aspartame. She commented

> "I've been told by three doctors specializing in allergy that no test has been developed as yet to test for aspartame. Since so many products on the market are sweetened with it, I feel it imperative that I know for sure if an allergy exists."

Case VIII-C-2

A 48-year-old clerical worker with a history of hay fever and adult-onset asthma consumed various aspartame soft drinks and four packets of an ATS daily for 11 months. Her asthma "worsened to the point of being life-threatening – that is, many emergency room visits, and two hospitalizations between October 1985 and July 1986."

Other symptoms developed while consuming aspartame. They included decreased vision in both eyes, severe dizziness, shortness of breath, palpitations, and attacks of rapid heart action.

She also suffered a grand mal seizure in March 1986 that required hospitalization. A second convulsion occurred three months later. She was seen by four consultants. Two CT scans of the brain and two electroencephalograms were normal. Phenytoin was prescribed.

Her complaints disappeared when she stopped all aspartame products. The patient stated, 'Since stopping the consumption of aspartame in July 1986, I have not had a single asthma attack."

II. Mouth and Throat Reactions

Aspartame reactions can affect the lips, mouth and swallowing. They are amplified in Chapter IX-D. Swelling of the tongue, mouth, pharynx and larynx associated with aspartame use was frightening among children.

Representative Case Reports

Case VIII-C-3

A 62-year-old woman experienced difficult swallowing as soon as she ingested aspartame. She stated, "I was eating a cereal and did not know that it contained aspartame. My throat became paralyzed and I could not swallow. My daughter asked if I had checked for aspartame. When I did check, that's when I realized I was using it." The daughter also suffered "throat paralysis" after ingesting aspartame.

Case VIII-C-4

A 60-year-old diabetic woman was asymptomatic on diet and small doses of glipizide. She found that "dietetic" pudding and candy containing aspartame predictably caused severe swelling and itching of her mouth.

Case VIII-C-5

A 23-year-old commercial banker consumed two cans of a diet cola, up to four glasses of aspartame-sweetened tea, and one glass of an ASD daily for three years. Reviewing her aspartame-associated symptoms, she indicated that pain in the mouth and difficult swallowing were "the very first thing, months before I realized the connection."

Other complaints included blurred vision in both eyes, ringing in the ears, difficulty with contact lens, marked sensitivity to noise, severe dizziness and unsteadiness, tremors, intermittent memory loss, tingling of the limbs, anxiety attacks with aggravated phobias, shortness of breath, palpitations, unexplained chest pain, bloody stools, a rash, and severe joint pains ("all over – the arms, legs, chest").

She was seen by two consultants. X-rays of the head, a CT scan of the brain, a barium enema, two sets of allergy tests, and special ear tests were not revealing. Her symptoms improved within four days after stopping aspartame products. Most had disappeared by the tenth day.

III. Tongue Reactions (See Chapter IX-D)

In addition to overt inflammation of the tongue, several aspartame reactors mentioned "loss of taste" and "burning" as highly troublesome symptoms.

Representative Case Reports

Case VIII-C-6

A 60-year-old housewife consumed four small bottles of diet cola, three glasses of an ASD, and two servings of dietetic gelatin daily. She developed marked irritation of the tongue which became "red and sensitive." Two consultants could find no cause. The only change in her diet or habits had been the use of these aspartame products. The problem promptly improved after avoiding them.

Case VIII-C-7

A 71-year-old man complained of a "general burning of the tongue" whenever he took small amounts of aspartame.

Case VIII-C-8

A 69-year-old man used aspartame in sodas, a tabletop sweetener, iced tea and chewing gum. Reporting loss of taste and headache as his major symptoms, he stated, "At that time, I was chewing 1 to 1-1/2 packs of aspartame gum a day. I went back to regular gum with sugar. In about a week, the symptoms were gone."

D. PHOTOSENSITIVITY

Aspartame products can cause or aggravate photosensitivity (reactions to sunlight). While a number of drugs and chemicals may induce this state, and also must be considered, individual aspartame reactors had convincingly determined its role in their cases. This subject also will be discussed under lupus erythematosus (VIII-E).

Representative Case Reports (also see Case VIII-E-2)

Case VIII-D-1

A woman who had carefully evaluated her condition wrote

> "I previously would break out in a rash whenever I did anything heat-related, such as sun bathing and exercising. It was as if my body was allergic to my own sweat. The big, usually oblong-shaped, and sometimes itchy welts would form on my arms and upper legs.

> "It was suggested that I avoid aspartame. I did so, and noticed major changes. I didn't seem as sluggish. Also, I steadily lost weight.

> "The big test came when I went to Pompano Beach over Christmas. The weather was wonderful – 80's and sunny. The five days I was down there, I sat in the sun hour after hour, reading and sipping rum and orange juice, just like I did in my 20s. NO WELTS! Three years ago, I was a lumpy itchy mess after a mere four hours in the sun. Only one thing changed: I had eliminated aspartame from my diet."

E. THE SYSTEMIC LUPUS ERYTHEMATOSUS ISSUE

Considerable concern has been expressed by anti-aspartame consumer groups (Chapter XXX), about an apparent correlation between widespread aspartame use and the rising frequency of systemic lupus erythematosus (SLE). Inasmuch as more than two million persons in the United States have been told they might have lupus erythematosus or a lupus-associated autoimmune condition, this association deserves careful consideration.

Lupus-like rashes, other systemic symptoms (especially joint pain), and even high titers of antinuclear antibodies (ANA) have been encountered in aspartame reactors. Photo-sensitivity (discussed in VIII-D) can be a prominent feature in both disorders. A diagnosis of SLE was considered in seven of the more recent 649 reactors in this series. All improved dramatically after stopping aspartame products.

352

The author had considerable reservation initially about including SLE as a manifestation of aspartame disease. After several astute health care professionals contacted me about this matter, based on <u>their</u> personal observations, the merit of this lead became evident.

> A nurse experienced marked improvement after avoiding aspartame products. She stated that two women "addicted" to diet colas with whom she worked in an emergency room had elevated ANA levels. One was diagnosed as having lupus; the other suffered unexplained excruciating joint pain.

Representative Case Reports

Case VIII-E-1

A 40-year-old female physician developed Hashimoto thyroiditis and a high titer of antinuclear antibodies. She had habitually consumed one liter of aspartame soft drinks daily. Other problems consisted of a severe optic neuritis, headache, memory loss, and menstrual changes. Her symptoms improved after stopping aspartame products, along with normalization of the elevated ANA titer.

Case VIII-E-2

A 57-year-old medical secretary suffered aspartame disease. Many of her manifestations were previously diagnosed as systemic lupus erythematosus. She had been seen in consultation by an allergist, two hematologists, two ophthalmologists, a neurologist, an internist, an endocrinologist and three dermatologists! Repeat ANA titers were elevated to 1:2,560 or higher.

She experienced pain in both eyes, marked photosensitivity (interfering with her ability to drive or travel), dry eyes, loss of hearing in both ears, unexplained facial pain, palpitations, pain of the tongue and lips, intense thirst, a painful violaceous rash of the eyelids, other eruptions, and thinning of the hair. Various diagnostic procedures had been negative – including skin biopsies of the lids and arms, a salivary gland biopsy, and various antibody studies.

The patient was told about aspartame disease by her pharmacist-son. Her daily consumption included up to 12 packets of an aspartame tabletop sweetener, one or two cans of diet cola, eight ounces or more of an aspartame yogurt, and other aspartame products (cereal, gelatins, gum, mints, juice cocktails). Her eyes began to improve within several days after avoiding aspartame products.

Possible Mechanisms

Another amino acid, N-canavanine (highly concentrated in alfalfa sprouts), has been identified with both the development of a lupus-like disease in monkeys, and the aggravation of pre-existing systemic lupus erythematosus in humans.

The lupoid and other inflammatory dermatoses induced by aspartame products may result from the generation of leukotrienes. These biologically active compounds are derived from arachidonic acid, and released from a variety of human cells (macrophages; monocytes; polymorphonuclear leukocytes; mast cells). There is a three fold rise of leukotrienes B_4 and C_4 and of 15-hydroxyeicosatetraenoic acid, along with other arachidonic acid metabolites, when macrophages are exposed to aspartame (Hardcastle 1997).

An additional hypothesis for the initiation of an autoimmune response by aspartame metabolites involves the "ambling" of proteins by formaldehyde (Chapter XXI) – thereby making them strange and antigenic to the person's immune system.

F. ADDITIONAL SKIN PROBLEMS

I. Acne Vulgaris

Acne vulgaris, referred to by young persons as "bad complexion," was caused or aggravated by aspartame products in several reactors.

Representative Case Report

Case VIII-F-1

A young paramedical worker began consuming various aspartame products daily – including diet bars, soft drinks, and an ATS in each of four cups of coffee. Her facial acne flared up, having been previously controlled by an oral or topical antibiotic. There was marked improvement within one week after avoiding aspartame.

II. Acne Rosacea

Reference was made earlier to an aspartame-induced eruption simulating acne rosacea. It may partly reflect chronic methanol toxicity (Chapter XXI).

Representative Case Report

Case VIII-F-2

A woman had suffered severe rosacea for seven years, along with an alarming rise of blood pressure. Her facial skin "felt like it was on fire." These problems failed to respond to treatment by dermatologists and allergists. In desperation, she stopped her "beloved" diet cola. "Within two days, everything changed. For the first time in seven years, my face was completely clear... Within just two weeks, my blood pressure came down to normal."

III. Loss or Marked Thinning of Hair

Considerable loss of scalp hair was prominent in 71 (6 percent) aspartame reactors. One woman commented, "I lost over half my hair volume before I realized that it was the diet cola making it fall out. After only a few days off the diet drink, I could comb my hair and it wouldn't fall out."

The hair follicles are highly vulnerable to illness, stress, metabolic injury, and various drugs and toxic substances. Aspartame should be considered among the latter.

Representative Case Reports

Case VIII-F-3

A 27-year-old housewife noted severe loss and thinning of her hair while consuming aspartame products. Other complaints included severe itching without a rash, intense headache, convulsions, a marked personality change, and difficult swallowing. She had a prior history of hay fever. Her symptoms disappeared within one month after stopping all aspartame products.

Case VIII-F-4

Hair loss was a major feature in this aspartame reactor. She stated, "My hair has been falling out in a strip from front to back on each side." Another prominent complaint was palpitations. She became symptom-free after avoiding aspartame products. "Now I can run my fingers into my hair, pull hard, and once in a while get one hair. Before quitting aspartame, I would get five or six hairs each time. Now my hair is obviously growing back."

IV. Other Hair Problems

The condition of alopecia areata refers to a patchy loss of hair from the scalp. Several persons implicated aspartame products as the cause – as in the case of a 34-year-old woman who developed the disorder within months after consuming aspartame.

Complete loss of body hair (alopecia totalis) occurred in several young male athletes consuming considerable diet sodas.

A few aspartame reactors emphasized the rapidity with which their hair turned gray after using aspartame products.

V. Nail Changes

Several aspartame reactors focused on splitting and discoloration of the nails.

- One woman stated, "My nails split down the middle, and my hair fell out. When I stopped all aspartame intake, my nails cleared up and the hair became healthy."
- A 32-year-old housewife who had consumed up to two liters of a diet cola daily for 12 years developed marked thinning of her hair and "fingernails so thin I can peel and bend them with no effort." She also had been studied for "mystery abdominal pain."

VI. Dryness of the Skin

Some aspartame reactors emphasized the dryness of their skin, with ensuing fissures (cracks), when they used large amounts of these products.

VII. Other Skin Problems

A. Exfoliative Dermatitis. The possibility of an aspartame reaction should be considered as causative or contributory in patients with this serious skin disorder who consume large amounts of aspartame.

356

Representative Case Report

Case VIII-F-5

An 18-year-old woman with a severe exfoliative eruption initially had been diagnosed as having psoriasis by several dermatologists. This eruption disappeared when she stopped aspartame products while pregnant because of concern for her fetus. It recurred after a subsequent pregnancy. On further questioning about aspartame use, she realized that a number of products being taken (such as gum and mouthwashes) did contain this chemical.

B. Recurrent Fungal (Monilial) Infections. Aspartame-related vulnerability to infection is considered in Chapter IX-H. Women with aspartame disease often complain of severe genital itching, and evidence a rash typical of monilial infection. Twenty-five (4 percent) of 649 reactors in the more recent series had these problems.

- A woman gave a ten-year history of aspartame reactions. She developed "a mouth full of canker sores" within 24 hours after using aspartame products, often coupled with "severe vaginal yeast infection." They recurred whenever she inadvertently ingested aspartame.
- Many women wrote me about experiencing severe genital itching and fungus infections after a syndicated medical columnist described their association with aspartame use. One correspondent with such "genital fire" also experienced visual problems, dizziness, fatigue, depression, hives, insomnia, intense thirst and joint pain.

C. Other Scalp Problems. A diabetic man had been afflicted with "scalp folliculitis" that could be controlled only partially with antibiotics for a decade. After discontinuing aspartame products, his scalp problem cleared and did not recur.

D. Impaired Sweating. Several reactors complained of markedly impaired sweat while using aspartame products. Case VIII-F-6 illustrates its severity.

This feature is consistent with the ability of aspartame to affect other secretory glands in the absence of customary contributory factors (e.g., hypothyroidism; drug side effects). The more prominent ones encountered clinically involve the eye and salivary glands, evidenced by dry eyes (Chapter IV) and dry mouth (Chapter IX-D).

Representative Case Report

Case VIII-F-6

A retiree had been disabled by aspartame disease until he became aware of it and discontinued aspartame, especially a tabletop sweetener. A major problem involved the virtual absence of sweat "even on the hottest days." He resorted to the purchase of a medical-grade Jacussi "to keep me going," soaking from 15-20 minutes at temperatures as high as 108 degrees! This complaint abated after avoiding aspartame. He wrote four years later, "I now sweat profusely when working outside."

E. **Additional Patient Experiences.** Individual aspartame reactors had other dermatologic problems.

- A 28-year-old woman with severe aspartame-induced joint pains also developed a "red sore face." A friend mentioned that it looked like a bad sunburn, even though there had been no sun exposure for weeks. Her face normalized after avoiding aspartame products.
- A 50-year-old woman suffered severe aspartame disease characterized by incapacitating"arthritis" and extreme cold intolerance. She noted an "ashen look of death-warmed-over" in describing her complexion while consuming two liters of diet cola daily. After discontinuing aspartame products, she observed, "I have color back, can think clearly, and have more energy."
- The concomitant complaint of an odor "like rubber burning" bothered several aspartame reactors. This symptom (possibly a methanol effect) disappeared after avoiding aspartame products.
- A 49-year-old woman was diagnosed as having systemic lupus erythematosus, and received prednisone which aggravated her condition. The diagnosis of CREST syndrome – a combination of skin calcification, the Raynaud phenomenon (see Chapter IX-C), esophageal dysfunction, and other skin changes – was later made. She died at the age of 51. This patient had consumed an average of five diet colas daily for 12 years.

VIII. Granulomatous Panniculitis

The fatty issues can be selectively irritated by aspartame and its metabolites, especially formaldehyde from the methanol precursor (Chapter XXI). Other physicians have documented this reaction, including Novick (1985), McCauliffe and Poitras (1991), and Downham (1992).

The 22-year-old woman reported by Novick developed nodular lesions over both legs during a two-month period. She had switched to an aspartame diet soda ten weeks previously. The lesions were consistent with erythema nodosum by microscopic examination. The nodules disappeared when she abstained from aspartame for one month. Within 10 days after resuming it, many more comparable nodules appeared They again completely resolved after avoiding aspartame. Similar lesions reappeared on her legs within 10 days after being challenged with pure aspartame (50 mg four times daily).

G. DUAL SENSITIVITY TO ASPARTAME AND MONOSODIUM GLUTAMATE (MSG)

Fourteen persons among the most recent 649 aspartame reactors in this series commented on the similarity of their reactions to MSG and to aspartame products. I reported this clinical phenomenon, and the apparent sensitization induced by one to the other, to a conference on "Adverse Reactions to Monosodium Glutamate" at the Life Sciences Research Office (Bethesda) on April 7, 1993.

As in aspartame disease, a great problem encountered by MSG reactors is their inability to ascertain the presence of MSG because of the "name games" used in labeling products. For example, it is a constituent of the hydrolyzed vegetable protein (HVP) – also known as protein hydrolysate – present in numerous products. They include soups, luncheon meats, gravies, sauces, candy, chewing gum, soft drinks, binders for drugs, and "flavors." Unfortunately, the ultimate detection of "hidden" MSG usually entails "trial by illness."

- Case III-1, a 31-year-old registered nurse, experienced her first convulsion within hours after ingesting two liters of an aspartame soft drink. Her ensuing sensitivity to MSG was dramatically evidenced by a seizure toward the end of a subsequent pregnancy. On returning from the obstetrician, she had stopped at a fast food establishment, and was served a hamburger prepared in broth containing MSG. The seizure necessitated delivery under anesthesia.
- A prominent businessman experienced attacks of intense anxiety, headache, paresthesias, chest discomfort, and a marked drop in blood pressure whenever he took minimal amounts of MSG. Even his cardiologist "panicked" during such a life-threatening reaction after the

patient had unknowingly ingested a small amount. Having also developed rectal bleeding following such re-exposure, he was impressed by the same reaction I had reported in aspartame reactors (Chapter IX-D).

Representative Case Reports

Case VIII-G-1

A 16-year-old girl developed severe symptoms that subsided when she avoided aspartame products. They included headache, tremors, confusion, seizures, and severe sensitivity to noise. Numerous studies were normal. She subsequently evidenced sensitivity to MSG, the ingestion of which induced severe confusion within one hour.

Case VIII-G-2

A 26-year-old woman with severe aspartame disease later found that MSG caused her "to feel drained, weak and mentally dull." MSG intake also reproduced muscle spasms comparable to those experienced with aspartame use.

Case VIII-G-3

An airline clerk volunteered the severe neurologic reactions to both MSG and products containing aspartame under an extraordinary coincidence – namely, while the author was making reservations to speak at the foregoing national meeting on MSG. After learning about the nature of this conference, the clerk stated

> "Let me tell you about the enormous problems of my ten-year-old son. He is highly allergic to MSG and to aspartame. He had recurrent convulsions that puzzled our pediatrician and consultants. Even though I raised the possibility of reactions to these additives, the doctors refused to believe it. But his third convulsion occurred right after consuming a small amount of MSG. He has totally avoided both of these chemicals since, and there have been no further convulsions."

General Considerations

Glutamic acid is a nonessential amino acid abundantly present in plant and animal protein. A sodium ion is added for the manufacture of MSG. It began to be produced in large quantities after 1958 by means of fermentation. Some of the flavorings and seasonings that contain this additive are Accent®, Zest®, Vetsen®, Subu® and Glutavene®. MSG is only effective as a flavor intensifier in its free state.

The amount of MSG in an average serving reconstituted from commercially available dry soup bases is about 735 mg or 0.735 gm *(Consumer Reports* November 1978, pp. 615-169). Glutamate levels increase proportionate to the quantity of MSG consumed.

An estimated 30 percent of persons in the United States are adversely affected by taking five grams or more glutamate daily (Kenney 1972, Reif-Lehrer 1976, Samuels 1991). Jack L. Samuels (1991) opined to the Federation of American Societies for Experimental Biology (FASEB) that at least 60 million persons in the United States have reactions of varying severity to MSG. Some experience the typical "Chinese restaurant syndrome" after ingesting soup (especially wonton) prepared with MSG.

Glutamate is a neurotoxin (excitotoxin). Its hydrolysis by chemicals or enzymes frees L-glutamic acid, which can be neurotoxic in the free state. Glutamate neurotoxicity also contributes to brain damage in severe hypoglycemia (Chapter XIV) and oxygen deprivation. The commonalities of aspartate and glutamate include binding to many of the same receptor sites, similar transport mechanisms, and interconversion via aspartate aminotransferase.

As with the D-forms of phenylalanine and aspartic acid (Chapter XXII), D-glutamate in processed food appears to cause or enhance adverse reactions to MSG (Jack L. Samuels, personal communication, August 16, 1995).

- The Ajinomoto Company abandoned its attempt to synthesize MSG without D-glutamic acid.
- Much of the research using L-glutamic acid employed commercial-grade MSG in which neither the presence nor amount of D-glutamic acid had been analyzed.
- Cooking probably increases the amount of D-glutamic acid.

Dr. John Olney

Dr. John Olney, a Washington University neuropathologist, raised the possibility that aspartic acid might interact with MSG, and thereby potentiate its neurotoxic effects, especially in children *(The Argus* [Rock Island, Illinois], May 6, 1986). He published considerable data about glutamate neurotoxicity.

- MSG destroys neurons withing the immature hypothalamus in minutes (Olney 1973).
- Liquid glutamine preparations pose a greater risk because of the associated high blood levels
- It is erroneous to assume that gastrointestinal absorption of glutamate in man is the same as in animals. In reality, humans absorb 20 times more.

Olney detailed his criticism of industry-sponsored research, including flawed studies and inaccurate reporting by "authorities"and "experts."

The recent finding that cells in the hypothalamus secreting a hormone called hypocretin (orexin) are absent in narcolepsy (Chapter VI-K) is consistent with their destruction by such a neurotoxin *(Nature Medicine* August 30, 2000). Indeed, the classic features of narcolepsy occur in genetically engineered mice that do not produce this hormone.

With reference to reactions in monosodium glutamate-placebo studies, confusion has been introduced because the placebos used in some of the "negative" studies contained aspartame! This fact was unknown to the investigators (Chapter XXXI).

H. THE MULTIPLE CHEMICAL SENSITIVITY (MCS) SYNDROME

Controversy persists concerning the MCS syndrome relative to harm from exposure to environmental chemicals. The related field of clinical ecology was discussed previously (Roberts 1990).

Clinical ecologists have amassed considerable evidence that the exposure of individuals who are sensitive to trace amounts of chemicals in common foods or indoor air can induce, and reproduce, a number of reactions. They include headache, dizziness, anxiety, confusion, memory loss, and severe gastrointestinal symptoms (especially in children). Examples of offending substances are corn, wheat flour, dyes, MSG and sulfites. The "sick building syndrome" resulting from indoor air pollution (Roberts 1984) provides another example.

Writers of fiction have tapped the subject of coexisting allergies as a basis for unexplained illness. One film focused on a man whose son deduced that his recurring blindness resulted from the combined effects of an addiction to tea and his exposure to the family cat.

There may be difficulty in distinguishing "sensitivity" from "toxicity." An important distinction is that the MCS syndrome is <u>not</u> associated with altered immunogobulins, as may occur with conventional "allergies." One explanation for the higher frequency of females with the MCS syndrome is their reduced efficiency in detoxification.

Callender (1991) suggested that the multiple chemical sensitivity-chronic fatigue syndromes represent variations of a toxic encephalopathy. In a study using SPECT scanning, 56 of 67 patients with well-defined chemical exposures evidenced decreased regional brain flow, especially in the frontal and temporal lobes and the basal ganglia. Several patients studied by PET scanning had reduced brain glucose metabolism involving the hippocampus, amygdala, putamen and thalamus.

Concomitant Aspartame/Pesticide Sensitivity

Several patients and correspondents emphasized their apparent sensitization to pesticides after having evidenced reactions to aspartame products. Although I initially considered these interrelations coincidental, the matter received more credence because of their impressive professional and academic backgrounds.

While only two cases are presented, other persons with aspartame disease provided vivid accounts. For example, one severe aspartame reactor stated in the hospital that she "almost died" as her home was being sprayed.

Representative Case Reports

Case VIII-H-1

A 24-year-old horticulturist had severe reactions to aspartame products, many of which improved after avoiding them. I saw her in consultation. In view of her extensive knowledge of pesticides and professional exposure, she submitted this requested account.

"Aspartame sensitized me to organophosphate pesticides (OPP), and possibly other chemicals as well. Before I consumed aspartame, I sprayed our orchard with OPP many times with no apparent ill effect. The onset of my sensitivity to OPP and my chronic 'stomach' pain from aspartame coincided. My body's ability to produce enough acetylcholinesterase seems to be greatly diminished.

"Before aspartame, I had high hopes and ambitions, and was fully capable of obtaining them. Now I just long for a normal life. I know aspartame has probably done irreparable damage to my mental faculties. When I totally avoid OPP (as well as aspartame), I think much more clearly, feel energetic, and almost feel like my old self, but my short-term memory still suffers.

"Avoidance of the truth about the connection between aspartame and OPP terrifies me. A Pandora's box has been opened, and the horrible effects may be much more widespread and devastating than previously realized. This connection may be a key to Multiple Chemical Sensitivity. The Gulf War set a perfect stage for an experiment testing the connection between severely overheated aspartame and OPP."

Case VIII-H-2

A 42-year-old professor of business management became permanently disabled from a severe medical disorder that resulted in the loss of her position and the need to file for bankruptcy. Her symptoms included decreased vision in both eyes, bilateral eye pain, ringing in both ears, severe headache, dizziness, drowsiness, marked mental confusion and memory loss, intense twitching (especially at night), unexplained facial pain, slurred speech, a dramatic change of personality, intermittent shortness of breath, rapid heart action, abdominal pain with diarrhea and bloat, severe itching and hives, marked thinning of the hair, swollen lips, difficult swallowing, intense thirst, marked frequency of avoiding (especially at night), the cessation of menses, severe joint pains, and a gain of ten pounds.

She had psychologic and psychiatric consultations, numerous x-rays of the gastrointestinal tract, and extensive allergy testing; all failed to define a cause. A SPECT study suggested "brain damage." There was a history of reactions to sulfites.

The problem initially was blamed on the pesticides used in farms and by aerial spray, along with outgassing of her new house. The role of aspartame disease was then raised by two persons: a friend with presumed multiple sclerosis and a neighbor with aspartame-induced headaches, each of whom had a significant remission after stopping aspartame products.

The patient was consuming large amounts of aspartame daily – up to eight cans of diet colas, four packets of a tabletop sweetener, gum and other products. Her symptoms improved after diligently avoiding both aspartame and pesticides.

Commentary

The contributory role of aspartame products in cross-sensitizing the population to other substances requires exploration. Several instances are cited

- A related insight derives from the behavioral cross-sensitization to cocaine after repeated low-level exposure to formaldehyde. Sorg et al (1998) relate this phenomenon to multiple chemical sensitivity in persons who manifest unexplained fatigue, irritability, problems with memory and concentration, depression, headache, muscle/joint pain, and gastrointestinal symptoms. They inferred limbic system sensitization as a mechanism.
- There has been a dramatic escalation of allergy to latex since the late 1980's, especially among personnel at hospitals and medical offices (*The New York Times* March 7, 1999, p. 27).

I. BROADER IMMUNOLOGIC PERSPECTIVES

The apparent cause-and effect relationship between use of aspartame products and various allergic manifestations may represent the tip of a large public health threat. Over half of our immunologically "primed" population currently consumes these products.

The following issues provide broader perspectives in this context.

- Multiple immunization procedures involving bacterial and virus material are mandated during infancy and childhood. In Massachusetts, for example, children receive up to 33 (!) doses of ten viral and bacterial vaccines by the age of five. This number is likely to increase as more vaccines are developed, coupled with the Immunization Association Act of 1965 that set up categorical programs whereby states receive federal funds for the purchase of expensive vaccines for public health clinics.

- Subsequent re-immunizations (as with tetanus toxoid and live measles vaccine) serve as chronic stimulants to the immune system.
- Noninfectious antigens can evoke heightened sensitivity, such as prolonged immunologic responses to one's sperm in vasectomized men (Roberts 1979, 1993d).

The apparent increased vulnerability of aspartame reactors to a host of environmental allergies (pollens, molds, dust, drugs, foods), irritants, and chemicals (e.g., formaldehyde) has been mentioned. Additionally, more than 1000 <u>new</u> chemicals are introduced each year. Interference with cellular immunity may ensue. Unfortunately, decades often lapse before physicians become aware of these biological consequences. This phenomenon is illustrated by the long-term effects of pentachlorophenol, a widely used pesticide whose toxicity the author has tracked over three decades (Roberts 1963, 1993b, 1990b).

The magnitude of severe allergic reactions to aspartame products undoubtedly exceeds that of persons with peanut allergy – estimated at less than one-tenth of one percent of the population *(The Wall Street Journal* September 2, 1998, p. A.1).

The extent to which <u>a hyperimmune population</u> has evolved is pertinent and disturbing.

- An increasing array of potentially antigenic substances can enhance the immune response, including many widely used drugs and their metabolites (Eisner 1972).
- Awareness of the hyperimmune state of Americans emerged from transplant studies. Professor G. Melville (John Hopkins University School of Medicine, personal communication 1977) noted the difficulty encountered in cross-matching kidney transplants and inducing acceptance, using the most sophisticated typing methods then available.

I. Immunization

Most Americans receive multiple immunizations involving both live and inactivated bacteria or viruses during infancy and childhood (see above). Such procedures create a hyperergic state.

366

- Some authorities argue against the ongoing excessive use of tetanus toxoid boosters for minor injuries (Edsall 1967, Peebles 1969). It has been shown that repeated immunization at intervals of less than five years leads to a qualitative change in antibody type and the development of skin-sensitizing antibodies.
- Revaccination with live measles vaccine augments immunity (Bass 1976).
- Persistence of high immunity follows many types of immunization. For example, 5,000 children up to the age of two years were given a single dose of live attenuated measles vaccine. They maintained a high level of protection when studied for antibody levels one decade later (Evans 1977). Indeed, the Medical Research Council advised against further injection of vaccine in such children.
- Linnemann (1976) expressed the need for caution relative to revaccination with live virus vaccines for protection against measles, rubella, mumps, vaccinia and poliomyelitis.
- White, Adler and McGann (1974) reviewed the possible adverse effects of repeated immunization in man. Some of the findings included depressed serum albumin and iron levels, elevation of the serum copper level, an increased erythrocyte sedimentation rate, relative lymphocytosis, and elevated serum hexosamine. Moreover, they reported the development of neoplastic disease of lymphoid origin (lymphosarcoma; myeloma; monoclonal gammopathy) in three individuals who had received from three to four immunizations.
- Chronic stimulation of the immunoglobulin-producing system in humans has been related to subsequent occurrence of plasma cell dyscrasias, autoimmune disease, amyloidosis, and rheumatoid arthritis. White et al (1974) commented on the possibility of continually stimulating a restricted population of immunoreceptor cells through repeated exposure to a single antigen or closely related antigens.

II. The Post-Vasectomy State

The immunologic aftermaths of vasectomy warrant questioning men with severe aspartame disease about a history of such surgery. The large numbers of entrapped spermatozoa and their phagocytosed or lysed fragments, resulting from obstruction to the vas deferens, may act as antigens. The author's clinical experiences and researches have been reviewed (Roberts 1979, 1993d).

- Ansbacher, Keung-Yeung and Wurster (1972) reported that eight of 15 men who had circulating sperm antibodies one year after vasectomy gave a history of allergy, compared to only three of 12 men in whom no sperm antibodies could be detected.
- Dr. Stephen Locke (personal correspondence), a physician correspondent, cited the case of a 34-year-old man with previously mild bronchial asthma who experienced marked intensification of his asthmatic distress following vasectomy. This was associated with recurrent attacks of typical erythema nodosum.

III. The Post-Tonsillectomy State

The long-term immunologic effects of tonsillectomy might influence reactivity to aspartame.

- Decreased immunity after tonsillectomy that predisposes to bulbar poliomyelitis has been long suspected.
- Graham (1973) reviewed some of the evidences linking tonsillectomy to subsequent cancer and lymphoma. A study performed by the New York State Department of Health Bureau of Cancer Control suggested that tonsillectomized persons appeared three times more likely to develop Hodgkin's disease.
- Dr. Rodrigo C. Hurtado (1974) emphasized the importance of the tonsils in cell-mediated immunity. Clinical data concerning increased rates of malignancy after their removal were provided.
- A significantly lower mean concentration of circulating gamma globulin has been reported in tonsillectomized adult females (Wingerd 1977). Dr. E. E. Sponzilli (1978) viewed this finding with alarm in terms of possible increased susceptibility to diseases involving the immune system and other disorders.
- Metcalfe-Gibson and Keddie (1978) invoked a similar consideration in analyzing the background of patients with several thyroid disorders believed to be autoimmune in nature – namely, Graves disease (Chapter IX-E) and Hashimoto's disease. In their analysis of 138 thyroidectomy cases, a history of tonsillectomy was obtained from 80 percent of those with Hashimoto's disease, and 66 percent of those with hyperthyroidism. (By contrast, a history of tonsillectomy could be obtained from only 10 percent of 75 patients in whom thyroidectomy had been performed for a colloid goiter).

IV. Associated Hypothyroidism

The frequency of hypothyroidism (underactive thyroid gland) in aspartame reactors manifesting allergic reactions (as Case VIII-B-16) merits attention. This influence may reflect the greater sensitivity of such patients to drugs and allergens, in part because they remain longer in the body.

The subject of hypothyroidism in aspartame reactors is considered in Chapter IX-E.

V. The Contributory Roles of Hypoglycemia and Diabetes

Interference with energy requirements appears to be a basic mechanism for some aspartame reactions. Accordingly, conditions that affect tissue metabolism could enhance the immunologic response. The frequent history of hypoglycemia (Chapter XIV) and of diabetes mellitus (Chapter XIII) in patients with aspartame disease, and the ability of these conditions to modify immune reactions, are relevant since such patients routinely use aspartame to avoid sugar.

I have conservatively estimated that one-third of the general population harbors the tendency to diabetogenic (functional) hyperinsulinism. The incidence is higher among Jews, Canadian Eskimos (Schaefer 1970), and persons with black or American Indian ancestry (Roberts 1964a, Stein 1965, Genuth 1967, Comess 1969).

The following observations are germane.

- Amelioration of chronic vasomotor rhinitis, bronchial asthma, recurrent dermatitis, and other presumed allergic disorders by a program aimed at preventing hypoglycemia has been repeatedly observed.
- Variations in clinical bronchial asthma, a prototype of the allergic state, have been correlated with charges in the blood glucose concentrations. More than six decades ago, Bray (1934) commented on the low fasting blood glucose concentrations in patients with bronchial asthma, and the frequency of hypoglycemia among children with asthma. Worne (1956) reported the intensification of infantile asthma as the blood glucose concentration falls.
- Hypoglycemia can enhance immune reactions. Abrahamson and Pezet (1951) asserted that hyperinsulinism can permit, if not induce, bronchial spasm and asthmatic attacks in individuals with allergic tendencies.
- There is a vast literature on the antigenicity of excess insulin (see below), and of diabetogenic hyperinsuhnism in various "autoimmune

disorders." They include recurrent thyroiditis, lupus erythematosus, myasthenia gravis, rheumatoid arthritis, and even juvenile-type diabetes mellitus (with ensuing destruction of the pancreatic islets.)

- Adamkiewicz (1963) reviewed the concept that hypoglycemia – whether from fasting, insulin administration or adrenalectomy – can potentiate anaphylactoid reactions, anaphylaxis, and the tuberculin reaction. In a similar vein, he found that the anaphylactoid reactions induced by glycogen were enhanced by insulin.

- While rats usually are highly resistant to horse serum or egg white anaphylaxis when antigen is administered without adjuvants, the mortality increases 60 percent by inducing hypoglycemia. Conversely, elevation of the blood sugar (by glucose, cortisone or epinephrine) tends to inhibit anaphylactoid reactions and the tuberculin reactions.

- Pieroni and Levine (1967) found an inverse correlation between glucose levels (both in experimental animals and in man) and susceptibility or reactivity to various pharmacologic, immunologic and physical stresses. These consisted of challenge with histamine, acetylcholine, serotonin, peptone, endotoxins, anaphylactic reactions, delayed-type hypersensitivity, irradiation, reduced atmospheric pressures, and cold stress. The agents or treatments employed to induce hypoglycemia included insulin, endotoxin, pertussis vaccine, beta-adrenergic blocking drugs, and adrenalectomy. These investigators commented: "It is proposed that a knowledge of the glycemic effect of an agent or treatment may be of predictive value in determining its influence on the response of an animal to these and other stress anoxae."

- Kraus (1964) noted that true anaphylaxis could be prevented in mice, and granulation tissue formation significantly depressed, by feeding glucose or inducing diabetes. Fatal anaphylaxis did occur in the diabetic or glucose-fed mice, however, when insulin was given one hour before a shock dose of egg albumin.

Antigenicity of Excessive Insulin

Many investigators have demonstrated that (a) persons with early maturity-onset diabetes release excessive amounts of biologically active insulin in response to glucose (referred to as "insulin resistance"), (b) autoantibodies are induced by exogenous insulin, eventually producing changes in cell membrane receptors and insulin resistance, and (c) heterogenous antibodies to insulin occur (Morse 1962; Deckert 1964).

Only a few of the evidences for the antigenicity of excessive insulin are listed.

- Karem et al (1969) reported a patient with insulin-resistant diabetes in whom autoantibodies were induced by exogenous insulin. Marked clinical improvement repeatedly occurred after stopping insulin, suggesting that her high levels of circulating antibodies contributed to maintaining insulin resistance.

- Foling and Norman (1972) demonstrated anti-insulin antibodies in a 42-year-old man with recurrent attacks of hypoglycemia, decreased glucose tolerance followed by reactive hypoglycemia, and elaboration of excessive insulin in response to glucose and meals. He had a history of allergic rhinitis, erythema nodosum, and a maternal background of rheumatoid arthritis.

- Ohneda and associates (1973) found antibodies to insulin in a patient with untreated chemical diabetes who suffered clinically from severe reactive hypoglycemia.

- High levels of antibodies have been induced experimentally by exogenous insulin, with the development of frank diabetes mellitus (Grodsky 1966, Toreson 1968).

- Nerup et al (1973) noted altered immunologic reactivity in one-third of diabetic patients by means of the leukocyte migration test.

- Eosinophilic inflammatory infiltrates have been documented in the pancreatic islets of infants born to diabetic mothers, and in children with acute-onset diabetes (Gepts 1965). This observation is consistent with an immunologic-related inflammatory response to excessive insulin.

- Makulu and Wright (1971) consistently produced an immune response in guinea pigs with a single injection of insulin.

- Egeberg et al (1974) demonstrated that inbred mice immunized with a single intracutaneous injection of a homologous pancreatic islet preparation developed sensitized lymphoid cells, and subsequently a condition resembling diabetes.

IX

OTHER DISORDERS

"No food additive should be used with blind reliance
that man will not or cannot react in an unpredicted way."
Dr. H. C. Hodge (1963)

A host of additional disorders occur in aspartame disease wherein the cause-and-effect relationship can be deduced by the relief following abstinence from such products, and their prompt recurrence after rechallenge. This experience reinforces the contention that aspartame disease is a "great mimic" or "great masquerader" in contemporary medical practice, especially illnesses lumped as "unexplained multiple-symptom syndromes."

Attempting to explain the bubonic plague to Philip VI of France, other than a freak alignment of Saturn, Jupiter, and Mars in the 40th degree of Aquarius, doctors at the University of Paris acknowledged that its cause might be "hidden from even the most highly trained intellects."

A. EAR PROBLEMS

Symptoms referable to the ears among aspartame reactors were often severe. In this series, they included the following:

"Ringing" or "buzzing" (tinnitus)	—	146 (12%)
Severe intolerance for noise	—	80 (7%)
Marked impairment of hearing	—	57 (5%)

Acronym Legend

ACB - aspartame cola beverage
ASD - aspartame soft drink
ATS - aspartame tabletop sweetener

Symptoms

A listing of the ways in which patients described ear symptoms illustrates both their severity and disability. They are amplified in the case reports. Additionally, the ear complaints among the initial 397 aspartame reactors who completed the survey questionnaire appear in Chapter XIX.

- Terms such as "ringing," "hissing," "buzzing," "humming," "like crickets," "whistling," "pulsating," "high-tension wire sounds," and "sounds like church chimes" were frequently used.
- A 49-year-old woman experienced severe ringing in both ears, marked sensitivity to noise, and "random fade-outs in my hearing."
- One patient felt "as if my ears were covered."
- In addition to "hearing problems in conversation," an aspartame reactor had such "severe pressure in my head" that he resorted to "equalizing the pressure by blowing my ear drums and holding my nose."
- A 51-year-old woman with aspartame disease developed hearing loss and extreme sensitivity to noise in both ears. She commented, "My children used to say that I had x-ray ears. Now I find I ask people to repeat quite often."

The precise relationship of the foregoing complaints to aspartame consumption occasionally could be documented. One individual noted the onset of his ear symptoms on April 2, 1986... the day he started drinking an aspartame soda.

The rapid ototoxicity of diet sodas is also illustrated by a 32-year-old certified public accountant in previous excellent health. She developed intense tinnitus after drinking several cans of an aspartame cola that had become "hot" in a storage area, requiring the addition of ice. Finding no cause, several ear specialists recommended that she "learn to live with it" when various drugs failed to help. Dramatic improvement occurred after learning about aspartame disease, and avoiding these products.

Representative Case Reports

Case IX-A-1

A 56-year-old patient had responded well to salt restriction and minimal medication for treatment of his hypertension.

He then presented with "ringing" in both ears, insomnia, "nervousness" and confusion that had progressed over a period of several weeks. As the comptroller of a major corporation, his unexplained confusion was alarming. No significant abnormalities could be detected on physical examination.

When queried about aspartame, the patient stated that he began drinking these beverages for the first time during the preceding month. All complaints regressed within three days after stopping them, and had not recurred two years later.

Case IX-A-2

A retired railroader first noticed a marked loss of hearing in the left ear during May 1986. The associated "humming" felt "as though I had caught cold." A hearing aid had been suggested when examination by several physicians failed to reveal any cause.

The patient chanced to read an article about aspartame disease that included brief reference to ear problems. He wrote, "I started using aspartame shortly after it came on the market, and have used it exclusively since. Rarely do I use sugar." Improvement followed the avoidance of aspartame products.

Case IX-A-3

A 30-year-old woman had been drinking several aspartame beverages for 17 months, averaging five or six cups or glasses daily. After ten months, she experienced ringing and pain in both ears along with dizziness. Antibiotic therapy failed to help. These complaints and a severe headache intensified over the ensuing six months. An audiogram evidenced considerable loss of hearing in the left ear. A CT scan did not reveal a tumor or other lesion. Otology and neurology consultants diagnosed Meniere's disease.

She then deduced that the aspartame sodas had caused these symptoms based on their predictable recurrence on rechallenge.

Case IX-A-4

A 36-year-old woman developed "buzzing in the ears," disorientation, and feeling "like a drug or alcohol is muffling the senses." She drank eight cups of hot tea daily, into each of which she placed an ATS packet. Other complaints included unsteadiness of the legs, drowsiness, marked memory loss, depression, severe nausea, frequent urination, and loss of appetite. Improvement occurred when she avoided all products containing aspartame. Her daughter had comparable reactions to aspartame products.

Case IX-A-5

A male aspartame reactor suffered ringing in the ears for two years. It was associated with dizziness, imbalance, sensitivity to noise, and motion sickness. He spent about $3,000 on various "negative" studies, including an MRI study of the brain.

After reading an article about aspartame disease, the patient abstained from all aspartame products. His dizziness and imbalance disappeared; only a minimum of tinnitus and sensitivity to loud noise persisted.

Case IX-A-6

A female aspartame reactor consumed six packets of a tabletop sweetener and considerable diet cola daily. She complained of hypersensitivity to noise, particularly on the telephone. "When talking on a cellular phone, a loud or distorted voice or sound would cause me to lose equilibrium, and get very dizzy and disoriented. Basically, I got the symptoms of motion sickness." Other reactions included impaired vision, depression, and recurrent yeast infections.

Case IX-A-7

A woman lost 35 pounds after completing graduate school by exercising and consuming sodas and many other products containing aspartame. She then experienced multiple complaints – including abdominal pain, diarrhea, headache, muscle cramps, severe fatigue, painful joints, cessation of her periods, lack of concentration, constant thirst and hunger, frequent urination, and marked irritability. Her most dramatic symptoms were "sudden deafness in one ear and tinnitus." Multiple physicians were consulted, but to no avail. She was told the problem was stress-related, and "I would have to live with tinnitus and partial hearing loss for the rest of my life."

The patient noticed that "fluctuations in my hearing and the humming in my ear seemed related to my consumption of diet soda." There was "immense" improvement of all symptoms within one week of abstinence. She commented, "It's almost like a miracle."

Commentary

In its evaluation of 13,000 surveys forms received from tinnitus sufferers, the American Tinnitus Association reported that more than a third replied to the possible cause of their distress as "Nothing known." Accordingly, it is apparent that few physicians suspect the possible contributory role of aspartame disease. For example, a 52-year-old stockbroker developed severe ringing in the left ear nine months after using an ATS. A physician attributed it "to my age, but the doctor gave me no reason."

The Better Hearing Institute emphasized the significant increase of <u>hearing loss</u> in persons from 40 to 60 years (T*he Palm Beach Post* June 14, 1999, p. D-4). Such impairment has been attributed to the exposure of "baby boomers" to loud noises variously from rock concerts, discos, power tools, leaf blowers, jet skis, motorcycles, etc. The possible primary or contributory influence of aspartame consumption, however, remains ignored.

Tinnitus and hearing loss were compounded in several aspartame reactors by the use of considerable <u>aspirin</u> to relieve associated headaches (Chapter V) or severe joint pain (Chapter IX-G).

Many of my patients with severe ear complaints also suffered severe <u>hypoglycemia</u> (Chapter XIV). The high energy requirements of the inner ear and acoustic nerves are pertinent.

The <u>potential damage to a fetus</u> from the mother's consumption of aspartame products (Chapter X), and the delayed manifestations (Chapter XI) can include hearing loss. Up to 2,400 children born every year are afflicted with impaired hearing, which might not be detected until they are two years or older.

B. EATING DISORDERS

"The belief in absurdities is bound to lead to the commission
of atrocities."
                    Voltaire

Our society is afflicted with problems concerning weight in the extreme. They range from anorexia and profound loss of weight to obesity... real or perceived. While many factors are operative in both, aspartame disease can play a major contributory role.

In the case of obesity, this association would seem paradoxic because aspartame products are widely touted for the loss or "control" of weight. A 1996 survey of 49 states and the District of Columbia by the Centers for Disease Control and Prevention indicated that more than two-thirds of persons 18 years and older were trying to lose weight or maintain weight loss (Serdula 1999).

Death statistics about cyclic loss and gain of weight offer a convincing indicator of the severe insult to the body that can result from arbitrary severe caloric restriction. Lissner et al (1991) reported on the increased total mortality from coronary heart disease in subjects participating in the Framingham Heart Study. When the data were analyzed for persons with considerable weight fluctuation, compared to those with stable weights, the risk of death among those having a fluctuating weight was about 50 percent greater for women, and nearly double for men – regardless of that individual's initial weight, blood pressure, smoking habits, cholesterol level, or degree of physical activity.

1. EXCESSIVE WEIGHT LOSS

Loss of appetite (anorexia) with a marked decrease of weight were striking features in 40 aspartame reactors (3 percent). Their weight loss averaged 21 pounds, ranging up to 80 pounds in Cases IX-B-1 and B-3. It can compare in severity to that encountered in classic anorexia nervosa.

Most persons in this category were women having extreme "fear of fat." They consumed considerable amounts of aspartame products, often in conjunction with strenuous exercise. Some continued using them even after being advised to the contrary because of probable aspartame disease. Such defiance became reinforced by the modest weight gain after they discontinued aspartame soft drinks (see Case XIX-3), and by withdrawal symptoms from aspartame addiction (Chapter VII-G).

Some physicians initially considered the diagnosis of diabetes mellitus in aspartame reactors who presented with considerable weight loss, intense thirst and frequent urination. For example, a 28-year-old woman lost 45 pounds after consuming two cans of an ACB and three packets of an ATS daily for five months. She wrote, "One of my first tests was for diabetes, but the test was normal."

On the other end of the age spectrum, aspartame disease should be suspected in older persons with "failure to thrive" during or after attempting weight loss. It is a risk factor in morbidity and mortality.

Representative Case Reports

Case IX-B-1

A 29-year-old mother of two children drank "enormous amounts" of an ACB, especially during the summer. She lost 80 pounds over a six-month period. At that point, she was unable to eat solid food, and refused supper because the food "smelled funny."

This patient sought help from numerous physicians for her many associated problems. They included "eye doctors, dentists, ear-nose-and throat specialists, psychiatrists, and at present an endocrinologist." The latter suspected porphyria, but could not document this diagnosis. She added, "I feel like a fool running to every doctor, but something is wrong and no one knows what it is."

She described her complaints in these terms:

> "Severe headaches, vision deterioration, shooting pains in my neck, throat pain, mood swings, dizziness, personality changes, complete memory losses, blackouts, extreme fatigue, crying for no reasons, and stomach pains. Some days I do not have even enough energy to pour a bowl of cereal for my children. Some days every little noise bothers me. I have severe suicidal thoughts. I never was depressed before, why now? I have two beautiful kids and a husband with a good job."

Case IX-B-2

A 41-year-old secretary lost 60 pounds (from 185 to 125) while drinking considerable ACBs daily. She also suffered intense headache and grand mal seizures.

Case IX-B-3

A 30-year-old licensed practical nurse consumed up to six cans of an ACB daily for six months. She weighed only 98 pounds after losing 80 pounds. The diagnoses of anorexia nervosa and "pernicious vomiting" were made. Other symptoms and disabilities included the following:

Decreased vision in both eyes
Recent "dry eyes" and difficulty in wearing contact lens
Ringing and marked sensitivity to noise in both ears
Severe headaches
Dizziness
Petit mal episodes without frank convulsions
Severe drowsiness
Marked mental confusion and memory loss

Tingling and numbness of the extremities
Slurred speech
Severe depression (attempted suicide on two occasions)
Extreme irritability and anxiety
Severe aggravation of phobias
Episodic shortness of breath
Palpitations
Severe nausea and diarrhea
Severe itching and a rash
Difficulty in swallowing
Intense thirst
Frequent urination, both day and night
Marked joint pains
"Low blood sugar attacks"
"Everything smelled bad"

The patient was treated by "at least 10 different doctors with at least 10 different diagnoses." The prescribed antidepressant drugs caused severe side effects. An allergist opined that she was "allergic to the 21st Century." She finally concluded, "All of my problems began with drinking diet cola."

Case IX-B-4

A 32-year-old businesswoman was seen in consultation for severe reactive hypoglycemia and depression. She was advised at the time to reduce her large intake of aspartame.

This patient returned three months later because of pleuritic chest pain. My nurses were appalled at her gaunt appearance after losing an additional 17 pounds. The pleurisy was diagnosed as a probable small pulmonary embolus secondary to thrombophlebitis in the lower extremities. Other complaints included severe leg cramps and a profound depression for which a psychiatrist prescribed tranylcypromine (Parnate®), a monomine oxidase inhibitor.

When asked why she had continued using aspartame, the patient replied, "I'm still too fat. I'd prefer to be a thin corpse!"

This attitude has been expressed by some patients with anorexia nervosa. One young woman stated, "I'd rather lose the weight and be happier with my life, even if it is shortened" (*Journal of the American Medical Association* 1999; 281:1126).

Case IX-B-5

A 39-year-old woman lost 72 pounds in eight months after beginning diet sodas. She also developed severe but unexplained emotional symptoms. She wrote

> "I broke down and told a friend that my wonderful husband who I've been with for 22 years, and my two kids, are ready to leave me because I'm making life hell for them at home. For the last three months, I have become a bitch to live with. I can't understand why I'm screaming for no reason at all. I am very down in the dumps and not wanting to be around family or friends. And the worst thing is I don't know why!"

Her husband chanced to read a feature about aspartame disease. She stated, "All the things that you listed as side effects sound like me!"

Commentary

A. Societal and Peer Pressures. The watch-your-weight motif common to these patients was unmistakable. Their use of aspartame products could be likened to a "culinary bypass" or "feeding without food."

- A line in the "Calorie Counter's Prayer" – written according to the style of the 23rd Psalm, and popularized by "Dear Abby" – read, "Thy diet colas, they comfort me."
- Ellen Goodman (1984) aptly regarded "the 5-pound overweight neurosis" responsible for the "lite blight" in food markets as one of the commonest afflictions in our food-disordered society. She jokingly theorized that it emerged after three-way mirrors were installed in the bathing-suit sections of department stores.

The number of overweight persons in the United States (over 100 million) approximates that of aspartame consumers. The widespread use of "nothingburger" foods and diet drinks as purported remedies has not gone unnoticed by cartoonists. Several capitalized on the theme, "What's left after the sugar, caffeine and carcinogens have been removed?"

Many factors reinforce the combination of severe caloric restriction and considerable aspartame consumption. They include the foregoing "fear of fat" by figure-conscious women in an image-oriented culture, peer pressure, and the virtual paranoia of some physicians when patients weigh more than their "desirable" weight as indicated by outmoded life insurance height-weight tables.

- An estimated six out of every ten American women fault themselves for being "overweight."
- An estimated one out of every four college-aged women has an eating disorder, largely due to societal pressures.
- The choice of a diet for persons fearing fat could be categorized as "the weighing game."
- George Balanchine, a foremost advocate of rail-thin dancers, stressed to his ballet corps, "I want to see bone." (Some contracts specifically stated, "Will lose five pounds before rehearsal starts.")

Men share this apprehension. A study cited by Ann Landers indicated that 78 percent of women weren't satisfied with their weight (35 percent wished to lose 25 pounds or more), and 56 percent of men would like to reduce weight (*The Miami Herald* August 17, 1987, p. C-2).

The tyranny of high-priced fashion emphasizes emaciation and "angularity," notwithstanding the greater appeal of women with natural curvaciousness for most men. It has been quipped that a model wanting to lose 20 pounds already would be considered five pounds underweight in the real world.

- A psychological study in 1995 revealed that 70 percent of women who spent three minutes looking at models in a fashion magazine felt depressed, guilty and shameful.
- The tragedy of this "think thin" phenomenon is reinforced by the fact that contemporary models weigh 23 percent less than average women, compared to only eight percent 20 years ago.
- Female undernutrition among young women due to an obsession with thinness has characterized the realms of dance and beauty pageants. For example, the body weight of Miss America winners declined by 12 percent from 1922 to 1999 (Rubinstein 2000).

These fears have been exploited commercially. Americans spend an estimated $20 billion annually on diet products and services.

- Fashion designers (see above) recognize that women believing they are thin are more likely to buy new clothes.
- The October 13, 1987 edition of *The Miami Herald* carried <u>four</u> large advertisements for weight reduction centers on the <u>same</u> page (C-2.) They began:

> "You lost weight. You look terrific!"
> "Your metabolism makes you thin."
> "Are you an overweight female?"
> "WOW! I lost 61 lbs. While eating two desserts a day!"

B. <u>**More on "Fear of Fat"**</u> Many women – even in the first decade – feel trapped by these attitudes. "Fear of fat" could be detected among **all** age groups in nearly 500 girls attending grades four through 12 at parochial schools in San Francisco according to a University of California study (*News/Sun-Sentinel* of Fort Lauderdale, November 1, 1986, p. F-1). Thirty-one percent of the nine-year-olds actively worried about being overweight or becoming fat!

A pathologic fear of fat is often imparted by parents, especially mothers. The ideal of skinniness became ingrained at the end of the baby boom following World War II. One manifestation was the progressive decrease in weight of Miss Americas during the mid-1950s.

Warped journalistic emphasis upon leanness contributed to this problem by equating thinness with "health." A cursory analysis of popular magazines aimed at women reveals that their front covers focus more on growing smaller than wiser. At least half the headlines indicate a preoccupation with weight. This is a variation of the theme attributed to the late Duchess of Windsor, "One can never be too rich or too thin."

> Dr. Adel A. Eldahmy (1987) averred the "toxic environment" for patients with eating disorders lies within the covers of fashion magazines... especially the androgynous, flat-chested and thin-hipped look referred to as the "little boy figure."

Psychiatrists, psychologists and epidemiologists are impressed by the extreme preoccupation of American women concerning weight. A psychologist in my community with an interest in eating disorders stated that she has yet to encounter an 18-year-old female satisfied with her figure.

The impact of television in transmitting related media images and values has been enormous. This is illustrated by the current high vulnerability of teenage girls in Fiji to anorexia and bulimia as they reject the traditional preference for robust body shapes (*Journal of the American Medical Association* 2000; 283:1409.)

Other attitudinal paradoxes exits. It is the general consensus that obese individuals seem less likely to commit suicide. Moreover, Dr. Domeena Renshaw (1987), Director of Loyola University's Sexual Dysfunction Clinic, concluded that obese women tend to have fewer sexual problems than females obsessed with thinness. The former try to come to terms with their body image, and are eager to date. By contrast, women with weight-loss disorders tend to have fewer dates, decreased sexual fantasies, and a lessened desire for sex. Some with anorexia and bulimia (see below) become so absorbed with their body image that they regard pregnancy as abhorrent.

C. <u>The Influence of Aspartame PR Campaigns</u>. The sophisticated advertising campaigns promoting aspartame products are discussed in other chapters. Producers realize the psychologic hangups about perceived weight-related threats to employment, health and social status. The PR implication becomes loud and clear: "Lose weight and join the fun crowd!"

My interviews with patients and an analysis of responses to the survey questionnaire (Section 4) indicate that half the aspartame reactors took such products "to control weight." The PR firms for businesses manufacturing and distributing aspartame products imply that consumers are able to eat the cake but not wear it. This is also the reasoning of physicians and dietitians who recommend low-calorie, no-caffeine, salt-free and cholesterol-free "lite" products containing aspartame. One aspartame product with alleged fat-burning attributes is promoted as a "metabolic enhancer."

While "disease-specific claims" are forbidden in the advertisements and labels of aspartame products, a pamphlet prepared for consumers in 1983 provided the manufacturer's direct answer to whether they help control weight: "Yes." A subsequent ad emphasized the caloric saving of 15,820 calories between ten pounds of sugar (18,080 calories) and the equivalent of 2,262 calories for a popular tabletop sweetener. There is one profound reservation: the dubious long-term (that is, one year and longer) effectiveness and safety of aspartame products taken to achieve weight loss.

D. **Biophysiologic Perspectives**. The prolonged use of hypocaloric foods and minimum-calorie beverages containing aspartame may cause or contribute to anorexia. Chemists, food scientists and "nutritionists" must recognize the potential harm of tampering with a satiety center that evolved over the millennia when famine posed a great threat to mankind.

- An astute researcher observed that the much-admired person who "can eat everything and yet remain thin" probably would have died in prior centuries when food was scarce.
- The Director of the FDA's Center for Food Safety and Applied Nutrition commented on the evolving gene-splicing technology capable of producing calorie-free chocolate cake: "You'll eat it and you're satisfied, and you starve to death with a smile on your face" (*The Evening Times* West Palm Beach, October 31, 1986, p. A-4.)

Most figure-conscious persons are oblivious to a related vital issue: the necessity of adequate fat. <u>Modest "obesity" constitutes a valuable reserve of energy</u>. This is particularly true for women, who need 12 percent to survive famine, compared to three percent for men. Moreover, greater body fat – that is, at least 20 percent body weight – is necessary for normal fertility and gestation.

> Females may be more vulnerable to arbitrary drastic caloric restriction because they mobilize more fat from adipocytes in the abdominal region and other depots than men (Leibel 1987). Conversely, such gender-related differences explain the greater tendency for men to accumulate fat in the abdominal region.

Long-term weight loss induced largely by aspartame consumption could be regarded as challenging "the wisdom of the body." Indeed, the underlying "thrifty gene" of diabetogenic hyperinsulinism that favors the deposition of fat (see below) constitutes a survival trait.

- Anthropologists have emphasized that "natural selection" favors obesity, especially for pregnant women and nursing mothers.
- Peter Brown and Melvin Konner (1987) of Emory University reiterated a theme similar to that presented in my earlier publications (Roberts 1964, 1965, 1971b) – namely, our ancestors survived famine because of their biologic endowment to store calories during times of relative

food surplus. This perception remains in developing countries (e.g., "fattening huts" in Africa for future brides), and among disadvantaged ethnic groups in the west.

E. Potential Concurrent Hazards. The hazards of malnutrition induced by the arbitrary severe reduction of calories has been recognized a long time.

- Seven decades ago, Dr. Morris Fishbein (1932) noted the increased rate of tuberculosis among adolescent girls and young women as a "craze for slenderization" swept the country. This led to the introduction of "propaganda" for replacing lean models by "hips, trains, and ruffles for the future mode."
- For women with existing or potential anorexia nervosa who are "dying to be thin," aspartame products could become "Eve's apple."

Persons who lose considerable weight through strict dieting and strenuous exercise risk other serious complications. I reviewed this subject (Roberts 1985), especially relative to abnormal heart rhythms (notably ventricular tachycardia) and pulmonary embolism (see Case IX-B-4). The changes in heart rhythm (IX-C-1) may reflect shifts of potassium, sodium and magnesium.

The paucity of carbohydrate and calories in aspartame products can contribute to depression (see Chapters VII and XXIII). It may reflect decreased serotonin synthesis and release (Lieberman 1987).

The adverse effects to a fetus whose mother intentionally loses considerable weight, or fails to gain weight, could be disastrous (Chapter X). This has become a nationwide problem among pregnant teenagers.

The excessive loss of amino acids has potential adverse nutritional effects. The D forms of amino acids (Chapters XXII and XXV) tend to be excreted more rapidly by the intestinal tract. Many weight-reduction formulas contain large quantities of these stereoisomers (Dr. Jeffrey Bada, personal communication, January 1987).

Erroneous diagnoses warrant mention. Marked weight loss in HIV-positive patients who consumed considerable diet sodas to avoid sugar (in the hope of preventing fungal superinfection) has been misdiagnosed as a manifestation of AIDS (see Case IX-H-6).

Other considerations are germane. This letter was received in May 1987 from the Health Committee Chairman of the National Association To Aid Fat Americans.

"In checking through my files, I found that I'd run across your work before in the form of a 1970 article on 'Overlooked Dangers of Weight Reduction.' Any doctor who challenges the orthodox assumption that weight loss is the panacea for all the ills of the obese is even more remarkable.

"In the course of my researches, I have become convinced that weight reduction may carry many more dangers than those outlined in your article. In fact, *there is hardly a single disease attributed to obesity which cannot be explained equally well as a consequence of chronic, repeated, or injudicious dieting.* The greater the number of dieters in a given population, the more hazardous obesity appears to be: thus, the obese members of a popular diet club show a higher rate of illness than do the obese members of a more generalized population like Framingham.

"On the basis of these and other facts, it seems logical to propose that dieting may be a major cause – if not **the** major cause – of morbidity and mortality in the obese." (Italics by the author)

2. ANOREXIA NERVOSA AND BULIMIA

The contemporary perils of anorexia nervosa and bulimia are compounded by the combination of "diet" foods and aspartame addiction (Chapter VII-G). The epidemic proportions of bulimia surfaced in December 1984 after singer Karen Carpenter died of heart arrest, and with its admission by actress Jane Fonda.

These eating disorders afflict from 10 to 15 percent of adolescent girls and young females in the United States (Health & Public Policy Committee 1986), and at least one in five college women. Their prevalence is indicated by the fact that 80 percent (!) of fourth-grade girls in one study had placed themselves on self-imposed diets.

A. Anorexia Nervosa. This disorder is characterized by extreme weight loss caused by not eating due to fear of becoming overweight. These individuals tend to distort their awareness of hunger and to deny fatigue when extremely active. Although they may appear healthy, most experience anxiety, depression and anger over misgivings about their body image.

B. Bulimia. Bulimia describes secretive binge eating followed by self-induced vomiting and/or the excessive use of laxatives and diuretics. (This combination of disorders has been termed "bulimorexia.") These persons often insert fingers down the throat after a meal or snack to induce vomiting, a habit that can cause rotting of teeth owing to repeated contact with the stomach's acid secretions.

The considerable use of aspartame products enhances the proneness of young women with insulin-dependent diabetes mellitus (IDDM) to bulimia (Stancin 1989).

Representative Case Report

Case IX-B-7

A 25-year-old graduate student in social work had anorexia nervosa and bulimia five years. She was successfully treated by a psychiatrist for recurrent major depression with tranylcypromine, a monoamine oxidase inhibitor.

This patient then began using aspartame products. She consumed six cans of ASD, eight packets of ATS, 2-3 glasses of presweetened tea, 2-3 glasses of an aspartame soft drink, and four sticks of aspartame gum daily. Her intense depression recurred, along with suicidal thoughts and "anxiety attacks." Other complaints included severe headache, extreme irritability, "red splotching" on the face, neck and chest, palpitations, shortness of breath, unexplained chest pains, and intense thirst. Elevation of the blood pressure was found for the first time.

She was seen by several consultants. Two CT scans of the brain and an electroencephalogram were normal. Her symptoms improved within two days after stopping aspartame, and returned within one day after two separate rechallenges.

Commentary

The _magnitude_ of anorexia nervosa and its complications is again underscored. About 500,000 Americans (mostly women) suffer from this disorder. For each decade of affliction, such individuals face a five percent risk of dying from heart problems, infection, and liver/kidney dysfunction. The disinclination of many insurance companies to continue payment for treatment may be superimposed.

Patients with anorexia nervosa or bulimia seem highly vulnerable to aspartame-induced neuropsychiatric disturbances, especially severe depression (Chapter VII). A Michigan psychologist sent this letter.

> "I thoroughly agree with your analysis that aspartame negatively influences health. Working with women who have psychological and physical deficits consistent with anorexia and bulimia nervosa, and who consume vast quantities of diet soda, led me to try an experiment. I requested that they eliminate the intake of diet soda for two weeks, substituting diluted fruit juice or water. I noted a clear improvement in their level of depression, as well as a sense of well-being. Primary caregivers and/or patients themselves also noticed a reduction in mood swings among individuals who were having uncontrolled episodes that could not otherwise be explained."

Aspartame reactors and their relatives made repeated reference to these disorders in the survey questionnaire. One described a niece who had required hospitalization for extreme anorexia and bulimia after "living on aspartame."

A vicious cycle can be established in weight-conscious young women preoccupied with dieting. Researchers at Wayne State University believe that anorexia may become a virtual physical addiction within three or four months (*Medical Tribune* October 8, 1986, p. 1). The behavioral manifestations of this "addiction to dieting" explain in part the failure of counseling.

Some of the cultural influences of young white <u>women</u> with anorexia nervosa were noted earlier. Although black women in the United States are nearly twice as prone to obesity as their white counterparts, studies of obese black teenage girls suggest that most have positive feelings about their appearance.

Young <u>men</u> also may become trapped into anorexia. In one scenario, they take wrestling or other sports in school, and are encouraged by coaches to lose weight in order to compete in lower-weight categories. Others are preoccupied with well-defined and minimal-fat muscles. The incidence of anorexia/bulimia in men is probably higher than previously suspected, based on deficient bone mineral density studies (Anderson 2000). About one of every six persons so afflicted is male.

Aspartame disease should be considered when the diagnosis "eating disorder not otherwise specified" (appearing in the diagnostic manual of the American Psychiatric

388

Association) is being entertained in an adolescent male. The problem in males has been compounded by distortion of the male body image in which there is preoccupation with overall muscularity without gaining fat ("the Adonis complex"). The concomitant view of weight gain as primarily a feminist matter contributes to the underdiagnosis of eating disorders in men.

The need for long-term studies is reiterated. Ryan-Harshman, Leiter and Anderson (1987) reported no alterations by phenylalanine and aspartame on feeding behavior, mood and arousal in males during short-term studies. But these results must take into consideration the selection of young men within the range of ideal body weight.

The treatment of anorexia remains expensive and frustrating for all, especially the struggle with perfectionism and low self esteem. Only one out of four patients "recover" at five years. The use of antidepressant drugs for concomitant depression cannot be expected to alleviate the basic eating disorder, concomitant malnutrition or aspartame disease. Accordingly, therapists and support groups ought to stress that the best "drug" for these individuals is a lifetime commitment to proper food and adequate calories if the serious effects of superimposed poor nutrition are to be avoided, and that the resumption of aspartame invites relapse.

Pertinent Experimental Observations

Drewnowski et al (1987) found that normal-weight bulimic patients and anorexia-bulimia patients prefer sweeter stimuli than control subjects; the pattern did not change following weight regain. This explains in part their tendency to binge with sweet or calorie-dense foods such as cookies and ice cream, and the high consumption of aspartame products.

Altered neurotransmitter function in the satiety center (Chapter XXIII) can contribute to the observed anorexia and severe weight loss. Blundell et al (1986) emphasized that aspartame's long-term effects on the appetite control system require clarification.

- Rogers and Leung (1973) demonstrated that rats markedly decrease their food intake while on a diet containing an excess of one amino acid.
- When aspartame was given to normal-weight and obese rats in place of sucrose to produce a 50 percent dilution of the diet, neither group increased its intake sufficiently to maintain energy requirements at baseline levels.
- Carbohydrates protect mice against aspartame-induced brain and hypothalamic damage (Fernstrom 1986).

- Other amino acids and neurotransmitters cause anorexia and promote weight loss by altering the central regulation of feeding. Ceci et al (1986) demonstrated such effects after administering oral 5-hydroxytryptophan to bulimic obese subjects.
- Phenylalanine is readily converted to tyrosine, a precursor for the brain's synthesis of catecholamines regulating food intake.
- Aspartame-altered dopamine metabolism, including blocking of dopamine D_2 receptors in the mesolimbic circuitry of the brain, can induce anorexia (Wang 2001).

Phenylalanine also releases cholecystokinin (CCK). This hormone can reduce food intake and stimulate insulin release (Chapters XXII and XXIV). There are two pools of cholecystokinin – one in the gastrointestinal tract; the other within the central nervous system. Ingested aspartame apparently stimulates the release of CCK when it arrives in the proximal intestine. More details concerning the biological and pharmacologic effects of cholecystokinin and its analogs, including effects on neuropsychiatric disorders, appear elsewhere (Reeve 1994).

- Rogers, Keedwell and Blundell (1991) suggested that aspartame might act as a cholecystokinin releaser to inhibit food intake by humans. These investigators were impressed by the fact that the amino acid sequence of aspartame is the same as the C-terminal dipeptide of cholecystokinin, a physiological mediator of satiety.
- Gastrin and CCK share the same five terminal amino acids, together with other structural similarities.
- Gourch et al (1990) found that a CCK pseudopeptide decreased food intake in free-feeding rats, and induced satiety comparable to that of CCK through both central and peripheral mechanisms.

3. OBESITY; PARADOXIC WEIGHT GAIN

A gain of considerable weight, as much as 80 to 100 pounds, occurred in 40 aspartame reactors. The term "paradoxic" conveys their initial intent to lose or "control" weight. The increase occurred with various aspartame products. Case IX-B-10 gained 60 pounds on a franchised diet plan containing aspartame. Abstinence from aspartame generally effects a significant loss of the undesired weight.

390

Even relatively small amounts of aspartame products may be conducive to weight gain, especially among children. Dr. Theron Randolph (1956) emphasized that small quantities of a specific excitant (e.g., various sugars, alcoholic beverages and monosodium glutamate) may effectively perpetuate "addictive eating and drinking."

- A 37-year-old woman experienced severe headaches, irritability, and a change in personality while consuming only one can of an ACB daily. She stated, "I was extremely hungry while drinking the soda."
- An aspartame reactor who was diagnosed as a "chemical diabetic" developed severe carbohydrate craving when using aspartame products. Commenting on the concomitant difficulty in losing weight, she stated

> "One of the most terrible things aspartame did was to render my body unable to tell me when I was full! I was never, ever full! I could eat and eat and eat and eat, and still have room for more food – at least that's what my brain was telling me!"

Huge amounts of aspartame products are being used by obese persons. According to current medical criteria based on body mass index, more than half of all Americans age 20 to 74 are overweight, while one-fifth whose body mass index is 30 or higher can be classified as obese.

Viewed in this context, the enormous corporate profits involved virtually guarantee opposition to the concept of aspartame-induced paradoxic weight gain (Section 7).

Representative Case Reports

Case IX-B-9

A successful businesswoman experienced headache, fluid retention, severe lethargy, depression, and frequency and discomfort of urination (day and night) while drinking aspartame beverages. She further anguished over an unexpected gain of 50 pounds.

> "I drank diet soda for the obvious reasons, to avoid both sugar and weight gain. The interesting thing is that I remember often thinking, 'My body knows that it is not sugar. It's not fooled,'

and I would go looking for the real thing. In other words, it did not accomplish my goal of finding a sugar substitute. I cannot be sure it increased my craving for sugar. No matter how much I exercised, eating light, etc., I could not lose even a pound. All of my symptoms disappeared after discontinuing aspartame."

Case IX-B-10

A 36-year-old housewife went on a franchised program for overweight persons.

"I ballooned up <u>60</u> lbs within a period of three years. I became very concerned as I am not a big eater. I read an article that made me think aspartame was my problem. I have been off it two weeks. I joined a diet center, and lost five pounds the first week."

Case IX-B-11

A 26-year-old North Carolina student majoring in landscape horticulture was seen in consultation for aspartame disease. In addition to severe abdominal discomfort and muscle spasms, she had developed intense hunger ("I became ravenous all of the time"), and gained <u>100</u> pounds (from 130 to 230) within one year! Several gastroenterologists could detect no stomach disease, and concluded that she was "too stressed." The patient added, "For the most part, I was scolded for being overweight. I have found doctors that hardly listen to a word I say, and treat me in a most patronizing manner."

Case IX-B-12

A 40-year-old woman gained <u>100</u> pounds while consuming considerable aspartame sodas and presweetened iced tea. She complained of marked memory loss, intense thirst, and cessation of her menstrual periods.

General Considerations

In a period of only seven years (1991 to 1998), the Centers for Disease Control and Prevention found a 50 percent (!) increase of obesity in all age groups and in all ethnic groups – namely, from 12 percent to 17.9 percent (Mokdad 1999). There has been a concomitant epidemic of childhood obesity.

The following facts underscore the importance of this subject in the present context.

- Two-thirds of adults in the United States are on diets to lose or control weight (Serdula 1999).
- Most overweight patients seen in consultation by the author consume considerable aspartame.
- Aspartame products have played a major role in our fat-enabling culture, with emphasis on the "snack well syndrome" using low-calorie foods and sodas.
- The American Cancer Society (1986) found that persons using artificial sweeteners gain more weight than those who avoid them.

Most patients with paradoxic weight gain fail to realize several vicious cycles that can culminate in the gain and maintenance of excessive weight. It is known that saccharin and other sweeteners in drinking water induce greater food consumption and obesity among experimental animals (Merkel 1979).

The paradoxic weight gain associated with aspartame use offers a valuable lesson in human physiology. It reflects metabolic defense when the body senses the need for more carbohydrate and calories as decreased energy threatens the needs of vital tissues. Accordingly, the biological regulatory systems of man tend to resist undereating strongly, but overeating weakly.

The use of considerable aspartame products by individuals who essentially eat only one meal a day, referred to as "forced feeding" (Roberts 1964, 1965, 1971b), invites further weight gain, especially if they consume more sugar and fat (which is considerable in many sweets). In essence, many persons who gain weight while using aspartame eat only one meal daily – akin to the experimental "gorging" that elevates free fatty acid and glucose levels, and induces obesity (Bortz 1969). (A cartoonist depicted two women at lunch, one lamenting that dieting always gave her an appetite.) These issues also apply to intermittent fasts.

Persons involved in assisting compulsive overeaters – whether professional therapists, support groups, or the spouse who purchases food – should emphasize both abstinence from aspartame products, and avoidance of quick-weight-loss diets. For most weight-conscious individuals, the avoidance of aspartame, refined sugar and white bread, coupled with prudent intake at meals and "scientific nibbling" (Roberts 1962), will prove helpful.

I have been impressed by the role of aspartame gum in persons with paradoxic weight gain, especially women. The most effective concentration of a gum base containing aspartame to increase hunger is 0.3 percent for females, and 0.5 percent for males (Tordoff

1990). The harmful attributes of aspartame gum, especially relative to altered brain function, were considered in Chapter II-E.

Given their intense zeal to lose weight, along with an unwillingness to accept their natural endowment stoically, many sophisticated individuals do not take kindly to the author's seemingly heretical views about <u>the nature of "acceptable" weight</u>. The problem is compounded by biased height-weight charts.

- A feature in *The Miami Herald* was titled, "Let Us Sing the Praises of Fat Women" (June 13, 1983, p. C-1). It provided perspective about the inherent value of a curvy silhouette for "cave mommas." The author asserted, "Pity. Thin may be in, but it's a mistake to think there is no limit. Ms. Nature is obviously miffed that we don't appreciate her thoughtful work."
- The editor of the literature review section in a periodical for health professionals regarded a report for supplementation with aspartame to enhance weight loss as "a lesson in distorting the data" (Gaby 1992). He pondered whether its conclusions were "manifestations of ignorance, wishful thinking or fraud."

The increased frequency of <u>early puberty</u> during the past decade, most notably as breast development in girls before the age of eight, may be a consequence of aspartame-related childhood obesity.

Hyperinsulinism and Related Metabolic Considerations

Insulin is essential for the deposition of body fat. Accordingly, weight gain can be regarded as reflecting an overinsulinized state (Roberts 1963, 1964, 1965, 1967, 1971). I have repeatedly emphasized this factor in obesity, especially among individuals with severe reactive hypoglycemia (Chapter XIV) who evidence proneness to diabetes ("decreased glucose tolerance"; "insulin resistance"). They secrete excessive insulin, and react to the ensuing hunger by consuming more sugar and carbohydrates.

The impaired conversion of phenylalanine to tyrosine in obesity (Brown 1973), with increased retention of phenylalanine, is also noteworthy. The significantly higher fasting plasma phenylalanine concentrations in obese persons (Caballero 1987), and the blunted response to carbohydrate intake (Felig 1969), reflect resistance to the effects of insulin on plasma amino acid levels.

There is experimental evidence that the administration of monosodium glutamate (MSG), a related amino acid, during the neonatal period results in increased body weight (Pizzi 1977), and alterations of pituitary, thyroid, ovarian and testicular function. These presumably reflect hypothalamic and endocrine injury (Chapter VIII-G).

Altered Satiety and Cephalic Responses

Another contribution to insulin hypersecretion is so-called reflex hypoglycemia, also termed the cephalic phase of insulin secretion. The taste or smell of sweet initiates a nerve-mediated reflex resulting in a pulse of insulin release that anticipates to the arrival of food. Aspartame can trigger this mechanism, causing intensified hypoglycemia and the deposition of fat.

There is an inherent link between sweetness and energy density. Blundell et al (1986) emphasized that it can be eroded when an intense sweetening agent is added to low-calorie foods for increasing palatability. Such disengagement disrupts a natural biological control system. Since greater palatability tends to enhance intake, a "reservoir" of residual hunger is created. Compensatory consumption of food has been observed with the administration of aspartame, saccharin and acesulfame-K, especially when consumed in liquid form (soft drinks) than solid form.

The cephalic responses that anticipate caloric intake also involve cerebral cholecystokinin and various neurotransmitters.

- Phenylalanine-induced hormonal changes include the release of cholecystokinin (Gibbs 1976), and increased norepinephrine concentrations in the hypothalamus (Leibowitz 1986).
- Brain levels of catecholamine neurotransmitters are increased after aspartame (Coulcombe 1986).
- The stimulation of insulin by phenylalanine, aspartic acid and other amino acids (Chapter XXIV) is pertinent to diabetogenic hyperinsulinism and contemporary dietary habits.

Aspartame-induced weight gain also probably involves the inhibition of carbohydrate-induced synthesis of serotonin, which blunts the craving for carbohydrates. This accounts in part for the increased consumption of sweets by aspartame users.

Aspartame-altered dopamine metabolism, including blocking of dopamine D_2 receptors in the mesolimbic circuitry of the brain, can lead to obesity. The availability of dopamine D_2 receptor is decreased in obese persons proportionate to their body mass index

(BMI) (Wang 2001). Indeed, dopamine deficiency may perpetuate pathological eating as a means to compensate for decreased activation of these circuits, representing a "reward deficiency syndrome."

C. HEART AND CHEST PROBLEMS

Patients with aspartame disease experienced various chest symptoms that improved or subsided after stopping these products. They include palpitations, rapid heart action (tachycardia), "shortness of breath," and atypical chest pain.

Among the first aspartame reactors who completed the survey questionnaire (Chapter XIX), 22 percent experienced palpitations ("heart fluttering"), 11 percent "rapid heart beat attacks," and 12 percent unexplained chest pains.

These reactions probably contribute significantly to the number of coronary arteriograms currently performed on patients having unexplained chest pain or cardiac arrhythmias with "panic attacks." The absence of demonstrable disease, coupled with failure to respond to anxiolytic therapy, should clue physicians to the possibility of aspartame disease.

Additionally, recent-onset or aggravated cardiac damage may be due to aspartame-induced cardiovascular reactions, especially when superimposed on high risk factors. The latter include hypertension, elevated lipid concentrations and excessive smoking. Case IX-C-5 illustrates potentially-fatal complete heart block in a hypertensive patient.

These complaints reflect physiologic disturbances induced by aspartame and its breakdown products (Section 5). For example, increased release of norepinephrine and dopamine can cause abnormal heart rhythms and elevation of the blood pressure.

1. ABNORMAL HEART RHYTHMS

Sixteen percent (193) aspartame reactors in this series experienced disorders of the heartbeat – including symptomatic palpitations ("fluttering"), and documented attacks of rapid heart action. Twenty-four (6 percent) of the initial 397 reactors who completed the questionnaire had one or two heart rhythm (Holter) monitor studies. Several striking instances are cited here and in the case reports.

- An aspartame reactor suffered repeated attacks of premature ventricular contractions while consuming three to four caffeine-free diet colas daily. He was taken to an emergency room "with caffeine-free diet cola in hand". The abnormal heart action dramatically subsided after avoiding aspartame, and was "almost a memory" a year later.
- One patient underwent unsuccessful radiofrequency ablation of areas in the heart before awareness of underlying aspartame disease.
- The possibility that aspartame products induced or aggravated "sick sinus syndrome" was raised by Case IX-C-4, who had no apparent cardiovascular risk factors. (In this condition, the heart rate may become very slow or fast, or both – with associated weakness and near-faint or actual syncope).
- Case IX-C-5 experienced transient complete heart block after drinking his **first** glass of an aspartame soda.

Sudden Death. I am repeatedly asked, "Can a severe aspartame reaction cause sudden death?" This has probably occurred – based on submitted case histories, the listing of "Death" by the FDA in its statistics for aspartame reactions, and unexplained fatalities among pilots and drivers (Section 6). ("The sweet hereafter" was conveyed in a cartoon with the caption: "Eat, drink, and be buried.") Persons with extreme sensitivity to monosodium glutamate (MSG) (Chapter VIII-G) harbor a similar fear.

Representative Case Reports

Case IX-C-1

A woman experienced "abnormal heart beat," difficulty in breathing, profuse sweats, and uncontrollable shaking the first day she used an ATS. Her symptoms intensified thereafter. They disappeared promptly after avoiding aspartame, only to recur when she ingested an unsuspected product. She reflected, "Doctors and hospitals couldn't tell me what was wrong. It took me a while, by my own detective work, to figure out what was causing the problems."

Case IX-C-2

A 52-year-old office manager developed severe eye symptoms after using up to three cans of aspartame soft drinks and seven packets of an ATS daily for three months. She also experienced attacks of rapid heart action, during which pulse rates up to 146 beats per minute were recorded.

Case IX-C-3

An 82-year-old female had been in good health until drinking an aspartame soda, followed by cardiac symptoms. "I had palpitations, flutterings, premature beats, and feelings that the heart was getting up and turning over. My doctor exhausted all the tests he could think of doing. Nothing seemed amiss. I was plagued with those symptoms around the clock, regardless of activity."

This patient wrote, "I then put 2 and 2 together, and came up with aspartame. All my symptoms disappeared two days after discontinuing the product and did not recur. To me, that sounds as if aspartame was the culprit."

Case IX-C-4

A 42-year-old business executive consumed about 12 cans of aspartame soft drinks a week. He developed "blackouts" that were "erroneously diagnosed as epilepsy for six months." He stated, "I became convinced of an aspartame relationship, but stopping its use did not stop my blackouts. I was finally diagnosed as having 'sick sinus syndrome,' and had a pacemaker implanted."

Case IX-C-5

A 73-year-old man had been under my care for modest hypertension and reactive hypoglycemia. He did well for three years on an appropriate diet, salt restriction and minimal medication. He was advised to abstain from aspartame products because of the tendency to hypoglycemic attacks.

The patient was seen on an emergency basis one morning after suddenly feeling "very drained." He had never experienced a comparable reaction. His pulse was noted to be slow and irregular, but he had no chest pain.

When examined, the patient's pulse was in the low 40s. Complete atrioventricular dissociation (heart block) and several two-second pauses were recorded. His random blood sugar was 67 mg percent. Feeling better after taking a snack, he pleaded to be observed rather than being hospitalized for the anticipated insertion of a pacemaker.

There was a remarkable aspect of his history. He had avoided all aspartame products, as suggested, until the previous night when he felt intense thirst at an event. The only beverage available was diet cola, which he drank for the **first** time.

The patient's rhythm spontaneously reverted to normal sinus while being observed in the office. No pacemaker was required. The foregoing symptoms did not recur over four years of subsequent observation.

Case IX-C-6

A 28-year-old woman started drinking diet sodas when she was 16. She experienced palpitations several months later. A consultant cardiologist indicated that her heart was "perfect," and she "should live to be 140." She avoided caffeine and smoking, and attempted to eat properly – but continued using diet sodas. Her palpitations persisted, coupled subsequently with slurred speech, confusion, depersonalization, mood swings, and "an acute anxiety and obsessive compulsive spectrum".

After finding references to aspartame-induced symptoms, the patient avoided these products. Dramatic improvement ensued. Two months after such abstinence, she became asymptomatic. "I cannot believe that I suffered needlessly for so many years (12) thinking that there was something wrong with me, such as a dangerous heart disease or psychological condition, and all along it was because of aspartame!"

2. ATYPICAL CHEST PAIN

The term "atypical chest pain" indicates chest discomfort that is not typical of either angina pectoris or aspartame-induced esophageal irritation (Chapter IX-D). Eighty-five persons (7 percent) had this complaint. Its severity is indicated by the fact that 33 of the reactors who initially completed the questionnaire were subjected to cardiac stress testing. (It proved normal in most instances.) A 29-year-old man stated, "I went through hell the last four years of my life with chest pains, anxiety, and thousands of dollars worth of treatment, only to find that stopping diet cola seemed to cure all my ailments."

This type of non-cardiac chest pain probably represents a form of visceral hyperalgesia having a central component (*The Lancet* 2000; Volume 356:1127-1128).

With the widespread availability of coronary care units, chest pain not attributable to coronary heart disease has crystallized as a major problem. Indeed, such patients now constitute up to half the admissions to such units (*The Lancet* 1987; 1:959-960). Confusion was introduced in several patients having severe aspartame disease who found that nitroglycerin placed under the tongue alleviated their chest pain.

The severity of aspartame-induced attacks of chest pain in children is illustrated by Case XI-4, a 13-year-old boy.

A Coronary Connection?

The question is properly raised, "Could aspartame reactions precipitate or aggravate existing ischemic (coronary) heart disease?" The histories of several reactors suggest a temporal relationship between beginning aspartame consumption and an ensuing heart attack.

Representative Case Report

Case IX-C-7

A 51-year-old businessman started taking one ACB and two packets of an ATS daily in September 1985. Diabetes had been diagnosed one month previously. He developed ringing in the ears, a marked decrease of vision in one eye, drowsiness, memory loss, and a change in personality. A heart attack (myocardial infarction) occurred during November.

Commentary

For perspective, the heart is essentially a muscular pump requiring considerable energy to function properly. Accordingly, angina pectoris could be a response to aspartame-induced hypoglycemia (Chapter XIV). The contributory role of hypoglycemia has been reviewed previously (Roberts 1964, 1965a,b, 1967a, 1971b).

- Glucose is a major source of energy for heart muscle (Shipp 1964, Weissler 1964, Kako 1965).
- It has been asserted that "the fundamental metabolic injury most commonly responsible for initiating ischemic heart disease in our society is myocardial glucopenia" (Roberts 1971b).
- The frequency with which diabetogenic hyperinsulinism is found in patients having ischemic heart disease (Albrink 1965, Keen 1965, Nikkilä 1965) further supports this concept.

Other clinical encounters are relevant, as in this instance.

A man with severe depression that had resisted psychotherapy and other treatment was found to have "a dangerously high level of CPK." It was interpreted by his physician as excessive production of this enzyme by the heart. He had been "addicted" to diet colas many years, drinking as much as a case daily.

After learning about aspartame disease, he suggested that both the depression and elevated CPK values had been aspartame-induced.

3. RECENT HYPERTENSION

Hypertension was found in 64 aspartame reactors (5 percent) who had not been known to have it previously. Several emphasized concomitant headache (Chapter V).

Cases of recent hypertension also appear in other chapters. Several patients were studied for suspected pheochromocytoma (an adrenal tumor producing epinephrine and norepinephrine) because of their dramatic acute hypertension (see Cases IX-C-10 and C-11).

Aspartame reactions can aggravate existing hypertension, notwithstanding the continued use of previously-effective medication.

The combination of phenylpropanolamine and aspartame in a number of "appetite suppressant" products may induce or aggravate hypertension and its complications. They include "maximum strength" appetite-control formulas and diet gums.

Representative Case Reports

Case IX-C-8

This woman always had normal, or even "low," blood pressure. An elevation was first recorded shortly after she began drinking an aspartame beverage. She also complained of headache. Her blood pressure promptly normalized after stopping this product, coupled with disappearance of the headache.

Case IX-C-9

A registered nurse whose blood pressure had been normal developed severe hypertension after drinking diet cola. Her readings rose as high as 280/160. Other symptoms included daily headache, confusion, and symptoms of hypoglycemia. These features improved dramatically after discontinuing aspartame products.

Case IX-C-10

A 41-year-old woman was treated for severe hypertension and diabetes. She had not used aspartame products previously. Hospitalization was required. Her condition improved on insulin, salt restriction, and prazosin (Minipress®), as evidenced by the virtual normalization of her blood pressure and blood glucose concentrations.

At her next visit, she complained of extreme sleepiness, fatigue, depression and intense sweats. The blood pressure had risen to 180/112 at home, and 180/102 in the office. Concomitantly, her fasting glucose concentrations (done by home glucose monitoring) were higher, averaging 160 mg percent. When I inquired about aspartame use, she stated that she began drinking considerable amounts of diet beverages on the recommendation of a hospital dietitian.

The problem was further confused by the finding of elevated plasma catecholamine levels – norepinephrine 1206 ng/l (normal 64-320); epinephrine 107 ng/l (normal 0-55); and dopamine 107 ng/l (normal 0-90). Subsequent extensive studies at two major university hospitals failed to document an adrenal tumor (pheochromocytoma) producing norepinephrine and epinephrine.

All aspartame products were discontinued. Her blood pressure declined to 155/90 within five days. Concomitantly, the morning blood glucose concentrations averaged 130 mg percent, while the afternoon glucose values ranged from 90-120 mg percent <u>without</u> a change in insulin dosage.

Case IX-C-11

A registered nurse began drinking an aspartame beverage shortly after it became available. Within several days, she experienced severe "blinding headaches" and elevation of her blood pressure to 240/150. Suspecting a pheochromocytoma, the physician promptly hospitalized her. All tests proved normal. Furthermore, her symptoms disappeared the week of hospitalization during which she did not consume aspartame.

She subsequently resumed the aspartame soda, with prompt recurrence of the same symptoms and hypertension. Her intolerance to aspartame was documented through a process of dietary eliminations. There has been no recurrence of symptoms or increased blood pressure after strict avoidance of aspartame products.

Commentary

Aspartame reactions induced or contributed to the hypertension in these patients through several probable mechanisms.

Increased brain phenylalanine can elevate norepinephrine levels (Chapter XXIII), becoming clinically manifest as hypertension (see Case IX-C-9). A comparable phenomenon has been demonstrated in spontaneously hypertensive rats.

Another plausible mechanism involves increased phenylalanine metabolites, especially dopamine, in the presence of excess insulin (Chapter XIV). Tourian (1985) demonstrated that insulin potentiates the synthesis of phenylalanine hydroxylase in tissue culture.

The documentation of essential hypertension in an insulin-resistant state associated with hyperinsulinemia (Ferrannini 1987), but independent of obesity, is germane because many aspartame reactors have reactive hypoglycemia (Chapter XIV). Furthermore, phenylalanine increases insulin release (Chapter XXIV). In the face of continued hyperinsulinemia, the down regulation of insulin receptors (and ensuing decreased insulin action), the increased reabsorption of sodium, and sympathetic stimulation can exaggerate hypertension.

Other clinical observations suggest a relationship between phenylalanine and tyramine (Chapter XXII). Severe hypertension may occur when increased tyramine (present in certain cheeses and alcoholic beverages) is consumed by persons taking monoamine oxidase inhibitors and cough-cold preparations or appetite suppressants that contain ephedrine, phenylephrine or phenylpropanolamine.

Patients consuming considerable aspartame have reported a craving for salt, as well as sugar and sweets (Chapter IX-B). This desire may be enhanced in those with severe hypoglycemia who have marginal "adrenal reserve." In conjunction with greater thirst, the increased sodium intake contributes to hypertension, excessive urine volume, and fluid retention (see below).

The hypertensive effect of aspartame might summate upon that of other drugs (both prescription and over the counter) that elevate blood pressure, such as phenylpropanolamine which has been incriminated in hemorrhagic stroke.

Patients receiving methyldopa (Aldomet®) for hypertension might be prone to accelerated hypertension after ingesting aspartame that could interfere with its action. For example, a 67-year-old female hypertensive aspartame reactor with three unexplained seizures had been taking methyldopa. It is also of interest that several patients with a prior idiosyncracy to methyldopa experienced severe reactions to aspartame. This occurred in Case VI-M-1, who also developed overt myasthenia gravis.

Patients with a <u>prior pheochromocytoma</u> should avoid aspartame products. This precaution is similar to their avoidance by persons with previous Graves disease whose condition can be exacerbated or simulated thereby (Chapter IX-E).

Experimental studies in both animals and humans suggest that repeated cycles of rapid weight loss and weight gain (Chapter IX-B) are conducive to hypertension. Although Kiritsy and Mahar (1986) reported a lowering of the systolic blood pressure in rats given aspartame (a response comparable to that with tyrosine in spontaneously hypertensive rats), they commented that an antihypertensive effect in this model cannot be transposed to humans.

4. SEVERE VASOMOTOR REACTIONS

Thirteen persons among the most recent 649 aspartame reactors in the present series evidenced striking peripheral vasomotor features. These included high or low blood pressure, intense flushing, "cold chills," coldness of the limbs, and severe sweats. A 49-year-old aspartame reactor described her major symptoms as "bouts of feverishness, sweat dripping down my face and body, and then shivering."

The severe vasomotor reactions in aspartame disease also were evidenced by <u>the Raynaud phenomenon</u> in several patients whose hands and feet became markedly discolored on exposure to cold.

The probable underlying mechanisms were discussed above under Hypertension.

<u>**Representative Case Reports**</u>

<u>**Case IX-C-12**</u>

A man suffered headache, palpitations, severe sweats and other symptoms suggestive of pheochromocytoma (an adrenal tumor releasing epinephrine and norepinephrine). Multiple studies, however, failed to corroborate this diagnosis.

He had been consuming considerable amounts of aspartame products. During my consultation, I pointed out that the phenylalanine in aspartame is converted to dopamine, epinephrine and norepinephrine, the effects of which might simulate such a tumor.

<u>**Case IX-C-13**</u>

A woman repeatedly experienced extreme coldness of the lower limbs, coupled with "a terrible anxiety attack," after consuming aspartame soft drinks. This reaction promptly recurred whenever she drank a soda not recognized as containing aspartame.

Case IX-C-14

A 50-year-old aspartame reactor with severe joint discomfort was also afflicted with extreme intolerance to cold. "I kept my thermostat at 75, sometimes 80, roasting my whole family out of the house!" She drank a two-liter bottle of diet cola daily, along with other aspartame products. Exposure to a cool breeze or a ceiling fan would cause her "to shake literally, sometimes uncontrollably." This symptom disappeared, along with the "arthritis," after avoiding aspartame products.

5. SHORTNESS OF BREATH

The frequency of "shortness of breath" (dyspnea) in patients consuming aspartame who did not have underlying heart or lung disorders was surprising. Specifically, 110 (9 percent) experienced this symptom. It predictably abated when they avoided aspartame products. For example, a 72-year-old woman reported, "My chest felt like it was stuffed," after using a ATS for two weeks. She "felt almost back to normal" within several days after stopping this product.

Several observations are noteworthy.

- Several aspartame reactors described the prompt onset of choking and shortness of breath after chewing aspartame gum ("choker gum"). This was mistaken for a "seizure" in one instance.
- One patient was observed to have swelling of the larynx.
- Decreased secretions in the upper respiratory passages, comparable to "dry eyes" (Chapter IV) and "dry mouth" (Chapter IX-F), may contribute to the pulmonary symptoms.
- An aspartame reactor developed severe choking while drinking a diet soda on a plane as it climbed to higher attitude.
- The occurrence of sleep apnea in aspartame users was discussed in Chapter VI-K.

The FDA noted receiving complaints of "difficulty breathing" from 112 consumers in its April 20, 1995 report.

The cause and significance of this feature remain puzzling. In the absence of asthma and other allergic features (Chapter VIII), the dyspnea presumably reflects neurotransmitter dysfunction within the brain's respiratory center.

Representative Case Reports

Case IX-C-15

A 40-year-old woman stressed that she previously did "not have any problems I cannot handle." She wrote:

> "Help! Last week I was fortunate to hear you on WWDB radio. I just came home from the hospital. I was in intensive care for two days. (They said I may have a clot on my lung.) After two days they said I did not have a clot, and did not know what was wrong with me. They gave me many tests.
>
> "My symptoms over the last three months have been shortness of breath (I get up in the middle of the night gasping), blurred vision, dizziness, headache, falling (I fell in Center City [Philadelphia], and when I came to, people thought I was drunk). I have been to many doctors, and they cannot seem to find what is wrong.
>
> "I called my family doctor when I heard you last week because I drank six to eight glasses of diet cola each day for three years. He said he would look into it."

Case IX-C-16

A 35-year-old woman developed "shortness of breath" that persisted. She consulted a number of physicians who variously told her that the cause was stress (despite an exemplary personal and professional life), atypical asthma, and a swollen larynx. Other symptoms included weight gain, hair loss, dizziness, irritability, fatigue, heavy menstrual bleeding, abdominal pain, and dryness of the skin. She also had hypothyroidism.

The patient probed every aspect of her diet and environmental contacts as her breathing problem intensified. She wrote, "Can you imagine my anxiety at waking up and still not being able to breath?" The only unusual aspect of her routine was the daily use of a gum flavored with aspartame. She wrote

> "I already spent a small fortune on tests that included asthma studies, upper/lower GIs, ultrasounds, x-rays, blood work, cholesterol, and heart, lung and gynecologic testing. I even considered seeing a psychiatrist. I then stopped using this gum, and felt relief almost immediately. I retested myself numerous times to see if I had really found the answer. I am completely assured that the aspartame caused <u>all</u> my problems. At one later time, I consumed a diet soda, not knowing that they had switched from saccharin to aspartame. Within the hour, I could not catch my breath."

Case IX-C-17

A female athlete had run from five to 13 miles daily for eight years without incident. Concerned about her weight, she began drinking diet sodas. She then experienced difficulty in breathing while on the treadmill. A physician diagnosed asthma. When numerous x-rays and other studies failed to reveal a cause, the issue of "stress" was raised... to her dismay. Other features included severe headache, memory loss, impairment of vision, numbness/tingling in the extremities, a rapid heart rate, and pain in the joints.

This patient happened to see a flyer on aspartame disease when she went to purchase a 24-pack of diet soda. As she read the convincing details, "I almost began to cry."

D. GASTROINTESTINAL REACTIONS

Gastrointestinal reactions to aspartame products can extend from the lips to the rectum. They included the following in this series.

Severe lip and mouth reactions (discussed in Chapter VIII)	54 (5%)
Difficult or painful swallowing	61 (5%)
Nausea	127 (11%)
Abdominal pain	125 (10%)
Severe diarrhea	106 (9%)
Associated bloody stools... 16	

In its April 20, 1995 report on 7232 "adverse reactions attributed to aspartame," the FDA received 647 complaints of nausea and vomiting, 453 complaints of abdominal pain and cramps, and 330 complaints of diarrhea.

Accordingly, gastroenterologists and other physicians must inquire specifically about aspartame use in patients who present with these features, especially when they fail to respond to conventional measures. The misdiagnoses have included hiatus hernia, peptic ulcer, gallbladder disease, inflammatory bowel disease (ulcerative colitis; regional enteritis or Crohn's disease), recurrent pancreatitis, diverticulitis, hemorrhoids, and exacerbations of the "irritable bowel syndrome" ("spastic bowel"; "nervous colitis.")

- A prominent Boston cardiologist requested further details from the FDA ("any technical information, research reports, etc.") in a letter dated April 26, 1984. He had encountered a patient suffering indigestion from aspartame that was sufficiently severe to mimic an acute ischemic vascular event.
- Case XI-4 illustrates the violent gastrointestinal reactions induced by aspartame products in children.

Severe gastrointestinal symptoms in aspartame reactors occasionally occurred during the early morning hours. Such timing might represent a delayed IgE-mediated hypersensitivity reaction to aspartame or its breakdown products, comparable to delayed urticaria or angioedema (Kulczycki 1987).

Involvement of Other Organs

Some patients believed that their aspartame-induced reaction was limited to the gastrointestinal tract. Inquiry about concomitant symptoms, however, indicated involvement of other organs.

Representative Case Report

Case IX-D-1

A 38-year-old business executive had gastrointestinal reactions during the 18 months she consumed three to four cans of an ACB daily. They included severe abdominal pain, intense nausea, diarrhea with bloody stools, and marked abdominal bloat. She also developed "dry eyes," had difficulty wearing contact lens, and gained 15 pounds. She described her experience in these terms.

408

"I was sick for over a year and a half as a direct result of ingesting aspartame. My reaction was, I believed, purely intestinal in nature... continual diarrhea and severe stomach upsets. A gastroenterologist put me through many upper and lower GI tests, several absorption-rate tests, and one particularly nasty 'string' test for parasites, but could not determine what was causing my nausea and diarrhea. He never questioned what I was ingesting.

"Becoming desperate, I started reading everything that remotely described my symptoms. With aspartame and food allergies both receiving media attention, I realized my symptoms appeared right after we moved into our new house, and approximately the same time aspartame was introduced into cola products. I immediately stopped consuming diet soft drinks. After ten days of uncomfortable withdrawal symptoms, I felt like a new person."

Costly Diagnostic Tests and Related Risks

The expense of x-rays, CT scans, MRI studies, endoscopy, and other gastrointestinal tests performed on aspartame reactors was often considerable (Chapter XIV).

The long-term consequences of such testing in themselves might be significant. They are especially disconcerting in the case of young persons exposed to considerable radiation from x-ray studies of the stomach, small intestine and large bowel for suspected peptic ulcer, Crohn's disease or ulcerative colitis.

Emotional Impact

The emotional response to aspartame-associated abdominal discomfort, other gastrointestinal complaints and weight loss (Chapter IX-B) was profound among some persons, particularly those having relatives who succumbed to gastrointestinal or pancreatic cancer.

A 55-year-old woman became petrified over recent bowel difficulty and rectal bleeding because her husband had died of colon cancer. A barium enema, sigmoidoscopy, and multiple blood studies were normal. Her symptoms improved within several days after stopping aspartame products.

Familial Incidence

The occurrence of similar gastrointestinal reactions among multiple members of the same family who had aspartame disease is illustrated in several of the case reports that follow (as Case IX-D-24) and in other chapters.

Representative Case Reports

Case IX-D-2

A 65-year-old advertising executive suffered severe diarrhea when she used an ATS "to sweeten everything that needed sweetening." Each of her daughters (who lived in different communities) also developed diarrhea after ingesting aspartame products.

Case IX-D-3

The dramatic onset of swallowing reactions in a mother and daughter is illustrated by the following correspondence.

"I was drinking aspartame hot chocolate two or three times a day. One evening while taking a walk, I was unable to swallow. It was as if my throat was paralyzed. I didn't mention it to my daughter because I didn't want to frighten her.

"Several days later, she related to me that she had been drinking a chocolate mix with aspartame every night, and that she couldn't swallow. Needless to say, I was much relieved to finally discover what was causing my throat to be paralyzed.

"We both stopped using the sweetener for a while, and then tried it once more with the same result -- inability to swallow. I'm sure the aspartame caused it because we have not had the problem since stopping it."

1. MOUTH, THROAT AND TONGUE REACTIONS

Reactions in the mouth to aspartame products varied.

- Aspartame reactors repeatedly mentioned <u>altered or lost taste</u> (see Case III-34-B).
- A "<u>bad taste</u>" in the mouth often accompanied aspartame-induced dryness of the mouth (see below).
- A 57-year-old woman with severe aspartame disease repeatedly developed <u>ulcers of the tongue</u> after chewing aspartame gum.
- <u>Vague mouth complaints</u> occasionally accompanied aspartame-induced "temporal lobe epilepsy," as the "disagreeably metallic taste" in Case III-34-A.
- <u>Acute swelling of the lips and tongue</u> was described in Chapter VIII.
- Case-IX-J-7 developed a <u>black tongue</u>, which gradually returned to healthy pink several months after discontinuing aspartame products.

Burning Tongue or Mouth

Aspartame reactors have repeatedly mentioned a "burning tongue" sensation after ingesting such products. It probably represents a protective mechanism involving the sweet taste buds on front of the tongue in response to toxins or an autoimmune inflammatory response.

- A male diabetic aspartame reactor had complained of "burning tongue" for several years. This symptom disappeared after avoiding aspartame products.
- A 50-year-old woman asked a columnist (see below) about her constant burning of the mouth and a salty taste (*Sun-Sentinel* May 5, 1999, p. E-2). The likelihood of aspartame disease was increased by other suggestive complaints.

Dry Mouth (also see Chapter IX-F)

Patients who complain of dry mouth or intractable oral sensations that remain unexplained after extensive dental, medical and neurological consultations (including cultures and allergy studies) warrant a trial period of abstinence from aspartame products (see Case IX-D-5).

The dry mouth caused by aspartame can have devastating effects on the teeth, gums and nutrition, especially when superimposed on a similar side effect due to many drugs prescribed for older persons (Parker-Pope 2000). Saliva has potent antibacterial and antiviral properties. Its absence invites overgrowth of such organisms and accelerated dental decay.

A diabetic woman with severe aspartame disease (dizziness, forgetfulness, diarrhea, a "schizoaffective disorder", and depression) also complained of dry mouth for which she used breath mints. There were multiple dental problems. "My dentist said he has never seen anyone have such a rapid deterioration of her teeth." In analyzing this problem, she found that the mints contained aspartame.

Swelling of Tongue; Difficult Swallowing

Syndicated physician-columnists receive many inquiries about unexplained swelling of the tongue or lips, and attacks of difficult swallowing (dysphagia) for which no cause could be found. Attributing the latter to hysteria ("globus") in an aspartame reactor represents a serious misdiagnosis.

Representative Case Reports

Case IX-D-4

A 72-year-old patient had attributed severe reactions of the lips and tongue to lipstick, even though these complaints persisted after avoiding it. This known aspartame reactor did not realize that the ginger ale she drank contained aspartame. The lip and tongue symptoms improved within one week after stopping it.

Case IX-D-5

The wife of a man who constantly chewed aspartame gum wrote

"He complained his gums hurt all the time, and his teeth would loosen and tighten up in his gums. So he stopped chewing the aspartame gum. Within one week he said his gums did not hurt anymore. He had a dentist appointment about two weeks after he quit chewing the gum. The dentist said that this was the best his gums had ever looked."

2. SWELLING OF THE SALIVARY GLANDS

The marked and reproducible swelling of the salivary glands after using aspartame products was impressive. This subject also will be considered under Excessive Thirst and Dry Mouth in Chapter IX-F.

412

Representative Case Reports

Case IX-D-6

A 28-year-old housewife noted swelling of her "glands located just under the jaw" on three occasions after ingesting aspartame beverages, puddings, gelatins and gum. Other complaints attributed to them included swelling of the lips and tongue, abdominal pain, severe nausea, diarrhea, ringing in both ears, dizziness, insomnia, depression, marked irritability, a personality change, attacks of rapid heart action, recent thinning of the hair, frequent urination during the day, less frequent periods, and joint pains. All subsided or improved within six weeks after avoiding aspartame products.

Case IX-D-7

A woman in her 60s reported the following dramatic enlargement of her submaxillary glands after drinking a six-ounce glass of aspartame cola.

> "I had an allergic reaction to a diet cola about a year ago. I drank a glass. About 15 minutes later, my saliva glands swelled.
>
> The knots in my neck were as large as golf balls. I went to the doctor. He said it was an allergic reaction to something I had eaten or drank. He gave me an injection of adrenalin and an allergy injection."

Case IX-D-8

A 36-year-old female claims representative became severely disabled by aspartame disease. The manifestations included decreased vision in both eyes, decreased hearing in both ears, marked impairment of memory, severe bloat, thinning of the hair, a facial eruption, and swelling of the salivary glands on each side. Dramatic concomitant enlargement of endometriosis lesions in her ovaries required surgery. She had been consuming considerable amounts of diet sodas, and aspartame-containing soft drink mixes, puddings, gelatins and gum.

It is of interest that her father also developed marked swelling of the salivary glands, altered hearing, and memory loss from the use of aspartame products.

3. ESOPHAGEAL PAIN

Severe irritation of the esophagus, manifest as painful swallowing and non-cardiac chest pain, occurred after consuming aspartame in 61 patients.

Representative Case Report

Case IX-D-10

A 51-year-old beautician had been treated for thrombophlebitis of the lower extremities. Her regimen included coumarin. The prothrombin time concentrations remained in the desired therapeutic range.

The patient experienced recurrent severe pain in the middle of her chest radiating to the back. Her blood pressure and electrocardiogram remained normal. The possibility of coronary artery spasm was raised, but an exercise stress test proved normal. A calcium-channel blocker, prescribed for suspect angina pectoris, had to be stopped because of side effects. A cardiology consultant then suggested that her discomfort represented esophageal irritation, particularly since it intensified during the night. Neither esophageal reflux nor a hiatal hernia, however, could be detected by x-ray studies.

The patient next presented with repeated bright-red rectal bleeding. When queried about aspartame use, she admitted to chewing aspartame gum, especially during work. The probability of aspartame-induced upper and lower gastrointestinal tract irritation was raised. There was no recurrence of chest pain or rectal bleeding over the ensuing several years of aspartame abstinence.

4. NAUSEA

In this series, 127 (11 percent) aspartame reactors experienced severe nausea, with or without other complaints. This symptom appears in many of the representative case reports. For example, a 48-year-old schoolteacher felt nauseated "immediately" after eating or drinking aspartame products.

5. ABDOMINAL PAIN; STOMACH AND BOWEL IRRITATION

Abdominal pain occurred in 125 persons (10 per cent) after ingesting aspartame. Nonspecific irritation of the stomach, small bowel, pancreas (see below), or combinations thereof, seemed the most likely explanation when other causes had been excluded. One patient stated: "It affected my stomach like I had drank a pint of gasoline."

Several patients (as Case IX-D-10) developed <u>gastric bleeding</u>, <u>intestinal bleeding</u>, or <u>both</u>, after drinking or chewing aspartame products.

Other reactors complained of <u>severe cramps</u> and "<u>gas</u>". Inasmuch as aspartame may cause dryness of the mouth, a similar influence on intestinal and pancreatic secretions might contribute to these symptoms.

Longstanding <u>constipation</u> and <u>other gastrointestinal complaints</u> were exacerbated by aspartame products. Paradoxically, an aspartame-sweetened effervescent "natural-fiber laxative" that is widely recommended for managing constipation and the "irritable bowel syndrome" was repeatedly incriminated (see Cases I-II and I-12). For example, a 68-year-old diabetic woman with no previous bowel complaints suffered "extreme" constipation on the <u>four</u> occasions she used aspartame products "in any form."

Longstanding <u>celiac disease</u> was aggravated by aspartame in a woman who had carefully avoided gluten.

<u>Unusual gastrointestinal disorders</u> warrant inquiry about aspartame use.

- Aspartame may have contributed to small bowel obstruction in a man hospitalized for probable aspartame disease. He experienced a seizure and other neurologic problems – including extreme weakness of the lower extremities, and difficulty in swallowing and speech – after recently consuming three two-liter bottles of an aspartame soda weekly. He underwent abdominal surgery to relieve "a kink in the loop of small intestine" nine days later.
- A 24-year-old woman developed progressive distention of the large bowel, diagnosed as "idiopathic megacolon" during the three years she consumed aspartame. Her absence of tears and minimal saliva were reminiscent of comparable features in other aspartame reactors.
- A 19-year-old student with unexplained severe upper gastrointestinal symptoms and associated chest pain had been seen by a number of physicians. She was found to have incomplete emptying of the stomach (gastroparesis). Other complaints included recurrent migraine, insomnia, dizziness and depression. She experienced marked improvement after avoiding aspartame products.

Aspartame reactors who had related gastrointestinal problems face further jeopardy when they use potentially harmful drugs for the relief of pain caused by aspartame products.

Ibuprofen and other nonsteroidal anti-inflammatory agents taken to relieve aspartame-induced headache and joint pain frequently cause gastrointestinal injury, most notably bleeding. Several experimental observations are germane.

- There is significant uptake of radioactivity by the gastrointestinal tract in adult rats 30 minutes after given aspartame labeled with a radioactive-carbon isotope (Matsuzawa 1984).
- Aspartame-induced inflammatory gastrointestinal reactions may result from the generation of leukotrienes, a group of biologically active compounds derived from arachidonic acid (Hardcastle 1997). These substances are released from a variety of human cells – including macrophages, polymorphonuclear leukocytes, mast cells and monocytes.

Needless abdominal surgery was performed in several patients with unrecognized aspartame disease. For example, recurrent nausea and pain persisted in Case IX-D-15 after her gallbladder had been removed until she became aware of being an aspartame victim.

Representative Case Reports

Case IX-D-11

A 42-year-old dentist was asked about aspartame use during routine questioning at his annual checkup. He replied, "I never touch that stuff anymore! Why, if I were to drink just one diet cola, my stomach would feel as if it had a brick in it!"

Case IX-D-12

A male aspartame reactor suffered several attacks of abdominal pain requiring hospitalization. Studies failed to reveal inflammation, ulcer or tumor of the stomach, duodenum or pancreas. In carefully analyzing his attacks, the patient realized that all occurred within one hour after ingesting aspartame. There has been no recurrence since avoiding products containing it.

Case IX-D-13

A 52-year-old insulin-dependent diabetic listed "gas and letting out air" as primary complaints ascribed to aspartame products. She wrote, "It is embarrassing to let gas out

416

when you are shopping or talking to someone." Other symptoms included headache and abdominal bloat. These features recurred when she retested herself with different aspartame products on several occasions.

Case IX-D-14

A 64-year-old man suffered intense pain in the upper abdomen, followed by black stools, shortly after he drank two large bottles of an ACB while working in the yard.

Case IX-D-15 A

The gallbladder was removed in this 38-year-old woman for recurrent nausea and abdominal pain. These symptoms – and others due to aspartame disease – persisted thereafter despite considerable medication (costing an average of $200 monthly). They disappeared within several days after stopping the many aspartame products she had been using.

Out of desperation, this patient fortuitously learned about aspartame disease when a friend entered her symptoms on the Internet, and found the condition listed!

Case IX-D-15 B

A college student was diagnosed as having the irritable bowel syndrome. She was an avid user of aspartame products – including soft drinks, a tabletop sweetener and gum. She stated: "Abdominal pain, embarrassing flatulence, and alternating diarrhea and constipation were a way of life for me. There were many occasions when I was awakened from a deep sleep by excruciating abdominal pain accompanied by cold sweats and nausea. Another disturbing problem I experienced was an uncontrollable, almost violent, craving for sweets. I worked very hard to stay thin, so I chewed a lot of sugarless gum to keep from putting fattening foods in my mouth."

She found reference to aspartame-induced gastrointestinal problems in the course of writing a research paper. There was dramatic improvement of her gastrointestinal symptoms after abstinence, along with a reduction of her "sweet craving."

This victim "experimented" with aspartame products on two occasions – once chewing aspartame gum for five consecutive days; the other time taking aspartame yogurt on five consecutive days. "At the end of both weeks, I experienced the same severe abdominal pains that I had in the past."

Case IX-D-16

An 85-year-old woman had been active and in good health. Her blood pressure was normal (115/60). Within several days after drinking two or three glasses of an lemony aspartame drink, her stomach "began to feel like it had a lump in it." She also developed a headache (unusual for her), and felt "nervous and fidgety." The blood pressure rose to 168/90.

Realizing that the only change in her diet had been the aspartame drink, she stopped it. The symptoms disappeared, and her blood pressure declined to 118/62.

6. PANCREATITIS

Several of my patients experienced attacks of intense upper abdominal pain shortly after consuming aspartame products that were probably due to inflammation of the pancreas. In view of its severity, none wished to be rechallenged for post-aspartame amylase levels, ultrasound imaging and other studies.

Several mechanisms may be operative. They include local irritation, pancreatic stimulation by the release of hormones in the gastrointestinal tract and brain, and the inspissation of pancreatic secretions.

- Pancreatitis has been reported in methanol poisoning (Bennett 1952, Monte 1984).
- Gastroenterologists use phenylalanine, with or without other amino acids, to stimulate the secretion of pancreatic enzymes. Go et al (1970) demonstrated that phenylalanine significantly increased pancreatic enzyme output in human volunteers. Moreover, an amino acid solution containing L-phenylalanine has been used to quantitate pancreatic exocrine secretion (Slaff 1984).

Significant radioactivity uptake by the adult rat pancreas occurs within 30 minutes after administering labeled aspartame (Matsuzawa 1984).

Representative Case Reports

Case IX-D-17

A 54-year-old registered nurse drank up to ten glasses of an aspartame soft drink, and four glasses of aspartame hot chocolate daily. She then suffered severe abdominal pain, nausea, bloody diarrhea and abdominal bloat. Other complaints included recurrent hypoglycemic attacks, visual problems, headache, dizziness, tremors, insomnia, confusion, memory loss, marked hyperactivity, tingling of the limbs, intense depression (with suicidal thoughts), extreme irritability, personality changes, palpitations, thinning of the hair, and joint pains.

This nurse attributed her "severe attacks of hypoglycemia and pancreatitis, which required frequent hospitalization," to aspartame. She explained

> "I feel that the pancreatitis was a direct result of aspartame use. I never used alcohol or drugs of any kind. The doctor could not find any explanation for it, other than the use of aspartame. The pancreatic pain began, along with the mental symptoms, following a vacation trip on which I consumed much more aspartame than while I was working. It was after consuming a large glass of aspartame on an empty stomach that I passed out and was rushed to intensive care."

Two sisters had aspartame disease characterized by severe depression, and attacks of hypoglycemia and anxiety.

Case XIII-D-18

A 62-year-old woman developed pancreatitis after drinking aspartame, with the subsequent onset of clinical diabetes. She attempted to get relief from the intense upper abdominal pain by pressing both fists against her abdomen as she paced the hospital halls. After deducing aspartame to be the probable cause, she literally demanded that it not be included in her "diabetic diet."

7. DIARRHEA

Diarrhea afflicted 106 aspartame reactors (9 percent). The stools were grossly bloody in 16.

Physicians should routinely inquire about aspartame use as a precipitating or aggravating factor in all patients with unexplained or refractory diarrhea, regardless of prior diagnoses. The latter include irritable bowel syndrome, regional enteritis (Crohn's disease), ulcerative colitis, and lactase deficiency.

> The review of chronic diarrhea in diabetes mellitus by Valdovinos et al (1993) made no mention of aspartame products under the category of "dietetic foods." These are widely used by diabetics to minimize sugar intake, but infrequently considered as a cause of diarrhea.

The problem of aspartame-induced irritable bowel syndrome is compounded by the prescription of newer drugs having their own formidable side effects.

Aspartame intake also must be considered in several noninfectious diarrhea syndromes that have surfaced. For example, collagenous colitis (characterized by the buildup of a collagen band at the mucosal surface of the colon) has become a relatively frequent cause of diarrhea in recent years. This disorder most often affects middle-aged or older women, and is coupled with joint complaints and thyroid disorders – features also found in aspartame reactors.

Representative Case Reports

Case IX-D-20

A 46-year-old male interior designer had mild colitis for three decades. Severe diarrhea was triggered by his daily consumption of aspartame sodas and up to five packets of an ATS. He became incapacitated because "I could not get out of the bathroom because of diarrhea and cramps." These complaints disappeared within one week after avoiding all aspartame products. He refused to rechallenge himself thereafter.

Case IX-D-21

A young woman consumed considerable aspartame colas the first summer they became available. Bloody diarrhea ensued, along with headache and dizziness. The diagnoses of "severe colitis and Crohn's disease" were initially entertained. Her symptoms disappeared, however, when she abstained from aspartame.

Her physician then told her that she was the <u>third</u> patient he had seen <u>that month</u> with comparable symptoms after ingesting diet colas.

Case IX-D-22

A 62-year-old patient with reactive hypoglycemia and hypothyroidism had longstanding constipation. She repeatedly experienced diarrhea, however, whenever aspartame was ingested.

Case IX-D-23

An 18-year-old college student suffered bloody diarrhea while drinking one liter of a diet cola daily. Associated complaints included abdominal pain, nausea, headache, dizziness, intense drowsiness, palpitation and marked thirst. The discomfort and diarrhea were sufficiently severe to force her to leave classes for the bathroom, and to miss many days of school.

The symptoms improved within ten days after stopping aspartame. She retested herself on one occasion, with prompt return of the diarrhea and abdominal distress.

Case IX-D-24

A 35-year-old woman developed diarrhea after drinking several cans of an ACB. Her 54-year-old mother also suffered diarrhea from this diet cola. Several weeks later, her husband had several bouts of diarrhea after consuming aspartame.

She offered these insights concerning the issue of "biological maximum intake" (Chapter XXVII).

> "Tolerance levels seem to vary. Only one or two cans of the
> soft drink affect my mother immediately. For me, it took more.
> If I had one glassful during the day, no problem. But after
> several throughout the day or for two days, the problem will
> begin."

Case IX-D-25

A 36-year-old man with prior ulcerative colitis and hypoglycemia had been attended for several years. His condition improved on a conventional diet and symptomatic measures.

The patient presented with recurrent diarrhea that had resisted sulfasalazine (Azulfidine®) prescribed by a gastroenterologist. He had been using an ATS and one can of aspartame soda daily. Improvement followed their cessation.

8. ABDOMINAL BLOAT

Many aspartame reactors complained of "severe bloat" while consuming aspartame products, particularly beverages. While this complaint is not infrequent among weight-conscious women, its frequency and severity seemed greater among aspartame sufferees.

In the absence of demonstrable gastrointestinal pathology (such as obstruction) and premenstrual changes, the bloat may be attributed to excessive ingestion of fluid from intense thirst, the swallowing of considerable air (aerophagia), the release of gas bubbles from carbonated drinks, and the altered gastrointestinal physiology mentioned earlier. Decreased mucosal resistance of the stomach associated with reduced estrogen also could contribute to the gastric distress of menopausal aspartame reactors.

Representative Case Reports

Case IX-D-26

A certified nutritionist was able to correlate the onset of abdominal pain, gas and bloat with her consumption of aspartame products by studying a food diary. She wrote

> "I confirmed this assumption by way of multiple trials and abstentions. Upon realizing the connection, I contacted the manufacturer, and was informed that the company would not take complaints."

Case IX-D-27

A professional woman was diagnosed as having "chemical diabetes" on the basis of a glucose tolerance test, and advised to avoid sugar. She avoided aspartame products thereafter because they induced her "diabetes symptoms."

Highly embarrassing gastrointestinal symptoms persisted. She described herself as "one huge gas bag, unable to control the noises coming from my body – sometimes noises that sounded like flatulence but were actually internal grumblings. When they would happen, my guts felt like they were dancing a jig inside my body." She initially regarded the problem as genetic.

A friend then noted that the non-dairy coffee creamer she was using contained aspartame. (There was no indication of its presence on the label.) Her bowel symptoms disappeared after stopping this creamer, as did the craving for carbohydrates.

9. ANAL DISCOMFORT

Interference with secretions of the lower gastrointestinal tract and rectal area can cause symptoms. One male reactor experienced "the burning after every bowel movement" until avoiding aspartame products.

> Case IV-19 complained of "constant soreness of the anus for which the doctor could find no cause." She suffered concomitant extreme dryness of the mouth, throat and eyes. These complaints promptly improved or disappeared after stopping the ATS she had been using. The anal difficulty, however, persisted several months. None of these symptoms recurred after resuming saccharin.

E. ENDOCRINE AND METABOLIC DISORDERS

The endocrine system consists of several "glands" that secrete hormones into the blood stream, which in turn influence growth and metabolism. This network includes the pituitary ("master") gland, the thyroid, the adrenals, the ovaries, the testicles, and the insulin-producing islet cells of the pancreas.

Profound disturbances affecting this interrelated system have resulted from the use of aspartame products. They are manifested in various ways, some discussed in other chapters – including the aggravation of diabetes mellitus and its complications (Chapter XIII), hypoglycemia (Chapter XIV), the thinning or loss of hair (Chapter VII-D), and diabetes insipidus associated with pseudotumor cerebri (Chapter VI-N). Existing underactivity of the thyroid and adrenal glands tends to create a vicious cycle in patients with aspartame disease.

There is increasing awareness of "endocrine disrupting chemicals" responsible for sexual, neurologic and immune dysfunction. Aspartame products should be added to this list.

Amino acids and synthetic peptides related to the chemical aspartame also have induced hormonal responses.

- N–methyl-DL-aspartate increases pituitary prolactin and gonadotropins in adult female rhesus monkeys (Wilson 1982).
- The administration of aspartate or glutamate to young mice causes hypothalamic lesions (Olney 1979).

The encounter of tumors involving the endocrine glands and related structures will be considered in Chapters XXIII-F and G. In this series, they include prolactin-secreting pituitary tumors (2 cases), unspecified pituitary tumors (2 cases), and a hypothalamic tumor.

- A female aspartame reactor who consumed six diet colas, considerable aspartame yogurt, and diet hot chocolate daily developed a pituitary tumor in 1992, which recurred three years later. Surgery followed by radiation therapy were performed on both occasions.
- Pituitary tumors were repeatedly noted in the Bressler Report (1977) Chapter XXVII) among the following female rats:

  No. M15CF – Pituitary adenoma
  No. H18HF – Pituitary adenoma
  No. K18HF – Pituitary adenoma
  No. M17LF – Marked enlargement of pituitary and both adrenals
  No. J30HM – Marked enlargement of pituitary

1. MENSTRUAL CHANGES

Menstrual changes were prominent in 76 women with aspartame disease. They largely reflect altered neurotransmitter function within the hypothalamus, pituitary and brain (Chapter XXIII).

A. Frequent Menses and Excessive Periods

Excessive menstrual bleeding, more frequent periods, or both, occurred in 34 women.

424

They may lead to invasive interventions – scraping (D&C), biopsy (see Case IX-E-6), or even hysterectomy... especially among women over 35. Stirrat (1999) editorialized on the enormity of unexplained excessive vaginal bleeding (idiopathic menorrhagia). He observed, "There is probably no other disorder for which so many powerful drugs are prescribed or more invasive surgery undertaken."

Others have reported a significant increase of menstrual cramps among women consuming aspartame (Reschevsky 1986). In most instances, previous pain-free menstrual rhythms resumed after abstinence from aspartame products.

Representative Case Reports

Case IX-E-1

A 31-year-old purser complained primarily of frequent menstrual periods while consuming two cans of an ACB, two packets of an ATS, and two glasses of presweetened iced tea daily. There was concomitant depression and anxiety. She wrote, "My menstrual cycle occurred approximately every 14-21 days, rather than 28 days. Since I have stopped using ANY products containing aspartame, it has never failed to occur exactly every 28 days." The same alteration of menses occurred within two weeks after aspartame rechallenge.

Case IX-E-2

A 36-year-old Ph.D.-analyst described her major reaction to aspartame in these terms: "My periods were so heavy and erratic that I couldn't go out during that week. I have found this to be true with other friends. When they stopped taking aspartame, the symptoms went away." Additional evidences of aspartame disease were severe dizziness, "epilepsy-like fits without convulsions," extreme irritability, and "anxiety attacks."

Case IX-E-3

A 17-year-old student described "severe menstrual bleeding" as her only overt reaction to aspartame sodas. She added, "If I accidentally drink aspartame, I start severe bleeding."

Her mother and father experienced aspartame reactions primarily manifest as "a scratchy feeling in the throat and coughing."

Case IX-E-4

A 29-year-old speech pathologist noted "mid-period spotting" while consuming two bottles of an ACB and five sticks of "sugarless bubble gum" daily. This problem ceased within several weeks after stopping aspartame products. No abnormality could be found by her physicians. Mid-period spotting recurred when she drank the ACB four months later.

Case IX-E-5

A 51-year-old housewife complained of "continuous periods." Other symptoms attributed to aspartame included severe headache, dizziness, palpitations, insomnia, marked memory loss, intense depression and anxiety attacks. She wrote, "After quitting all foods sweetened with aspartame, my periods became normal again within a few weeks."

Case IX-E-6

A 49-year-old athlete had excessive menstrual bleeding about every two weeks one summer. It began several weeks after drinking considerable aspartame-sweetened iced tea and diet drinks. She also developed severe hives. These problems disappeared during the winter.

Both conditions recurred the following August when she again consumed more aspartame. A uterine biopsy proved normal. On learning that other women had attributed menstrual problems to aspartame, she discontinued such products with ensuing normalization of her periods

B. Diminished or Absent Menses

The menses diminished dramatically, or stopped, in 42 aspartame reactors. Instances of absent menses are also described elsewhere (see Case III-15).

Others encountered this problem. A nutritionist in Silver Springs (Maryland) told me of three patients, ages 18 to 21, who lost their periods after consuming considerable aspartame. One recycled in six months, but the others still had not.

This phenomenon reflects in part the stimulation of pituitary prolactin (Chapter XXIV).

426

Representative Case Reports

Case IX-E-8

A 45-year-old interior designer had no menstrual periods two weeks after beginning to consume "diet food meals" and four cans of an ACB daily. She also complained of abdominal bloat. Concomitantly, her two teenage daughters stopped menstruating. When aspartame was suspected as the cause, normal menses resumed in all three women within one month after stopping these products.

Case IX-E-9

A 39-year-old woman had regular periods until she drank an eight-pack of aspartame cola (each containing 16 oz) over three days. Her period was delayed three weeks for the first time. The menses normalized when she switched back to a regular cola beverage. A similar menstrual irregularity occurred several months later when she retested herself with the diet cola.

Case IX-E-10

A 43-year-old woman experienced cessation of her menses as the apparent sole reaction to aspartame beverages. It occurred two months after drinking up to six cans of diet drinks daily.

Case IX-E-11

A 26-year-old woman consumed one can of an aspartame soda and one packet of an ATS daily for several months. Her previously-normal periods stopped. She also suffered severe bloat, headache, dizziness, marked depression, irritability, personality changes, and frequent urination at night.

Case IX-E-12

A 30-year-old housewife had been drinking six glasses of aspartame-sweetened tea daily when she experienced decreased vision with pain in both eyes, severe headache, dizziness and intense thirst. The change in her periods, however, was most bothersome.

> "My menstrual cycle was disrupted and my gynecologist could
> find no reason for this. I stopped using the iced-tea product and
> my cycle became normal. The severe headaches also ceased.
> I tried the product again, and these symptoms recurred."

Case IX-E-13

A 34-year-old teacher lost her periods after consuming two cans of an ACB and aspartame hot chocolate daily for two months. She complained of abdominal bloat, decreased vision in both eyes, recent "dry eyes," sensitivity to noise in one ear, headaches, severe dizziness, unsteadiness of the legs, insomnia, mental confusion, marked memory loss, depression with suicidal thoughts, extreme irritability, anxiety with aggravated phobias, personality changes, swelling of the legs, intense thirst, joint stiffness, and a gain of 15 pounds. She neither smoked nor drank alcohol. Her prior medical background was not remarkable aside from being slightly overweight.

Her menstrual periods returned after discontinuing aspartame products. Concomitantly, the other complaints subsided. When she resumed these beverages the following year during hot weather, her periods again disappeared. They had not returned 1-1/2 years later.

Case IX-E-14

A 35-year old businesswoman lost her menstrual periods approximately six months prior to contacting me. In addition, "my hair suddenly and rapidly began turning gray and thinning." Other problems were severe confusion, memory loss, marked irritability, fluid retention, weight gain and depression. These features improved after discontinuing her daily intake (two liters) of an aspartame soda.

Case IX-E-15

An aspartame reactor summarized her menstrual problem as follows:

> "I developed a strange illness about two years ago. Although it seemed related to my menstrual cycle, and the symptoms suggested endometriosis, endometriosis could not be found. I used to drink a lot of diet drinks. When I quit taking any aspartame for two weeks, I had my first real period in two years!"

Case IX-E-16

A 19-year-old woman developed anorexia at the age of 12 after she began drinking diet cola. Her menses ceased thereafter. Her physician prescribed Provera – initially as pills,

428

and subsequently by injection. The patient then decided to avoid all aspartame products. She wrote, "Remarkably enough, after one week without aspartame, I discovered my amenorrhea was suddenly 'cured.' "

2. DECREASED SEXUALITY; INFERTILITY

Decreased Libido and Impotence

Many possible causes for these problems are recognized. Nevertheless, I was impressed when such concerns were volunteered by astute aspartame reactors, both male and female, in whom no gross psychological affliction was apparent.

Decreased sexuality also occurred in the wake of debilitating aspartame-associated complaints, especially severe depression and headache. For example, both spouses in one marriage had severe aspartame reactions. The wife stated, "I am so sick from headache that my mate and I have had no sex life at all." Similar information surfaced in replies to the survey questionnaire (Section 4), generally in the portion dealing with the personal impact of aspartame disease.

The travesty of ascribing decreased sexuality in older male aspartame reactors to "the normal aging process" will be discussed in Chapter XV.

> Barbara Mullarkey (*Wednesday Journal of Oak Park & River Forest* March 26, 1986, p. 37) described a 75-year-old California physician who substituted an ATS for sugar when diabetes was suspected. He had enjoyed regular sexual activity until then. Within ten days, he experienced "a complete and total loss of libido." His prior sex life returned within six weeks after avoiding aspartame.

An article in the August 1999 issue of *New Woman* Magazine asserted that aspartame can be an aphrodisiac. While this alleged property was attributed to phenylethylamine (PEA), PEA is a minor pathway of phenylalanine metabolism in normal human subjects (Stegink 1984, p. 81).

Infertility

The issue of aspartame-associated infertility was initially minimized. This attitude had to be revised in the face of striking evidence thereof -- most notably, pregnancy among previously infertile couples in whom at least one spouse had aspartame disease. For example, a female aspartame reactor had been unable to conceive for ten years while drinking diet colas. After avoiding all aspartame products, she became pregnant and gave birth to a healthy boy.

The matter of <u>aspartame-induced premature menopause</u> also was raised.

> A 31-year-old woman had been on a fertility program for considerable time without success. She consumed 2-3 liters of diet sodas daily for over eight years. When increased doses of fertility drugs proved ineffective, coupled with a high FSH level, the diagnosis of "early menopause" was made.

The concept that aspartame constitutes an "endocrine disrupting chemical" was mentioned earlier. Some suspect that aspartame has contributed to the continuing decline of sperm counts over the past two decades. The observation of testicular atrophy among animals in the Bressler Report (Chapter XXVII) is relevant.

3. HYPOTHYROIDISM; THYROIDITIS

Persons with hypothyroidism are "sticking out their necks" – an expression used by Mary Shoman (2000) – in consuming aspartame owing to their greater vulnerability to its adverse effects.

Triiodothyronine and thyroxine are the two most active thyroid hormones. Since they derive from tyrosine, a link to phenylalanine (Chapter XXII) exists.

Hypothyroidism, whether spontaneous or due to previous thyroid surgery, was known to exist in scores of aspartame reactors. This was the case for 22 who completed the initial survey questionnaire (Section 4). The association is significant for several reasons.

- <u>Thyroid disease occurs with greater frequency among patients having diabetes and reactive hypoglycemia</u> (Roberts 1969a, 1971b), who routinely are advised to avoid sugar.
- <u>The effects of drugs and chemicals tend to be greater and more prolonged among hypothyroid individuals</u> (Chapter VIII).

- Any interference by aspartame with thyroid production, release or action during pregnancy and early infancy could have drastic consequences. Hypothyroidism early in life can severely retard growth and mental development (Sokoloff 1967).

- The intellectual deterioration of persons with unrecognized hypothyroidism can be devastating. For example, Case VI-L-2, an 18-year-old college student with previously undiagnosed hypothyroidism, evidenced profound intellectual deterioration, narcolepsy, headache, and severe reactive hypoglycemia after using aspartame products. Several maternal relatives had a goiter. The diagnosis of hypothyroidism had been overlooked prior to my consultation, as indicated by markedly elevated thyroid stimulating hormone (TSH) levels. Her response to aspartame abstinence, an appropriate diet, and replacement thyroid hormone was gratifying.

- Less replacement thyroid may be required when aspartame products are avoided. For example, a male aspartame reactor had longstanding treated hypothyroidism. After stopping aspartame products, he noted, "My replacement thyroid dose, which had been steadily increasing the last few years, dropped by 30 percent. My doctor was quite surprised, and had no other explanation for it."

Aspartame disease might cause or contribute to thyroiditis, an inflammation of the thyroid gland (see Case IX-E-16). This possibility was raised in a 43-year-old female aspartame reactor who experienced severe pain on swallowing after consuming aspartame, followed by transient thyroid overactivity.

Thyroiditis is commonly considered an autoimmune phenomenon. Several reports are germane.

- The sustained immunologic challenge from chronic methanol intake, with the release of antigenic formaldehyde (Thrasher 1988), is reviewed in Chapters VIII and XXI.

- Fudenberg and Singh (1988) reported diminished thyroid function, antibodies to thyroid constituents, and T-lymphocyte dysfunction in a majority of patients whose headache and aberrant cognition were triggered or exacerbated by chemical stress.

Representative Case Reports

Case IX-E-15

A 39-year-old clerk became severely incapacitated because of impaired vision. She had developed a cataract at the age of 36, requiring removal of the lens in one eye. Other complaints included ringing in one ear, severe headache, dizziness, insomnia, confusion, marked memory loss, numbness of the upper extremities, depression, anxiety attacks, phobias, palpitations, unexplained chest pain, a recent rise of blood pressure, marked swelling of the legs, recurrent hypoglycemia attacks, and a gain of 50 pounds. She had used considerable aspartame sodas and a tabletop sweetener for over a decade.

Replacement thyroid was prescribed for hypothyroidism at the age of 33. She subsequently became aware of the probable association of many symptoms with aspartame use.

> "Since discontinuing use of aspartame, I have had less water retention, less craving for sweets, <u>no</u> palpitations (I used to have them at least every other day), no hypoglycemia episodes, no lightheadedness, no dizziness, and my memory and thought processes seem sharper. I was a real basket case."

Case IX-E-16

A 40-year-old female physician developed severe optic neuritis with marked loss of vision, headache, decreased menses, and memory loss after drinking one liter of aspartame soft drinks daily for eight years. She also evidenced Hashimoto thyroiditis – with a TSH level of 29 (normal up to 5), and a high titer of antinuclear antibodies (ANA). Most of her symptoms improved after stopping aspartame products, coupled with normalization of the ANA titer.

4. HYPERTHYROIDISM (GRAVES DISEASE); PSEUDOHYPERTHYROIDISM

Six persons with aspartame disease developed <u>hyperthyroidism</u> (Graves disease; "overactive thyroid"), an unexpected association reported earlier (Roberts 1997). Indeed, persons who use considerable aspartame are literally "sticking out their necks" (see above) because of the potential for developing an overactive goiter.

- Through serendipity, I encountered two biologically unrelated step-sisters who suffered severe aspartame disease, and then developed Graves disease.

- Five persons contacted the Aspartame Consumer Safety Network after concluding that the use of these products contributed to the onset of Graves disease (personal communication, November 1991).

Comparable complaints occurred in four additional *patients with previously treated Graves disease* who suffered from aspartame disease.

Two points are stressed. First, *physicians should interrogate patients with recent Graves disease about aspartame consumption*. If being used, these individuals ought to be observed for a possible spontaneous remission after stopping aspartame before definitive interventions (radioiodine treatment; surgery) are recommended (see Cases IX-E-17 to 22).

Second, *unexplained palpitations, tachycardia, "anxiety attacks," headache, weight loss, hypertension, and other features occurring in patients with prior Graves disease warrant* specific *inquiry about aspartame use when the diagnosis of recurrent hyperthyroidism is entertained* (see Cases IX-E-22 to 26).

Representative Case Reports

Case IX-E-17

A 34-year-old university professor (environmental studies) developed classic primary hyperthyroidism after using considerable amounts of products containing aspartame – specifically, 4-5 cans of a diet soda daily, four liters of a diet cola weekly, 3-4 servings of diet ice cream a day, and other products (gelatin; gum; breath mints). Such consumption for attaining "the mean fit look" also reflected her added capacity as a supervisor of aerobics classes. She had enjoyed excellent health until then.

The patient suffered severe sweats and attacks of sinus tachycardia (up to 180 beats per minute). Other suggestive aspartame-related features included recent headaches, bilateral decreased vision, dry eyes, tinnitus, severe dizziness, tremors, "numbness and shooting pains in the arms and legs," confusion and memory loss, slurred speech, extreme swings in mood (including thoughts of suicide never experienced previously), personality changes (almost to the point of leaving her husband and children), a paradoxic gain of weight despite her physical activity, itching, abdominal pain, thinning of the hair, menstrual problems, and swelling of the lips, tongue and eyes. She then evidenced a goiter clinically.

She had been adopted by a couple unrelated to her parents. Her biological mother was diabetic.

The patient received propranolol and propylthiouracil. Radioiodine therapy was then recommended because hyperthyroidism persisted. Inasmuch as no search for "an environmental trigger" had been attempted, this keen educator opted for a delay in order to review the events preceding her illness. She regarded a doctor's suggestion that her condition had been caused largely by stress as "a copout."

The only plausible pertinent factor was the use of considerable aspartame. Her extreme fatigue, headache, swelling of the eyes, depression, tachycardia and several other symptoms abated within several days after abstaining from these products. Her thyroid studies progressively improved, and normalized within three months.

An "accidental retest" from drinking aspartame-sweetened tea promptly precipitated most of her symptoms. There was no recurrence over the ensuing two years notwithstanding the cessation of all medication, continuing a full academic teaching schedule and aerobics instruction, and rearing three children.

Case IX-E-18

This 39-year-old woman developed Graves disease subsequent to that of her step-sister (Case IX-E-17). She was an insulin-dependent diabetic who began using aspartame products to avoid sugar. Shortly thereafter, her blood glucose concentrations became highly erratic, coupled with loss of urinary bladder control that was ascribed to diabetic neuropathy.

The patient sought advice from her step-sister when the diagnosis of hyperthyroidism was made. A comparable clinical remission ensued after abstaining from aspartame products, along with striking improvement of her diabetes control and bladder function. These observations are consistent with my repeated experience that aspartame products can cause loss of diabetes control, and aggravate or simulate diabetic retinopathy and neuropathy (Chapter XIII).

Case IX-E-19

A 43-year-old woman began ingesting two cans of diet cola, one liter of another aspartame soda, one glass of a dietetic mix, and one serving of aspartame gelatin daily. She did so for two years to avoid sugar because of noninsulin-dependent diabetes. Multiple symptoms five months later resulted in the loss of her job. They included palpitations, tachycardia, unexplained chest pains, severe headache, dizziness, two grand mal seizures, paresthesias, slurred speech, "anxiety attacks," swelling of the tongue, and painful swallowing. The diagnosis of Graves disease was subsequently made.

The patient then chanced to read an article citing comparable complaints in persons having reactions to aspartame products. Her symptoms improved within weeks after avoiding them, and then disappeared. They recurred one month after resuming aspartame, coupled with neck discomfort and difficult swallowing (dysphagia) attributed by her doctor to "an overactive thyroid."

Case IX-E-20

A 54-year-old woman consumed increasing amounts of aspartame products, including 15 packets of a tabletop sweetener in hot drinks daily. She had been energetic until her health "mysteriously deteriorated with a bewildering number of symptoms so varied and strange that it didn't make sense." She did not smoke or drink alcohol.

A diagnosis of Graves disease was made. She received methimazole and propranolol, with improvement of her tachycardia.

The patient's other symptoms during the previous year included fatigue, anxiety, headache, "fuzzy mind," depression, recurring abdominal pain, tinnitus and insomnia. She initially gained weight despite "light eating habits" until losing it once the hyperthyroidism became overt.

The contributory role of aspartame products was suspected by her daughter who had rarely used aspartame products. She stayed with the patient for four days at the onset of treatment for Graves disease. After adding the tabletop sweetener and drinking diet colas, the daughter experienced "extreme irritability which felt totally irrational and uncontrollable," depression, tremors, panic attacks and difficult breathing. These symptoms disappeared when she returned to her own home – only to recur shortly after purchasing the tabletop sweetener. "Then it clicked." She and her mother promptly improved after abstaining from aspartame products.

Case IX-E-21

A Belgium correspondent with typical Graves disease became asymptomatic within two months after avoiding aspartame products. She had been "stubborn enough to convince my doctors to wait for some months" before instituting treatment after she made "the aspartame connection." By nine months, her tests had totally normalized without further intervention.

Case IX-E-22

A nurse drank as many as three 2-liter bottles of diet cola daily for several years. Hyperthyroidism was diagnosed, and she received two courses of radioiodine treatment. Her symptoms persisted, however. They included depression, headache, joint pains and "fibromyalgia." Her sister (a registered nurse) then informed her about aspartame disease when she also developed anxiety, tachycardia and suicidal thoughts. These promptly regressed after abstaining from aspartame.

Case IX-E-23

A 44-year-old executive developed headache, blurred vision in both eyes, and irritability ("being short with my staff and clients.") These complaints began six months after consuming 2-3 cans of diet soda and chewing five sticks of aspartame gum daily. They abated after he avoided such products, only to recur on eight separate challenges. A subtotal thyroidectomy for Graves disease had been done in 1963.

Case IX-E-24

A 49-year-old realtor had been treated for Graves disease five years previously. She experienced palpitations, severe dizziness, intense nausea, and an unexplained rise of blood pressure after ingesting three cans of diet cola and other aspartame products daily. Her symptoms disappeared within one month after stopping them. They promptly recurred on three separate challenges.

Case IX-E-25

A 43-year-old nutritionist had been treated for Graves disease 20 years previously. She developed severe depression and visual problems within two weeks after consuming 8-10 glasses of an aspartame soda daily. These complaints disappeared within two days after avoiding the beverage. She refused to ingest it again on a trial basis.

Case IX-E-26

A 59-year-old writer had undergone two partial thyroidectomies for Graves disease three decades previously, and then received radioiodine therapy. She suffered severe headaches, abdominal pain, bloat and diarrhea after beginning to ingest diet colas, a tabletop sweetener (5-6 packets daily), and other aspartame products. Her complaints subsided within two days after avoiding them, only to recur within 30 minutes on two challenges.

436

<u>Commentary</u>

The possibility of spontaneous remission in patients with Graves disease always must be considered when evaluating the clinical course and therapeutic response. This appeared unlikely in the present context, however, because of the prompt and dramatic improvement following cessation of aspartame products, and the <u>predictable</u> precipitation of symptoms on rechallenge. The concomitant subsidence of other aspartame-induced symptoms is noteworthy.

The occurrence of Graves disease in these patients while consuming aspartame products is explainable by the cumulative effect of several factors. They include (a) voluntary severe caloric restriction, (b) increased energy demands relating to excessive exercise and other physical activity, and (c) metabolic derangements caused by aspartame and its metabolites. The latter involve changes in satiety, neurotransmitter dysfunction, alterations of hormonal homeostasis (insulin; growth hormone; glucagon; cholecystokinin) by the amino acid components of aspartame and their stereoisomers (Chapter XXIII and XXIV), and the effects of <u>free</u> methanol, a metabolic poison (Chapter XXI). The author previously emphasized the precipitation of Graves disease and thyroiditis following voluntary severe caloric restriction (Roberts 1969, 1985), especially with increased physical activity.

The vulnerability of two step-sisters to hyperthyroidism (Cases IX-E-17 and E-18) may have been influenced by their family and past history of diabetes mellitus. Diabetics are known to have an increased tendency to develop thyropathies. Describing conjugal Graves disease, Ebner et al (1992) commented, "It is possible that the phenotype for Graves disease is expressed only in the presence of a critical combination of genetic and environmental factors."

5. BREAST TENDERNESS (GYNECOMASTIA)

Several women experienced tenderness in one or both breasts following the ingestion of aspartame products. It subsided when they were avoided. An estrogenic influence, comparable to that causing excessive menstrual bleeding (see above), is probably operative.

Inasmuch as aspartame was designed as a drug, it is pertinent that at least 34 drugs can cause breast enlargement.

6. HYPERPARATHYROIDISM

The finding of elevated parathyroid concentrations in two aspartame reactors was unexpected. The binding of aspartame to calcium-ion receptors, discussed in Chapter IX-G, suggests one plausible mechanism.

Persons consuming considerable aspartame sodas also risk the calcium-depleting influence of the considerable phosphoric acid in an acid medium therein through impairment of calcium absorption. Moreover, the increased excretion of urinary calcium after aspartame intake, associated with a rise of blood calcium (Nguyen 1998), may be triggered by phosphate activation from its amino acids.

Representative Case Reports

Case IX-E-27

A 51-year-old woman sought consultation for persistent cramps in the legs and back spasms. She had been on Synthroid (0.075 mg daily) for spontaneous hypothyroidism, and Premarin (0.3 mg daily) for menopausal symptoms. Other complaints included confusion, memory loss, disequilibrium, depression, awakening with shortness of breath, and fluid retention. The physical examination was not remarkable except for a blood pressure of 160/92. Her parathyroid hormone assay (rechecked), performed because of a marginally elevated blood calcium level, was elevated at 491 (normal 0-340).

The patient related her problems caused by the use of aspartame, and stopped such products. There was virtual complete relief from her symptoms within one week! The blood pressure declined to 140/90. Her parathyroid hormone level normalized at 49.

The clinical improvement continued when next seen in February 1986. In the interim, her hair had grown back and the "eyebrows are full." Her blood pressure was now 130/84. A repeat parathyroid hormone level in June 1986 was normal. She remained well, and was playing tennis when next seen two years later.

Case IX-E-28

A 53-year-old woman (FDA Project #2964) consumed two cans of aspartame sodas and four packets of an ATS for 3-1/2 years. She experienced depression, severe fatigue (no longer having the energy to play golf and tennis), memory loss, hair loss, "spasms in the chest," insomnia, elevation of blood pressure (175/105), headache, impaired speech, esophageal spasms, nausea, lethargy, dizziness, bloat, a facial eruption, considerable gain in weight, and possible seizures.

The patient was found to have elevated concentrations of <u>both</u> thyroid and parathyroid hormones. Her symptoms promptly improved one week after stopping all aspartame products. The blood pressure and hormone levels subsequently normalized.

F. FLUID DISTURBANCES

Many aspartame reactors complained of intense thirst, dry mouth, fluid retention, and urinary difficulties. Identifying aspartame products as a prime contributory factor not only afforded them prompt relief, but also obviated interventions with inherent risk and considerable cost.

1. INCREASED THIRST AND DRY MOUTH

Intense thirst in the absence of marked sweating or hot weather was experienced by 126 (11 percent) aspartame reactors. Many complained of concomitant "dry mouth" (Chapter IX-D) or a nonspecific "sore throat." One perceptive engineer-patient volunteered that "aspartame seems to create thirst, not quench it." A possible clue to the intense thirst generated by aspartame products is the oft-observed habit of carrying bottled water in public.

Two aspartame reactors who complained of "thick saliva" also developed parotid gland enlargement or tenderness (Roberts 1993c).

Weiffenback et al (1987) demonstrated that taste impairment is not a necessary consequence of salivary gland dysfunction among patients with "dry mouth" caused by the absence of saliva. Accordingly, such individuals may come to prefer the taste of aspartame in satisfying their chronic thirst... with perpetuation of the sicca (dry eye–dry mouth) syndrome (Chapter IV).

The intense thirst also may be mediated by aspartame–increased production of endorphins (chemicals resembling morphine) within the brain.

Dry mouth (xerostomia) tends to be more severe among the elderly, and persons who have various disorders or take drugs that decrease salivary flow (Sreebry 1987). The ensuing complications include severe inflammation of the tongue, lips and mouth, superimposed yeast (Candida) infection, and problems related to impaired speech, taste, mastication and swallowing.

The dry mouth caused by aspartame can have devastating effects on the teeth, gums and nutrition, especially when superimposed on a similar side effect of the many drugs prescribed for older persons (Parker-Pope 2000). Inasmuch as saliva has potent antibacterial and antiviral properties, its reduction favors the overgrowth of organisms and accelerated dental decay.

The convincing basis for such an association is twofold: the gratifying and relatively prompt improvement of xerostomia following avoidance of aspartame products – usually within several days; and its recurrence shortly after resuming aspartame, even inadvertently.

Some experimental observations are pertinent. Matsuzawa and O'Hara (1984) found significant uptake of radioactivity in the salivary glands of adult rats within 30 minutes after administering a radioactive-carbon-labeled isotope. This finding is relevant to the swelling and irritation of the salivary and sublingual glands encountered in patients with aspartame disease (Chapter IX-D).

Representative Case Report

Case IX-F-1

A 34-year-old insurance agent indicated that her major reaction to aspartame products was severe and constant thirst. Other complaints included phobias, decreased hearing in both ears, and unexplained attacks of shortness of breath. She retested herself on four occasions, with recurrence of these symptoms in one day. Various studies, including a glucose tolerance test, were normal. She remained asymptomatic after avoiding aspartame products for one month.

Possible Insights Concerning the Sjögren Syndrome

Sjögren syndrome is characterized by reduced or absent secretions from the salivary and lacrimal (tear) glands. These individuals suffer dryness of the mouth and "dry eyes" (Chapter IV). The "lipstick-on-teeth" sign (that is, lipstick adhering to the upper front teeth) reflects a lack of saliva. An estimated two percent of the adult population has this disorder.

Large amounts of water are consumed by such persons in order to moisten their lips and mouth. When aspartame drinks are used, a vicious cycle can ensue.

Aspartame reactions might identify some persons who are prone to Sjögren's syndrome. This matter assumes added significance in light of evidence that up to one-fourth of patients manifest serious brain dysfunction (Alexander 1986). In this regard, a previous analysis of 39 aspartame reactors with "dry eyes" who completed the initial questionnaire revealed that 15 experienced intense thirst, 11 had mental confusion, 22 complained of marked memory loss, and 20 had severe depression.

2. FLUID RETENTION; "BLOAT"

Aspartame reactors evidenced disturbances of water metabolism in ways other than increased thirst. In this series, 100 (11 percent) complained of marked "bloat" (Chapter IX-D), 143 (12.5 percent) swelling (edema) of the lower limbs, and 126 (11 percent) increased frequency of urine.

Women with reactive hypoglycemia who are subject to premenstrual fluid retention (the premenstrual syndrome; PMS) seem more vulnerable to these features of aspartame disease. They frequently experienced severe tension, depression, headache and behavioral changes while consuming aspartame. The psychological impact of edema occasionally was profound.

- Case VI-14, a 39-year-old woman with reactive hypoglycemia and migraine, developed marked swelling of the legs and a severe polyneuropathy as a result of "addiction" to an ACB. She complained, "I take great pride in my appearance. I had great legs. Now I look like hell and am out of tone."

- An aspartame reactor wrote

  "I used to get swollen legs at work after drinking diet pop. I stopped drinking it even though the doctor said it was PMS. Since then, I have avoided aspartame, and no longer have a problem."

Persons who ingest considerable aspartame also may develop a craving for salt. Their greater sodium intake, in conjunction with marked thirst, contributes to fluid retention, excessive urine volume, and possibly hypertension (Chapter IX-C).

Representative Case Reports

Case IX-F-2

A female executive wrote

> "The worst thing I noticed was that I was bloated all of the time, especially at night when I awoke and would have to make six trips to the bathroom. I went to doctors several times to see if I had a bladder infection, but they did not diagnose anything.
>
> "Why do I blame aspartame? Because I only really drink diet drinks in the summer, and the symptoms disappear when I stop drinking them. I have not touched any for about three weeks and I feel great. The bloating is gone, and I have lost three pounds without starving myself."

Case IX-F-3

A secretary began consuming aspartame sodas when they became available in 1983. Her legs then swelled by as much as three inches (!) at the calves, with associated pain. She also "got a lot of kidney infections." Medical evaluation, however, failed to reveal evidence for a renal-tract infection or other disorder.

A friend subsequently told her that "aspartame can cause swelling." Her symptoms disappeared after avoiding it.

Case IX-F-4

A 46-year-old woman focused chiefly on her abdominal distress. In four trials, it predictably recurred within one day after ingesting aspartame beverages. She wrote, "When I drink two glasses of diet drinks, I feel bloated and have diarrhea the next day." These symptoms also recurred whenever she drank a product not suspected of containing aspartame.

Related Physiologic Considerations

Aspartame can alter water metabolism through several possible mechanisms.

442

- Excessive fluid intake due to intense thirst (see above).
- Altered neurotransmitter physiology in the brain and hypothalamus (Chapter XXIII) influencing thirst and water metabolism.
- Effects on insulin and carbohydrate metabolism (Chapters XIII and XIV). It is known that excess insulin ("the hyperinsulinized state") and hypoglycemia favor the migration of both water and sodium into cells (Yannet 1939; Roberts 1964a,b, 1965a, 1966b). As a case in point, fluid retention – including facial edema, dependent edema, and pulmonary edema – has occurred shortly after diabetic patients first receive insulin (Shaper 1966).
- Aspartame-associated weight loss (see above). Wolff (1959) emphasized that homeostatic reactions to starvation involve not only fat and carbohydrate metabolism, but also the renal control of water and electrolytes.
- Reversal of the normal diurnal pattern of urine volume (see below) in patients with diabetogenic hyperinsulinism (Roberts 1964, 1966b, 1967d).
- Increased or inappropriate antidiuretic hormone activity. Mandell et al (1966a) demonstrated an antidiuretic hormone-like effect shortly after the onset of REM sleep. This could reinforce the tendency to edema, especially in persons with narcolepsy (Chapter VI-K) wherein prompt REM activity during sleep is characteristic.
- The metabolic disturbances associated with severe depression, a prominent feature in many patients with aspartame disease (Chapter VII-B). Shaw and Coppen (1966) investigated the distribution of water and potassium in depressive illness. They reported a relative deficiency of total body potassium, a low concentration of intracellular potassium, and a relative increase of intracellular water.

3. URINARY COMPLAINTS

This section is properly preambled with the premise that frequent urination, coupled with intense thirst, may represent "the wisdom of the body" in attempting to rid itself of poisons and potential carcinogens (Michaud 1999).

Many callers asked about urinary bladder problems during talk-show interviews.

Frequency

In this series, 126 aspartame reactors (11 percent), both male and female, complained of increased frequency of urination during the day, the night, or both.

The prodigious consumption of diet drinks, especially those containing caffeine (a diuretic), accounts in part for their large volumes of urine, as well as fluid retention. Additionally, amino acids and a high-protein diet increase renal blood flow and the glomerular filtration rate through several mechanisms (Klahr 1988).

Urgency and Bed-Wetting

Children and adults with aspartame disease have suffered extreme urgency and bed-wetting specifically related to use of these products. A popular columnist relayed such an experience in the case of a husband whose problem with urgency promptly stopped after avoiding diet sodas (Ann Landers, *Los Angeles Times* May 15, 2000).

Severe Burning on Voiding

Other persons experienced recurrent severe burning on voiding (dysuria) while consuming aspartame products. This symptom may reflect irritation of the urinary bladder and urethra by aspartame or its breakdown products.

- The D-forms of aspartic acid and phenylalanine are poorly metabolized in the body, at least half being excreted in the urine (Dr. Jeffrey Bada, personal communication, March 1988). The associated markedly acidic urine also might cause discomfort.
- The loss of lubricating secretions in the urethra among aspartame reactors – akin to "dry eyes" (Chapter IV) and "dry mouth" (Chapter IX-D) – could be another basis for symptoms on urinating.

The relationship of these complaints to aspartame use was established by their subsidence when these products were stopped, and recurrence after resuming aspartame. For example, Case IX-F-6 promptly developed marked frequency of urination and bladder discomfort after rechallenging herself three times.

Representative Case Reports

Case IX-F-6

A 40-year-old nuclear medicine technologist suffered marked frequency of urine during the day, and had to void up to four times at night. On one occasion, she became incontinent of urine during sleep. Other symptoms included marked thirst, severe depression, and "a general feeling of ill health." She was seen by three physicians and consultants. "Enlarged red blood cells" were found.

444

This patient had been consuming diet colas and sodas, and up to ten packets of an ATS daily. She deduced an association with aspartame because these symptoms regressed within three days after stopping such products. When she retested herself on three separate occasions, the complaints returned within "several hours to overnight" – even with a single diet soda or one packet of the ATS. She wrote

> "If I hadn't stopped using aspartame with benefit, my next referral was to a urologist for urethral dilation, as suggested by my gynecologist. Fortunately, I noticed a severe increase in symptoms after two cans of diet soda, and began to research it on my own."

Case IX-F-7

A 31-year-old sales representative drank two cans of a diet cola daily. Her primary symptoms were intense frequency and pain on urination at night, which disappeared after avoiding aspartame. They predictably recurred within five days whenever she retested herself.

Case IX-F-8

A 62-year-old construction foreman noted marked "burning of the urine" and a headache after ingesting one can of diet cola daily. A urologist recommended prostate surgery. Both symptoms disappeared as soon as he discontinued this product, and had not recurred after five months observation.

Case IX-F-9

A 64-year-old woman required several doses of insulin daily to control her diabetes. She fared relatively well until the summer of 1986 when she increased her intake of aspartame soft drinks and tea to ten glasses a day. Severe "burning," frequency of urination, and poorer diabetic control ensued. Her blood sugar levels (monitored by home testing) continued to rise even after the insulin dosage was increased. She also experienced visual difficulty (initially thought to represent a complicating retinopathy), leg cramps and depression.

The urinary symptoms and other complaints subsided within several days after stopping aspartame. Concomitantly, her blood sugar concentrations declined, enabling a reduction of insulin.

Case IX-F-10

A 53-year-old printer suffered "almost instantaneous" severe lightheadedness and pains in the face, abdomen and chest when he drank small amounts of a diet cola. He volunteered, "I urinate a lot also."

Case IX-F-11

A woman with severe aspartame disease had a urethroplasty performed for urinary bladder complaints. Her "bladder burning" and other symptoms disappeared when she stopped drinking diet colas.

Case IX-F-12

A woman suffered from "interstitial cystitis." Her symptoms promptly subsided after avoiding aspartame products. She added that her daughter also experienced a "hyper attack" of bladder irritation, and "couldn't stop urinating" until aspartame was avoided.

Commentary

Various underlying or associated problems have to be considered as the cause of urinary complaints in these patients. They include

- High permeability of the urinary bladder epitheliuim to urine components, leading to the infiltration of T cells, B cells, plasma cells, neutrophils, and mast cells
- Infection (bacterial, fungal) of the urinary tract or prostate (see Cases IX-H-2 and IX-H-3)
- Impaired function of the urinary bladder with diabetic neuropathy or stroke
- Greater urinary output due to increased fluid retention (see above)
- Increased urine volume associated with aggravated diabetes (Chapter XIII), as in Case IX-F-9

Some of the mechanisms for more frequent and greater urination were discussed in the preceding section. One is a reversed diurnal excretion of urine volume in patients with hypoglycemia (Roberts, 1964b, 1966b, 1967d), characterized by consistently greater 12-hour "night" volumes than 12-hour "day" volumes. This disorder reflects acquired disturbances involving the kidneys, hypothalamus, anterior pituitary and posterior pituitary. In most instances, the author could find no appreciable influence by daytime recumbency, cessation of smoking, ovariectomy, dietary modification, season of the year, or glucocorticoid administration.

Local reflex mechanisms within the mouth or oropharynx may contribute to aspartame diuresis. Their innervation involves visceral sensory afferent fibers of the trigeminal and glossopharyngeal nerves. The activation of oropharyngeal receptors by cold liquids has been shown to inhibit the release of vasopressin (antidiuretic hormone) independent of osmotic or gastric factors (Salata 1987).

G. JOINT AND MUSCLE COMPLAINTS

Joint discomfort (arthralgia; arthropathy) and aching of the muscles and ligaments are prevalent in the general population, along with several major forms of arthritis (osteoarthritis; rheumatoid arthritis; gout). They may be caused or aggravated by many influences. The use of aspartame products should be added to this list (Roberts 1991). I have repeatedly encountered professors of rheumatology who were totally unaware of aspartame disease.

The frequency and severity of otherwise-unexplained joint pain among 163 (14 percent) aspartame reactors in this series were impressive. Their considerable aspirin intake intensified other complaints attributable to aspartame disease – especially dizziness, ringing in the ears, and hearing loss. Gastric irritation (particularly severe bleeding) occurred when they resorted to ibuprofen and related non-steroidal anti-inflammatory drugs.

The subject of atypical pain in aspartame disease was considered in Chapter VI-H.

1. GENERAL CONSIDERATIONS

Magnitude of the Problem

The enormous medical and economic ramifications of these aspartame-induced problems can be inferred from the estimate that two-thirds of the adult population currently consumes products containing this chemical. These facts are germane.

- The extent of severe arthritic pain in the United States population generates a market for analgesics exceeding 10 billion dollars annually.

- The Centers for Disease Control reported a high incidence of "chronic joint symptoms" in seven states during 1996 (*Morbidity and Mortality Weekly Report* 1998; 47:345-351). Furthermore, a large portion of persons in whom a doctor had diagnosed "arthritis" did not know what type they had.

Age

The disappearance of joint pain and muscle discomfort came as a welcome surprise for "older" patients when they avoided aspartame products for other aspartame-induced problems. They had assumed that joint discomfort, stiffness of the hands and aching were part of the "aging process."

At the other end of the age spectrum, aspartame-induced arthritis and "palindromic rheumatism" can affect children.

> The mother of a 7-year-old girl with insulin-dependent diabetes joined a group of parents with children juvenile diabetes. After comparing notes, she wrote, "We noticed that a number complained of joint aches and pains. After stopping aspartame, their symptoms usually left."

Gender

The preponderance of women with aspartame disease in this series (Chapter II-H) is replicated in the FDA's data base. These observations are pertinent.

- A number of women indicated that their joint pains persisted longer than most other aspartame-related symptoms.
- Three reactors emphasized the virtual total disappearance of joint pain during subsequent pregnancy, a theme reminiscent of rheumatoid arthritis remissions while pregnant.

Related Diagnostic Considerations

The aggravation of longstanding arthritic problems from aspartame use was encountered. For example, a 51-year-old woman emphasized that her chronic hip pain (a) predictably intensified whenever she drank aspartame beverages, and (b) improved within three days after avoiding them.

448

There were many instances of "diagnosis by ordeal" from aspartame rechallenge.

> An aspartame reactor had been diagnosed as having "polyarthritis of unknown cause." She discovered that the use of aspartame caused her symptoms, especially when adding it to tea. She later rechallenged herself. "Twenty minutes after I took the first sip, the large vertebra at the base of my neck started zinging with pain." This also occurred when she inadvertently ate frozen yogurt containing aspartame.

The misdiagnosis of "seronegative rheumatoid arthritis" was made in several instances. Some aspartame victims with presumed rheumatoid arthritis received gold injections and even were subjected to surgery.

> A man underwent synovectomy of the right knee at the age of 31 because of marked joint swelling and difficulty in walking. He then received injections of a gold compound every other week. His aspartame intake included 6-8 diet colas and several packages of gum daily. Improvement was experienced after avoiding these products.

The misdiagnosis of gout had been made in young adults with aspartame disease. For example, a 26-year-old man consumed up to four cans of diet cola daily. He developed marked pain and swelling of a foot, which was diagnosed as gout. His problem persisted until he chanced to read about aspartame disease. All joint symptoms subsided within several weeks after discontinuing aspartame products, and did not recur.

The simulation or aggravation of systemic lupus erythematosus by aspartame disease was considered in Chapter VIII. Seven aspartame reactors among the most recent 649 persons in this series evidenced the typical facial rash in conjunction with joint pain. Several had high antinuclear antibody (ANA) titers.

> A correspondent experienced marked improvement of aspartame disease after avoiding these products. She volunteered that two women "addicted" to diet cola with whom she worked in an emergency room had elevated ANA levels. One was diagnosed as lupus erythematosus; the other suffered excruciating pain in her joints.

These observations offer intriguing insights concerning other rheumatologic disorders or diagnostic enigmas considered elsewhere. They include the Sjögren syndrome (Chapter IV), and the systemic symptoms in women with silicone breast implants (Chapter XXVII-F). Some of the underlying mechanisms will be discussed at the end of this section.

Recent erudite discussions of patients with severe arthritic complaints did not mention the possibility of aspartame disease as a primary or contributory cause. For example, the *Journal of the American Medical Association* (2000; 283:524) focused on a 55-year-old woman with rheumatoid arthritis receiving prednisone who had a poor response to oral and intramuscular gold, methotrexate, penicillamine, hydroxychloroquine sulfate, and cyclosporine. The aspartame issue seemed relevant in view of her history of insulin-dependent diabetes mellitus, the Sjögren syndrome, and "gastritis."

Corroboration By Non-Physicians

Callers to talk shows on which the author was being interviewed often emphasized joint pains and back discomfort while taking aspartame products.

- A young man indicated that he had suffered intense back pain for three years, especially on arising. No cause could be found. His pain totally subsided when he abstained from aspartame products. On joking that he do the indicated scientific experiment ("Why don't you see if resuming diet sodas will cause a recurrence of the back pain?"), he retorted, "I did... and the pain came back even worse!"
- A woman called about her 6-year-old niece. The girl suffered severe migrating joint pains that had been diagnosed as "palindromic rheumatism." Her discomfort disappeared shortly after aspartame products were discontinued.
- A male aspartame reactor experienced pain in the joints, headache, eye discomfort and impaired short term memory. These features ceased when he discontinued aspartame products, along with associated fatigue. He summarized his feelings on the matter: "The stuff was a nuisance and pain in the neck, literally."

A correspondent with visual problems had been treated with Precise Corneal Molding (PCM) by an ophthalmologist. This patient's symptoms improved after modifying his diet and avoiding aspartame sodas. As an aside, he wrote, "I also suggested to my wife that she quit diet drinks. She did so, and noticed that her joints no longer gave her pain."

450

Appreciation

The gratitude for relief of joint pain is illustrated by a 52-year-old woman who became pain-free after going "cold turkey" off diet sodas. An appointment with a rheumatologist had been scheduled. She wrote, "I now can open jars, grasp the handles on plastic grocery bags, and sleep through the night without waking up with frozen fingers which are extremely painful to straighten from their clenched position."

Patients with "miraculously cured arthritis" following the cessation of aspartame products volunteered in national and international efforts warning of aspartame disease (see Cases IX-G-11 and G-23).

Professional Skepticism

Most rheumatologists have categorically denied an association between these disorders and aspartame. Their reasons – as dissenting reviewers of manuscripts submitted to prominent journals – included "absence of controls," "failure to study subjects in a prospective double-blind fashion," and "lack of objective or quantifiable observations" (e.g., joint scans). Its ultimate validation resides in the subsidence of joint discomfort after stopping aspartame products, and prompt recurrence on their resumption... intentional or inadvertent.

2. "ARTHRITIS"

Inquiry about aspartame use is warranted in patients who present with unexplained joint pain or the exacerbation of conventional arthritic disorders. If this history is obtained, a brief trial of aspartame avoidance is warranted before ordering expensive studies, consultations and potent drugs. Prompt and persistent improvement, coupled with recurrence on aspartame rechallenge, needs no further justification for medical "doubting Thomases" by aspartame sufferees (see Case IX-G-16).

The reports of multiple aspartame reactors (see Case IX-G-15) highlighted the precipitation of similar rheumatic complaints by different aspartame products.

In view of the severe joint manifestations encountered in aspartame disease, considerable caution is urged about using aspartame products for the treatment of osteoarthritis, as recommended on the basis of a single case (Edmundson 1998).

Representative Case Reports

Case IX-G-1

A 55-year-old secretary developed "arthritis," aching of the legs, and other symptoms (memory loss, dizziness, depression) several days after drinking an aspartame tea mix. Her complaints subsided within one week after avoiding this product. She wrote

> "On August 8, my body ached from my toes to my neck. I felt as though I had arthritis in my whole body. It hurt to move an arm or even my hand. Since that time, I have not touched anything sweetened with aspartame, and have experienced no unusual aches, memory loss or dizziness."

Case IX-G-2

A 45-year-old telephone technician used two packets of an ATS daily for three weeks. He became markedly impaired during this time because of "severe joint irritation. I had less than 1/4 my normal strength." These complaints improved within one day after stopping the product. He retested himself on <u>three</u> occasions, each time suffering return of joint pain by the next day.

Case IX-G-3

This female aspartame reactor "began to have pains in all my joints resembling arthritis three months after beginning to drink diet colas." A trial of various medications by several consultants failed to provide relief. The role of aspartame beverages became suspect when her joint pains disappeared after avoiding them. She described these pains and associated eye symptoms in a letter to Senator Howard Metzenbaum supporting his proposed Aspartame Safety Act (Section 7).

Case IX-G-4

Richard J. Sabates, M.D., a 40-year-old physician (Board-certified in internal medicine), called to express thanks for my article on aspartame-induced joint pain published in the *Townsend Letter For Doctors* (Roberts 1991d). He had suffered prolonged severe aching of many joints, and underwent numerous studies by rheumatologists in Miami and elsewhere (including the Mayo Clinic) when no cause could be uncovered. His pains disappeared <u>within three days</u> after stopping aspartame products.

Dr. Sabates subsequently wrote a book titled, *The Preventive Diet*. The following excerpts from the first chapter (reproduced with permission of Dr. Sabates) are relevant.

452

"The pain continued to plague me. From my right shoulder, the pain shifted to my left shoulder. I had more x-rays, this time chest x-rays. I had more blood drawn, and again, all tests proved negative. I resigned myself to the possibility that I had some sort of hidden cancer. I remembered being depressed and not being able to concentrate on my work. I had to clap my hands in the morning just to get the feeling back. At that time, I thought my symptoms of depression were caused by my inability to cope with this terrible affliction. I had no idea that all my symptoms may have been the result of some illness.

"Eight months had passed since the start of my arthritis. My research uncovered an article in a publication call *The Townsend Letter*, written in May, 1991. I read an article titled, 'Joint Pains Associated with the Use of Aspartame,' written by H. J. Roberts, M.D., of West Palm Beach, Florida. In his introduction, he referred to the fact that his article had been turned down for publication in the *Journal of the American Medical Association*. With much interest but very little hope, I read Dr. Roberts describe 58 cases of multi-articular arthritis associated with the use of Aspartame (NutraSweet). All symptoms subsided after the patients discontinued using this artificial sweetener. The pain returned when he reintroduced Aspartame... I reread Dr. Roberts' article, and started to believe that maybe Aspartame could be the cause of my arthritis.

"I nearly fell off my chair when I read this. This must be it. Full of renewed hope, I stopped my daily yogurt and called Dr. Roberts in West Palm Beach. The doctor spoke to me at length and told me his frustrating story of trying to alert the community about the Aspartame problem he uncovered. He had tried to publish his article not only in JAMA, but also in three other publications Each turned him down.

"My improvement was a lot slower than I wished, but little by little the pains became less intense and I began to engage in all my previous normal physical activities. Small tasks such as combing my hair, and raising and lowering the glass of my car window to throw a coin in the Turnpike toll became very significant milestones in my life. Two months after... all my pains had disappeared, though I was still troubled by my left eye.

"I started my Aspartame-loaded diet as a test, consuming colas, yogurts, gelatins and ice creams. It was with a mixture of happiness and sadness that I woke up the very next day with the familiar throbbing pain, this time in my shoulder."

Case IX-G-5

A 59-year-old salesman experienced intense pain of both wrists and knees that could not be diagnosed. He wrote, "The wrist pain made even writing uncomfortable. A deep knee bend was a lesson in agony." He also developed severe blurring and decreased vision in the left eye (which two ophthalmologists could not explain), daily headache, dizziness and imbalance. The patient consumed three cans of diet soda and up to 6 packets of an ATS daily, along with aspartame breath mints. He chanced to read one of my publications on aspartame disease, and then avoided all aspartame products. After seven weeks, he was "ninety-seven percent pain free." The headache and dizziness also disappeared within two days. In addition, "After three weeks of not using aspartame, I have regained over sixty percent of the vision I had lost."

Case IX-G-6

A 62-year-old supervisor consumed up to eight packets of an ATS in coffee, one glass of an aspartame hot chocolate, and two servings of aspartame puddings or gelatin daily for four months. He stated, "<u>All</u> my joints ached <u>all</u> the time." Other complaints included "loss of vision" in one eye, sensitivity to noise in both ears, severe headache, marked drowsiness, tingling of the limbs, unexplained facial pains, extreme irritability, unexplained chest and abdominal pains, extreme irritability, unexplained chest and abdominal pains, and a weight gain of 30 pounds. These features subsided within five weeks after stopping aspartame. They recurred within eight hours on <u>two</u> retesting trials.

Case IX-G-7

A 78-year-old man had been treated since 1958 for hypertension, and reactive hypoglycemia associated with a prior gastrectomy. He presented on an emergency basis with severe pain in the right elbow. I suspected an attack of gout or local infection. The condition subsided within several days of conservative therapy. His fasting blood sugar was

156 mg% on August 3, 1987, and 146 mg % on August 10, 1987. A midafternoon blood glucose concentration, however, was only 65 mg %. The uric acid, sedimentation rate, and studies for rheumatoid arthritis were normal.

The patient was asked about aspartame use. He stated that he began drinking large amounts of diet root beer and cola recently. These were discontinued, and replaced by interval snacks. There had been no recurrence when seen three months later. A repeat fasting blood sugar in one week was 118 mg %.

Cases IX-G-8 and IX-G-9

A 29-year-old research chemist returned to England after having worked three years in Switzerland. She resumed drinking two diet sodas daily. (These products had not been readily available in Switzerland.) She developed severe pain in the joints requiring anti-inflammatory medication. Other complaints included migraine headaches, flushing of the face, indigestion, mental confusion, and marked fatigue. Chancing to read about aspartame disease, she stopped these products. Within a week, her knee joints and back were much improved. The headaches, "hot flashes" and red face also left, and her energy felt restored.

Mentioning this experience at her physician's office, the nurse indicated that she had had "the same problems with aspartame – and then with MSG." Although diagnosed as rheumatoid arthritis, the nurse found aspartame to be the culprit when she went on an exclusion diet. The chemist added, "Now she has all movement and no pain anymore in her joints."

Case IX-G-10

A 50-year-old woman developed severe "arthritis" while drinking two liters of diet cola daily, along with other aspartame products. Her joint pain and extreme weakness reached the point where "I had to hold a cup of coffee with both hands. I couldn't open a car door from the inside, and I had to crawl up our stairs to use the bathroom because my legs were too weak." Other prominent symptoms included extreme cold intolerance and severe weight loss. There was loss of joint discomfort and a remarkable regain of strength when she stopped all aspartame products.

Case IX-G-11

A 41-year-old mother of three children described her "miraculous recovery from aspartame poisoning." This occupational therapist had been sick for five years, beginning shortly after the birth of her youngest son. She wrote

"When I was at my worst, I suffered from extreme joint pain in the lower parts of my body, and began to have symptoms suspicious of multiple sclerosis. It got to the point where my oldest son (age 12) would come to my room to hug me in the morning, and I would cry from the pain or ask him not to hug me. Since my recovery after avoiding aspartame products, I have begun to share my story with people all over the world."

Case IX-G-12

This patient experienced discomfort in his right knee and left shoulder during the fall of 1995. He was treated for "migratory bursitis." The pains recurred every several weeks, and then intensified in the spring of 1996. Anti-inflammatory drugs were only partially effective. A rheumatologist subsequently placed him on ibuprofen and chloroquine daily; these medications did not help. He "began to feel that I might be crippled with this disease for life."

Desperate for relief, he began searching the Internet. When the subject of diet was raised, he realized that he had been "addicted to diet colas." His joint pains were reduced "to a manageable level" after quitting them. There was improvement of his short-term memory and energy at the end of the day, and a spontaneous loss of ten pounds in two months. His condition progressively improved to the point he could resume exercising and playing squash.

Case IX-G-13

A 35-year-old diabetic patient consumed aspartame products "in mass quantities." Severe arthritic and neuropathic symptoms, particularly of the shoulder and hip, precluded working for two years. After avoiding all aspartame products when his fiancee read about aspartame disease, these symptoms improved dramatically... including his extreme fatigue.

Case IX-G-14

A 52-year-old woman experienced "debilitating joint pain," especially of the fingers and wrists. She was to be seen in consultation by a rheumatologist. (Her father had suffered from arthritis.) Her son then informed the patient about joint pain reported in aspartame disease. She later wrote

"I went 'cold turkey' off diet sodas about five weeks ago, and am now totally pain-free! I can open jars, grasp the handles on

456

plastic grocery bags, and sleep through the night without waking up with 'frozen' fingers which were extremely painful to straighten from their clenched position. I'll NEVER consume aspartame again!"

Case IX-G-15

A homemaker used peppermint mints containing aspartame to freshen her breath.

> "After a few weeks of consuming a six-pack a week, I started to have aches in my back and shoulders which got worse. It also started to affect my neck area. Finally, it became so intense I was going to the doctor to find out what my problem was. About the same time, I happened to read the packaging and discovered the ingredient aspartame. Having heard various discussions about this sweetener, I decided to eliminate the breath mints. After five or six days, there was no more shoulder pain!"

> "About March of this year (1997), without thinking about it, someone offered me hard candy. I accepted it. A few days later,

> the shoulder and neck aches returned, but were much more intense. When I discovered the candy was 'sugar free,' I immediately stopped it. Again, the pain left."

Case IX-G-16

A publishing executive was afflicted with "an undiagnosed rheumatological condition my doctors have been trying to figure out for almost a year." She had been placed on prednisone and Plaquenil®. She could not convince her rheumatologist to omit at least one of the drugs after learning about aspartame disease, and experiencing improvement by avoiding aspartame. The patient had been drinking considerable diet cola, now referred to as "The Stuff."

3. "FIBROMYALGIA"

The "fibromyalgia syndrome" describes a type of soft tissue rheumatism characterized by widespread muscle pain, but without demonstrable inflammation in muscle tissue. In addition, there may be joint pain, fatigue, weakness, stiffness, poor concentration, and subjective numbness or tingling.

More than 80 percent of persons in the United States suffering this affliction are women. Their misery is evidenced by the willingness of some to undergo "decompression" of the brain for presumed "posterior fossa compression." A severe aspartame reactor emphasized "my whole body's SCREAMIN' MEEMEES," which she defined as "every bone ached like a toothache, every muscle spasmed, and every joint ached."

A diagnosis of fibromyalgia was made in 27 persons among the most recent 649 aspartame reactors in this series, generally after conventional tests failed to uncover other rheumatologic disorders. In their review of fibromyalgia, Quintner and Cohen (2000) asserted that "it is a label so easily abused as to have become meaningless" – as was the case with its antecedents (muscular rheumatism; fibrositis; neurasthenia).

Several instances of <u>familial</u> aspartame-induced fibromyalgia are illustrated by Cases IX-G-20 and G-21.

Aspartame reactors manifesting fibromyalgia may require several months of aspartame abstinence before marked symptomatic benefit. The possible explanations include serotonin deficiency and chronic methanol poisoning (Chapter XXI).

Representative Case Reports

Case IX-G-18

A correspondent elaborated on her pains caused by products containing aspartame that were previously diagnosed as "fibromyalgia" and "myofascial pain." She was amazed that small amounts – namely, "one little tablet in a cup of tea about five days a week" – could induce this reaction.

This reactor also described comparable difficulty experienced by several friends whom she attempted to warn, but to no avail. She wrote, "Hard to believe being slim is more important than having less pain. We can lead them to water, but we can't make them avoid drinking aspartame."

Case IX-G-19

A young woman training as an occupational therapist "suffered horribly from hip and lumbar pain, and morning immobility." The discomfort even precluded proper toileting. A diagnosis of fibromyalgia was made.

After reading an article about aspartame disease, she avoided such products. "Something magical happened" during the fifth week, She progressively became pain-free, more mobile, and was able to discontinue her own physical therapy.

Cases IX-G-20 and IX-G-21

A 30-year-old woman experienced "extreme" joint pain that promptly improved, and then disappeared, after stopping aspartame products. Other symptoms of aspartame disease included "excruciating headaches far worse than any migraine," confusion, memory loss, dizziness and fatigue. These features also promptly improved after aspartame abstinence, and had not recurred in five years.

Her mother (age 64) and a sister (age 43) suffered severe joint pains diagnosed as fibromyalgia. In addition, they were afflicted with depression, insomnia and diarrhea. These complaints quickly improved after avoiding aspartame. Her 4-year-old daughter also developed severe headache after ingesting aspartame.

Case IX-G-22

A female health professional was diagnosed as having fibromyalgia. She recounted her experience.

> "I was a heavy aspartame user, drinking about two liters of diet soda daily since this stuff hit the market. My symptoms: screaming leg pain mostly at bed time, especially as intrascapular tearing pain; heart palpitations nearly daily, but no cardiac involvement according to testing; joint pain (no swelling or articular deterioration); nightmares; evening rashes; slowed speech; forgetfulness; depression; moodiness; vomiting; and loss of about eighty percent of my strength. I previously could press over 800 pounds at a gym. That went down to less than 50 pounds.

> "Within the first three days after stopping aspartame, the fog has nearly lifted and my toes are coming back. There is now pain where there previously was numbness. It was so great to feel that this is reversible."

Case IX-G-23

A woman diagnosed as fibromyalgia stated that she had "such severe pain I could barely make it to work. I couldn't remember anything. I had to close my business and take a job." Other problems included depression (including contemplation of suicide), marked personality changes, and muscles so tight that I couldn't get up in the morning." She had consumed considerable aspartame. ("I drank diet sodas all day, and everything I put in my mouth was filled with it.")

A "miracle" ensued after stopping aspartame products. She reported two months later, "I have no muscle pain now. My mind is clearer and my memory better. I haven't had restless legs since I went off this stuff. I have had only one migraine headache. My energy level is much higher. I have been exercising three-five times a week. I am not depressed. My PMS is less severe. I can sleep through the night, and there is little or no muscle stiffness in the morning."

The proof of her affliction with aspartame disease occurred several weeks later when she ate fresh strawberries at the home of a neighbor. A severe migraine attack ensued, along with feeling "horrible all day." On investigating the matter, she found that the neighbor had sprinkled the fruit with an aspartame tabletop sweetener.

Insights from the Eosinophilia-Myalgia Syndrome (EMS)

The hazards of ingesting single amino acids, with or without neurotoxic contaminants, are underscored by the eosinophilia-myalgia syndrome following use of L-tryptophan. Its clinical manifestations included severe joint and muscle pain, fatigue, a rash, peripheral edema, polyneuropathy, grand mal seizures, and a striking elevation of the eosinophil count in the absence of infectious or neoplastic disease.

The long-term followup of such patients, predominantly women, is pertinent. Sack and Criswell (1992) observed or followed 22 EMS patients. Marked fatigue, weakness and myalgia remained in all. Their commentary merits repetition in view of the potential toxicity of excessive phenylalanine and aspartic acid (Chapter XXII).

> "What of the future? Could a situation similar to EMS occur with even more devastating consequences? We say yes, for the following reasons. First, the general public, and probably many physicians, regard food constituents as 'natural' and hence safer than synthetic compounds. This was clearly the case with L-

tryptophan, because in 1989 an estimated 2% of American adults were using this agent. Second, the FDA, though long concerned with the safety of substances, has not been successful in controlling their use. In the 1970s, the FDA removed amino acids (including L-tryptophan) from the 'generally regarded as safe' category and classified them as 'food additives.' As such, amino acids can be used to significantly improve the biological quality of the total protein in a food containing naturally occurring protein..., but it is illegal to use such supplements to 'treat or prevent' an illness. Yet this is precisely how consumers were using L-tryptophan before the recognition of EMS. Third, the FDA has not introduced new regulations to prevent similar events from occurring again."*

4. POLYMYALGIA RHEUMATICA

Several of my patients with polymyalgia rheumatica, a generalized "aches and pains" disorder, experienced aspartame disease. They had been under good control with small doses of corticosteroids (cortisone-like drugs) until suffering severe flareups after ingesting aspartame products. Improvement followed aspartame avoidance.

5. MUSCLE CRAMPS

Spontaneous severe cramping of muscles in the legs and hands was a significant complaint by 28 of the most recent 649 aspartame reactors in this series.

Representative Case Report

Case IX-G-24

A 42-year-old patient had been treated for hypothyroidism. Concerned about a modest gain in weight, she began consuming considerable aspartame products – including at least four diet sodas daily; and a "weight loss nutritional supplement." Her fingers repeatedly went into spasms within 10-15 minutes after ingesting diet cola. Other aspartame-related complaints included urinary bladder irritation, visual difficulty, numbness of one hand, severe fatigue (notwithstanding an adequate dose of Synthroid®), and recent elevation of the fasting blood glucose level.

---

*©1992 *Southern Medical Journal*. Reproduced with permission.

Commentary

Others have reported this phenomenon. For example, a Miami physician stated that he had been playing tennis 30 years without experiencing small muscle cramps. When this problem occurred one year previously, the only change he could determine was having added aspartame to coffee and using diet drinks. His cramping ceased when he stopped these products. (*Cortlandt Forum,* October 1990, p. 44).

Several metabolic and toxic mechanisms by which aspartame and its metabolites irritate skeletal muscle are discussed below and in Section 5. The roles of hypoglycemia (tissue glucopenia) and the hyperinsulinized state (Chapter XIV) in severe leg cramps have been described in previous publications (Roberts 1965, 1973).

6. POLYMYOSITIS

The diagnosis of polymyositis was made or considered in several patients with aspartame disease who suffered severe muscle weakness. Skeletal muscle is affected in this presumed autoimmune process. It occurs in women twice as often as men. The disorder is termed dermatomyositis when a characteristic skin rash exists.

Representative Case Report

Case IX-G-25

An 18-year-old woman began using aspartame sodas and an aspartame tabletop sweetener in her coffee. Shortly thereafter, she developed an extensive rash that was initially diagnosed as psoriasis. Subsequent marked weakening of her muscles caused slumping of the shoulders. Tests for lupus erythematosus were negative. Her CPK level was over 900. A rheumatologist made the diagnosis of polymyositis and prescribed prednisone.

When the patient became pregnant, she was advised to avoid aspartame products. Her CPK level normalized during the pregnancy. Shortly after delivery, she resumed aspartame sodas. The CPK level rose dramatically. The same sequence of events occurred during her next pregnancy.

A cousin relayed an article about aspartame disease that mentioned "tissue damage," causing her to avoid aspartame products. Her CPK declined from over 250 to 75. When it then rose to 100, she discovered that her gelatin contained aspartame.

My first followup revealed that this patient remained in a prolonged remission for two years. The muscle weakness then recurred along with "scleroderma" of the hands and feet, and the Raynaud phenomenon (Chapter IX-C) on exposure to cold. Although still attempting to avoid aspartame, she did not realize its presence in various products being used – notably mouthwashes and gum. Steroid treatment was suggested, but she refused pending the results of total aspartame abstinence. In a second followup five months later, the patient stated that the features of polymyositis had gone.

7. PATHOPHYSIOLOGIC MECHANISMS

The mechanisms involved in aspartame-induced rheumatologic disorders probably include direct effects of its three components (phenylalanine; aspartic acid; methanol), altered neurotransmitter metabolism, decreased tissue substrate due to the combination of increased insulin release and decreased food intake by persons attempting to lose weight, and immunologic reactions to aspartame or its metabolites, perhaps acting as haptenes (Chapter VIII). Only several aspects are considered here. It is likely that chronic methanol poisoning (Chapter XXI) plays a role. The methyl alcohol derived from aspartame is detoxified to formaldehyde, and then to formate or formic acid.

The conjugation of formaldehyde with human serum albumin (F-HSA) forms a new antigenic determinant. Symptomatic patients chronically exposed to formaldehyde develop anti F-HSA antibodies and elevated Tal cells (antigen memory cells), consistent with sustained immunologic stimulation (Thrasher 1988).

A simplified hypothesis for initiation of an autoimmune response involves the "ambling" of proteins by formaldehyde, thereby making them strange to the person's immune system, and serving as antigens. Additionally, an increase of leukotrienes, 15-hydroxyeicosatetraenoic acid and other arachidonic acid metabolites has been found when macrophages are exposed to aspartame (Hardcastle 1997).

Abnormalities of calcium and phosphate metabolism (Chapter IX-E) may be contributory.

- The affinity of aspartame for calcium (Matsuzawa 1984) suggests its preferential distribution in bones and joints.
- Aspartame has been shown to be bound to a human Bence-Jones dimer, as determined by x-ray crystallography of the ligand protein complex (Edmundson 1998). Moreover, dipeptide-binding proteins require the calcium ion, which may enhance the binding of aspartame to the Bence-Jones dimer.

• The calcium-depleting influence of considerable phosphoric acid present in the acid medium of aspartame sodas (Wyshak 2000) could contribute to the rheumatologic complaints of aspartame reactors.

H. INCREASED SUSCEPTIBILITY TO INFECTION

Susceptibility to infection appears to be increased in aspartame disease, reflecting altered tissue metabolism and immunologic changes.

This problem becomes compounded when <u>diabetes control</u> is adversely affected (Chapter XII). Superimposed infection, especially in the urinary tract, can create a vicious cycle of insulin resistance. The prostate gland is unique because its chief substrate is fructose, not glucose.

Similarly, aspartame reactors with <u>reactive hypoglycemia</u> (Chapter XIV) suffered recurrent bacterial infections of the sinuses and bronchi, and herpes simplex of the lips notwithstanding medical treatment and preventive measures (see Case IX-H-1). Paradoxically, they were consuming considerable aspartame to avoid sugar. Once aware that these products could aggravate hypoglycemia, clinical improvement followed their cessation.

<u>Vaginitis</u>. The recurrence of vaginitis in aspartame reactors is noteworthy. One aspartame reactor suffered "severe vaginal yeast infections" whenever she consumed aspartame products, generally within one day. It may be a consequence of decreased vaginal lubrication, similar to "dry eyes" (Chapter IV) and "dry mouth" (see above).

<u>Yeast Infections</u>. Patients with diabetes or hypoglycemia who have aspartame disease are prone to superimposed yeast (Candida) infection. Recurrent fungal skin infections are discussed in Chapter VIII.

<u>Concern Over Recurrent Infection</u>. Patients with prior serious infections that had required considerable treatment become concerned about delayed complications, when in fact their new symptoms represented aspartame disease.

A woman had suffered severe Lyme disease. She later experienced "strange reactions to diet drinks" that included severe headache, marked tremors and gastric complaints. She was concerned about recurrence of the infection until realizing that her symptoms disappeared on weekends when "I don't drink this stuff."

464

Simulation of Infection. Aspartame reactions may simulate infection. Several aspartame reactors developed chills and fever as a vasomotor response (Chapter IX-C) shortly after consuming aspartame. One female patient experienced chills and a subsequent fever of 101° when she ingested a single glass of an aspartame soft drink mix daily for three days. A battery of studies proved normal.

Extensive Testing for Suspected Infection. Patients with aspartame disease have been investigated for other infections that did not exist.

- "Chronic infectious mononucleosis" was repeatedly considered. Large sums were wasted on testing for the Epstein-Barr virus in the case of persons with chronic fatigue, sweats, weight loss, headache and joint discomfort who proved to be aspartame reactors.
- Others needlessly anguished over the fear of having HIV infection when their complaints could not be explained.
- Aspartame disease has simulated Lyme disease, especially its rheumatologic and neurologic features. Case IX-G-4, a physician, had seen many consultants for these complaints. Aspartame also appeared to activate Lyme disease in several instances.

Representative Case Reports

Case IX-H-1

A 59-year-old engineer had been treated for longstanding reactive hypoglycemia. He evidenced a severe hypoglycemic reaction after the third hour of a glucose tolerance test as his blood glucose concentration precipitously declined. His longstanding rhinitis responded to an appropriate diet, allergic precautions, hyposensitization, and other measures.

This patient then began suffering more frequent and severe respiratory infections, including an attack of maxillary sinusitis. Several allergists and nose-and-throat physicians recommended surgery for a deviated nasal septum, which was performed. His severe "allergies" and bronchitis then recurred. Several antihypertensive drugs were later added because of lightheadedness, a "humming" in the ears, and elevated blood pressure.

When seen for another attack of bronchitis and sinusitis, he was queried about aspartame use. He admitted to taking considerable quantities because of "my sweet tooth." Gratifying improvement occurred within several weeks after avoiding all aspartame products.

His daughter also had a marked intolerance to aspartame products.

Case IX-H-2

A 64-year-old man presented with persistent low back pain. He also complained of recent headache, decreased vision, marked fatigue and leg cramps – symptoms not mentioned during the many years under my care. When queried about aspartame, he admitted to using considerable amounts of an ATS daily. His prostate was found to be swollen and tender. The prostatitis responded promptly to antibiotic therapy. His other symptoms disappeared after avoiding aspartame products.

Case IX-H-3

A 58-year-old man had repeated attacks of prostatitis for one year for which he took maintenance trimethoprim and sulfomethoxazole (Bactrim®). A urologic consultant could find no overt cause.

The hint that aspartame might be contributory was raised when he presented with other suggestive complaints – namely, unexplained severe headache, dizziness, depression, increasing visual difficulty, confusion, and a profound loss of memory. He stated, "My memory is so bad that if I am cooking something in the kitchen, I'm likely to forget about it." Additional symptoms were "dry eyes," drowsiness and marked irritability.

In view of his longstanding symptomatic reactive hypoglycemia, this patient had avoided sugar. In its place, he drank two cans of an ACB and three glasses of aspartame-sweetened iced tea daily. Within one week after stopping these products, he felt markedly improved. There were no further attacks of prostatitis over the next four years.

Case IX-H-4

A 74-year-old retired realtor developed a number of aspartame-associated complaints. They included fever, "open sores on my back," headache, sleepiness, heartburn, itching, dizziness, lack of coordination and "dry eyes." All subsided within three days after discontinuing the ATS she had been using daily, coupled with progressive healing of the sores.

Commentary: Relevant Reports

Other reports suggest a relationship between aspartame use and infection.

466

- Dr. Woodrow Monte (cited by Reschevsky 1986) requested a Federal District court to issue a temporary restraining order prohibiting the continued use of aspartame as a food additive. In the affidavit, he cited a 12-year-old child who developed brain abscesses after consuming aspartame. Monte hypothesized that changes in the brain caused by aspartic acid, one of its amino acids, had lowered resistance to bacterial invasion.

- In 1977, Searle Laboratories reported three outbreaks of infectious diseases among rats receiving the diketopiperazine metabolite of aspartame (Chapter XXV) that required penicillin treatment.

Commentary: Contributory Mechanisms

Some of the possible mechanisms involving an increased tendency to infection in aspartame disease are listed.

- Increased phenylalanine appears to alter cell-mediated immunity. This is evidenced by the enhanced immunity noted in both animals and humans placed on phenylalanine restriction (Norris 1990).

- In turn, elevation of the serum phenylalanine by infection (Wannemacher 1976) can contribute to a vicious cycle. The phenylalanine/large neutral amino acid ratio increases in acute infection by as much as 50 percent.

- A diet high in D-forms of the amino acid stereoisomers (Chapter XXV), as well as one inadequate in protein, might impair the function of white blood cells, macrophages and antibody-immune systems.

- Fudenberg and Singh (1988) found T-lymphocyte dysfunction in a majority of patients with problems triggered or exacerbated by chemical stress. T-lymphocytes recognize conventional antigens as short peptide fragments that are bound on the heavy chain of major histocompatibility complex molecules (Sissons 1993). These peptides are anchored by amino acid residues at critical points in the peptide sequence. (As another point of reference, some researchers believe that butyl nitrite, [known on the streets as "poppers"] weakens the body's ability to ward off virus infections, including the HIV virus.)

- The occurrence of "dry eyes" and dryness of the mouth in aspartame disease was described in Chapters IV and IX-D. Other chemicals and drugs have caused or simulated the Sjögren syndrome, including its characteristic immunologic features (Oxholm 1986). These were noteworthy with epirubicin, which interferes with DNA synthesis in proliferating cells and influences cells of the immune system.

Dr. Joyce Marshall (personal communication, September 1999) observed that aspartame seems to work as an adjuvant in mass vaccination, thereby intensifying disease or complications among immunized persons, especially involving Mycoplasmas. She further noted the following:

- Some vaccines for children contain formaldehyde. (Triple antigen DPT may have formaldehyde, mercury and aluminum phosphate.)
- Aberrant responses to such vaccines could result in demyelination, epilepsy, autism, allergies and aberrant behavior when compounded by the effects of aspartame.

Commentary: Possible Relationship to Selected Infection

The emergence of several epidemics or near-epidemics of infection during recent years raises the contributory role of an altered immune system caused by widespread aspartame consumption. Several areas that warrant such study are listed here and in Chapter XXVII.

Rheumatic Fever. A dramatic resurgence of rheumatic fever ("the red plague") due to Streptococcal infection occurred after 1984. Contrasting with its prior characterization as a "slum disease," serious outbreaks were reported among members of affluent families (*Newsweek* December 22, 1986, p. 60). Similarly, two-thirds of children with acute rheumatic fever (including cardiac involvement) coming from affluent backgrounds did not have a history of preceding respiratory infection. (Streptococcus usually could be cultured from their siblings.)

Chronic Epstein-Barr Virus Infection. This infection causes infectious mononucleosis (also referred to as "Yuppie Flu"). It has commanded much attention in recent years. The symptoms include recurrent fever, sore throat, aches and pains, and debilitating fatigue.

Acquired Immune Deficiency Syndrome (AIDS). Persons with AIDS often consume aspartame to avoid sugar. This is pertinent in view of (a) the preponderance of females among aspartame reactors, (b) their apparent greater vulnerability to more severe and fulminant AIDS, and (c) evidences for aspartame's influence on the immune system (see above and Chapter VIII). (Aspartame disease may be misdiagnosed as AIDS, especially its unrecognized neuropsychiatric, ocular and gastrointestinal symptoms.)

The author has encountered patients with HIV infection whose primary presenting complaints appeared to be aspartame reactions. They began or intensified after switching to aspartame products when gastrointestinal, perianal and other symptoms were ascribed to aggravation of a fungal infection by sugar intake. In a related vein, desperate patients with HIV infection relentlessly pursue methods to bolster their immune system. Concerned about yeast superinfection, they avoid sugar and use considerable aspartame, coupled with the ongoing (but erroneous) belief that saccharin causes cancer.

Representative Case Report

Case IX-H-6

A 38-year-old engineer sought further consultation from the author (as an endocrinologist) for a dermatitis of the perianal area that had resisted treatment by three dermatologists and other physicians. He was known to be HIV-positive. When the possibility of diabetes with a superimposed fungus infection was raised, he abstained from sugar and began consuming at least one liter of aspartame beverages daily.

The local lesions became more painful. They were accompanied by considerable abdominal cramping, a 20-pound weight loss, decreased vision in both eyes, intense drowsiness after eating, and severe hypoglycemic attacks (especially if he delayed lunch). When seen two weeks after avoiding aspartame products, he felt much improved relative to the dermatitis and other complaints.

I. INTERFERENCE WITH DRUG ACTION

The author's clinical observations indicate that aspartame products can alter the action of important drugs. They include coumarin (Coumadin®), phenytoin (Dilantin®), antidepressants, other psychotropic agents, propranolol (Inderal®), methyldopa (Aldomet®), thyroxine (Synthroid®), and insulin (Chapter XIII). This phenomenon is illustrated in many case reports presented in other sections.

It is also likely that some herbs interact with aspartame. Noting numerous herb-drug interactions, Fugh-Berman (2000) stated, "Health care practitioners should caution patients against mixing herbs and pharmaceutical drugs."

General Considerations

Aspartame may either reduce or potentiate drug action by various mechanisms. A few of the possibilities are listed.

- Alteration of the blood proteins to which drugs attach.
- Alteration of drug receptors on cell membranes.
- Changes in the sites at which impulses are transmitted along nerves and to muscle.
- Metabolic abnormalities in the elderly that are known to enhance their vulnerability to drug reactions (Weber 1986). This problem increases in the case of persons taking multiple drugs ("polypharmacy") prescribed by several physicians.
- Interference with drug action by amino acids and protein. An example is the erratic therapeutic effects when patients with parkinsonism who were controlled on levodopa began to use aspartame products (Chapter VI-J). The antagonism of levodopa by dietary protein presumably reflects impaired transport from serum across the blood-brain barrier by neutral amino acids (Pincus 1986).

The <u>methanol</u> component of aspartame (Chapter XXI) might interact with compounds containing ethanol. Examples include the hypoglycemic sulfonylureas, metronidazole (an antibacterial drug), and allopurinol (commonly used in the treatment of gout). In his review of this subject, Posner (1975) emphasized that such interactions pose "an important area for careful clarification."

Drug Reactions After the Cessation of Aspartame

The phenomenon of increased sensitivity to a drug after the removal of some interfering factor is known to clinicians. Examples include severe insulin reactions in diabetics after cure of an infection, and bleeding from coumarin after terminating a drug that influenced its binding to carrier proteins. This type of encounter probably reflects an increase in the "free" forms of such drugs. It occurred, for example, when patients on maintenance coumarin or phenytoin avoided aspartame.

A. Coumarin (Coumadin)

Coumarin is commonly prescribed as an anticoagulant ("blood thinner") for the treatment or prevention of serious problems caused by thrombosis (clot formation) and embolism (the migration of a thrombus). The vascular beds frequently affected include the coronary arteries, the carotid arteries, the inner lining of the heart (endocardium) in patients with heart attacks or irregular heart action (atrial fibrillation) from which embolism to the 7brain or lower extremities may originate, and veins in the lower extremities and pelvis that are frequent sites for pulmonary emboli.

This form of therapy constitutes a major commitment for physicians, particularly the need for continually monitoring the prothrombin time. Patients may bleed if the anticoagulant effect becomes excessive. Conversely, the loss of desired anticoagulation invites recurrence of thrombosis or embolism.

The likelihood of interference by aspartame was raised in patients who had been maintained on coumarin for extended periods without difficulty. Unexpectedly, their prothrombin times approximated the control values (meaning a loss of anticoagulant effect), coupled with recurrent thrombophlebitis or angina pectoris.

Representative Case Reports

Case IX-I-1

An 82-year-old woman had received coumarin for two reasons: recurrent transient cerebral ischemic attacks ("small strokes") due to embolism from the carotid arteries, the heart, or both; and severe thrombophlebitis in the lower extremities with multiple attacks of pulmonary embolism. A registered nurse administered her medication daily.

The patient's prothrombin time, monitored every 3-4 weeks, had remained stable a long time. It was found to be only 14 seconds (control, 13 seconds) on August 19, 1986. Several days thereafter, she developed severe pain in the lower extremities and exquisite tenderness over the deep veins, consistent with recurrent thrombophlebitis. The dosage of coumarin was increased.

On direct inquiry, it was determined that she recently began to use aspartame products. These were discontinued. Three days later, blood was noted in the urine. At that time, her prothrombin time had returned to the therapeutic range – namely, 21 seconds. Coumarin was withheld several days. The failure of urinary bleeding to recur when coumarin was then resumed probably reflected a return of full anticoagulation after the loss of aspartame interference.

Case IX-I-2

A 72-year-old woman had been treated with coumarin for longstanding angina pectoris and thrombophlebitis. Her prothrombin times generally ranged between 19.5-22 seconds.

The patient then developed unstable angina pectoris and rapid heart action (tachycardia) for which she was hospitalized. No precipitating cause could be determined. At the time, little significance was paid to the slight decrease of her most recent prothrombin time (17 seconds). Even though the dosage of coumarin was increased, the prothrombin time then declined to 15 seconds.

The occurrence of other complaints suggesting aspartame disease raised the question as to whether aspartame also had influenced the prothrombin time. They included severe "burning and swelling" of the lips and tongue, headache, increased visual difficulty (despite recent cataract surgery and prescription glasses), marked "nervousness," and unexplained nausea. Although she initially denied using aspartame, the "diet" ginger ale she drank did contain it. The prothrombin time rose to 22 seconds (control, 12 seconds) one week after stopping aspartame. During this time, her intense fatigue and lip-tongue reactions subsided.

B. Phenytoin (Dilantin) and Other Antiepileptic Drugs

Phenytoin is a key drug in managing epilepsy. When convulsions are associated with or aggravated by aspartame products (Chapter III), the patient confronts several dilemmas. First, the dose of phenytoin is likely to be increased, possibly to the point of toxicity (see Case III-35). Second, other anti-epilepsy drugs may be added, thereby increasing the potential for side effects. Third, the continuation of these drugs in high doses could result in "rebound" toxicity after stopping aspartame.

The apparent potentiation of valproic acid (Depakene®; Depacote®), another antiepileptic drug, was personally reported to the author by a 51-year-old man who drank considerable diet cola daily. When his physician increased the dose, he became comatose and required hospitalization.

Representative Case Report

Case IX-I-3

A 28-year-old man suffered seizures after a head injury while serving in the Marines. As a civilian, his convulsions unexpectedly increased despite multiple anti-epileptic medications, causing him to lose his job.

The patient's mother noted that he "acted like he was intoxicated." She expressed concern over his large consumption of aspartame sodas. Shortly after discontinuing them, he had to be taken to an emergency room for phenytoin intoxication – presumably representing the rebound phenomenon.

472

C. Antidepressant Drugs

Aspartame may interfere with the action of important drugs used to treat depression, particularly <u>imipramine</u> (a tricyclic antidepressant). Others have made similar observations.

Walton (1986) described a 54-year-old woman with recurrent major depression who had been well controlled on a maintenance dose of 150 mg imipramine at bedtime. She subsequently experienced marked behavioral changes, manic behavior characterized by inappropriate euphoria and flighty ideas, and a grand mal seizure. It was then learned that she had been drinking considerable aspartame-sweetened iced tea for several weeks prior to the seizure. All evidence of manic activity subsided within four days after stopping aspartame and the addition of lithium. Her depression recurred, however, two months later. Imipramine was resumed at the previous dosage with no recurrence of severe depression or mania over the ensuing 13 months.

The <u>monoamine oxidase inhibitors</u> (MAOIs), another group of antidepressant drugs, can have additional adverse effects when aspartame is consumed. These include phenelzine (Nardil®), isocarboxazide (Marplan®), and tranylcypromine (Parnate®).

It is pertinent that hypertensive crises have occurred in patients so treated after they consumed foods and beverages containing tyramine and tryptophan. This response probably represents vasospasm caused by amino acid-derived sympathomimetic substances such as norepinephrine and tyramine (Chapters IX-C and XXIII).

The serotonin-elevating action of <u>fluoxetine</u> (Prozac®) for treating depression could be counteracted by aspartame. It can block tryptophan entry into the brain, thereby inhibiting synthesis of serotonin (Chapter VII).

A Minnesota physician called to inquire about a possible interaction between Prozac and aspartame. He had suffered depression for which Prozac was prescribed, but without much benefit until he avoided aspartame. At that point, the drug proved helpful.

D. Propranolol (Inderal)

The occurrence or aggravation of benign ("essential") tremor by aspartame was described in Chapter VI-J. This condition usually can be controlled with small or modest doses of propranolol. Several patients and correspondents stressed that their tremor intensified after consuming aspartame – even with increased dosage of propranolol – and improved when they avoided such products.

E. Thyroid Replacement Therapy

The increased susceptibility of hypothyroid to aspartame (Chapter IX-E) has been repeatedly emphasized. Conversely, there may be interference with the activity of thyroid replacement therapy.

Case IX-I-4

An aspartame reactor had been taking thyroid hormone several years. After avoiding aspartame products, he noted "My replacement thyroid dose, which had been steadily increasing for the last few years, dropped by 30 percent. My doctor was quite surprised, and had no other explanation for it."

F. Female Hormone Replacement Therapy

Patients with aspartame disease expressed firm convictions about interactions involving female hormone replacement therapy.

Representative Case Report

Case IX-I-5

A 40-year-old saleswoman consumed considerable diet sodas and other aspartame products, especially during the summer. She supplemented her description of reactions in the survey questionnaire with a two-page analysis of major changes when taken in conjunction with Premarin/Provera®. They included cloudy vision, dizziness, tenderness and tingling of the feet, joint pains, numbness of the lower limbs, headache, "foggy thinking," confusion, slurred speech and extreme fatigue. She took as many as 18 ibuprofen tablets daily to obtain relief of her constant pain. Extensive neurologic studies – including electromyography, nerve conduction studies, x-rays and MRI scanning – failed to reveal a cause.

Considering a possible connection to the hormonal therapy, she reduced Premarin by half and quit Provera. There was considerable relief from the joint pain and muscle aches within two days, along with cessation of her neuropathic symptoms. After then avoiding all aspartame products, she wrote, "I felt IMMEDIATE relief within two days of what remained of the lumbar ache, muscle aches, foggy thinking, dizziness, and cloudy vision. All these improvements continue in the week since. Walking seems less of an effort; hip pain improved."

G. Methyldopa (Aldomet)

There have been references to enhancement of seizures and other disorders in patients receiving methyldopa for hypertension who also consumed aspartame. Seven of the initial 397 reactors completing the questionnaire were taking this drug when they experienced aspartame disease. Maher and Kiritsy (1987) demonstrated that aspartame administration decreases the entry of methyldopa into rat brain.

Representative Case Report

Case IX-I-6

A 67-year-old retired hypertensive woman had been treated with methyldopa. She experienced three unexplained seizures while drinking one can of diet cola and eating various aspartame puddings daily. The convulsions stopped when she avoided aspartame products, as did her sensitivity to noise and attacks of rapid heart action.

H. Analgesics

Lidocaine (Xylocaine®) is an important drug used for local anesthesia and the treatment of ventricular arrhythmias in intensive care units. Alterations of its pharmacology by aspartame require study.

Kim et al (1987) reported that the intraperitoneal administration of aspartame significantly reduced the 50 percent convulsion dose of lidocaine. They indicated that PKU patients and asymptomatic PKU heterozygotes may be more sensitive to the toxic effects of this and related local anesthetics.

Nikfar et al (1997) noted that aspartame increased morphine analgesia in the early phase (wherein saccharin had no effect), and further enhanced morphine analgesia during the late phase. The sister of a heavy diet cola consumer related the apparent potentiation of morphine by aspartame while he continued drinking it in an intensive care unit after a heart attack. This interaction became evident when the aspartame was stopped, coupled with halving the insulin required for managing his diabetes.

J. BLOOD AND LYMPH NODE DISORDERS

Bone marrow and lymph nodes, the organs chiefly responsible for blood cells, are highly vulnerable to toxic substances. For example, aplastic anemia and leukemia may occur after treatment with potent drugs, or exposure to pesticides and other chemicals in the environment (Roberts 1984, 1990b). Aspartame products could be another cause of disorders therein.

A. Bone Marrow and Blood Changes

Aspartame disease may be evidenced by changes involving red blood cells, white blood cells and platelets. The aspartame reactors reported below and elsewhere evidenced either anemia, a striking elevation of the white blood cell count suggestive of leukemia, or markedly decreased platelet counts (thrombocytopenia).

- A patient with recurrent "histiocytic leukemia" following aspartame ingestion (Case IX-J-1) offers an intriguing clue to the so-called histiocytosis syndromes in children (*The Lancet* 1987; 208-209). The Langerhans cell in histiocytosis is a dendritic cell derived from the bone marrow.
- Many drugs and other substances have been implicated in "immune thrombocytopenia."
- Case IX-F-6 mentioned the finding of "enlarged red blood cells." Deficiency of folic acid or its altered metabolism (see below) causes macrocytic (large red blood cell) anemia, while deficient absorption of vitamin B_{12} can result in a similar anemia.
- Patients with pernicious anemia may be more vulnerable to aspartame. For example, a 51-year-old woman with severe aspartame disease gave a history of treatment for documented pernicious anemia as her only significant past medical history.

Representative Case Reports

Case IX-J-1

A 10-year-old girl began consuming various aspartame products at the age of eight, initially during summer weekends. She developed marked swelling of one shoulder which then involved the neck. Her arm almost tripled in size. There was no history of allergies or aspirin use existed. The patient also evidenced a high fever, pleural effusion (fluid in the lung cavity), striking enlargement of both the liver and spleen, and a precipitous decline of the platelet count to 1,000 per cubic mm (normal, 150,000 or higher). A striking increase of histiocytes was found in her bone marrow. Several "liver enzymes" were markedly elevated – i.e., SGOT 3,080 units/L (normal, up to 50); CPK 30,000 units/L (normal, up to 50).

Numerous physicians and consultants saw this child. Most diagnosed histiocytic leukemia. The patient received large doses of prednisone.

Dramatic clinical improvement and virtual normalization of the foregoing blood changes occurred when the mother closely monitored her diet and eliminated additives. The prednisone was then stopped.

The patient subsequently ate several bowls of an aspartame cereal. Marked swelling of the checks developed, coupled with recurrence of the aforementioned features. When aspartame was discontinued, the swelling receded without prednisone.

Several months later, the girl was given aspartame chewing gum without the mother's knowledge. Swelling of her entire body, recurrent enlargement of the liver and spleen, a dramatic increase of bone marrow histiocytes, and severe pain in many joints ensued. Total abstinence from aspartame again effected the disappearance of her symptoms and blood abnormalities within six months. At the time of my last discussion with her mother, the child had minimal enlargement of the liver, and was receiving prednisone in low doses only intermittently.

This patient had two sets of head x-rays, three CT scans of the brain, two spinal punctures, four bone marrow studies, two electroencephalograms, two heart monitoring studies, two barium enemas, and a host of other studies. Her mother estimated the medical costs at $750,000!

Case IX-J-2

A 62-year-old man developed severe gastrointestinal problems while ingesting aspartame products. He developed "an erratic blood count, with red and white cell imbalance, and platelets off some." He received "cortisone" for six months when his condition was diagnosed as "an immune deficiency problem."

His daughter suffered intense abdominal pain, a bleeding peptic ulcer, severe headache, and repeated grand mal convulsions when she used aspartame products. A granddaughter had phenylketonuria (Chapter XVII) at birth, and subsequently manifested severe learning deficiencies.

Case IX-J-3

A 61-year-old personnel director began drinking diet colas at the age of 59, and consumed up to one liter daily. His platelet count declined to 54,000/cu mm thereafter. He also became concerned over "forgetting to perform things for which I was responsible." Other complaints included "double vision," severe sensitivity to light, headache, dizziness, two convulsions, "fits without convulsions," marked sleepiness during the day, insomnia, slurred speech, and a nonspecific rash. Extensive studies failed to uncover a major medical problem.

His symptoms improved within 10 weeks after avoiding aspartame, although some problems with vision, memory, sleep and "concentration" persisted. There was an **immediate** exacerbation during one retest trial. After avoiding all aspartame products, the platelet count had increased to 75,000/cu mm at the time of his subsequent correspondence.

Case IX-J-4

A registered nurse developed hypertension and a platelet count under 30,000 during her third pregnancy. Neither of these features had been noted in previous pregnancies. She began using diet colas after the birth of her second child. Other symptoms included severe headache, depression, loss of hair, and symptomatic reactive hypoglycemia.

Her symptoms dramatically improved after avoiding aspartame products. Concomitantly, the blood pressure and platelet count normalized.

Case IX-J-5

A 41-year-old woman consumed diet cola for 14 years. She experienced many symptoms of aspartame disease for three years, including headache, visual problems, severe aching of the joints, numbness of the left hand, and easy agitation. Her white blood cell count was only 460 (normal 4000-10,000), for which no other cause could be determined.

478

B. Lymph Node Enlargement

Enlargement of the lymph nodes (lymphadenopathy) occurred in several aspartame reactors without the finding of another convincing cause. This featured differed from the striking salivary gland enlargement in other with aspartame reactors (Chapter IX-D).

Representative Case Reports

Case IX-J-7

A mortgage broker began drinking diet cola in January 1995. She developed markedly enlarged glands in the neck ("the size of golf balls") one year later, along with a constant sore throat. These features persisted despite considerable doctoring. Subsequent symptoms included blurred vision, migraine headaches, severe joint and muscle pains, constant diarrhea with bloody stools, ringing in the ears, palpitations, night sweats, "a tongue as black as black leather," a 30-pound weight gain, and "incapacitating" chronic fatigue. Various suggested diagnoses – including carbon monoxide poisoning, fibromyalgia, lupus erythematosus, and Epstein-Barr infection – could not be confirmed.

The patient was "absolutely in shock" on learning about aspartame disease. Improvement proved gratifying after discontinuing aspartame products. The tongue returned to a normal healthy pink state. The enlarged glands in her neck decreased within several months.

Case IX-J-8

A 44-year-old loan officer experienced headache, drowsiness, hyperactivity, severe tingling, irritability, personality changes, palpitations, a recent elevation of blood pressure, abdominal pain, itching, hives, other rashes, marked frequency of urine, and joint pains. These symptoms were provoked "immediately" on three retesting trials with aspartame products.

His son also had aspartame disease. It was primarily evidenced as "noncancerous lumps under the arms" and a rash.

C. Altered Folic Acid Metabolism

Aspartame may deplete important nutrients related to folic acid. Folic acid assists in eliminating the formic acid derived from methyl alcohol degradation (Reitbrock 1971). It tends to decrease with higher methanol concentrations (Chapter XXI). In view of the rarity of low blood folate levels in contemporary clinical practice, this finding could prove a clue to aspartame disease.

Aspartame-induced decrease of folic acid could have clinical significance, especially anemia and birth defects.

> A physician in the State of Washington noted anemia in a patient who ingested large amounts of aspartame sodas, and suspected folic acid deficiency. He found the blood methanol level to be elevated. Unfortunately, the tube sent for a folate level broke in transit after he started replacement therapy.

There has been a recent impressive decline in neural-tube following the fortification of grain products and vitamin formulations with folic acid, coupled with an associated increase of median serum folate concentrations. This decline might be less evident, however, among pregnant women who consume aspartame products that can deplete folate levels as methyl alcohol is metabolized.

K. LIVER DYSFUNCTION

The vulnerability of patients with pre-existing liver disease to aspartame was noted in the introduction of this section. These disorders include hepatitis, cirrhosis (Case IX-K-5), hemochromatosis (iron storage disease), and the liver dysfunction complicating many infections and drug reactions.

Several aspartame reactors without known liver disease evidenced marked elevation of blood aminotransferases ("liver enzymes"). They are variously referred to as alanine aminotransferase (ALT; SGPT), aspartate aminotransferase (AST; SGOT) and glutamyl transpeptidase (GGT). (Serum levels of ALT and AST in normal persons are less than 35units/L. In Case IX-J-1, a 10-year-old girl, the SGOT was 3,080 units/L. One such aspartame reactor had been told, "Your liver is pickled."

Monte (1984) made reference to such an association. Taylor (1996) also raised the issue of liver toxicity caused by aspartame in a 51-year-old man who evidenced repeated jaundice.

General Considerations

In a recent National Health and Nutrition Examination Survey, 2.6 percent of the United States population surveyed had elevated serum ALT for which no cause of chronic liver disease could be found (James 1999). Even though 70 percent of the adult population consumes aspartame products, aspartame disease was not suspected as a likely causative or contributory cause. It is of historic interest that Dr. Misael Uribe (1982) expressed concern that the FDA had not adequately considered the potential toxicity of aspartame in patients with liver disease shortly after its forthcoming release was announced.

Persons with cirrhosis of the liver are at increased risk because they may be unable to metabolize aspartame and its breakdown products adequately (Jagenberg 1977; Heberer 1980; Dhont 1982).

The possibility of aspartame toxicity should be entertained in patients diagnosed as having **nonalcoholic steatohepatitis**. This liver disorder has become a common liver disorder in North America, and can progress to cirrhosis (James 1999). Its frequent features of persistent fatigue, upper abdominal discomfort, diabetes and hyperlipidemia are also encountered in aspartame disease.

Obese persons and diabetic patients who consume considerable aspartame appear to be at higher risk for the development of chronic nonalcoholic steatohepatitis, especially when addicted to such products (Chapter VII-G). The term "nonalcoholic" is misleading in this instance because aspartame contains ten percent methyl alcohol.

Admittedly, it may be difficult to single out precise symptoms attributable to aspartame products in patients with liver disease. Yet, few physicians considered the contributory role of aspartame to hepatic changes among patients in this series. Some even were hostile to the idea (see Case IX-K-3).

By contrast, astute persons and various consumer groups submitted related observations to the FDA. The husband of one patient, an attorney, became irate over the absence of any warning labels on aspartame products for persons with liver disease.

Representative Case Reports

Case IX-K-1

A 68-year-old housewife described how she became "incapacitated" from aspartame products in these terms: "My eyes would not focus. I had confusion, dizziness, depression, insomnia and memory loss. I could not drive or leave the house alone." Other complaints included severe nausea, diarrhea, marked thirst, considerable frequency of urination, and attacks of hypoglycemia. Her "liver reading" (presumably the ALT) rose from 44 to 264. It declined to 78 after she avoided aspartame. Although her physician assumed it was due to "drinking," the patient empathically stated that she <u>never</u> drank alcoholic beverages.

Case IX-K-2

A prospective blood donor was surprised, and angered, when a blood bank would not accept her blood because several liver enzymes (SGOT and SGPT) were markedly elevated. She consulted a gastroenterologist. He confirmed the finding, and by exclusion diagnosed hepatitis C infection. Abdominal ultrasound studies and other tests were normal. Aside from advice to stop her modest drinking, the only other treatment option offered was interferon. She declined the latter because of its inherent severe side effects.

Her tests remained unchanged over the next two years despite total abstention from alcohol. She would not kiss persons for fear of transmitting the presumed infection.

A friend commented that aspartame products could harm the liver. As personal proof, she pointed to the normalization of her own blood studies after discontinuing diet sodas. The patient thereupon discontinued such products – including the seven packs per day (!) of aspartame chewing gum. A dramatic decline of her liver enzymes ensued.

Overwhelmed by this experience, she reported her case to the FDA and criticized its approval of aspartame as "total disregard for human health and safety."

Case IX-K-3

A man had consumed 24-60 ounces of diet sodas daily for a year while on "a very low calorie diet." He experienced numbness of the left hand, left foot, face, and then the right hand. Two MRI studies and other neurologic tests were normal. His liver enzymes, however, were elevated (GGT 350; SGOT 150); repeat testing confirmed these abnormalities. A CT scan of the liver and an ultrasound study of the abdomen were not revealing.

This patient was scheduled for consultation with a gastroenterologist. Learning about aspartame disease in the interim, he stopped aspartame products, and consumed considerable filtered water "in an attempt to flush my liver." Repeat liver tests evidenced progressive declines of the GGT to 15, and of the SGOT to 50. The gastroenterologist disregarded these observations, and criticized the patient's inference about aspartame being a possible cause.

482

Case IX-K-4

The 28-year-old manager of an architectural firm, and mother of a six-month child, had markedly elevated liver enzymes for four years, the cause of which eluded multiple physicians. Her AST, ALT and alkaline phosphatase levels averaged 200, 200 and 1100, respectively. The bilirubin levels remained normal.

She never used drugs of abuse or smoked, and had not ingested alcohol for three years. No birth control pill was used since the age of 21. Numerous studies for hepatitis and HIV viruses, and for various auto-immune diseases were negative. In addition to multiple CT scans and an MRI study, two liver biopsies proved normal.

The patient had "practically lived on" diet cola for ten years... "drinking more than water or any other beverage." This soda was avoided during pregnancy.

After reading about aspartame disease, she stopped all diet products. There was a prompt and striking decrease of all the enzymes, which progressively normalized with no other interventions.

Case IX-K-5 (FDA Project # 3898; Courtesy, Dr. Linda Tollefson)

A 76-year-old woman with longstanding cirrhosis died in progressive "liver coma." In his correspondence to a consumer advocate, her husband indicated that she had been "in pretty good health" until October 1983 when an elevated blood glucose concentration was found. Tolbutamide and diet were prescribed. In an attempt to avoid sugar, she used four packets of an ATS daily in coffee, cereal and desserts.

The patient evidenced dramatic clinical deterioration within two weeks. It was manifest by indifference to her surroundings, forgetfulness, slurred speech, dizziness, impaired vision, loss of interest concerning food and her favorite television programs, and a change in gait. She made irrelevant statements as if hallucinating. Her condition deteriorated to the point of becoming incontinent and bedridden. A diagnosis of "hepatic encephalopathy" was made.

Related Biochemical Aspects

Deterioration of brain function in patients with severe liver disease has been attributed to the <u>retention of phenylalanine and other amino acids</u> (Fischer 1971). Striking changes in amino acid metabolism are known to occur in liver disease – particularly the hydroxylation rates of phenylalanine, tyrosine and tryptophan. The elevated phenylalanine concentrations in patients with cirrhosis rise significantly after protein consumption (Fernstrom 1979).

Methanol poisoning (Chapter XXI) creates another serious problem in patients with liver disease. The enzymes alcohol dehydrogenase and aldehyde dehydrogenase are involved in methanol metabolism. The considerable alcohol dehydrogenase activity of the liver decreases when it is diseased.

One mechanism may be the production of tumor necrosis factor (TNF)-*a*. It is an early event in many types of liver injury that triggers the release of other cytokines, and then the destruction of liver cells.

A vicious cycle involving aggravated hypoglycemia also can occur. Contributory causes include the tendency to "hepatic hypoglycemia" among persons with severe liver disease (owing to difficulty in storing and metabolizing glycogen), aspartame-induced hypoglycemia (Chapter XIV), the use of glucose-lowering drugs for control of diabetes, and the failure of diabetics receiving such drugs or insulin to take interval feedings. For example, the physician who prescribed tolbutamide for Case IX-K-4 "said nothing about diet."

Hemochromatosis (iron storage disease; hepatic iron overload; bronze diabetes) might be aggravated in its pre-cirrhotic stage by aspartame consumption (see Case XIII-1), especially through insulin stimulation (Chapter XIV). Related features of insulin resistance – in addition to hyperinsulinemia – are increased body mass, elevated lipids, and abnormal glucose tolerance.

The separate entity of primary hepatic iron overload differs from genetic hemochromatosis because transferrin saturation is normal, as is the frequency of the HLA A3 genotype (Ferrannini 2000). It has been suggested that insulin's primary action in stimulating glucose transport is coupled with a redistribution of transferrin receptors to the cell surface where they mediate extracellular iron uptake.

SECTION 3

HIGH-RISK GROUPS

"What the American people don't know can
kill them."
> Fred Friendly
> (former president, CBS News)

"By far the most mutagenic agents known to man
are chemicals, not radiation. And in this regard,
food additives rather than fallout at present levels
may present a greater danger."
> Dr. Richard Caldecott (1961)

"Every specialist, whatever his profession,
skill or business may be, can improve his
performance by broadening his base."
> Dr. Wilder Penfield

GENERAL CONSIDERATIONS

Several groups of persons other than those with phenylketonuria or PKU (Chapter XVII) are at higher risk for reactions to aspartame products, even when taken in modest amounts. Foremost are pregnant women, infants and young children, patients having diabetes mellitus, "reactive" hypoglycemia and eating disorders, and individuals with a past history of migraine, epilepsy, alcoholism or drug abuse.

There is an imperative need for such perspectives. It was underscored by testimony given to the United States Senate Committee on Labor and Human Resources on November 3, 1987. FDA Commissioner Frank E. Young indicated that 60 percent of diabetics, 50 percent of persons attempting to lose weight, and 50 percent of women of childbearing age were consuming aspartame products – compared to 35 percent of the total population.

As the author's database expanded, it became obvious that additional groups are at increased risk for aspartame disease.

- Older persons are more vulnerable to medical and intellectual or behavioral deterioration while consuming aspartame (Chapter XV). Moreover, the possible acceleration of Alzheimer's disease by such products (Roberts 1995b) has been raised.
- Relatives of aspartame reactors appear more vulnerable (Chapter XVI).
- Persons with chronic liver disease (Chapter IX-K) and severe renal disease (Pickford 1973, Jones 1978, Stonier 1984) are at increased risk because of their inability to metabolize or excrete aspartame and its breakdown products. The high phenylalanine concentration in uremic patients is attributed to impaired phenylalanine hydroxylation (Fürst 1980). Garibotto et al (1987) demonstrated a disproportionately greater increase of arterial whole blood phenylalanine levels than of other amino acids among patients with chronic renal failure who ingested an amino acid mixture.
- A history of prior allergies was relatively common among aspartame reactors (Chapters VIII and XIX)
- Hypothyroidism (underactive thyroid function) existed or was uncovered in 44 patients with severe aspartame reactions (Chapter IX-E). Conventional doses of drugs are known to have exaggerated pharmacologic effects in hypothyroid patients. It is therefore not surprising that they may evidence higher and/or longer concentrations of aspartame (which was originally developed as a drug), and its breakdown products.

486

- Patients with <u>iron-deficiency anemia</u> have an impaired ability to convert phenylalanine to tyrosine. The heightened phenylalanine concentrations found by L-(^{2}H$_5$) phenylalanine loading were intermediate between normals and heterozygotes for phenylketonuria (Lehmann 1986). The presence of an iron molecule in the enzyme phenylalanine hydroxylase might partly explain the elevated phenylalanine concentrations in persons with iron-deficiency anemia after a phenylalanine load. When their iron status was normalized, the response to phenylalanine challenge normalized.

- Patients with a <u>prior pheochromocytoma</u> (an adrenal tumor producing epinephrine and norepinephrine) should avoid aspartame products. This precaution is similar to their avoidance by persons with previous Graves disease whose condition can be exacerbated or simulated.

- Persons with <u>various enzyme deficiencies affecting the metabolism of neurotransmitters</u>, both congenital and acquired, might have adverse responses to aspartame. For example, <u>congenital dopamine beta-hydroxylase deficiency</u> manifests itself as chronic failure of the autonomic nervous system. (Dopamine derives from phenylalanine.) The abnormalities include severe orthostatic hypotension, skeletal muscle hypotonia, and recurrent hypoglycemia. Very low amounts of dopamine beta-hydroxylase exist in up to four percent of the population, presumably reflecting an inherited autosomal recessive trait. In one patient, neither epinephrine nor norepinephrine were detectable in the plasma, urine or cerebrospinal fluid (In 'T Veld 1987), whereas excessive concentrations of dopamine were found in body fluids.

These high-risk groups assume considerable importance relative to the need for educating both consumers and health professionals about the potential threat posed by aspartame products.

Possible Misdiagnosis of PKU

Persons in several categories risk being misdiagnosed as PKU heterozygotes because of increased fasting phenylalanine-tyrosine ratios and post-load phenylalanine-tyrosine ratios. They include <u>pregnancy</u> (Yakymyshyn 1972), <u>malnutrition</u> (Antener 1981), <u>obesity</u> (Brown 1973), <u>infection</u> (Wannemacher 1976), <u>leukemia</u> (Wang 1961), and women taking <u>oral contraceptive drugs</u> (Landau 1967; Rose 1970; Craft 1971).

X

PREGNANT WOMEN

"The fetus has a unique position legally and medically. It
does not choose many of the things that are imposed
upon him. Hence, he deserves more protection by some
public spokesmen than his mother can provide for him."
Dr. Karlis Adamsons (1973)
(Professor of Obstetrics and Gynecology,
Mount Sinai School of Medicine)

A pregnant woman should abstain from aspartame products to avoid potential damage to herself and her fetus.

Most obstetricians do not appreciate the potential damage to a fetus from consumption of aspartame products during pregnancy, and their delayed manifestations. Some of the neurological, psychological and behavioral problems were considered in Section 2.

Promotion and Disinformation

Many pregnant women and physicians who had inquired about the safety of aspartame products during pregnancy did not receive adequate or truthful information in the author's opinion. Moreover, their use was often encouraged.

- Ads focusing on "blue ribbon babies" underscored the safety of diet sodas and other foods sweetened with aspartame for "eating well during pregnancy."
- A major aspartame producer asserted on the Internet that it is "a trusted choice during pregnancy and while breast feeding."

Acronym Legend
ACB - aspartame cola beverage
ASD - aspartame soft drink
ATS - aspartame tabletop sweetener

487

- A nationally syndicated physician-columnist summarily dismissed products containing aspartame as a factor causing problems for children and pregnant women *(Sun-Sentinel* March 12, 1999). He stated to a concerned mother: "Neither you nor your children are in danger from aspartame."

Warnings

The author's publications and lectures to professionals have raised doubts among some obstetricians. One told a patient, "Aspartame can burn a baby's brain."

There have been analogous warnings about other products. A remark by Horace Greeley might apply to pregnant women who relish aspartame products: "Those who cheer today will curse tomorrow."

- A TV ad urging pregnant women not to use drugs ended with the voice of a child saying, "Mommy, don't!"
- In a prophetic statement, Dr. John W. Olney (cited by Honorof 1975) wrote the FDA, "Unless the FDA acts decisively, aspartame could be another thalidomide tragedy in the making."
- *Pravda,* The Russian paper, reported a warning from the Novosibirsk State Medical Academy that substitution of phenylalanine for sugar in bubble gum may be hazardous for pregnant woman and their children because retardation, delayed growth, and nervous system disorders might result (January 30, 2001). Blond and blue-eyed persons were regarded as being at higher risk due to possible deficient enzyme activity involving the metabolism of phenylalanine.

SYMPTOMATIC ASPARTAME DISEASE

Many unsuspecting women who completed the questionnaire indicated that they had taken aspartame during pregnancy. Some developed nausea, dizziness and other symptoms shortly after using these products. Paradoxically, they considered themselves fortunate because such reactions served as a clear warning to avoid them... at least during pregnancy.

Aspartame-induced hypertension was discussed in Chapter IX-C. The National Institutes of Health expressed concern that the rate of pre-eclampsia (pregnancy-associated hypertension) rose by nearly a third during the 1990s.

Convulsions were among the most alarming aspartame reactions during pregnancy. Walton (1987) reported two pregnant women with aspartame-induced seizures.

Representative Case Report

Case X-1

A young mother called during my interview on a Fort Wayne talk show. She experienced a headache shortly after drinking diet sodas. While doing so on one occasion as she nursed, her child convulsed within minutes. There were no further seizures after she avoided aspartame products.

Altered Maternal Appetite and Weight

Aspartame can reduce appetite and cause weight loss (Chapter IX-B). While many women seek to remain slim during pregnancy, this effort could be harmful. Aspartame-associated failure to gain adequate weight might be disastrous for a fetus, especially among pregnant teenagers. Several mothers attributed the low birth weights of their babies to aspartame use during pregnancy.

These reports are relevant.

- Studies at the University of Washington indicated that expectant adolescents who gave birth to normal-weight infants gained an average of 34.2 pounds during pregnancy. This compared to an optimal gain of 24-28 pounds for older women. The greater gain in weight among the former group probably blunts a number of factors that might adversely influence the outcome of pregnancy, including relative immaturity and marginal nutrition (Rees 1986). Conversely, pregnant teenagers whose weight gain was significantly less tended to have underweight infants.
- A study of 2,000 young women indicated that failure to gain enough weight in the first and second trimesters represents a major cause of low birth weights (*The Palm Beach Post* November 22, 1991, p. A-6).

MATERNAL-FETAL PHENYLALANINE CONCENTRATIONS

Brain growth is maximum during the third trimester of pregnancy and the first year of life. Consequently, elevated phenylalanine concentrations (see below) are likely to cause harm at these critical periods.

The National Collaborative Study for Maternal PKU recommended that blood phenylalanine levels not exceed 6 mg percent during pregnancy. Yet Matalon et al (1987) detected higher concentrations in 14 percent of normals, and in 35 percent of PKU carriers who took 100 mg aspartame/kg/day. High concentrations of phenylalanine inhibit specific ATP-sulfurylase activity and decrease the synthesis of sulfatides required for proper development of myelin in the central nervous system at this critical time (Hommes 1987).

Dr. Louis J. Elsas, II (Professor of Pediatrics, Emory University School of Medicine) emphasized the neurotoxicity of excess phenylalanine in his statement for the Labor and Human Resource Committee of the U.S. Senate on November 3, 1987. Both the acute and chronic ingestion of aspartame (34 mg/kg/day) resulted in two- to five-fold increases of maternal blood phenylalanine concentrations. They may be magnified up to sixfold in a developing fetus because of its concentration by the placenta. Accordingly, a maternal phenylalanine level of 150 µmol/L could reach 900µmol/L in developing fetal brain cells... a concentration sufficient to kill them in tissue culture. Irreversible brain damage also might occur in the rapidly growing post-natal brain (children up to 12 months). These changes are manifest in adults by slowing of the electroencephalogram and prolongation of cognitive function tests. Dr. Elsas suggested, "Declare an immediate moratorium on the addition of aspartame to more foods, and remove it from all low-protein beverages, foods, and children's medications."

Other investigators corroborate these warnings.

- Dr. William Pardridge (*Congressional Record-Senate* 1985, p. 5495; 1986) emphasized that elevated blood phenylalanine levels constitute a high risk for the developing fetus.
- Pitkin (1984) demonstrated a significant accumulation of radioactive-carbon-labeled phenylalanine in the fetal circulation of primates after administering this tracer intravenously to the mother.
- Plasma phenylalanine levels in normal pregnant women (averaging 3-5 µmol/L) could double after ingesting phenylalanine-containing foods (Pitkin 1984). Were they to take "potential abuse concentrations" of aspartame (100-200 mg/kg body weight), the levels would be even higher – with fetal phenylalanine levels twice those of the mother.

NEUROLOGICAL AND BEHAVIORAL ABNORMALITIES IN OFFSPRING

Many women who had consumed aspartame during prior pregnancies anguished over its possible contributory role in the neurologic problems afflicting their children.

- The children of several who drank diet colas during the relevant gestation had a severe attention deficit disorder (Chapter VI-G).
- "During my pregnancy, I was The Aspartame Queen. My child was born with a neurological condition."
- The mother of a 9-year-old daughter with neurological problems and an arachnoid cyst was "an adamant diet cola drinker" from conception until the sixth month of pregnancy when she learned about aspartame reactions.
- The dual complications of aspartame-associated brain damage and blindness in a fetus are suggested by a case report submitted to the FDA (Project # 1716). The mother consumed two diet sodas daily during pregnancy. Her child was blind in both eyes and manifested brain damage since birth (courtesy, Dr. Linda Tollefson, September 2, 1987).
- The youngest child of a woman who ingested considerable diet cola during that pregnancy expressed remorse for having done so. Her son evidenced failure to thrive, petit mal and grand mal seizures, and subsequent emotional immaturity.

A relationship clearly exists between increased maternal-fetal phenylalanine concentrations (see above) and ensuing adverse effects in the brain.

- A fivefold increase in the plasma phenylalanine concentration (as from 50 to 250 µmol/L) can cause impairment of brain function in a developing fetus or child (Pardridge 1986).
- The IQ of babies born to mothers with 250 µmol/L increments in the blood phenylalanine level is significantly lower (Levy 1983; Kirkman 1984).
- Mahalik and Gautieri (1984) reported that aspartame administration to mice during late pregnancy delayed the achievement age for visual placing in the offspring.
- Lewis et al (1985) demonstrated that slightly elevated maternal phenylalanine and tyrosine blood levels resulting from theadministration of aspartame to rats prior to conception resulted in microcephaly and lasting behavioral problems. These problems, entailing hyperactivity and learning difficulty, were noted earlier.

The risks to infants whose mothers consume aspartame while breast-feeding will be discussed in Chapter XI.

Representative Case Reports

Case X-2

A 42-year-old woman had consumed two to three cans of aspartame sodas more than 11 years, including while pregnant. She developed a number of symptoms attributable to aspartame disease – namely, headache, dizziness, a seizure, abdominal pain, intense itching, pain in multiple joints, and progressive gain of weight.

Her daughter exhibited attention deficit disorder, and a "mild encephalopathy of unknown origin" along with "language dysfunction," anger, mood swings, immune problems, and chronic yeast/sinus infections. The mother added that she also drank aspartame-containing beverages while nursing.

Case X-3

A 21-year-old "aspartame addict" consumed numerous diet colas daily during her pregnancy. She was found to have gestational diabetes, her blood glucose concentration once being 600 mg percent. Although placed on a strict diet, she did not avoid diet cola. Her son was autistic and "very nonverbal." When pregnant five years later, she did not consume diet sodas and had a normal boy.

Other Contributory Mechanisms

Additional adverse effects of aspartame, discussed elsewhere, are appropriate for mention.

- The methyl alcohol of aspartame (Chapter XXI) poses a unique problem during pregnancy. It is known that ethyl alcohol taken during gestation can influence the subsequent behavior and intelligence of children. For example, a 14-year study of 1,500 women and their offspring, conducted by the Department of Psychiatry and Behavioral Sciences at the University of Washington, indicated that children born to mothers who drank alcohol during pregnancy had shorter attention spans and slower reaction times... independent of the "fetal alcohol syndrome" *(The Palm Beach Post* January 17, 1987, p. A-1.

- Hypothyroidism early in life can retard somatic growth and mental development (Sokoloff 1967). Accordingly, any interference with thyroid function by aspartame (Chapter IX-E) during pregnancy could have comparable consequences.

- There is experimental evidence that the blockade of N-methyl-D-aspartate (NMDA) glutamate receptors by drugs during late pregnancy can result in neurodevelopmental disorders *(The Lancet* 1999; 353:126).

THE ISSUE OF BIRTH DEFECTS

Any reasonable doubt concerning the safety of a drug, additive, or amino acid "supplement" during pregnancy MUST be investigated.

Mention was made of "clueless" aspartame victims who had children with birth defects, and later connected these issues. The scoffing by physicians of such a carefully considered idea profoundly shocked these intelligent persons

The author has received many poignant case histories about severe birth defects from mothers who consumed aspartame products during pregnancy, and even from parents who did so at the time of conception. These "anecdotes" serve as constructive insights for the initiation of valid epidemiologic studies in the hope of sparing others comparable anguish.

- A young couple consumed considerable amounts of aspartame. Their first child had multiple congenital defects, and died three days after birth. I was not aware of this until the husband returned for a visit because of aggravated reactive hypoglycemia. His symptoms promptly abated after avoiding aspartame. The wife, a diabetic, did likewise. When seen two years later, the patient proudly displayed a picture of his "completely healthy" 9-week-old son.
- The daughter of a heavy consumer of diet sodas was born without a uterus. The mother suffered intense migraine. After learning about aspartame disease, she avoided these products – with "almost immediate" relief of her headaches. She reflected, "I am inclined to believe that aspartame was the cause of my daughter's birth defect. It doesn't make me feel good knowing that what I consumed may have caused the problem, but it makes a lot of sense."
- A London dietitian reported that her daughter had been born unable to swallow or speak, and still could not do so at the age of two. She added, "I am a dietitian, and have always felt uneasy with the amount of diet cola I drink!"
- A husband wrote, "We tried to conceive for five years, but with great difficulty. We have had three pregnancies, all of which resulted in

miscarriage at different stages. During the 20th week of the last pregnancy, the fetus was diagnosed with hypophosphatasia, a rare and lethal deformity. My wife and I had chewed a pack of sugarless gum daily for approximately 10 years."

- A professional correspondent who had personally suffered aspartame disease was impressed by the occurrence of esophageal defects in the babies of women consuming aspartame products during pregnancy. Pursuing this association, he found an increased number of operations for such disorders at his institution.

- One aspartame complainant requested a Federal District Court to temporarily restrain the use of aspartame as a food additive. The request followed discovery of gross abnormalities in the fetus of a woman who consumed several aspartame products daily during early pregnancy (cited by Reschevsky 1986).

- Another birth defect attributed to aspartame use during pregnancy is craniosynostosis. In this condition, the bones of the skull close prematurely, causing the head and facial features to be severely misshapen – at times with decreased brain size (microcephaly). The mother of such a patient "drank a ton" of aspartame iced tea during the last trimester.

- The mother of three children switched to diet sodas when told she had borderline diabetes during her first pregnancy. The child, a girl, had learning disabilities and attention-deficit disorder. She continued using diet drinks during her second pregnancy. The child, a boy, was born with a "rare birth defect" and suffered seizures. Her third baby was also born with a heart defect; she required surgery at two days of age. In addition to developing overt diabetes, this woman gained weight ("even though I had not changed my eating habits"), and suffered anxiety/panic attacks, headaches, impaired vision, memory loss, and personality changes. Her anxiety attacks improved after avoiding diet sodas.

The dangers to a fetus posed by chemicals and drugs provide added perspective.

- It is axiomatic that a fetus should not be exposed to methyl alcohol (Chapter XXI). The teratogenic potential of formaldehyde formed during its metabolism has been documented. Similarily, the decline in neural-tube defects following fortification of grain products with folic acid might be less evident among pregnant women who consume aspartame products due to the ensuring depletion of folate levels (Chapter IX-J-C).

- The tragic birth defects attributed to thalidomide and to doxylamine succinate (used for treating nausea during pregnancy) received international attention.

- Congenital malformations and central nervous dysfunction afflicted the infants of mothers who had used psychoactive drugs (such as the benzodiazepines) during gestation (Laegreid 1987).

- There is considerable scientific evidence that the fetus can suffer serious effects from pesticides and other chemicals at lower levels of exposure than adults.

Representative Case Report

Case X-4

A 34-year-old teacher ingested two cans of an ASD, one or two packets of an ATS, one glass of presweetened iced tea, one glass of another aspartame beverage, and two bowls of cereal containing aspartame daily for two months. Such consumption began immediately prior to conception, and continued during the first two months of pregnancy. During this time, she experienced severe headache, lightheadedness and foot numbness.

Fetal malformations were suspected on the basis of repeat ultrasound studies, and confirmed by amniocentesis. Her pregnancy was terminated at the 18th week. An autopsy revealed deformed limbs, unusual skin changes, and chromosomal abnormalities consistent with Turner's syndrome. She offered these recommendations concerning the regulation of aspartame: "Don't use if pregnant!" Her husband also consumed aspartame. His complaints included headache, insomnia and depression.

Mechanisms

Many of the mechanisms mentioned earlier could be operative in aspartame-associated birth defects. The concentration of methanol-derived formaldehyde in DNA is considered in Chapter XXI.

The following information is germane.

- Pregnancy itself tends to impair the conversion of phenylalanine to tyrosine (Yaymyshyn 1972).
- Cleft lip and cleft palate occur more often in persons having PKU and hyperphenylalinemia (Tocci 1973).

- Folic acid deficiency caused by formic acid (Chapter IX-J) is conducive to birth defects.
- Exposure in early pregnancy to folic acid antagonists, including some common drugs, may increase not only neural-tube defects, but also cardiovascular defects, oral clefts, and urinary tract defects (Hernandez-Diaz 2000).
- Aspartame can alter human diploid cells in culture, with a corresponding decrease of mitochondrial activity (Kasamaki 1993).
- Brunner et al (1979) continuously exposed rats to aspartame before conception, and for three months after birth. They reported delays in eye-opening, surface-righting, swimming development, forward quadripedal locomotor development, hypoactivity, and delayed auditory startle. Decreased brain weight and lower cerebellar olfactory granule cell counts were found.
- Products from the browning reaction (Chapter XXV) caused by the reaction of amino acids and sugars during cooking include a variety of DNA-damaging agents that may be highly mutagenic and even carcinogenic (Abelson 1983).

RELATED CONSIDERATIONS

In his 1910 analysis of premature senility, Arnold Lorand emphasized that persons so afflicted may be "the victims of the immoderation of their ancestors." He emphasized that pregnant woman should avoid "anything that may prove fatal to the foetus or influence its nutrition," especially the use of drugs.

A pressing need exists for corporate-neutral studies to determine whether the incidence of chromosomal abnormalities and congenital deformities is increased among women who consumed aspartame at the time of conception and during pregnancy. This also applies to the female fetus because all the ova (eggs) she will ever have are vulnerable to genetic damage. Suggestive experimental data exists. The tragedy involving Case X-4 underscores this issue.

Dr. Robert H. Moser (1969) wrote in *Diseases of Medical Progress*: "Our reverses have been minor when contrasted to our advances, but negative effects cannot be ignored or derogated... the thalidomide disaster indicated how expensive it can be."*

---

*From Moser, R.H.: *Diseases of Medical Progress: A Study of Iatrogenic Disease.* 3rd Edition, 1969. Courtesy of Charles C Thomas, Publisher, Springfield, Illinois.

There is experimental evidence that exposure *to chemicals and other adverse influences during pregnancy can affect subsequent generations independent of genetic factors.*

Gauguier et al (1990) rendered rat dams (F-0) hyperglycemic during the last week of pregnancy by a continuous glucose infusion. The females born of these rats (F-1) exhibited glucose intolerance and impaired insulin secretion in adulthood. They were mated at three months with males born of control dams. The F-2 newborns of F-1 hyperglycemic dams evidenced the main features of newborns from diabetic mothers – namely, hyperglycemia, hyperinsulinemia and macrosomia – with subsequent hyperglycemia and defective insulin secretion as adults.

Neuroscientists increasingly are impressed by <u>the importance of extragenetic factors on brain architecture and development</u> (Barnes 1986). Neuronal activity and brain circuitry (such as synaptic connections) can be profoundly influenced during embryonic development by malnutrition, chemical factors, drugs and toxins. This has been impressive in the microanatomy of neuronal connections to and within the visual cortex, as evidenced by the inability of nerve cells to migrate at the proper time and along the correct pathways. Other than phenylketonuria (Chapter XVII), the author is not aware of published studies by geneticists concerning the effects of aspartame in familial disorders characterized by severe brain damage.

- A gene regulating the production of aspartocyclase, an enzyme that controls the amount of N-acetylaspartic acid, is lacking in children with <u>Canavan disease</u>.
- Patients afflicted with <u>the fragile X syndrome</u> evidence hyperactivity, autistic features and intellectual impairment, particularly boys who inherit this trait. Although previously thought to be rare, it has emerged as the second most common form of mental retardation (after Down's syndrome or mongolism).

XI

INFANTS AND CHILDREN

"We owe our children a set of good habits, for habit is to be either their best friend or their worst enemy, not only during childhood, but through all the years."
George Herbert Betts (1868-1934)
(Fathers and Mothers)

"The chemicals we ingest may affect more than our own health. They affect the health and vitality of future generations. The danger is that many of these chemicals may not harm us, but will later do silent violence to our children."
Senator Abraham S. Ribicoff (1971)

Aspartame reactors and their relatives have decried the promotion of aspartame products for infants and children as "crimes against humanity." Clinical and scientific observations bolster this assertion.

The author's data on the adverse effects of aspartame in infants and children warrant two conclusions. First, nursing mothers ought not consume aspartame while breast-feeding. Second, parents should try to minimize the consumption of aspartame products by their children... and grandchildren. These issues are poignantly demonstrated by the occurrence of seizures in a suckling infant as its mother drank an aspartame soda.

Acronym Legend
    ACB - aspartame cola beverage
    ASD - aspartame soft drink
    ATS - aspartame tabletop sweetener

Others concur. The European Union banned the addition of aspartame in any food consumed by infants (Directive 96/83/EC).

Of the 397 aspartame reactors in the initial survey, eight were less than 10 years, and nine were 11-20 years.

The vulnerability of children to aspartame neurotoxicity is reinforced by many observations. For example, the density of synapses in the human cerebral cortex reaches its maximum at the age of three years, concomitant with peaking of the cerebral metabolic rate between 3 and 4 years (Huttenlocher 1990).

Methanol Exposure

The adverse effects on a fetus of excess phenylalanine and aspartic acid during pregnancy (Chapter X) and in infancy are considered below and elsewhere.

The hazards of methanol exposure to an infant from the breast milk of a mother drinking aspartame sodas or using other aspartame products can be profound. The level of alcohol dehydrogenase activity during the first year of life is less than 50 percent of that in adults (Pikkarainen 1967). Moreover, there is evidence for impaired neurologic development among children exposed to alcohol through breast milk (Little 1989).

GENERAL CONSIDERATIONS

Consumption of Aspartame by Children

The magnitude of aspartame consumption was described in the Overview. These supplemental observations are relevant.

- Nearly 40 percent of children up to the age of nine regularly drink soft drinks containing artificial sweeteners according to National Center for Health Statistics.
- Parents frequently give toddlers diet sodas at famous theme parks.
- A physician expressed concern over repeatedly observing second- and third-grade children standing at bus stops with diet colas in their hands (*The Palm Beach Post* August 14, 1998, p. A-4.).
- A survey for the Department of Agriculture by National Analysis Inc. indicated that one- to three-year-old children consume about two ounces soft drinks daily. Inasmuch as only 25.4 percent of the 312 children so tested drank any soft drinks, the mean consumption for those ingesting carbonated beverages was actually <u>seven</u> fluid ounces.

Concerning the maximum allowable daily intake (ADI) of 50 mg/kg body weight (Chapter XXVII-D), approximately five servings of an aspartame pudding by a 50-pound child, or equivalent servings of other aspartame products, amounts to 50 mg/kg.

"Sweet Innocence"

Without a widespread educational or regulatory effort, it is unlikely that the current enormous consumption of aspartame by children will decrease.

- The lasting impact of television commercials was encapsuled in the quip that children learn their NBCs and CBSs before their ABCs.
- In one television advertisement, a little boy refers to aspartame as "the good stuff."

The children-at-risk theme is compounded by a national disgrace: the prevalent "fear of fat" among young children, especially in affluent families and communities (Chapter IX-B). This morbid obsession about weight gain was discussed at length in *Sweet'ner Dearest* (Roberts 1992a). For example, one-third of children under ten years of age <u>actively</u> worry about becoming fat!

Nutritional Deficiencies

It is the general consensus that regular and diet soft drinks have limited nutritional value for children. The tendency of teenagers to substitute them for milk incurs the added problems of reduced calcium, vitamin A, vitamin C and riboflavin intake. Other considerations are the erosion of tooth enamel by acidic cola beverages (even when devoid of sugar) and increased fractures (Wyshak 2000).

The hazards of absent or limited food intake by children before going to school become compounded when they take aspartame sodas as "breakfast." Some surveys indicate that as many as 30 percent of school-age children do not eat anything at home prior to school (*Sun-Sentinel* March 4, 1999, p. B-9).

The use of aspartame-sweetened foods and beverages by young children incurs two other risks: a life-long preference for sugars and sweets rather than "good nutrition," and aspartame addiction (Chapter VII-G).

Corporate Promotion and Bias

Corporate-sponsored studies concluding that aspartame is safe for infants and children require scrutiny of their protocols and data (Section 7). These should indicate the manner of processing and delivering aspartame drinks and foods – such as specific reference to the dates of manufacture, duration of storage, and maintained temperature of soft drinks supplied in coded bottles.

- A professor of pediatrics disclaimed any adverse effects of aspartame products on child behavior in a lecture. When the writer asked about the method of preparation and the temperature of the aspartame drinks administered, he was unaware of these details.

- The conclusion by Wolraich et al (1994) that neither aspartame nor sucrose affect the behavior and cognitive function of children is diametrically opposite to longstanding observations by the writer and others.

- The data on problems relating to sugar intake, and the ensuing hyperinsulinized state, were summarized in a clinical and metabolic reevaluation of reading disability (Roberts 1969b). Concomitant clinical problems (e.g., hyperactivity and unrecognized narcolepsy due to recurrent cerebral glucopenia), and the need for preventing severe nocturnal hypoglycemia in children were emphasized. (Striking improvement in reading, hyperactivity, drowsiness and growth problems often followed the institution of a proper diet and supportive measures.)

Lack of Awareness by Pediatricians

Many pediatricians remain unaware of aspartame disease. An unexpected encounter at a large pediatrics seminar illustrates the point.

A visiting professor of pediatrics emphasized the safety of breast milk while discussing the management of infection. He challenged the audience to name any substance consumed by breast-feeding infants that increased risk.

When the author mentioned aspartame, he threw up his hands in disbelief and exclaimed, "Oh, give me a break!"

As the parents of two chemically sensitive children, Ken and Jan Nolley (1987) stressed the serious shortcomings of pediatricians and other physicians in this realm, along with the limited reliability of diagnostic procedures. They added, "These patients apparently were quite accurate in their accounts to physicians, even in the face of contrary prevalent medical opinion."

Needless Exposure to Radiation

Many of the young aspartame reactors in this series were exposed to radiation for diagnostic purposes (see Case XI-3). Such studies included x-rays of the stomach, small intestine and large bowel for suspected peptic ulcer, Crohn's disease or ulcerative colitis (Chapter IX-D), and the entire gamut of radiologic studies for suspected brain lesions (Chapters II, V and VI).

Family Tribulations

Case III-20 illustrates the anguish among families of children with aspartame-induced convulsions and other reactions. This ordeal became compounded when multiple children in the same family (see Cases III-22 and III-23) suffered seizures after aspartame use, especially in the case of mothers who consumed aspartame during pregnancy and while nursing.

Unrecognized Sources of Aspartame and Phenylalanine

Parents and physicians generally do not realize that many over-the-counter and prescription drugs intended for use by young children contain aspartame. These include tasty suspensions (especially in cherry and grape flavors), and chewable tablets of antibiotics or analgesics. Correspondents repeatedly express concern over the frequency with which vitamin products used by children contain aspartame. Finding calcium supplements that do not contain aspartame poses a special problem for the parents of young children having milk intolerance. Locating aspartame-free acetaminophen for children usually requires much diligence, but such products can be found (Chapter XXXIV).

Iatrogenic (doctor-induced) problems also are caused by the administration of phenylalanine to infants.

- Puntis et al (1986) emphasized the serious nature of neurotoxic hyperphenylalaninemia in newborn babies give intravenous solutions of amino acids. It may be exacerbated by the addition of breast milk. One such child evidenced cerebral atrophy and delayed motor development at one year.

- Walker et al (1986) found high plasma phenylalanine concentrations in two newborn babies during total parenteral nutrition (TPN). Their studies indicate that combined intravenous phenylalanine-tyrosine loads are probably excessive for sick infants because of immature livers. They urged re-evaluation of the phenylalanine content of amino acid mixtures used on pediatric units owing to the inherent neurotoxicity.
- Evans et al (1986) found different phenylalanine concentrations in commercial solutions used for TPN of newborns. They suggested monitoring infants receiving this therapy, especially when premature, to maintain phenylalanine concentrations at 200-500 μmol/liter.

ADVERSE EFFECTS

Children can evidence aspartame disease in a variety of ways. Headache, convulsions, rashes and asthmatic breathing were considered in earlier chapters. The dramatic onset of seizures in children shortly after consuming aspartame products is illustrated by Case III-21b, a two-year-old boy. Similarly, a 6-year-old boy had been well until he vomited and was given a popular pediatric acetaminophen product. A fatal seizure followed for which no abnormality could be found at autopsy.

Severe aspartame-induced reactions have occurred among children in a special context: Halloween. They were handed aspartame candy and gum by well-meaning neighbors who wished to avoid giving sugar "treats." Headache, vomiting and severe tremors were the most frequent symptoms.

There may be considerable associated anxiety. An increasing concern of children having frequent headache is shared by their parents: the possibility of a existing brain tumor (Chapter XXVII-F).

Abnormal Behavior (Chapter VII-D)

Irritability, aggression, hyperactivity ("the need to keep moving"), crying, whining, impulsivity, slurred speech, and learning problems have been associated with or aggravated by the use of aspartame products. Some concerned teacher-correspondents attributed the increased frequency of attention deficit/hyperactivity disorder (Chapter VI-G) and declining school grades to their widespread consumption. These changes have been variously referred to as "Jekyll and Hyde behavior" and "the Halloween effect."

The following experience of <u>Dr. Miguel Baret Daniel</u> in the Dominican Republic (personal communication, November 19, 1999) underscores the adverse mental effects of aspartame in children.

> "I have been working with a pediatrician giving nutritional support to children with diabetes. Since cow's milk has a specific protein that can cause diabetes, especially in children, I removed milk from the diet of 360 children studying in public schools in my country. These 360 children were not diabetic, but I removed the milk for prevention. The pediatrician started noticing that a considerable number were having what I call a kind of "brain allergy" – showing abnormal restlessness, lack of concentration, irritability and depression. In the beginning, I suspected it was happening because of the extreme heat we were having those days. But then the weather changed, and the situation didn't get better. So, I took a look at their diet and discovered that ALL of them were drinking a lot of one kind of concentrated juice sweetened with ASPARTAME. They drank about 6 oz twice a day.
>
> "I talked to their parents, and asked them to impress upon the children that they should not drink that juice anymore for a while. The results were as astonishing. Their symptoms disappeared within 4-5 days in ALL of them!"

There is increased concern that <u>the reflexive prescription of psychotropic drugs</u> for children manifesting behavioral and neurological problems has created a "generation Rx." A dramatic increase in prescribed psychotropic medications for preschoolers (ages 2 to 4 years) occurred between 1991 and 1995, based on analysis of the ambulatory care records from two state Medicaid programs and a salaried group model health maintenance organization (HMO) (Zito 2000). The majority were for stimulants – methylphenidate (Ritalin) in 90 percent. The other frequent ones were clonidine and neuroleptics.

- The *Congressional Record-Senate* (1985a, p. 5495) cited the erratic behavior of a four-year-old boy who drank an aspartame soft drink over a three-week period. His behavior normalized within 24 hours after stopping this product. A violent recurrence ensued within 30 minutes after rechallenge two weeks later.
- Severe behavioral changes in a five-year-old boy consuming aspartame were noted in a subsequent *Congressional Record-Senate* report (1985b).

- A young mother told the author that her autistic child became extremely agitated whenever he consumed diet sodas. She pleaded that parents having "exceptional" children should not allow them to use aspartame products.

The following extraordinary coincidence is germane.

> Waiting to be interviewed on March 11, 1987 by Irv Homer, a popular talk-show host on Philadelphia Station WWDB, I was shocked to hear in the national news of the death of four teenagers who died from carbon monoxide poisoning in a locked car "suicide pact." The announcer asked, "Why did they do it?" Shortly after my interview began, the host sought an example of aberrant behavior by children consuming aspartame. I replied: "Although I don't know the circumstances involved or their nutritional habits, the deaths of the four teenagers just mentioned could qualify. And since aspartame reactions tend to occur in families, the fact that two were sisters would increase my suspicion."

Reference was made in Chapter VII to increased <u>criminal behavior</u> by young children and teenagers. Many sociological factors are operative in adolescent violence. They include prolonged conflict at home, difficulties in communication with parents, the ineffectiveness or absence of parental discipline, exposure to substance-abusing parents, and violence shown on television. To these must be added the possible contributory role of aspartame disease in view of the massive advertising campaigns for these products specifically directed to children.

Attention-Deficit/Hyperactivity

The attention-deficit/hyperactivity disorder was discussed in Chapter VI-G. Many concerned parents and teachers have attributed its increase to the consumption of aspartame products. Their effects, coupled with inadequate sleep due to late television viewing, aggravate fatigue and impaired attention. Sally Dunday, Director of the Hyperactive Children's Support Group (personal communication, October 21, 1999), reinforced the author's implication of aspartame as a contributory factor.

Aspartame Addiction

A number of parents have been appalled by the "addiction" of their children to aspartame sodas and other products. This phenomenon is detailed in Chapter VII-G.

Cognitive Problems

The deterioration of intelligence and learning skills in aspartame reactors, as evidenced by slippage in school performance, was discussed in Chapter VI-L. It may take a generation or longer to ascertain the full extent of this problem.

Levy and Waisbren (1987) regarded the assertion by Pardridge that "a 10.5-point drop in the IQ of babies born of mothers with 250μmol/L increments in the blood phenylalanine level" as an incorrect interpretation of their data. Admittedly, it has not been definitively determined whether the effects on brain function of elevated maternal phenylalanine levels follow a linear or threshold pattern. On the other hand, Pardridge (1987, p. 206) emphasized that the 10 mg/kg aspartame intake referred to by Levy and Waisbren as "large amounts of aspartame" could be consumed at one sitting by a 50-pound child drinking a **single** can (12 ounces) of such a beverage!

Depression and Suicide

Aspartame-induced depression and suicidal thoughts (Chapter VII-B) have been discussed previously, as were oft-associated anorexia nervosa and bulimia (Chapter IX-B). The following points warrant emphasis.

- An estimated ten percent of teenagers suffer significant depression.
- The relation between "junk food" and depression in children seems convincing.
- The superimposition of aspartame-induced emotional reactions upon existing social and medical problems among children and teenagers could have tragic consequences.
- The rate of suicide among teenagers, especially white males, is increasing. This was underscored by the 1986 annual *Morbidity and Mortality Weekly Report*.

Several aspartame reactors expressed concern about a link between aspartame consumption and suicide in young persons.

- A 62-year-old woman experienced depression and suicidal thoughts while consuming an aspartame beverage. She also suffered a marked decrease of vision in both eyes, insomnia, severe tremors, ringing in the ears, facial pains, slurred speech, personality changes, shortness of breath, palpitations, diarrhea, abdominal bloat, itching and severe joint pains. There was improvement within six days after discontinuing aspartame. Two sisters, a grandson, a brother, and her husband also suffered from disorders that promptly improved or disappeared after avoiding aspartame products. She wrote:

> "I think that aspartame is at the bottom of many suicides in teens. They get much more than most adults, and anything is enough to set them off in a depression. Someone needs to check the teenage suicidal tendency and see how much (aspartame) they consume."

- A 43-year-old attorney attributed severe depression to aspartame. His niece also suffered depression and menstrual changes while consuming such products. He pleaded, "Please research as many suicides as you can regarding quantity consumed prior to the act. Also child abuse: Watch in particular the teen suicide situation!"

Gastrointestinal Reactions

The severe gastrointestinal reactions in children associated with aspartame use are illustrated by the ordeal of Case XI-5.

Hypothyroidism

The presence of aspartame or increased phenylalanine (especially its D-stereoisomer) in maternal milk, pediatric formulas and other products fed infants may adversely affect thyroid development. The first two weeks after birth can be critical in this regard. It is known that bottle-fed infants are more prone to develop thyroid pathology (notably hypothyroidism) than breast-fed controls.

There are close biochemical relationships between phenylalanine, tyrosine and the major thyroid hormones. Accordingly, elevated phenylalanine and tyrosine concentrations in the milk of lactating mothers (Baker 1984) might influence a neonate's thyroid function.

The children of mothers with hypothyroidism (particularly if unrecognized) and other thyroid disorders (Chapter IX-E) are likely to be at greater risk.

One in 3,000-4,000 infants have congenital hypothyroidism. There are few symptoms and signs at this early period. The disorder can have drastic consequences, however, relative to physical and mental retardation (Sokoloff 1967). These infants also have a higher incidence of congenital heart disease, non-cardiac malformations, and the respiratory distress syndrome (Fernhoff 1987). They probably reflect insults during embryonic life that concomitantly disrupted thyroid gland development, perhaps from a maternally-derived immunoglobulin crossing the placenta during the second and third months.

Allergies

The aggravation of allergies in children by aspartame (Chapter VIII) should be cause for concern. They include hives, other rashes, and asthma.

The increased frequency and severity of asthma during the previous decade is pertinent. For example, asthmatic children may suffer attacks when prescribed chewable tablets that contain aspartame.

Obesity

Childhood obesity has assumed epidemic proportions, especially in the large northeast cities. More than 20 percent of American children are overweight, representing a doubling over the past two decades. The contributory role of aspartame (Chapter IX-B) must considered along with decreased physical activity.

The striking increase of soft drink consumption (both sugar- and artificially sweetened) by adolescents has been invoked as one reason for this concomitant rise of obesity. A possible explanation is the less complete compensation at subsequent meals for energy consumed in liquid than solid form (Chapter IX - B-3).

Children having a compulsion to gorge food because of medical disorders should avoid aspartame products. They include the Prader-Willi syndrome.

Other Disorders

Fruit-flavored drinks pose another risk for young children: severe decay of the front teeth caused by highly acidic drinks that are constantly sipped from a bottle rather than being served in a cup.

The encounter of patients with <u>sleep apnea</u> attributable in part to aspartame use (Chapter VI-K) suggests caution with these products, especially relative to the sudden infant death syndrome (SIDS).

An aspartame reaction should be considered when entertaining the diagnosis of "<u>benign paroxysmal vertigo of childhood</u>" in which there is no loss of consciousness.

Aspartame disease must be considered when the "<u>chronic fatigue syndrome</u>" (CFS) in children remains unexplained.

There is concern about the recent rise of <u>early puberty</u> among girls before the age of eight, most notably as breast devolvement. It may be triggered primarily by aspartame-associated hormonal influences and childhood obesity.

Representative Case Reports

Case XI-1

An 8-year-old girl experienced severe headache daily. Concerned over the constant need for aspirin, her mother planned to obtain medical consultation. The child then stated that the headaches **predictably** occurred ten minutes after chewing gum containing aspartame. They promptly ceased when the gum was avoided.

Case XI-2

A 7-year-old girl suffered severe diarrhea shortly after drinking an aspartame soda. It promptly recurred on each of the four subsequent occasions she drank this product, necessitating absence from school.

Case XI-3

A 2-1/2 year-old girl had been drinking up to six cans of an ASD and two glasses of another ASD daily when she experienced a "focal seizure" involving the right side of her body lasting 45 minutes. Extensive studies – including two sets of head x-rays, a CT scan and an MRI study of the brain, and two electroencephalograms – were normal. When reports of comparable aspartame-induced reactions were found, it was concluded that the seizure was due to aspartame. The child's mother had aspartame-induced headache.

Case XI-4

A 13-year-old girl was diagnosed as having hypoglycemia at the age eight years. She avoided sugar, and used considerable diet soda and an ATS as substitutes.

The patient complained of severe abdominal pain, nausea, dizziness ("could hardly hold the head up"), headache, severe mood changes, and difficulty with vision ("everything was very blurred"). She developed an extensive rash over the body and face, with "blistered cheeks and sores on the face that would get real red. The blisters would go away in a few days, but came back again." Her mother also noted a craving for aspartame products.

The child underwent numerous studies, including gastrointestinal X-rays. Only nonspecific enlarged gastric folds were found.

The mother happened to view a talk show on which aspartame disease was discussed. She called her daughter's physician to mention this possibility. "He said he had never heard of it."

The child improved within several days after avoiding aspartame products. A dietitian then placed her on a diet containing aspartame, which precipitated a recurrence of symptoms within two days. Aspartame products were totally avoided thereafter. The mother stated, "She was a different child. You just would not believe the difference it made. We have got to put a stop to this on the market."

Case XI-5

The following correspondence was received from a mother who wished to "share our nightmare experience" concerning her son's ordeal.

> "Our son, D__, age 13, had been very ill since November 1986. Initially, his severe chest pains were diagnosed as an ulcer. Tests for a hiatal hernia proved inconclusive. Tagamet® was prescribed, but the pain continued and increased.

> "Upper GIs were done. EKGs were done. A gastroscopy was done, as were sonar tests for a possible gall bladder problem. Countless stool samples also were run.

> "His pains in both the chest and abdomen continued. His heart beat became irregular on occasion, especially after strenuous

exercise. This pain became nearly constant, and was there upon rising in the morning. It became acute after meals. Severe attacks followed exercise. Breathing became constricted during the attacks. Difficulty in swallowing on occasion brought him great fear. During severe bouts, the hands and feet were like ice, and all color was drained, leaving him nearly white as a sheet.

"Doctors at this point said it was psychological. They insisted that because of "puberty" and "stress", D,____ could not cope, and probably needed counseling. God was merciful to us. He pressed upon me the word aspartame.

"We are a family with diabetes problems (my husband and oldest son), and are also battling Candida due to excessive antibiotics. Therefore sugar has been stricken from our diet. In retrospect, now that D____'s ordeal is over, I can readily see how the attacks were directly associated with the increased consumption of aspartame. The attacks during exercise often were on the heels of a meal in which diet drinks were used.

"Other members of my family experience headache and stomach distress from aspartame, but never such severe symptoms as those disabling D____. Having removed ALL items containing aspartame from his diet, the pains ceased."The sad note of all this is that even when I was totally sure aspartame had caused our nine-month nightmare, the doctors would not believe me. The usual response was, 'I've never heard of that!'

"The tragic thing is that for diabetics and such there is little alternative. Very subtly, the other non-nutritive sweeteners have been replaced by aspartame dietetic items.

"After we discovered the cause of D____'s pain, we also learned of another young teenager who experienced similar problems, though not as severe. She recovered promptly after stopping diet colas."

OTHER PERTINENT ASPECTS

Neurotoxin Exposure

Infants should be protected against exposure to neurotoxins, such as aspartame. Experimental studies support this assertion. For example, administration of the neurotoxin capsaicin to neonatal rats during a critical period results in permanent loss of 85-93 percent peripheral C fibers innervating the spinal cord (Jansco 1978).

Longevity Prospects

The projection of research pertaining to the greater longevity of underfed experimental animals onto the nutrition of young children must be challenged. It has been asserted that aspartame "sweetens your life without shortening it." In the author's opinion, the opposite seems more likely.

The United States is blessed with an adequate supply of affordable good food. Yet, some concerned parents purposefully underfeed their children in a well-meaning attempt to prevent coronary heart disease, cancer and other degenerative disorders, coupled with using noncaloric sweeteners.

Transgenerational Considerations

Aspartame-related fatigue, depression and abnormal behavior in the mothers of infants can affect the mental and behavioral development of their children. For example, it has been shown that the flatness and less melodic tone of a mother's voice – rather than perky, high-pitched adult "baby talk" – tends to decrease an infant's attention to new learning opportunities.

The daughter of Case X-2, a woman with aspartame disease who consumed these products during pregnancy and while nursing, was afflicted with attention deficit disorder and a "mild encephalopathy of unknown origin." Other features included "language dysfunction," marked anger, mood swings, and immune problems manifested by recurrent yeast and sinus infections.

Myelin Synthesis

High concentrations of phenylalanine in infancy can interfere with the synthesis of myelin. They inhibit specific ATP-sulfurylase activity within the central nervous system (Hommes 1987). This issue is relevant to the simulation or aggravation of multiple sclerosis by aspartame (Chapter VI-D).

Development Defects (see Chapter X)

Women who consumed aspartame products during pregnancy and delivered children with birth defects later correlated these facts, especially when children they carried during subsequent aspartame-free pregnancies were normal. Their inability to convey this constructive "anecdotal" opinion about aspartame disease to physicians proved frustrating.

The Maternal PKU Collaborative Study (Waisbren 2000) convincingly indicated that insufficient maternal control of PKU prior to or early in pregnancy – that is, plasma phenylalanine levels less than 10 mg/dL – increases the risk for developmental problems.

Seizures (Epilepsy)

Aspartame-induced seizures, considered in Chapter III, resulted in enormous apprehension when children were so affected.

Several experimental observations are germane.

- Maher and Pinto (1987) noted that the administration of aspartame to immature mice lowers the threshold to seizures induced by pentylenetetrazole.
- Aspartic acid and its derivatives or analogs, such as N-methyl-D-aspartate, have a powerful convulsant effect when injected into the cerebral cortex and other brain structures (Turski 1984).

Effects of Related Amino Acids

There is evidence that related amino acids administered during the neonatal period can have life-long repercussions. Pizzi et al (1977) gave two- to 11-day-old mice monosodium glutamate (MSG). This resulted in reproductive dysfunction (both in females and males), fewer pregnancies, smaller litters, reduced fertility among males, and increased body weight. The decreased size of pituitary, thyroid, ovaries and testes presumably reflected hypothalamic and endocrine dysfunction.

Deficiency of key enzymes involved in the metabolism of related amino acids can result in childhood leukodystrophy of the brain and severe psychomotor retardation. Hagenfeldt et al (1987) reported on a male infant who excreted large amounts of N-acetylaspartate in his urine, attributed to deficient aspartoacyclase activity. The high cerebrospinal fluid/plasma concentration ratio of N-acetylaspartate indicated that this substance originated in the brain.

CONCERNS EXPRESSED BY ASPARTAME REACTORS AND OTHERS

Responses to the Survey

Many persons with aspartame disease who completed the survey questionnaire (Chapter XIX) volunteered extreme concern for children consuming aspartame products. The following examples illustrate these feelings that repeatedly invoked "I shudder to think.."

- A patient with severe reactions remarked, "If aspartame can have such a profound effect on an adult, it is frightening to think of what it may be doing to children."

- A 28-year-old woman with two convulsions and numerous other aspartame-associated complaints asserted, "I'm terrified of the problems with aspartame in our country's kids."

- An aspartame reactor anguished, "Where is it all going to end? I shudder to think of the effects of chemicals being put into children's bodies. Their lives surely will be shortened."

- A 33-year-old registered nurse who suffered multiple severe aspartame reactions observed, "I think it is frightening to see all the foods available with aspartame that the children and youths are eating. Who knows what the long term effects will be?"

- A 31-year-old female aspartame reactor stated, "So many children are raised drinking and consuming products containing aspartame that we may never know the impact on their lives."

- A 62-year-old home economist with severe aspartame reactions opined, "Substances such as aspartame should never be allowed in products to be consumed by children. All advertising, especially on TV, should carry a warning about the possible damages caused by aspartame."

- A 36-year-old female real estate broker with aspartame-induced headache, dizziness and anxiety attacks wrote, "I shudder to think of its longterm effects on children."

- A 27 year-old aspartame reactor with violent headaches commented, "Aspartame started out as a diet product. Now it is in children's vitamins, breakfast cereals and soft drinks. Children are better off with natural sugar than aspartame. Many are too young to realize that they react adversely to these products, and their parents don't realize it, either."

- A 56-year-old homemaker attributed her prior severe dizziness, mental confusion, depression, and recent elevation of blood pressure to aspartame. She anguished:

"I think of the many children whose parents are feeding aspartame to them in the form of cereal, gelatin, soft drinks, etc. It is quite alarming, as children do not understand symptoms. If aspartame damage is cumulative, what will happen to these children?"

Concern of Grandparents

Grandparents repeatedly expressed their concern for grandchildren who were allowed to drink aspartame sodas.

A grandmother visited her 12-year-old grandson only once or twice a year. Having been "a very bright child when three or four years old," she was shocked to discover his learning disability. The response of his parents was even more disturbing. "They shrugged at my reprimand for allowing him to drink diet colas all through the day – even for breakfast! I can't help but believe that these sodas are the cause of his problem."

The dismay over grandchildren with congenital deformities and other disorders is great. For example, a man wrote concerning his grandson born with spina bifida, "We give him food and drinks with aspartame to help keep his weight down. Our family doctor says your ideas are wrong. Who do we believe?"

Physicians and Other Professionals

Physician-investigators have expressed apprehension comparable to that of the author.

- Dr. Louis Elsas of Emory University asserted, "...there's no reason why a child less than six months old should be taking aspartame" (*Congressional Record-Senate* 1985b).
- Dr. William M. Pardridge regarded children from seven to 12 years as being at a higher risk for aspartame reactions because of their lower body weight (*Congressional Record-Senate* 1985a).

A professional who had worked five years at a pre-kindergarten school expressed horror over the encouraged use of aspartame products. This was reinforced by her personal reactions to such products.

516

The Press

A journalist had followed "the aspartame story" for several years. She anguished over the enthusiasm with which high school coaches in her community encouraged their players to avoid sugar and to substitute aspartame products... a nationwide trend.

Proper Labeling: An Analogy to Reye's Syndrome

Reye's syndrome describes an acute illness, primarily among children, that is characterized by severe deterioration of the brain and liver. The fear of this disorder by parents in the 1970s and 1980s compared to that over poliomyelitis before vaccines were introduced. For a considerable period, its relationship to aspirin use was regarded with skepticism, particularly in the absence of evidence for a dose-related response.

Aspirin was then determined to cause or risk Reye's syndrome. Such causation was further evidenced by the striking decline of Reye's syndrome after appropriate labeling of aspirin-containing products.

Based on the observations and research in infants and children, it is believed that comparable labeling of aspartame products used largely by children – concerning aspartame disease – is reasonable (see Chapter XXVII-B).

One solution to circumventing aspartame exposure in pediatric preparations is splitting or grinding the "adult" aspartame-free tablet into halves or quarters, and giving the desired amount in juice, cereal, apple sauce, ice cream, or another acceptable carrier.

Senator Howard Metzenbaum

Senator Howard Metzenbaum stated his concern relative to aspartame consumption in a news release dated March 3, 1986: "We cannot use America's children as guinea pigs to determine 'safe' level." He expressed alarm over the large amounts of aspartame being taken by young people in everything from soft drinks to vitamins and cold remedies (*The Philadelphia Inquirer* March 4, 1986, p. A-4).

The Senator's anxiety heightened with the subsequent failed passage of his bill to label the aspartame content of products. The manufacturer reassured a member of his staff concerning the safety of aspartame for children who consumed large amounts (*Congressional Record-Senate* 1985a, p. S5491).

XII

PRIOR ALCOHOLISM; ALCOHOL USE

"Man does not die, he kills himself."
Seneca

Some aspartame reactors with prior alcoholism volunteered that their "withdrawal" symptoms after stopping aspartame products were more severe than when going "cold turkey" from alcohol. This is a cardinal feature among persons with aspartame addiction (Chapter VII-G). Such individuals intuitively began consuming more sugar and other carbohydrates under these circumstances.

Additional observations link problems associated with the use of both aspartame and alcohol.

- Persons having a history of prior abuse of alcohol, drugs, or both, seemed more vulnerable to aspartame reactions.
- Several aspartame reactors stressed the exacerbation of seizures and other complaints after consuming alcohol <u>and</u> an aspartame beverage. Moreover, some nonalcoholic patients suffered aspartame reactions, especially convulsions (Chapter III), after drinking a small amount of alcohol.
- The severe symptoms from drinking small or moderate amounts of alcohol after reactors had discontinued aspartame is reminiscent of others who developed allergies to multiple substances. An example is dual sensitivity to monosodium glutamate (MSG) (Chapter VIII-E) following an initial reaction to aspartame. The specific alcoholic beverage (as wine), or some preservative or other ingredient therein, might have triggered the subsequent attacks.

<u>Acronym Legend</u>
    ACB - aspartame cola beverage
    ASD - aspartame soft drink
    ATS - aspartame tabletop sweetener

- The methyl alcohol in cheap "house" wines may summate upon the effects of methanol in aspartame (Chapter XXI).
- The reactivity of aspartame with certain aldehydes (another class of flavoring compounds) has been demonstrated for ethanol (Hussein 1984).
- Severe visual deterioration, including transient blindness diagnosed as optic neuritis (Chapter IV), occurred in the **same** person – but on different occasions – following excessive intake of either aspartame or alcohol. (The vast majority of persons with aspartame disease who had visual problems, however, consumed little or no alcohol.)

Representative Case Reports

Case XII-1

A 47-year-old woman sought consultation for increasingly severe problems over the previous 1-1/2 years, during which time she consumed large amounts of aspartame. She began the day by drinking three cups of coffee to which an ATS was added. She then ingested 10-12 glasses or cups of aspartame-sweetened beverages, and ate considerable aspartame pudding.

This patient gave a history of alcoholism and excessive amphetamine use decades earlier. (The amphetamines were taken for extreme fatigue and weight reduction.) She joined Alcoholics Anonymous 20 years previously, and had taken only a single social drink in five years. She was now happily married.

Her main concern was increasing confusion and memory loss over the past year... especially because she prided herself on a "photographic memory." During this time, she also suffered severe headaches ("never a problem before"), hearing difficulty ("as if my ears were covered"), lightheadedness with "staggering," vertigo on lying down ("the room was actually spinning"), attacks of severe nervousness and agitation, intense hunger, a craving for sugar and sweets, muscle cramps, pains in the legs and thighs, aching and stiffness of various joints, an elevation of blood pressure (for the first time), and marked intolerance to cold. Dryness of the eyes (Chapter IV) became so bothersome that she now required one bottle of artificial tears a week.

Another distressing symptom was severe depression. The patient thought of committing suicide on several occasions, but had the good fortune of belonging to a circle of caring friends.

The family history was pertinent. Both patients had been alcoholic. Her mother was "a potential diabetic," and her nephew a juvenile diabetic.

After learning of the possible cause or aggravation of similar problems by aspartame, she promptly stopped all such products. She emphasized that <u>the ensuing "withdrawal symptoms" were far worse than those experienced after discontinuing alcohol or amphetamines</u>.

This patient was seen by the author in consultation. Her initial blood pressure was still 130/102 shortly after "the aspartame connection" had been deduced. When rechecked several weeks later, it had normalized. She weighed 148 pounds. There was a large café-au-lait spot over the left wrist... a frequent finding in patients with diabetogenic hyperinsulinism (Roberts 1964, 1965c, 1971b).

A subsequent glucose tolerance test (after consuming an adequate diet) indicated a diabetic-type response, followed by severe symptoms suggestive of "hypoglycemia" – especially acute fatigue, headache and hunger. The test had to be stopped at the fourth hour. Her condition improved when fed.

	Glucose (mg %)	Insulin (μU/ml)
Fasting	133	10.3
½ hour	223	68.6
1 hour	212	118.0
2 hours	162	80.6
3- ½ hours	93	----
4 hours	90 (clinical reaction; test stopped)	

On a regimen of an appropriate diet, supportive measures and continued aspartame avoidance, her symptoms improved. She no longer needed artificial tears. An entire subsequent visit was devoted to discussing her lifelong "fear of fatness" (Chapter IX-B). Within one month, she felt well enough to travel with a volunteer church group doing relief work in Haiti.

Case XII-2

A 52-year-old administrator had a "drinking problem" for ten years prior to 1976, but never drank alcohol thereafter. She had been subject to "low blood sugar attacks" since 1981. There was an intolerance to aspirin, tranquilizers, and nonsteroidal anti-inflammatory drugs.

520

The patient experienced severe ear symptoms, drowsiness, slurred speech, marked depression, a change in personality, and intense thirst within one to two hours after ingesting modest amounts of aspartame. She wrote

> "I reacted to aspartame from my first or second ingestion. The reaction was so dramatic that it took only four to five instances for me to determine the cause, and halt the intake. I felt with aspartame in my system just like I did years ago when drinking alcohol, like my brain was drugged. I felt hopeless and helpless. The complete personality change was totally like my drinking days."

She offered this poignant commentary.

> *"Having suffered from active alcoholism and knowing now the three-part disease I believe it to be (mental, physical and spiritual), as well as the effect on me if I were to take that first drink, I wonder about how many recovering alcoholics have gotten back into problems and/or active drinking after ingesting aspartame, and suffered the reactions I did."*

Case XII-3

A 32-year-old female author experienced severe headache, marked drowsiness, insomnia, unexplained facial pain, extreme irritability, palpitations, abdominal pain with nausea and diarrhea, severe bloat, marked thinning of the hair, intense thirst, more frequent menstrual periods, aggravated hypoglycemia, "dry eyes" with difficulty in wearing contact lens, and allergic-type sinus problems. Her craving for sweets led to "binging on sugar products." The symptoms promptly improved within two or three days, and disappeared in one week, after discontinuing the two cans and a two-liter bottle of diet cola she drank daily. They promptly recurred within two days after one rechallenge. A sister had comparable aspartame-associated problems.

This patient gave a history of both alcohol and marijuana abuse. She commented on the similarity of her reactions to aspartame products and those during such prior substance abuse.

Case XII-4

A 42-year-old dentist consumed two cans of diet cola and six packets of an ATS daily. He experienced decreased vision in one eye, ringing in both ears, severe headache, dizziness, marked mental confusion, facial pains, slurred speech, depression, irritability, nausea, pain on swallowing, and a loss of feeling over the left side of his fact. Two sets of x-rays of the head, three CT scans and one MRI study of the brain, an electroencephalogram, cerebral angiography, and a lumbar puncture during two hospitalizations were normal. He improved after avoiding aspartame. The patient noted that comparable severe attacks had been precipitated by drinking a glass of wine or "anything with alcohol."

Case XII-5

A 31-year-old teacher suffered attacks of severe headache, dizziness, and pain in both eyes after consuming an ATS or aspartame soft drinks. Her symptoms promptly recurred within one day during three subsequent rechallenges. They also returned if she consumed "very little" of an alcoholic beverage.

Case XII-6

A 37-year-old manager experienced decreased vision, marked sensitivity to noise, severe headache, dizziness, memory loss, insomnia, depression, facial and limb pains, a change in personality, and severe nausea after consuming up to four liters of an aspartame soft drink daily for several weeks. These symptoms improved when his mother suggested that he discontinue the product after she viewed a program on aspartame disease. Some numbness and tingling or pain still persisted over one side of the face and in the limbs. The ingestion of wine would <u>predictably</u> exaggerate his pain and numbness one year after stopping aspartame.

Case XII-7

A 28-year-old woman had multiple convulsions, severe headache, marked memory loss, a change in personality, intense itching, and difficulty in swallowing while consuming two cans of diet cola and three packets of an ATS daily. She emphasized, "I was mixing alcohol with pop that had aspartame." Her consumption of alcohol was described as "moderate." The complaints disappeared within one month after eliminating aspartame.

Case XII-8

A woman checked herself into a hospital rehabilitation center for alcoholism at the age of 27. A period of 14 years of abstention from alcohol ensued, only to be replaced by aspartame disease. She stated, "The problem was that when I sat the bottle of brandy down, I picked up the diet cola and drank it in the place of all liquids."

After switching to diet colas, this active person experienced severe fatigue, easy agitation, numbness of the left hand, marked pain in the muscles and joints, difficulty in vision, headache, and "loss of at least half my hair." Many physicians and consultants were seen, but none paid attention to the heavy consumption of aspartame. Her condition was variously diagnosed as fibromyalgia, depression, and possible hepatitis C. The white blood cell count was only 460. Studies for lupus erythematosus, Lyme disease, and other conditions proved normal. She learned about aspartame disease in June 1999, at which point she discontinued diet sodas with benefit.

RELATED PERSPECTIVES ON ALCOHOLISM

The projected frequency of aspartame disease in the general population raises important related public health considerations about alcoholism. Recent data indicate that 13 percent of American adults have been diagnosed as being alcoholic at some time during their life, and about six percent of adults actively combat this disease at any given time

The Role of Hypoglycemia ("Low Blood Sugar Attacks")

Most alcoholics and many persons with aspartame disease are prone to severe reactive hypoglycemia (Chapter XIV). This explains in part their habitual use of considerable sugar and sweets (Roberts 1971 b), and their prodigious use of sweeteners. The author has
successfully helped many patients abstain from alcohol by insisting on the avoidance of sugar, and taking food every 3-4 hours... day and night.

Excessive aspartame consumption by alcoholics with severe hypoglycemia places them in added jeopardy through severe aspartame reactions, deprivation of calories, the epileptogenic effect of small amounts of alcohol in persons with aspartame-induced seizures,
and the potential cumulative effects of aspartame and disulfiram (Antabuse®). Concerning caloric curtailment, alcoholics tend to have greater energy requirements because of increased microsomal enzymic activity related to the oxidation of ethyl alcohol (Jhangian 1986).

The Problem of Female Alcoholics

The preponderance of females among aspartame reactors was discussed in Chapter II. Up to two percent of American women are active alcoholics, often as a "hidden agenda."

The frequency and severity of aspartame reactions are likely to be exaggerated among women who drink moderate to large amounts of alcohol.

In the author's experience, most alcoholic women resorted to alcohol (fermented sugar), rather than food, to alleviate their severe symptoms of unrecognized hypoglycemia. A vicious cycle ensued wherein the action of alcohol interfered with the enzymes in the liver required for transforming stored starch (glycogen) into body sugar (glucose).

Another pertinent element is weight control for obesity, real or perceived (Chapter IX-B). Figure-conscious women who are alcoholic may consume large amounts of aspartame, thereby intensifying the complications of both hypoglycemia and alcoholism. Furthermore, ravages of the latter – including liver disease, malnutrition, traffic-related deaths, high blood pressure, and bearing children with birth defects or mental retardation – tend to be more severe for various reasons, including decreased body water. In point of fact, the mortality rate for female alcoholics may be more than four times higher than for alcoholic men.

Superimposed Disulfiram-Methyl Alcohol Toxicity

The consumption of considerable methyl alcohol from consuming "abuse doses" of aspartame might have disastrous effects for alcoholic patients who use maintenance disulfiram (Antabuse®) to control their affliction. Prior manufacturer data indicated that about 400,000 persons took the trademarked product at any given time, and at least as many who used the less expensive generic form. Disulfiram can compound the problem by slowing the degradation of **methyl** alcohol present in aspartame (Chapter XXI).

Chronic Methanol Toxicity

The important issue of chronic methyl alcohol poisoning caused by aspartame consumption is relevant. It will be discussed in Chapter XXI.

Genetic Factors

Genetic variations in the gene(s) for alcohol dehydrogenase that alter the rate of alcohol metabolism appear to have clinical significance (Hines 2001). They may explain the observed familial nature of aspartame disease (Chapter XVI), and the severity of methanol effects in reactors having a slow rate of oxidation.

XIII

DIABETES MELLITUS

"As their highnesses traveled, they were always
making discoveries, by accidents and sagacity,
of things which they were not in quest of."
        Horace Walpole (1754)
        (alluding to fairy tale, *The Three
        Princes of Serendip*)

Patients with diabetes mellitus and "potential" diabetes currently consume large amounts of aspartame products with the enthusiastic approval of their physicians and dietitians. A popular aspartame tabletop sweetener containing less than one gram of carbohydrate and four calories per packet is widely recommended as a "free exchange." Multicolored ads for other aspartame products focusing on diabetes appear in professional journals and lay publications.

Observations involving 118 diabetic aspartame reactors (10 percent) in this series suggest the need for caution. They indicate that *aspartame may adversely influence control of diabetes, precipitate clinical diabetes, and aggravate or simulate complications referable to the eyes, kidneys and peripheral nerves.*

Such concern is reinforced by a report from The Centers for Disease Control indicating a dramatic rise of diabetes among the adult population – from 6.5 percent in 1998 to 6.9 percent in 1999. Moreover, it involved almost every demographic category (race; age groups). The CDC projected that the number of Americans so afflicted will increase from 16 million to 22 million in 2025.

The initial 60 diabetics who completed the questionnaire fell into the following categories (Roberts 1990).

Acronym Legend

        ACB - aspartame cola beverage
        ASD - aspartame soft drink
        ATS - aspartame tabletop sweetener

Group A - 18 patients with untreated diabetes who developed
high fasting blood glucose concentrations (greater than
140 mg %)
Group B - 25 patients on insulin and diet
Group C - 17 patients on oral drugs and diet

The following clinical encounters deserve attention, and will be amplified in the ensuing discussion.

- Aspartame reactors being treated with insulin or an oral drug sometimes could not decide if they were experiencing a reaction to insulin or to aspartame.
- Several insulin-dependent diabetics seemed more prone to aspartame-induced convulsions – both grand mal (see Case III-24) and petit mal (see Case III-25).
- Insulin resistance and diabetic control tended to improve **promptly** after avoiding aspartame products.
- Questions arose about missed or doubled dosages of insulin or oral drugs due to aspartame-induced confusion (Chapter VI).
- A few of my diabetic patients (not included in this series) had abstained from aspartame before I queried them about its use because they already had concluded that it aggravated their condition.
- Aspartame addiction (Chapter VII-G) compounded the problem when diabetics used these products to get their "sugar fix."

A. PRECIPITATION OF CLINICAL DIABETES

Several patients whom the author had followed for years evidenced a prior diabetic response ("decreased glucose tolerance") by glucose tolerance testing – that is, their blood glucose concentrations after drinking a glucose load exceeded 200 mg percent. On an appropriate diet, the fasting blood sugar (FBS) concentrations remained normal (115 mg percent or less) or only slightly elevated. Their subsequent elevated values (hyperglycemia), along with weakness and other symptoms of diabetes, proved puzzling until it was ascertained they used aspartame products. Clinical and biochemical improvement occurred when such products were stopped.

In addition, some patients with longstanding reactive hypoglycemia were found to have fasting hyperglycemia for the first time after consuming aspartame (see Cases XIII-2 and XIII-3). Their FBS values then normalized after abstinence.

Three aspartame reactors developed diabetes after attacks of apparent aspartame-induced pancreatitis (Chapter IX-D). Case XIII-4 illustrates this sequence.

Representative Case Reports

Case XIII-1

A 47-year-old man with hemochromatosis or iron storage disease had been attended several years. (This condition is also known as "bronze diabetes" because iron deposits in the pancreas can damage the islet cells that product insulin.) When seen in July 1986, his FBS had risen to 159 mg percent. On direct inquiry, he stated that he had been drinking considerable aspartame sodas. The FBS declined to 97 mg percent three weeks after abstinence.

Case XIII-2

A 75-year-old woman had documented reactive hypoglycemia; her blood glucose declined to 45 mg percent during a prior glucose tolerance test. She presented in September 1986 with recurrent conjunctivitis over the past 1-1/2 years. Three ophthalmologists prescribed local antibiotics without benefit.

This patient had been consuming large amounts of pudding and other products containing aspartame. The FBS was now 143 mg percent. The hemoglobin A_1C concentration (an indicator of sustained blood glucose elevations) was 14.3 (normal 4-6). After stopping aspartame, her FBS progressively dropped to 119 mg percent within one month. Concomitantly, the hemoglobin A_1C decreased to 6.1.

Case XIII-3

A 78-year-old man had been treated since 1958 for reactive hypoglycemia associated with a prior gastrectomy. He developed an unexplained arthropathy involving the right elbow that was not gout. (The uric acid concentration was normal.) This attack subsided within several days of conservative therapy. His FBS was found to be repeatedly elevated – 156 mg percent on 8/3/87, and 146 mg percent on 8/10/87. A midafternoon blood glucose concentration on 8/10/87, however, was only 65 mg percent. When asked about aspartame use, he stated that he recently had been consuming large amounts of diet root beer and diet cola. These were discontinued and replaced by his customary interval snacks. A repeat FBS one week later was 118 mg percent.

Case XIII-4

A 62-year-old beautician began drinking aspartame soft drinks and presweetened tea to lose weight. She subsequently experienced severe abdominal pain "under the rib cage on the left side." It became so intense that she pressed both fists against the abdominal wall seeking relief. Bicarbonate of soda afforded no benefit. There also was intense nausea, severe abdominal bloat, and blood in the stools.

Two months after the onset of aspartame use, a physician found her FBS to be 435 mg percent. It had been normal (100 mg percent) one year previously. She craved sweet cider while consuming aspartame.

A diagnosis of pancreatitis was made. The patient continued to suffer these symptoms while receiving cimetidine (Tagamet®) and an antacid in the hospital. She then deduced that her problems might be related to aspartame in her "diabetic diet," and demanded it be discontinued. Thereafter, "my hurting left and my sugar was regulated."

This patient had a history of asthma, hypoglycemia attacks, and allergy to penicillin. Her children also were aspartame reactors – a daughter suffering abdominal distention and eye-ear problems, and her son aspartame-induced headaches.

B. LOSS OF DIABETES CONTROL WHILE ON INSULIN THERAPY

Twenty-three diabetic patients among the first 551 aspartame reactors had been controlled for considerable periods on diet and one or several doses of insulin daily. Subsequently, they were found to have a persistent increase of the blood glucose concentration (by home glucose monitoring) in the absence of intercurrent infection or other problems conducive to loss of control. Inquiries about aspartame revealed a moderate or large intake of diet sodas and foods. Shortly after avoiding aspartame products, their glucose concentrations generally declined, enabling a reduction in dosage of insulin.

The vicious cycle of poor diabetic control with superimposed aspartame-associated infection and resistance to insulin was described in Chapter IX-H.

The experiences of couples in whom both spouses were diabetic proved impressive. Cases XIII-16 and XIII-17 illustrate such an "aspartame duet."

Comparable problems in controlling diabetes surfaced in the form of questions sent syndicated medical columnists. For example, a diabetic asked Dr. Neil Solomon if there was a relationship between starting to drink diet soft drinks and difficulty in controlling his blood sugar *(The Miami Herald* October 8, 1986, p. D-2).

Insulin-dependent diabetic patients may have another superimposed problem of biotechnology: the increase of side effects from genetically-engineered recombinant human insulin. They include arthritic complaints, weight gain, and reduced hypoglycemia awareness.

Representative Case Reports

Case XIII-5

A 61-year-old woman required hospitalization for readjustment of her insulin dosage due to the loss of diabetes control even though she adhered carefully to a "diabetic diet" and other measures. She also had been experiencing intense dizziness, headache and progressive loss of memory. Considerable aspartame products were being used as part of the recommended diet.

The patient then discovered her intolerance for aspartame products.

> "A nurse told me about listening to you on radio station WWMR-FM, and gave me the gist of your comments on aspartame and its side effects. My diabetes is under better control since I have completely stopped using anything with aspartame. I am feeling better. The dizziness is gone. The headaches are fewer, and I think my memory is keener than it was even though it has only been three weeks."

Case XIII-6

A thin young woman with insulin-dependent diabetes described the severe exacerbation of her visual and neuropathic symptoms, along with loss of diabetes control, while consuming aspartame products. Her insulin requirement had increased to 110 units daily. When she avoided aspartame, the visual and neuropathic symptoms disappeared, and the insulin dosage could be decreased to 12 units daily.

Case XIII-7

A 59-year-old diabetic man had required 20 units of an intermediate-acting insulin daily for many years. His insulin requirements more than doubled when "my sugar ran out of control" after consuming three liters of diet cola daily.

Case XIII-8

A 12-year-old diabetic boy required multiple hospitalizations while consuming considerable aspartame. He was twice admitted in diabetic coma. The physicians at a university hospital encountered considerable difficulty in stabilizing his insulin dosage during the periods aspartame was taken.

Case XIII-9

A 46-year-old interior designer had maintained good control of insulin-dependent diabetic for three decades. He then consumed several aspartame soft drinks and up to five packets of an ATS daily. "At that point, my diabetes went haywire, and I had terrible insulin reactions." Control of diabetes reverted to its previous status within one week after stopping aspartame products.

Case XIII-10

A 45-year-old obese woman required hospitalization for uncontrolled diabetes. She improved on an appropriate diet and split doses of insulin, with virtual normalization of her fasting and random blood glucose values over several weeks. Prior to that time, she had not consumed aspartame products.

In a subsequent visit, the patient complained of extreme sleepiness, fatigue, depression and intense sweats. Her FBS concentrations now ranged up to 160 mg percent, and the blood pressure had risen to 180/112. When asked about aspartame use, she stated that she began drinking considerable amounts of diet sodas on the advice of a dietitian. Five days after stopping all aspartame products, without any change in insulin dosage, the FBS values averaged 130 mg percent and the afternoon glucose values ranged from 90-120 mg percent. Concomitantly, her blood pressure declined to 155/90.

Case XIII-11

This 80-year-old active diabetic had been controlled on diet and tolbutamide (Orinase®) for several years. She then was shifted to insulin because of elevated blood glucose concentrations that persistently exceeded 200 mg percent. The dosage of insulin had to be increased over the ensuing eleven months from 12 units to 28 units. Her FBS on 8/14/86 was 230 mg percent. She also experienced severe headaches.

This patient happened to hear my discussion about aspartame disease, and stopped using it. The headaches promptly disappeared. Her FBS declined to 101 mg percent within two weeks, at which point the insulin dosage was reduced.

Case XIII-12

An elderly diabetic woman had been doing well on 10-12 units NPH insulin before breakfast, and 6-8 units NPH before her evening meal. The FBS progressively rose to 209-214 mg percent over the next five months, notwithstanding several increases of the insulin dosage. No infection or other contributory factor could be uncovered. Within five days after discontinuing aspartame, her FBS declined to 110 mg percent, and the insulin dosage reverted to her prior requirements.

Case XIII-13

A 48-year-old insulin-dependent diabetic began using aspartame products to avoid sugar. She reported, "It increased my blood sugar, making it necessary to take an extra shot of insulin to counteract it." Associated nausea and extreme irritability interfered with her performance as a teacher. She had a longstanding allergy to penicillin. Her daughter also experienced severe nausea and dizziness after ingesting aspartame.

Case XIV-14

An insulin-dependent diabetic described her problems with aspartame in these terms:

> "When using this sweetener, I have increased blood sugar, and more difficulty controlling the diabetes. It also caused a more rapid heart beat. I am fighting to get this sweetener out of everything! There is not a diabetic 'treat' I can have because they are loaded with this sweetener. That includes diet pop."

Case XIII-15

A 67-year-old insulin-dependent diabetic woman presented with severe headache, leg pains, and lightheadedness. These complaints disappeared after avoiding aspartame for three weeks. The previously unexplained rise of her FBS (from 130-165 mg percent to 313-331mg percent) declined to 131mg percent. The blood glucose concentration after breakfast now did not exceed 191 mg percent.

Case XIII-16

A husband shifted to diet colas when diabetes was diagnosed, and "got used to the taste" in the transition from regular cola. Symptomatic retinopathy with retinal bleeding subsequently developed. He also suffered severe joint pain, and nonhealing of a sore. Learning about aspartame disease, he discontinued such products. "Within a month, the numbness in my hands was gone, the sore on my right index finger healed (and has not come back), and my joints don't hurt anymore."

Case XIII-17

The diabetic wife of Case XIII-16 had been unable to maintain her blood glucose level below 200 mg percent for several years despite exercise and trying to lose weight. Observing the beneficial affect of aspartame avoidance in her husband, she also abstained. Within two weeks, she lost fifteen pounds, coupled with a decline of her blood glucose to 152 mg percent.

C. POOR CONTROL ON ORAL DRUGS FOR DIABETES

More than a score of non-insulin-dependent diabetics who were being treated with oral hypoglycemic drugs unexpectedly manifested high morning and afternoon blood glucose concentrations while consuming aspartame drugs.

Representative Case Reports

Case XIII-18

A 67-year-old diabetic woman had been maintained relatively well on diet and tolazamide (Tolinase®). Her blood glucose concentrations increased during August 1986 – the morning values ranging from 180-247 mg percent, and the afternoon values up to 248 mg percent. During this period, she was taking two to three diet colas and other aspartame products daily. Fungal involvement of a thumb (reflecting loss of diabetic control) also developed.

The patient then stopped aspartame. She felt much improved one week later. The nail infection already had begun to improve. Her serial FBS values were now 108, 106, and 108 and 82 mg percent. The pre-supper values were 198, 64, 94, and 82 mg percent.

Case XIII-19

A prominent engineer sent the following letter to Aspartame Victims and Their Friends.

"I am a Type II (adult onset) diabetic. I am normally able to keep my blood sugar under reasonable control with the use of oral medication.

"When an aspartame tabletop sweetener first appeared on the market, I purchased the pre-prepared packets to use in place of the saccharin sweetener I had been using. I had concern about saccharin due to its reported carcinogenic effects.

"Very shortly after beginning aspartame, my blood sugar jumped to 268, then to 351, 321 and 333 over a period of 18 days. Suspecting that this sweetener might be the cause of the rapid rise in blood sugar, I discontinued its use. My blood sugar dropped back to 200 in six days. I am still controlling it within an acceptable range three years later.

"The doctor to whom I was going at the time of this surge ridiculed the idea that such a small amount of aspartame could trigger this dramatic effect in my blood sugar. I changed doctors shortly thereafter. I am personally convinced that the usage of aspartame was the cause of my high blood sugars.

"I have definite knowledge of one Type I diabetic on insulin who was using the same tabletop sweetener and monitoring his blood sugar. When he visited his doctor, the test (as run by the laboratory) showed his blood sugar to be out of control.

"I try to avoid aspartame in any form, and am very disturbed by its presence in so many products."

Case XIII-20

A 51-year-old stockbroker began consuming one can of diet cola and two packets of an ATS daily after diabetes was diagnosed. Even though he conscientiously followed a diet and took tolbutamide, there was difficulty in controlling his blood glucose concentrations. He also developed marked ringing in the left ear, "distorted vision" in the left eye (attributed to "macular degeneration of unexplained cause"), severe drowsiness, memory loss, and a marked personality change.

Case XIII-21

A 48-year-old truck driver saw the author in consultation for poorly controlled diabetes, intense neuropathic discomfort of the feet and left hand, and progressive blurring of vision. The latter had been attributed to "some oozing in the right eye." His FBS on tolbutamide was 278 mg percent; a random blood glucose was 178 mg percent. The total serum cholesterol (normal, up to 225 mg percent) was 321 mg percent, the HDL cholesterol only 20 mg percent (normal, over 35 mg percent), and the triglyceride level 1,468 mg percent (normal, up to 160 mg percent).

The patient was drinking four diet sodas daily. He had not ingested alcohol for several years. Striking improvement of vision was noted within less than one week after stopping aspartame, especially the absence of a blur while driving. His FBS declined to 146-163 mg percent within one week. Concomitantly, the blood pressure decreased from 150/100 to 134/84. There was subsequent improvement of the neuropathic symptoms, and a lowering of his cholesterol to 192 mg percent, and triglyceride to 273 mg percent.

D. REACTIONS TO INSULIN AND ORAL DRUGS

Many diabetics noted a greater tendency to insulin reactions/hypoglycemia while using aspartame products.

Insulin

Several diabetic patients unequivocally attributed more frequent and severe insulin reactions to the use of aspartame. A contributory factor in some may have been marked confusion and memory loss (Chapter VI-C), causing them to repeat doses of insulin or to forget their interval feedings.

Representative Case Reports

Case XIII-23

A 41-year-old housewife developed insulin-dependent diabetes at the age of 22. Its control had become a problem the previous five years because of frequent and severe insulin reactions. Her husband at times had to force-feed her. This posed a considerable challenge inasmuch as aggression and "complete obstinance" characterized her attacks. Concomitant problems included weight gain, bloat, fluid retention, marked personality changes, and a striking loss of short-term memory.

She consumed considerable amount of aspartame products – including sodas, (averaging two liters daily), hot drinks, chewing gum, mints, and diet hot chocolate.

Case XIII-24

A 36-year-old woman with insulin-dependent diabetes (25 years) initially had denied any contributory role of aspartame products because she felt that the negative allegations were "reactionary." Moreover, a dietitian told her they were "perfectly safe." As a result, "I just went wild eating it in everything." She wrote

> "My blood pressure went from difficult to horrible. My appetite was running rampant. I was waking up with 500 blood sugars, and also going to lows of 35-40. No one could figure out what was wrong with me. I didn't want to have sex with my husband. I even began having hot flashes. I had some minor tingling, which I always passed off as 'just one of those diabetic things.' I was gaining weight, feeling uncoordinated and spacey, and felt like hell.

> "I then remembered the correspondence about aspartame, and decided to give it up as a trial. The next day, my blood sugars were perfect, as they have been now for almost two weeks. It is uncanny. I am so beside myself with glee I can hardly stand it. My insulin dosage has gone from 37 units to 17 units daily. I have, simply put, been reborn."

Case XIII- 25

A 37-year-old woman was diagnosed as having diabetes seven years previously. She then began using aspartame products. There was a strong family history of diabetes.

The patient experienced many unexplained symptoms. Her family physician and endocrinologist initially attributed them to her diabetes medication. They included confusion, loss of memory, anxiety attacks, unexplained chest pains, headache, dizziness, joint pains, weight loss, and drastic declines of the blood glucose concentration... at times with loss of consciousness. Her family had to stay with her constantly, and feed her frequently. She wrote, "Without warning, I was fine one minute, and the next minute the room would be spinning and I was looking for a place to lay down. It was like being in a dream or fog. I even had to leave work."

She stopped all aspartame products when a friend sent her an article about aspartame disease. Dramatic improvement ensued. "I haven't had to leave work due to blood sugar levels dropping. My loved ones haven't had to feed me or be with me. I haven't had to drive in a mental fog. I haven't had nearly as many headaches, joint aches or dizzy spells."

Case XIII-26

A businessman expressed appreciation for being informed about the probable role of aspartame disease relative to his problems with diabetes and memory loss.

> "I am a diabetic who consumes large amounts of sugar-freebeverages containing aspartame. For about three months, I have been experiencing a loss of memory the following ways:
>
> a.   About five days per week I will forget if I ate lunch that day. When I get home in the evening, I will be ravished, but I don't know if or what I ate. This is dangerous for a diabetic on insulin who should be eating three meals on time to balance the insulin dosage.
> b.   I will see people I've known for years, but I cannot remember their names."

Case XIII-27

A 21-year-old insulin-dependent teacher suffered more frequent insulin reactions (both at work and home) while consuming 15 or more cans of aspartame colas daily. He stated, "When we cut down on aspartame, I stopped having so many reactions."

Oral Drugs

Type II diabetic patients who did not receive insulin by injection also experienced more frequent and severe hypoglycemic attacks while consuming aspartame products.

Representative Case Report

Case XIII-28

A diabetic woman had been controlled on diet and tolazamide. During the two years she consumed aspartame, her FBS values decreased. She then suffered grand mal seizures and transient paralysis on one side. Swelling of the mouth and tongue also occurred on two occasions after taking aspartame. Her condition stabilized on the prior regimen after avoiding aspartame, with no recurrence of the seizures or mouth reaction.

E. REAL OR SIMULATED DIABETES COMPLICATIONS

Diabetic patients who react to aspartame products face an additional major problem: the aggravation or simulation of diabetes complications – namely, neuropathy, retinopathy, and nephropathy (kidney involvement). In turn, failure to recognize aspartame disease invites needless or hazardous treatments, including eye (laser) surgery.

Erroneous Diagnoses

The role of aspartame disease relative to visual impairment (Chapter IV), headache (Chapter V), dizziness (Chapter VI-B), limb pain (Chapter VI-H), and diarrhea (Chapter IX-D) became evident when these symptoms abated after aspartame products were discontinued.

- Cases IV-25 to IV-29 reported striking and prompt improvement of blurred vision and eye pain after stopping aspartame.
- Case I-29 had prompt improvement of severe difficulty in focusing after abstinence from aspartame, proving she did not have a suspected symptomatic retinopathy.
- A diabetic who drank four liters of aspartame sodas daily complained of severe changes in vision. An ophthalmologist reassured him that there was no demonstrable retinopathy. fter reading about blindness in an aspartame reactor, he stopped such products... with marked improvement.

- 75-year-old physician (reported by Barbara Mullarkey in the *Wednesday Journal of Oak Park & River* Forest March 26, 1986, p. 37) had enjoyed regular sexual activity. Within 10 days of using an ATS for recently diagnosed diabetes, he noted "a complete and total loss of libido." This might have been ascribed to diabetic neuropathy except for the fact that his vigorous sex life returned within six weeks after avoiding aspartame.

- A diabetic woman developed agonizing pains "from my knees to my ankles which I was not able to handle." They began shortly after drinking two cans of an aspartame beverage. Other symptoms included "large sores over my head, face and back, plus I was on the verge of fainting and sick all the time." At the insistence of a physician-daughter, four specialists saw her for a presumed diabetic neuropathy. The provoking cause could not be determined. The patient then "took it upon myself to cut out the soft drinks. I was immediately normal with the exception of my leg pain."

- Case IV-1, a 66-year-old diabetic man, had been controlled with diet and an oral hypoglycemia drug. He then experienced temporary "loss of vision" and pain in both eyes, as well as "dry eyes" requiring the frequent use of artificial tears. Other complaints included severe drowsiness, decreased hearing in both ears, itching, and "red blotches." These features subsided after stopping aspartame, but promptly recurred during one rechallenge. He abstained from these products thereafter because "I was afraid I'd go blind."

Aggravation of Diabetic Complications

Repeated reference was made in previous chapters to the aggravation or simulation of diabetic retinopathy (Chapter IV) and diabetic neuropathy (Chapter VI-E) in aspartame disease. Mention of this subject on talk shows predictably evoked calls from diabetic patients about the onset of severe complications when they began using aspartame products after having been in "good control."

The metabolic stress superimposed upon diabetics by aspartame disease can be intensified when kidney failure coexists, as in Case XIII-21. (See Introduction to Section 3.)

The aggravation or simulation of neurologic complications by aspartame was considered in Chapter VI and elsewhere. Suspicion about the diagnosis of multiple sclerosis in a diabetic consuming considerable aspartame is paramount. Terms such as "diabetic dementia" and "diabetic encephalopathy" should raise suspicion about aspartame disease in the case of patients who consume these products. The variety of other misdiagnoses included "polyradiculoneuropathy" and the Guillain-Barré syndrome.

Hemochromatosis (iron storage disease; bronze diabetes) might be aggravated in its pre-cirrhotic state by aspartame through the stimulation of insulin (Chapter XIV). This association is suggested by Case XIII-1. In addition to hyperinsulinemia, other evidences of insulin resistance include obesity, elevated lipids, and abnormal glucose tolerance. The primary action of insulin in stimulating glucose transport appears to be coupled with a redistribution of transferrin receptors to the cell surface where extracellular iron uptake is mediated (Ferrannini 2000).

Representative Case Reports

Case XIII-29

A 50-year-old surgeon with diabetes began consuming considerable amounts of diet soda. He had to give up surgery and driving when his vision deteriorated to 20/100 in both eyes. Laser therapy was administered to one eye. Once he discontinued diet drinks, his vision improved to 20/30 and 20/40, and his blood sugar values were generally normal.

Case XIII-30

During an interview on Philadelphia Station WWDB, the mother of a 20-year-old diabetic woman called. She stated that a hemorrhage in one eye of her daughter had caused virtual blindness notwithstanding careful control of diabetes with insulin, and severe impairment was beginning in the other eye. This mother had pleaded with her to reduce or stop the considerable use of diet sodas, but to no avail. She then wrote

> "My suspicions that aspartame might be responsible for losing her sight in the left eye were raised. I realize that most people, including many physicians I have spoken to, will blame this on her diabetes. But they have also admitted to me that her problem as a diabetic who is very well controlled under the care of a diabetologist, and with regular visits (every six months) to an eye surgeon, is very unusual.

> "It all happened so quickly. We are suffering from shock even though it has been almost a year since she lost all central vision.

One reason for our panic is that now she is experiencing blurring, etc. in her right eye. I was even afraid to mention any suspicion about aspartame to family or friends as I thought they would think me grasping at straws or just a 'hysterical' mother."

Case XIII-31

This case, reported to Dr. Richard J. Wurtman of Massachusetts Institute of Technology, is part of the public record.

The patient had longstanding diabetes with renal failure. A kidney transplant was unsuccessful, necessitating hemodialysis. She subsequently died at the age of 37.

Four months prior to her death, she began consuming increasingly large amounts of aspartame-sweetened tea and lemonade. Her mother tried to dissuade her from doing so after reading about aspartame reactions. The patient, however, insisted that "it was safe because the F.D.A. had approved it." Within two months, she experienced severe muscle spasms, slurred speech, difficulty in swallowing, inability to control the limb muscles, and seizures.

The attending physician stated that he did not know enough "to make a judgment" about the possible contributory role of aspartame. The parents thereupon went to the hospital library, and found an article by Dr. Wurtman on aspartame-induced seizures which they handed to the physician. The mother subsequently wrote, "I honestly believe that the aspartame may have been the cause of her seizures. Surely any one with kidney failure would be at high risk."

Increased Triglyceride and Cholesterol Concentrations

Elevated blood triglyceride and cholesterol concentrations are commonly found in patients with diabetes. Indeed, they may serve as clues to this underlying metabolic disturbance.

A large literature exists concerning the impaired ability of diabetics with insulin resistance to metabolize a glucose load – as reflected by their increased insulin concentrations after meals, and associated triglyceride elevation.

Aspartame can evoke or aggravate hypertriglyceridemia and hypercholesterolemia, as in Case XIII-20. The problem may be compounded when high-fiber laxatives containing aspartame are recommended because they reduced blood cholesterol levels in short-term studies

Case II-2 evidenced clinical diabetes for the first time after more than two decades under the author's care. She recently began drinking large amounts of aspartame beverages. Concomitantly, her triglyceride levels rose to 1,284 mg percent and 1,616 mg percent (normal, up to 160 mg percent), and her serum cholesterol to 354 and 349 mg percent (normal, up to 225 mg percent).

These metabolic aberrations could be viewed as reflections of compensatory, albeit inefficient, mechanisms whereby the body attempts to provide basic energy needs for vital organs (Roberts 1964, 1967b, 1964c, 1971b). The superimposed adverse effects of aspartame are discussed in Section 5.

Many diabetic patients conducted "self-experiments" with aspartame products, and independently confirmed my observations.

A woman with type I diabetes decided to "experiment with the use of aspartame from time to time to satisfy my own curiosity about its effects on my body." She stated "Invariably, if I use aspartame – just one or two diet sodas per day and a few sticks of aspartame gum – my former symptoms of aspartame poisoning return with a vengeance. My blood sugars go haywire. Only one tiny unit of insulin would drop my blood sugar over 100 points in under half an hour, sending me into a series of hypoglycemic reactions. Rebound into high blood sugars followed. The tingling along my spine and under my breast bone, which had disappeared after I gave up aspartame, returned. And my menstrual periods, which had been very irregular prior to giving up aspartame but came every 28 days for three days like clockwork after giving up aspartame, came on two weeks early, then three week early, two days after re-introducing aspartame into my diet."

GENERAL CONSIDERATIONS

Public Health Ramifications

The Centers for Disease Control and Prevention reported a striking 33 percent rise in the incidence of diabetes nationally between 1990 and 1998. While various factors were incriminated (most notably overweight, stress, fast foods and less exercise), the possible contributory role of aspartame products was apparently not considered.

Consumption of Aspartame and Sugar By Diabetics

FDA Commissioner Dr. Frank E. Young testified as to the United States Committee on Labor and Human Resources on November 3, 1987 that 60 percent of diabetics were using aspartame products, compared to 35 percent of the total sample population. Yet, Farkas and Forbes (1965) concluded there was "...no basis for generalizing on the effect that the use of non-caloric sweeteners has or will have on adherence to a carbohydrate-restricted diet by patients with diabetes in the age range of 40 to 70 years."

There has been a paradoxic rise in the consumption of **all** sugar products over the past two decades, concomitant with the dramatic increased use of artificial sweeteners. The Department of Agriculture noted that the per capita consumption of sugar in 1985 was 130 pounds, compared to 118 pounds in 1975. (The consumption of artificial sweeteners, including aspartame and saccharin, rose from 6.2 pounds in 1975 to 17.0 pounds in 1985.) Many diabetics add aspartame to coffee or tea, which they then proceed to take with cake, pie or ice cream.

Diabetics use aspartame as soft drinks and tabletop sweeteners because they are told it contains "no sugar," a reference to sucrose (table sugar). They fail to realize, however, that the first ingredient listed in a popular ATS is "dextrose with dried corn syrup."

The excessive use of aspartame products helps explain the proneness of women with insulin-dependent diabetes mellitus (IDDM) to bulimia (Stancin 1989). Such behavior involves self-induced vomiting, the taking of laxatives, diuretics and enemas, and even the intentional reduction of insulin in order to lose weight (Chapter IX-B).

Legal Ramifications

The problems considered in this chapter have potential legal ramifications. Special mention is made of pregnant women, children, older persons, epileptics, and other high-risk groups. Several examples are cited.

- An insulin-dependent diabetic who suffered seizures after using an ATS sued the manufacturer for alleged breach of an "implied warranty" that these sweeteners were "fit for ordinary use" (*The Grand Rapids* Press March 6, 1986, p. C-6).
- Aspartame-related hypoglycemia may have caused or contributed to the "dead-in-bed syndrome" in diabetics with hypoglycemia unawareness.

542

Diabetes: A Brief Overview

Diabetes mellitus is a chronic disease in which there is insufficient insulin – total or relative (resistance to insulin action) – for deriving adequate energy from ingested food. It tends to be familial.

There are more than ten million diabetics in the United States, but less than half have been formally diagnosed. Most (85 percent) do not require insulin, and are termed "Type II." Paradoxically, many persons in this category, especially when overweight, release considerable insulin after taking sugar or a meal, and then experience reactive hypoglycemia ("low blood sugar attacks"). I have used the term diabetogenic hyperinsulinism (see Introduction and Chapter XIV) to describe this transitional phase (Roberts 1964,1965,1966, 1967, 1968, 1971b, 1973). The remaining 15 percent are referred to as having "Type I" insulin-dependent or juvenile-type diabetes.

Most diabetics desire sweets. This may represent an inborn characteristic, an acquired habit, or both.

- A survey of 500 diabetic patients conducted in West Germany (cited by Horwitz 1983) revealed that only 84 could abstain from sweets.
- A comparable situation exists among juvenile diabetics. Court (1976) found that 72 percent of mothers used artificial sweeteners in preparing the meals of their diabetic children to achieve compliance.

The hazards of aspartame for diabetics require further clarification in light of statistics concerning premature mortality. The years of potential life lost (YPLL) increased only for the categories of diabetes mellitus and chronic obstructive pulmonary disease in the *Morbidity and Mortality Weekly Report* (December 1986 Supplement.)

Mechanisms of Aspartame's Diabetogenic Potential

The adverse metabolic, hormonal, toxic and other undesirable effects of aspartame and its components are detailed in Section 5. Many could contribute to the aggravation of diabetes and its complications. They encompass the wasting of insulin, impaired insulin-stimulated glucose transport, increased growth hormone and glucagon release after phenylalanine administration, other effects of its amino acids (see below), and additional pharmacologic activities. Another mechanism whereby aspartame-induced stimulation of insulin could aggravate diabetes involves the generation of insulin receptor antibodies capable of blocking the access of insulin to liver receptors (Dozio 2001).

With reference to aspartame-induced insomnia (Chapter VI-F), sleep debt has a detrimental impact on carbohydrate metabolism and endocrine function – including decreased glucose tolerance, and altered thyrotropin and cortisol concentrations (Spiegel 1999).

Some of the scientific observations that pertain to the effects of aspartame and its amino acid components on insulin release, other hormones, and metabolism are briefly reviewed.

- Phenylalanine and aspartic acid might enter the brain of diabetics more readily due to altered permeability of the blood-brain barrier. They could then aggravate fetal development during gestational diabetes in conjunction with elevated sorbitol concentrations because of increased polyol metabolism (Eriksson 1986) – conducive to eye and neurologic complications.

- Limited insulin reserves could be further depleted by pancreatitis (Chapter IX) or phenylalanine-induced pancreatic stimulation (Chapter XXIV). This and other amino acids, as well as protein, increase insulin and blood glucose levels. Years ago, Conn and Newburgh (1936) demonstrated comparable elevations of the blood sugar in diabetic patients consuming either dextrose or beefsteak.

- Schusdziaria et al (1981) reported that digested gluten elicited a more rapid and significantly greater rise in postprandial (after a meal) peripheral vein insulin and glucagon levels than undigested gluten.

- Wahren et al (1972) found accelerated splanchnic uptake of amino acids in diabetic patients (24 hours after withdrawal of insulin), compared to healthy controls. This increase was most notable for phenylalanine, glycine, serine, threonine, methionine and tyrosine.

- Awata et al (1990) noted the high frequency of aspartic acid at position 57 of the HLA - DQ β-chain in Japanese patients with insulin-dependent diabetes mellitus.

- Another influence of phenylalanine and its analogs on glucose and insulin metabolism involves the binding and activation of glucose-dependent insulinotropic polypeptide (GIP) receptors by the photoactivable p-benzyl-L-phenylalanine (Yip 1999). GIP, an important regulator of insulin release, also increases the binding affinity of the insulin receptor as well as insulin action on target tissues.

Sardesai et al (1987) concluded on the basis of experimental data that aspartame may adversely influence the control of diabetics. They found that a single dose of aspartame administered to both normal and streptozotozin-induced diabetic rats increased liver tryptophan oxygenase by 12 percent. Furthermore, aspartame decreased blood and brain tryptophan, and increased serum glucose and glucagon in the diabetic animals. The chronic administration of aspartame to both groups also resulted in increased tryptophan oxygenase activity, hyperglycemia, and a further rise of glucose in the diabetic animals.

Insulin/Hypoglycemia Reactions

The subject of hypoglycemia reactions in aspartame disease and the mechanisms involved will be considered in Chapter XIV.

Excessive insulin may be released by aspartame through a reflex mechanism involving the cephalic phase of insulin release. This is exaggeration of normal physiology relative to anticipating the arrival of food. It could result in hypoglycemic symptoms, or aggravation of diabetes mellitus when the binding of more insulin at cell membranes creates "insulin resistance."

Severe caloric restriction and other forms of metabolic stress in noninsulin-dependent diabetics increases the release of endorphins and enkephalins. These endogenous peptides with opiate-like activity have been shown to have important glucose-regulating effects in humans – notably, significant increases in plasma insulin and glucose concentrations (Giugliano 1987). Such effects can also lead to clinical hypoglycemia and insulin resistance.

Diabetic patients who receive increased doses of insulin for "tight control," as occurred while using aspartame, are at greater potential risk for the adverse cerebral consequences of hypoglycemia. This problem is compounded by reduced release of counterregulatory hormones (epinephrine; growth hormone; cortisol; glucagon) in response to severe hypoglycemia. These altered counterregulatory hormonal thresholds in well controlled Type II diabetics, even at normal blood glucose concentrations (Spyer 2000), can further compound complications by aspartame-induced hyperinsulinemia.

- Widom and Simonson (1990) demonstrated that diabetic patients may develop cognitive impairment before the onset of symptoms attributable to the release of epinephrine and norepinephrine.
- Amiel et al (1991) reported a threefold increase in the incidence of both severe and asymptomatic hypoglycemia among diabetic patients treated intensively with insulin. Furthermore, they are more likely to develop EEG abnormalities during hypoglycemia.

Criticism of Related Research (see Chapter XXVIII)

The administration of aspartame as capsules to evaluate its effect on diabetic control, rather than "real world" products, is relevant. This introduces the deficiency of not invoking the cephalic phase of insulin release associated with the taste of sweet (see above). If insulin production is already strained, such superimposed stimulation could result in a state termed "high-output failure of insulinogenesis" (Roberts 1964, 1965).

Professional Confusion and Disagreement (see Chapter XXVIII)

Many physicians and other health care professionals disagree with the author's concern about aspartame use by diabetics.

- Filer and Stegink (1989) reviewed aspartame metabolism in diabetic subjects, and concluded "aspartame may be safely ingested at projected levels of use." (These investigators received considerable corporate support.)
- John D. Fernstrom, Ph.D. (1987) opined that the "pros" of aspartame in improving the quality of life for "millions of diabetics in the population" far outweigh "any imagined cons" of this and related products. He argued against wasting effort by "being obsessive about something that isn't really there."
- Dr. F. Xavier Pi-Sunyer, a physician-representative of the American Diabetes Association, reaffirmed this organization's approval of the safety of aspartame – both for diabetics and the general population in testimony given a U.S. Senate hearing on November 3, 1987. He asserted that there had been no significant input from physicians concerning problems in managing diabetics related to aspartame use. Moreover, he expressed concern over the unwarranted anxiety created by this hearing, and objected to spending any more money for research "already done."

Furthermore, most physicians accept the assertion by diabetologists that aspartame is harmless for diabetics.

- Horwitz and Bauer-Nehrling (1983) concluded that there is "no evidence of alteration of diabetic control because of aspartame ingestion."
- Visek (1984) stated that aspartame does not interfere with the basic treatment of diabetic patients.

- Stern et al (1976) followed 43 non-insulin-dependent diabetics at two centers. They were given either two capsules of aspartame three times daily with meals, or a comparable placebo, for 90 days. These investigators stated that "diabetic control was unaffected by the chronic administration of these substances."

The author's interpretation of the fasting blood sugar (FBS) concentrations in the subgroup of patients treated and followed at the Jewish Hospital and Medical Center of Brooklyn, based on the published data, differs from this assessment. The FBS values at one, five, nine and 14 weeks for the 9-10 patients given aspartame were 115.7, 116.2, 136.5, and 134.9 mg percent, respectively. The FBS values for the placebo group (ranging in number from 10 to 11) at one, five, nine and 14 weeks were 88.9, 107.2, 117.7, and 95.5 mg percent, respectively. The P values at one, five, nine and 14 weeks were 0.10, >0.50, >0.40, and >0.10, respectively.

- Nehrling et al (1985) gave aspartame and an identical-looking placebo containing corn starch to insulin-dependent and non-insulin-dependent diabetics in a randomized, double-blind study over an 18-week period. Three capsules were taken with each meal (total of 9 capsules daily). They concluded that adverse reactions were no more common with aspartame. These investigators, however, did not compare the corn starch with an inert non-carbohydrate placebo (e.g., alanine). Moreover, one subject developed severe diarrhea while receiving aspartame. (It disappeared when the aspartame was discontinued, and recurred after rechallenge.)
- The inclusion of monosodium glutamate (MSG) in presumed placebos raises another problem.

Resistance

The author asserted in many publications and written testimony to Congress that the current wholesale ingestion of aspartame products constitutes a perceived "imminent public health hazard," especially for diabetics. Yet the FDA and the American Diabetes Association (ADA) continue to express the <u>unequivocal</u> opinion that aspartame is "completely safe" for diabetics.

As a case in point, it has been virtually impossible to present these observations at national meetings of diabetologists and other physician groups. For example, the ADA (of which I had been a member for over three decades) refused to print an **abstract** of adverse reactions encountered in 58 diabetic patients that was submitted for its 1987 annual meeting. *Clinical Research* subsequently published (1988;Vol. 3:489A).

The following letter indicates the resistance this subject provokes. The correspondent, a 60-year-old diabetic woman with many ailments, had a sister and multiple relatives who suffered severe reactions (including convulsions) to aspartame products, but defended their use.

> "How in the world can someone take a product that is relied upon by diabetics to live, and make it bad? This was a big hoax. I just wonder how many people are depriving themselves of a pleasure just because someone scared them into not using it (an aspartame tabletop sweetener). The American Diabetes Association approves its use."

Patient Input

Diabetic aspartame reactors have expressed severe disapproval over the continued recommendation of aspartame products by the American Diabetes Association. Some averred that this is tantamount to helping diabetics die.

Patients have expressed this attitude in dramatic <u>confrontations with doctors</u>, even resorting to ridicule (see Case XIII-19). For example, a diabetic patient with aspartame reactions was dismissed by her physician, "a diabetes specialist," when she became irate over his lack of knowledge or interest on the subject – especially after providing him considerable information on aspartame disease obtained from the Internet.

The virtual unconditional approval of aspartame products by endocrinologists astonished <u>parents of diabetic children</u> when they learned the adverse effects of this chemical. For example, the outraged mother of a 9-year-old diabetic boy stated, "His endocrinologist backs aspartame 1001 percent, and highly recommends diet sodas. When I questioned any side effects from drinking so much, he assured me that the boy would have to drink over 100 cans/bottles of diet soda a day for the rest of his life to have any damaging side effects."

XIV

HYPOGLYCEMIA

"But the interesting thing – or better, the tragedy – is that the most dangerous things we do, and our most dangerous items, provoke no fear at all. We decide caveat emptor when, but only when, it is convenient to do so."
                    Dr. John B. Thomison (1983)

Seventy-four aspartame reactors specifically attributed the aggravation of previously-diagnosed reactive hypoglycemia ("low blood sugar attacks") to using aspartame products. Other aspartame reactors who returned the survey questionnaire undoubtedly were similarly affected, but did not realize they had this disorder.

Most patients in this category had clinical and laboratory evidence for reactive hypoglycemia, with or without diabetic responses (decreased glucose tolerance), by glucose tolerance testing. Prolonged elevations of the plasma insulin to a glucose load were the rule. The attacks precipitated by such testing were sufficiently severe in some patients to necessitate terminating the study (see Cases XII-1 and XIV-1), particularly when there was a history of seizures (see Cases III-1 and III-2).

The subject of diabetogenic hyperinsulinism has been discussed in the introduction and Chapter XIII. Its presence may be suggested prominent café-au-lait spots and other pigmentations (Roberts 1964 a-d; 1965c; 1966b;1967b,d; 1969a;1971b) that are often found in such patients – as in Case VI-L-2, a college student with aspartame-induced intellectual deterioration.

Acronym Legend
        ACB - aspartame cola beverage
        ASD - aspartame soft drink
        ATS - aspartame tabletop sweetener

REPRESENTATIVE CASE REPORTS
(also see Cases III-1, VI-L-2, XII-1)

Representative Case Reports

Case XIV-1

A 36-year-old businesswoman initially was seen in consultation during March 1985 for unrecognized severe reactive hypoglycemia. She responded promptly to an appropriate diet and other supportive measures. The results of her initial glucose tolerance test were as follows:

	Glucose (mg %)	Insulin (µU/ml)
Fasting	55	3.6
1/2 hour	154	27.9
1 hour	229	52.0
2 hours	110	110
3 hours	86	----
3-1/2 hours	31 * (attack; test stopped)	----

The patient presented a year later with multiple complaints. They included recurring intense hunger, lightheadedness, headache, leg cramps, difficulty with contact lens, and a tendency to increased bruising. Another physician found a modest anemia and elevated triglyceride concentration. She had been drinking diet cola and chewing aspartame gum in the interim.

In view of the predictable recurrence of her symptoms several hours after eating, and previous elevated glucose concentrations at one hour, a second glucose tolerance test was done. She experienced intense headache, lightheadedness, and "the jitters" after the third hours, at which point the test was stopped. The results were as follows:

	Glucose (mg %)	Insulin (µU/ml)
Fasting	76	3.8
1/2 hour	176	29.4
1 hour	199	81.7
2 hours	140	46.6
3 hours	53*(attack; test stopped)	----

550

There was striking improvement within two weeks after avoidance of aspartame products.

Case XIV-2

A woman wrote about her grandson who suffered a convulsion at the age of 2-1/2 years. He had been taking one glass of an aspartame drink and two packets of a tabletop sweetener daily for two weeks. The child was hospitalized when his "blood sugar dropped to 'zero', and IVs were required."

Case XIV-3

A 40-year-old woman had been diagnosed as having reactive hypoglycemia nine years previously. She religiously adhered to her diet because "a slip would produce my feelings of headaches, dizziness, faintness, depression, and many other symptoms that people with this problem experience."

She summarized her reactions to aspartame.

> "All went well until my soft drinks began to contain aspartame as an additive.
>
> "This summer has been exceptionally hot in the area where I live. I was drinking several cans a day of aspartame soft drinks and colas when I began to experience side effects that had me feel as I did before my condition was diagnosed and then gave up sugar.
>
> "Deep depression, extreme nervousness, dizziness, diarrhea, and severe headaches were a daily occurrence.
>
> "I finally began to pay attention to what I was consuming. After halting the intake of diet drinks, I felt much better within a week. I can personally say that aspartame is dangerous for me."

Case XIV-4

A 54-year-old registered nurse consumed up to ten glasses of an ASD and four glasses of aspartame-sweetened hot chocolate daily. Recurring hypoglycemic attacks ensued. She also suffered intense abdominal pain, nausea, bloody diarrhea, and severe abdominal bloat.

Other complaints included blurred vision, recent "dry eyes," severe headache, dizziness, tremors, insomnia, confusion, memory loss, marked hyperactivity, tingling of the limbs, intense depression with suicidal thoughts, extreme irritability and anxiety, a personality change, the aggravation of phobias, attacks of shortness of breath and palpitations, marked thinning of the hair, and severe joint pains.

She underwent extensive evaluations by four physicians, and was hospitalized four times. The costs were estimated at $15,000 out of her own pocket, and $35,000 for the insurance carrier.

Two sisters also experienced aspartame reactions – chiefly manifest as depression, anxiety and hypoglycemic attacks.

This nurse lost her job and became incapacitated "by severe attacks of hypoglycemia and pancreatitis [see Chapter IX-D], which required frequent hospitalizations." She wrote

> "I am 95% certain that aspartame reactivated my hypoglycemia symptoms, which I had not had in over 10 years. I also feel that the pancreatitis was a direct result of its use. I have never used alcohol or drugs of any kind. The doctors cannot find an explanation for it other than the use of aspartame.
>
> "The pancreatic pain began along with the mental symptoms following a vacation trip on which I consumed much more aspartame than while working. It was after consuming a large glass of aspartame soda on an empty stomach that I passed out and was rushed to intensive care. I've been through three years of agony."

Case XIV-5

A registered nurse decided to lose weight after the birth of her second child, and began drinking diet cola. Developing symptoms suggestive of hypoglycemia, she was found to have blood glucose concentrations "in the 40s." Reactive hypoglycemia was confirmed by glucose tolerance testing. Other symptoms included daily headaches, photosensitivity, marked loss of hair, a "foggy" feeling, recent hypertension, and a marked decline of her platelet count (under 30,000). Dramatic improvement occurred after stopping aspartame products.

552

Case XIV-6

A 49-year-old woman consumed large amounts of aspartame products in an unsuccessful attempt to lose weight. She developed headache, depression, profuse sweating, unquenchable thirst, and "episodes of disorientation." Concerned that she was developing diabetes, a diabetic friend monitored her blood glucose levels with a home glucose monitor. The values were consistently low – "usually in the 50s and 60s, even after I had eaten."

HYPOGLYCEMIA - A CLINICAL OVERVIEW

A vast literature exists on hypoglycemia and diabetogenic hyperinsulinism (see Introduction; Chapter XIII). The author has observed and studied many patients with documented "reactive" hypoglycemia – also known as "functional hyperinsulinism" – with or without decreased glucose tolerance (proneness to diabetes mellitus). The clinical findings, diagnostic criteria, high and sustained plasma insulin responses to a glucose load, and other tests, are detailed in prior publications (Roberts 1964 a-e;1965 a-c;1966a,b;1967 a-d; 1968; 1969b; 1971b; 1973).

Importance of the Disorder

Severe reactive hypoglycemia assumes considerable importance in the context of aspartame disease.

- It is a **common** affliction in the general population, conservatively estimated as existing in one out of three adults.
- The nervous system requires an adequate and continual supply of glucose for proper function (see below).
- Hypoglycemia can be a <u>direct</u> cause of accidents by altering the attention, perception, coordination and appropriate motor responses of drivers or pilots (Roberts 1971 a, b; 1999) (Section 6).
- Hypoglycemia/hyperinsulinemia precedes or accompanies many important medical, neurologic and psychiatric disorders.
- If unchecked for prolonged periods, the individual's pancreatic islet cells that make insulin can be depleted, culminating in overt diabetes mellitus (Chapter XIII).
- Hypoglycemia is treatable by corrective diet and simple supportive measures.
- The carcinogenic potential of chronic hyperinsulinemia is considered in Chapter XXVII-E.

- The striking increased mitogenicity of insulin glargine and other insulin analogs over human insulin (Berger 2000) assumes considerable relevance relative to brain, prostate and other tumors.

In evolutionary perspectives, diabetogenic hyperinsulinism represents a biological endowment for surviving hunger and famine. It became accentuated over the past century by radical changes in diet and habits (Roberts 1964, 1971b). The "western" diet is characterized by a reduction in complex carbohydrates (chiefly as cereals and vegetables), and a marked increase of simple sugars (Hodges 1965).

Manifestations of Hypoglycemia

Attacks of hypoglycemia are commonly manifest by these features: (1) profound cyclic weakness ("draining of my strength"; "sapping of my energy"; "late morning slump"; "afternoon letdown") that occurs several hours after eating; (2) associated tremors, nervousness, headache, sweats, and intense hunger with a craving for sugar; and (3) the prompt subsidence of these features after ingesting food or caloric sweets. A young woman made this analogy concerning her desire for sweets under these circumstances: "It's like sugar is dope."

Hypoglycemic attacks tend to intensify prior to lunch and during the latter part of the afternoon and evening. This is attributable to the effects of activity, and the accelerated release of insulin as the day progresses. The latter phenomenon may be demonstrable only by the method of **afternoon** glucose tolerance testing (Roberts 1964d; 1968).

Hypoglycemia often presents with an array of neurologic and psychiatric features. They include tremors, dizziness, true vertigo, double vision, "pins and needles" (paresthesias), muscular weakness, inability to think or speak properly, convulsions, psychopathic behavior, disorientation, total confusion, amnesia, overt psychotic features (e.g., paranoia, mania, depression), delirium and unconsciousness. The nervous system manifestations tend to follow certain patterns for a given individual, being polysymptomatic in most but occasionally monosymptomatic. Haier (1988) reported a correlation between cerebral glucose metabolism and psychological function.

Adverse Effects of Glucose Deprivation on the Brain and Nerves (Neuroglucopenia)

The ravages on the brain of recurring severe hypoglycemia, especially when unchecked (as during the night), are readily understood in the light of these facts: (a) the brain is almost totally dependent upon an adequate supply of circulating glucose for normal function; and (b) neither the nervous system nor the body can store glucose and readily - available carbohydrate for more than one day.

The following observations amplify these issues. They tend to be compounded in aspartame disease.

- The developing central nervous system is highly susceptible to the ravages of energy deprivation (Laatsh 1962). This is believed to account for the frequency of narcolepsy (Roberts 1964 a-e; 1971 a,b), reading disability (Roberts 1961b), migraine and related headaches (Roberts 1966b,c), and abnormal behavior (Roberts 1969b) in young persons with severe hypoglycemia.

- Certain neurologic manifestations are importantly influenced by biochemical and enzymic differences within specific areas. In turn, they are rendered more vulnerable to hypoglycemia (Roberts 1966b,c). For example, the concentration of glucose-6-phosphate dehydrogenase activity is four times greater in heavily myelinated central tracts than in lightly myelinated ones (McDougal 1961, 1964.)

- The adverse effects of glucose deprivation on the central nervous system are enhanced by water retention within nerve cells and myelin. It may result from excessive ingestion of fluids in the wake of aspartame-induced thirst (Chapter IX-F), hormonal influences (especially estrogens and birth control drugs), and the hyperinsulized state itself (Roberts 1966b,c). Water and sodium are known to migrate into nerve cells following hypoglycemia or the experimental removal of glucose from a perfusing environment (Yannet 1939; Stern 1949; Krebs 1951.)

- The consequences of combined glucose deprivation and water retention ultimately may disrupt the functional and anatomic integrity of myelin (the sheath that "insulates" nerve fibers). A vicious myelin-destroying cycle might ensue (Roberts 1966b,c). The frequency with which an initial diagnosis of "multiple sclerosis" was made in many aspartame reactors (Chapter VI-D), especially weight-conscious young women, is germane.

The body's compensatory responses for minimizing the nervous system insult of severe hypoglycemia through the release of counterregulatory hormones invite additional complications. For example, the secretion of large amounts of epinephrine ("adrenaline") and norepinephrine can induce severe tremors, sweats, rapid heart action, and elevation of the blood pressure. Moreover, their effects might be cumulative. Stosky and Shamoom (1986) demonstrated that excessive epinephrine induced by hypoglycemia persists during maximum exercise, being proportionate to the intensity and duration of such activity.

ASPARTAME-INDUCED HYPOGLYCEMIA

Clinical Observations

Many influences can aggravate hypoglycemia or precipitate hypoglycemic attacks in nondiabetics. They commonly include severe caloric restriction and the missing of meals by weight-conscious persons, fever, the use of oral contraceptives ("the pill"), various drugs (including aspirin), and unaccustomed exercise (especially in hot weather.) Aspartame should be added to this list.

Despite his longstanding interest in this subject, the author remained baffled by the failure of patients with hypoglycemia to respond – or continue to respond – to diet and other conventional measures in the mid-1980s. Their cessation of aspartame products often solved this puzzle. Unbeknown to me at the time, several patients with severe hypoglycemia had concluded that aspartame made them ill, and resumed sugar-containing products or took saccharin. When sugar was taken in small amounts, along with adequate protein and fat, most fared well.

The desire for sweetness, whether an inborn or acquired trait, poses a challenge for most persons with reactive hypoglycemia. Paradoxically, they should avoid sugar (sucrose) because it stimulates insulin secretion and can precipitate an attack. The appeal of a popular ATS resides in its being advertised as containing no sugar.

Patients with aspartame disease emphasized the difficulties they encountered when hospitalized, especially for surgery. Foremost, hypoglycemic attacks occurred when they were not fed or did not receive intravenous glucose prior to and following surgery. Second, the "full liquid" diet prescribed pre- or postoperatively often contained aspartame, thereby precipitating or compounding their symptoms.

Vicious Circles

Several vicious circles involving aspartame may be generated by the consumption of excessive calories, sugar intake, the habitual use of large amounts of aspirin, caffeine, nicotine and alcohol, and various drugs taken to combat headache, fatigue, sweats, tremors and other symptoms. For example, testosterone enhances insulin biosynthesis and secretion, as demonstrated by the hyperinsulinemia encountered in hyperandrogenic syndromes.

Aspartame reactions are better understood in this context. They represent not only deranged physiology (especially within the brain), but also the impact of hypoglycemia insults inflicted on weight- and fashion-conscious persons. Of special interest are the severe reduction of carbohydrate and calories, and forced feeding (eating only one meal a day) when coupled with vigorous exercise. Some of the catastrophic consequences include attacks of rapid heart action (paroxysmal tachycardia), angina pectoris, convulsions, nonthrombotic stroke, multiple sclerosis, various thyroid disorders, and severe personality changes.

As noted, the brain is almost totally dependent upon an adequate supply of glucose for proper function under ordinary circumstances. When aspartame is substituted for carbohydrate or food in persons having diabetogenic hyperinsulinism, it and other vital organs may be deprived of glucose. They then do what car engines do when running out of fuel... make warning noises or stop.

Mechanisms

I. Reflex Hypoglycemia. Intense sweetness without sugar invites "reflex hypoglycemia." The cephalic phase of insulin release initiated by introducing food or sweet in the mouth is neurally mediated. It "prepares" the body to receive glucose and other nutrients. This occurs before the blood glucose increases. The afferent limb of this reflex involves olfactory, visual, taste and oropharyngeal receptors (Proietto 1987). The vagus nerve mediates its efferent limb.

Powley and Berthoud (1985) emphasized the critical nature of this cephalic phase because it represents the first rapid physiological response to food. It is influenced by color, appearance, flavor, aroma and texture. This phenomenon also has been demonstrated in rats using water sweetened with saccharin. The insulin response could be correlated with the concentration of saccharin solution.

A NutraSweet Company scientist noted that the cephalic reflex increased insulin release in mice after tasting aspartame at The First International Meeting On Dietary Phenylalanine and Brain Function (Washington, D.C., May 9. 1987).

II. Aspartame-Induced Insulin Release. Studies by Melchior et al (1991) indicate the impressive rise of both insulin and beta endorphins after aspartame consumption. They administered two chocolate drinks – one sweetened with 50 g sucrose; the other with 80 mg aspartame – to 10 subjects of normal weight who averaged 21.7 years. Plasma beta endorphin concentrations were more elevated after the aspartame drink than after sucrose or fasting, while insulin increased as much after the aspartame drink as with sucrose. The beta endorphin rise after aspartame may represent increased insulin secretion or a direct effect of aspartame on the liberation of beta endorphins.

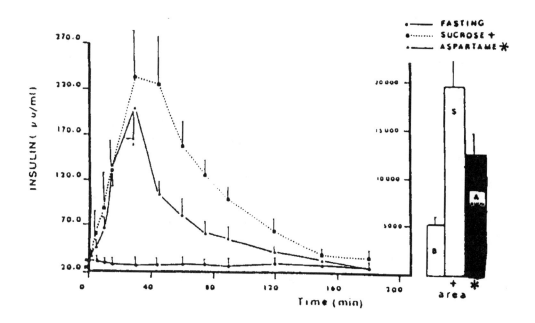

Figure XIV-1

Insulin concentrations under three conditions (mean ±SEM). The rise after sucrose and aspartame was different from fasting. The sucrose and aspartame responses were comparable.

Melchior, J.C., Rigaud, D, Colas-Linhart, N., et al. Immunoreactive beta-endorphin increases after an aspartame chocolate drink in healthy human subjects. *Physiology and Behavior* 1991; 54:941-944. Reproduced with permission of Elsevier Science

558

III. The Insulin-Glucose Effects of Amino Acids. A number of investigators have conclusively shown that insulin secretion is stimulated by certain essential amino acids – both when given individually, and as mixtures (Chapter XXIV). The released insulin then facilitates utilization of amino acids in protein synthesis within cells. Concomitantly, blood glucose and free fatty acid concentrations decline.

These observations are germane in view of the phenylalanine and aspartic acid components of aspartame.

- Floyd et al (1966) demonstrated that elevated blood levels of insulin are induced in healthy persons following the intravenous administration of phenylalanine, being exceeded only by arginine, lysine and leucine. Such stimulation did not depend on the presence of leucine or increased blood glucose concentrations. (Leucine-induced hypoglycemia is a well-known phenomenon.)
- The marked increase of plasma insulin after ingestion of phenylalanine drinks by healthy men is further elevated when the amino acid is ingested with carbohydrates (van Loon 2000).
- Phenylalanine and arginine have a synergistic effect on insulin secretion when given to humans (Floyd 1970). (See Figure XXIV-1) This is not a reflection of increased blood glucose or glucagon concentrations.
- Schmid et al (1989) demonstrated a 3.6-fold greater insulin response among obese subjects given an infusion of amino acids (including phenylalanine and aspartic acid) than lean subjects.
- A dramatic rise of circulating insulin and growth hormone concentrations occurs both in pre-term infants given an infusion of essential amino acids (Figure XXIV-3), and in adults (Reitano 1978).
- Phenylalanine and its analogs influence the binding and activation of glucose-dependent insulinotropic polypeptide (GIP) receptors (Yip 1999). GIP is not only an important regulator of insulin release, but also increases insulin receptor binding affinity and the effect of insulin on target tissues.

IV. Methanol. The effects of methanol are reviewed in Chapter XXI. Even in small amounts, it may exaggerate hypoglycemia by delaying the release of epinephrine as a protective counterregulatory mechanism, as has been shown with non-intoxicating doses of ethanol (Sood 2001).

XV

OLDER PERSONS; ALZHEIMER'S DISEASE

"For this effect defective comes by cause."
Shakespeare
(*Hamlet* 2:2:103)

A host of neuropsychiatric problems due to aspartame disease affect older persons, especially confusion and memory loss (Chapter VI-C), tremors (Chapter VI-J), and seizures (Chapter III). The burden on health care facilities and costs has increased because of seizures in old age (Stephen 2000).

Bender et al (1999) reported that excess obesity-related mortality declined with age at all levels of obesity in a large cohort of obese persons. Accordingly, vigorous attempts by "older" persons to reduce through severe caloric restriction and aspartame intake may be counterproductive.

Astute correspondents projected the public health problems associated with aspartame-induced confusion and memory loss, based on their own reactions.

- An attorney wrote: "I can't help but wonder how many other people are being injured by cognitive impairment from aspartame without even realizing what is happening to them."
- An affected couple underscored the subtle nature of aspartame-induced memory loss: "My wife and I both quit drinking diet-anything. We actually threw out some cooking stuff that had aspartame in it. Now after eight weeks, we feel much better, have more energy, and my memory has returned to even better than before. That's hard to comprehend since I never knew it was going."

560

GENERAL CONSIDERATIONS

The aspartame-is-everywhere dilemma (Chapter 1), and the vigorous promotion of aspartame products to health-conscious older persons, ought to be cause for concern.

> A radio commercial for an aspartame product (heard on July 23, 1986) featured the voice of a woman **insisting** that the husband put it in her elderly mother's tea. She repeatedly prevented him from informing the mother that "the two teaspoons of sugar" weren't the <u>real</u> thing.

Consumer Reservations

Older persons may prefer higher concentrations of a mixture of essential amino acids (Murphy 1987). Yet, many intuitively reject aspartame products. This reflects their distrust of "artificial" foods, and the side effects experienced on sampling them... especially "the strange chemical taste."

An Alzheimer Connection?

This chapter later amplifies the author's concern that aspartame products might initiate or accelerate Alzheimer's disease (AD). Many patients and correspondents have provided impressive histories about themselves or relatives that document the simulation of "early" Alzheimer's disease by aspartame disease.. A number also gave striking family histories of AD.

> There have been references in mythical legends to nonalcoholic drinks severely impairing memory. One is the "magic draught of forgetfulness" drunk by Siegfried in Wagner's *Goetterdaemmerung,* causing the hero to forget his beloved wife Brunnhilde. In plotting this act, Hagen uttered
>
> "Recall the drink in yon shrine, and doubt not him who gained the charm. The hero for whom thou burn'st fondly 'twill bind to thy heart. Did now but Siegfried come and taste of the wonderful draught, that he'd seen a woman ere thee – or e'er a woman had neared, would wholly pass from his head."

Premature Aging

Comparable problems with memory among younger aspartame reactors at times were attributed to "premature aging" and prodromal AD (Chapter VI-C). Of the 397 initial reactors completing the questionnaire, 73 (18.8 percent) were 50-59 years, and 48 (12.1 percent) 60-69 years.

The need for considering exposure to aspartame and other neurotoxins before making a diagnosis of "premature aging" is paramount. Such exposure may explain why some younger individuals develop "older-person diseases." This experience of a man with aspartame disease illustrates the issue: "I was a 7-year drinker of diet colas. I quit drinking them 45 days ago, and cannot believe how great I feel now! My doctors and friends had told me that it was old age creeping in. I am only 56."

The following reactors who were less than 60 provide other examples.

- An 18-year-old man experienced severe confusion when he drank two liters of an aspartame beverage daily.

- A woman was concerned about her husband who consumed 2-3 two-liter bottles of diet drinks daily. She stated, "He was always complaining to me that he thought he was getting senile because he couldn't remember anything."

- The memory of a 59-year-old man deteriorated while consuming three liters of diet colas daily. His physician-son expressed concern about "early Alzheimer's disease."

- A 40-year-old professional speaker experienced "disorientation and couldn't remember things" within minutes to an hour whenever she drank an aspartame cola.

- A housewife in her 50s described her reactions after seeing an article about my research on aspartame disease in the *Saturday Evening Post.* She also cited other friends who had comparable memory loss and headache, including a married couple (both teachers).

"When this article came to my attention, I was so excited that I cried. After several years of using an aspartame tabletop sweetener and having headaches, depression, memory loss and zombie-like behavior, I was so relieved to know that there are others like that.

"It is awful to forget your Social Security number and phone numbers. I couldn't converse with others because I couldn't use words properly. All self confidence went down the drain. There was such a zombie-like state that I couldn't feel excited even when my granddaughter was born.

"About two years ago, I read an article in a local paper that stated aspartame could cause headaches and memory loss. It scared me. Needless to say we threw away all of this aspartame sweetener.

"I have regained a lot of my memory, and no longer feel depressed or like a zombie!

"About two months ago, I accidently consumed the same sweetener, and had a nauseous headache and feeling of anxiety. I knew immediately what was wrong. I read the label, and there was aspartame. Boy, was I angry!

"Please continue to speak out against this poison. **A mind truly is a terrible thing to lose.**"

- A 50-year-old secretary had been drinking up to three cans of diet cola daily. She complained of decreased vision, ringing in the ears, headache, extreme irritability and unexplained chest pain. She wrote, "I felt my problem of eyesight, head pains and irritability were perhaps just 'getting on in years.' But after stopping the diet cola, the head pains are gone, and the irritability has decreased."

Aggravation of Existing Alzheimer's Disease

Aspartame products can aggravate the problems of persons afflicted with probable AD. The following patients illustrate this issue.

Representative Case Reports

Case XV-1

The author had doctored a 76-year-old man for 13 years for an organic brain syndrome of the Alzheimer type. His studies were normal – including serum vitamin B_{12} and folate levels, and endocrine tests. Various supplements had not helped.

A dramatic change had occurred when next seen. He previously looked forward to going to a day-care center, but now could hardly get out of bed. (He was receiving no medication.) The physical examination and laboratory tests remained unchanged. Direct questioning revealed that he had been using aspartame puddings and gelatin, and diet cola.

Abstinence from aspartame products was urged. He improved considerably in both appearance and activity when rechecked 10 days later... a fact noted by persons attending him. His wife volunteered, "I think, for the record, you should know that aspartame makes him jumpy and impatient."

Case XV-2

A 66-year-old retiree consumed 6-8 cans of diet cola daily for one year. He described his problem as "procrastination, sedentary, memory loss, bad mental attitude about myself, itchy skin, headaches, depression, and inability to coordinate my thought." He also noted marked thinning of the hair, frequent urination (day and night), slurred speech, and suicidal ideas. These symptoms improved <u>within one week</u> after stopping aspartame. He explained

> "I did notice changes taking place, but I attributed them to the aging process, and even commented that I was perhaps going through 'male menopause.' Then one night, I was watching TV when an exposé on aspartame was being aired. The symptoms narrated were just the things I was experiencing. I stopped using the product at once, and my problems started to clear up."

Case XV-3

A retired boilermaker listed "marked memory loss" as his sole complaint. It improved shortly after stopping aspartame, and disappeared by four months. He wrote this retrospective letter.

> "I was drinking an aspartame soda in large amounts since it came out in the summer of 1983. For the last six or seven months, I found I was losing my presence of mind. My short--term memory was bad. I did stupid things due to lack of alertness, and my eyes were very sensitive to sunlight. Does this sound like an aspartame problem? I am age 70, 160 lbs, in good health, and had no problem at all until this came about."

Case XV-4

A 71-year-old saleswoman remained active and enjoyed fishing. Being "health conscious," she began to use one packet of an aspartame tabletop sweetener daily. She then experienced severe headaches, intense drowsiness with a desire to fall asleep (even at the

564

wheel), unsteadiness on her feet, marked memory impairment, unexplained chest pains, heartburn, severe nausea, itching, "open sores," dry eyes, and an extraordinary loss of energy.

> "My judgment was affected a number of times while driving. I would drive across the center line without being aware of it until I would notice an approaching car. I couldn't understand what was happening to me. I have always been an excellent driver. Once I drove into a ditch and was not conscious of actually doing it. The sleepiness and feverishness increased to the point where I had to lie down every day! I am an avid fisherman, and the thought of not being able to go fishing was very disturbing to me."

After reading an article about aspartame disease, she eliminated the product. There was marked improvement within three days. Her sores healed in three weeks. She became convinced of aspartame's role after the following rechallenge.

> "I discovered a can of an aspartame soft drink in my refrigerator about three weeks later. Being thirsty and thinking that one can wouldn't affect me, I drank it. About 20 minutes later, I became so sleepy that I had to lie down.

> "There is no doubt in my mind that aspartame is the culprit. If aspartame affects me so drastically, there must be thousands of other people who are affected and don't suspect aspartame as the cause. It frightens me to think of the serious accidents I could have been involved in as a result."

SELECTED CLINICAL FEATURES OF ASPARTAME DISEASE IN OLDER PERSONS

Dry Mouth

Aspartame-induced dry mouth (xerostomia) was described in Chapter IX-F. It can be compounded in older persons by the many drugs that reduce saliva. The ensuing problems include severe inflammation of the tongue, lips and mouth, superimposed yeast infection, accelerated dental caries, and further impairment of speech, taste, mastication and swallowing.

Fatigue

Many older persons in this series suffered "severe fatigue." Aspartame disease should be considered before ascribing it to "the tired man syndrome " in a retiree consuming these products.

Aggravation of Diabetes and Hypoglycemia

Older persons who suffer aspartame disease often evidence impairment in metabolizing a glucose load and/or increased insulin levels. The associated aggravation of diabetes and hypoglycemia are discussed in Chapters XIII and XIV.

Depression

Aspartame-associated depression with suicidal thoughts (Chapter VII-B) is serious in the elderly, particularly after the death of a spouse. Dr. Robert H. Willis (1987) reported that nearly all first-time suicidal attempts by persons over the age of 60 are successful, compared to only one in 100 attempts by adolescents.

Cardiac Complications and Stroke

Cardiac events (Chapter IX-C), stroke, or both, occurred in older patients after they began consuming aspartame products. Most were NOT included in this series because of previous attacks or associated risk factors (e.g., hypertension; elevated cholesterol concentrations; vascular disorders elsewhere) even though the clinical sequences suggested precipitation by an aspartame reaction.

Representative Case Report

Case XV-5

An active 89-year-old housewife was hospitalized ten days for her first myocardial infarction (heart attack). The hospital course was uneventful. The evening after returning home, she ate some aspartame gelatin brought over by a neighbor. She felt "trembly" shortly thereafter, but had no chest discomfort or pulse abnormality. The next morning, she used an aspartame tabletop sweetener. Within minutes, she experienced numbness over the face and body, and then drooping of one side of her face with marked "drooling."

The possibility of a cerebral embolus was entertained, but she had received heparin, and was taking dipyridamole (an anti-clotting drug). Her electrocardiograms that day and the next were stable. The patient was treated symptomatically, and advised to avoid aspartame products. Her neurologic features had disappeared the following day.

Insomnia

The frequency with which older persons experienced "insomnia" (Chapter VII-F) and had bad ("negative") dreams, even essentially happy individuals, ought to be respected as a defensive signal by the brain. These nightmarish experiences may be provoked by food (glucose) deprivation, decreased oxygen, neurotoxin exposure, and combinations thereof... as is often the cause with aspartame users.

ASPARTAME AND AGISM

Agism is a pernicious system of destructive and false beliefs about the elderly. A prime illustration is the frequency with which unrecognized aspartame reactions were reflexively ascribed to "old age."

Agism and the Medical Profession

Physicians often harbor negative beliefs about the elderly, in large measure because their exposure to robust and productive older persons was limited. Many hold the cultural stereotype of older individuals as senile and cantankerous "wrinkled babies."

Agism is an undesirable attitude among doctors for another reason: it stifles communication with older persons. A vicious cycle then occurs when they become reluctantto see young doctors after repeated encounters of indifference or hostility. The same may apply to nurses.

> While attending a patient on the emergency floor of a local hospital, the author read a poem that had been posted by a staff nurse on the bulletin board. Titled, *Just A Little Mixed Up*, it was written by "A. Nonny Mouse." (I could not locate either the poet or the periodical in which it appeared.) The first stanza read
>
> > "Just a line to say I'm living, That I'm not among the dead; Though I'm getting more forgetful, and mixed up in the head."

Having practiced in a "retirement community" more than four decades, I am impressed by the vitality of many retired individuals. Accordingly, the rebound of "senior citizens" from severe fatigue, confusion and other complaints after stopping aspartame products (as Cases XV-2 and 4) had a great impact. Paradoxically, the striking decline in mentation among some younger aspartame reactors continued long after other symptoms subsided.

> Case III-13 developed gross personality changes, headache, and grand mal convulsions at the age of 41 while consuming aspartame. She had no further seizures or headaches after avoiding aspartame products. This patient later wrote, "I feel the sharpness in my mind became dulled. Although some might say that could be attributed to age, I don't believe one ages so fast in one year's time."

Erroneous Diagnoses

The tendency by physicians, the media and support groups to equate "memory loss" with Alzheimer's disease (see below) must be resisted.

> An ad in *The Miami Herald* (September 30, 1986, p. A-14) carried the heading ALZHEIMER'S in bold capital letters. It began: "If you or a loved one are experiencing memory loss, then you are invited to contact _____ . Our programs are conducted by board certified neurologists with extensive experience in the treatment of Alzheimer's disease, stroke and general aging." This was clearly an industry-sponsored solicitation for "clinical trials" of drugs not yet approved for AD.

Concomitant aspartame-induced depression (Chapter VII-B) can create another vicious cycle when older persons erroneously label themselves as "senile."

Aspartame disease should be suspected in older persons who "fail to thrive," especially during or after attempted weight loss. It is a documented risk factor in morbidity and mortality. This general term describes an unexplained decrease in function or metabolism in excess of that expected in an age-matched cohort. It has been encountered with alcoholism and drug effects.

The presumed "normal aging process" has been invoked to explain decreased sexuality in older men. Case XV-2 initially regarded his problem as "the male menopause."

568

Similarly, the impotence of some diabetic men with aspartame disease has been wrongly attributed to <u>diabetic neuropathy</u>.

> Barbara Mullarkey *(Wednesday Journal* March 26, 1986, p. 37) cited the case of a 75-year-old physician who discontinued sugar when diabetes was suspected. Until then, he had enjoyed regular sexual activity. He noted "a complete and total loss of libido" within ten days after substituting an aspartame tabletop sweetener. His sexual desire and performance returned within six weeks after stopping this product. He wrote
>
> > "Many people may not think this is an effect of aspartame. People my age might simply blame it on old age or an underlying illness, keep right on taking aspartame, and be resigned to a sexless old age. Younger people might blame it on the stresses and strains of everyday living. But the very abrupt onset and gradual disappearance just about rule out any other cause. The release of aspartame in the presence of so much unfavorable evidence calls for an explanation by the FDA, and that explanation better be good."*

Added Commentary

The author's views on agism were expressed in an editorial titled, "Medical and Ethical Guidelines for Managing the Elderly Ill," published by the *Journal of the Florida Medical Association* (Roberts 1982). The following excerpts are germane.

> "Primary care physicians increasingly are confronted with the challenge and complex responsibility of managing older persons over prolonged periods. When they develop superimposed illnesses and emergent disorders, a host of ethical – as well as medical – considerations often are introduced. An attitude of diagnostic or therapeutic nihilism is not infrequent once patients have been categorized as 'vegetables.'

"Over the years, I have adopted some guidelines for my own orientation to this situation. Hopefully, they may be useful to others.

1. A physician must remain alert to the coexistence or development of other conditions in other patients, especially if amenable to treatment.
2. A physician must encourage handicapped patients to function within the prudent limits of their tolerance – whether in the realm of work, hobbies or sexuality.
3. A physician must respect the body's inherent power for functional improvement before labeling any disorder as 'hopeless.'
4. A doctor must resist pressures against diagnostic or therapeutic intervention from the patient or the family that are based upon 'quality of life' misperceptions if he deems such professional efforts to be warranted.

"Doctors must not allow themselves to be diverted from the reasonable pursuit of a potentially treatable disorder by the foregoing quasi-ethical arguments when they are not truly convinced the situation is hopeless. I have witnessed enough worthy contributions by 'senior citizens' after their salvage through proper medical care that I feel compelled not to ignore their potential remaining value to society."*

RELATED PATHOPHYSIOLOGIC CONSIDERATIONS

The functioning human brain must be regarded with awe. It is greater than any computing machine. Its surface alone contains more than 100 trillion(!) interconnections. My observations (Roberts 1995) reinforce those of others who believe that it is defeatist to equate Alzheimer's disease (AD) with inevitable age-related loss of neuronal function.

Alterations of major neurotransmitters by aspartame and its components (Chapter XXIII) are relevant to disturbances of both memory and behavior in the elderly. Furthermore, the influx of large amounts of these amino acids poses a problem in light of their sharply decreased requirements with increasing age (Stegink 1984).

*© 1982 *Journal of the Florida Medical Association.* Reproduced with permission.

570

The deterioration of "benign senescent forgetfulness" warrants greater attention. It occurs in the wake of deficiencies or dysfunction of neurotransmitters (Chapter XXIII), and altered glucose metabolism within the hippocampus (a central relay area) and the temporal and parietal regions (Mozar 1987). The corticolimbic system, notably the hippocampus and amygdala, is importantly involved in recent or fact-declaratory learning.

Vulnerability to Energy Deprivation (Cerebral Glucopenia)

Decreased glucose uptake in multiple areas of the AD brain, especially within the hippocampus, has been shown by positive emission tomography (PET) scanning. This probably reflects both causation and secondary injury. Three considerations are central to the vulnerability of brain function in older persons – especially when they reduce calories, go too long between meals, and consume large amounts of the excitotoxin aspartame.

- More than 98 percent of the brain's energy is derived from body glucose under normal circumstances.
- Many older persons have impaired glucose metabolism or actual diabetes.
- They are more susceptible to severe lowering of the blood (and brain) glucose concentration resulting from decreased absorption, liver dysfunction due to various causes, and increased insulin secretion. (Aspartame-induced hypoglycemia was discussed in Chapter XIV.)

Numerous observations indicate intensification of the hyperinsulinized-diabetic state in later years.

- The high frequency of reduced glucose tolerance in elderly "normal" persons has been documented by many investigators. It was found to be 77 percent by Streeten et al (1965), 53 percent by Chesrow and Bleyer (1954), 75 percent by Brandt (1960), and 100 percent by Gottfried et al (1961).
- Hayner and co-workers (1965) emphasized the age factor among criteria for diagnosing diabetes. In a study of responses to a 100 gm glucose load ingested by 2,983 individuals over the age of 16, the one-hour blood glucose values steadily shifted toward higher concentrations proportionate to increasing age through the seventh decade. The regression slope approximates 13 mg/100 ml per decade.

- Circulating insulin levels are higher ("insulin resistance") in the elderly subjects – both fasting and after repeated injections of glucose (Streeten 1964, 1965).

- Zeytinoglu, Gherondache and Pincus (1969) analyzed the results of five-hour oral glucose tolerance testing and simultaneous serum insulin concentrations in elderly nondiabetic subjects (20 males and 20 females), ranging in the age from 68 to 91 years. According to the author's criteria, there was evidence of reactive hypoglycemia – especially by the four and five-hour values – in at least 23 of the 40 subjects.

- The data of Streeten et al (1965) are consistent with diabetogenic hyperinsulinism in an older group. Specifically, the mean serum insulin concentrations (μU/ml) while fasting, and 20 minutes after three successive intravenous loads of 50% glucose solution, were 305.9, 417.5, 364.2 and 563.7, respectively. Comparable values for normal young subjects, were 230.9, 261.0, 295.7 and 322.0 μU/ml, respectively.

The Cumulative Adverse Effects of Hypoglycemia on Nervous System Function with Aging

An accelerated loss of brain neurons after the fifth decade due to decreased tissue glucose (glucopenia) can be superimposed upon prior loss of these cells. This cumulative insult increases the probability of functional error in terms of both perception and response.

The death of nerve cells is characterized by failure to respond to stimuli, and a loss of ability to synthesize protein owing to exhaustion of their RNA. Cellular aging appears to be a consequence of molecular changes within the biological information system – namely, the manner in which DNA-based information is transcribed onto RNA, and ultimately translated into enzymic protein (Samis 1968).

Drugs and Chemical Vulnerability

Adverse drug reactions (ADR) associated with metabolic abnormalities and impaired kidney function contribute to the vulnerability of the central nervous system in older persons. Weber and Griffen (1986) correlated ADRs in this age group with the net number of prescribed drugs. Superimposed aspartame disease enhances their plight.

THE ASPARTAME-ALZHEIMER CONNECTION

Aspartame consumption may accelerate, and possibly initiate, Alzheimer's disease (AD). The details appear in *Defense Against Alzheimer's Disease* (Roberts 1995b). Accordingly, caution about its use is warranted from physicians, dietitians, and hospital/nursing home personnel.

The urgency of this matter is indicated by the enormous projected estimates of symptomatic Alzheimer's disease within the next two decades (see below). Furthermore, Dr. Joseph Foley (1987), Chairman of the National Institutes of Health consensus panel on Differential Diagnosis of Dementing Diseases, emphasized: "Our first obligation is not to allow the remediable to get out of hand."

"Benign senescent forgetfulness" and senile dementia of the Alzheimer type (SDAT) probably represent a continuum reflecting basic pathophysiologic processes (Brayne 1988). A diagnosis of "mild cognitive impairment" (MCI) could be the "slippery slope" to AD. (An estimated 12 percent of such persons progress to full-blown AD annually.) This perspective assumes significance in the present context as aspartame disease accelerates this process "to the right."

AN OVERVIEW OF ALZHEIMER'S DISEASE

Alzheimer's disease (AD) is an affliction that first appeared early in the 20th Century (Roberts 1995b). The contributory intake of dietary excitotoxins and of exposure to numerous environmental neurotoxins increased dramatically after 1950. They stemmed from technical achievements, such as changes in the manufacturing of monosodium glutamate (MSG) and aluminum, and economic factors. These perspectives are pertinent.

First, *Alzheimer's disease is believed to represent one type of brain reaction to cumulative metabolic, hypoxic and neurotoxic insults.*

Second, *a cascade of dietary, societal and technologic changes spawn a vicious neurodegenerative cycle. Their impact may be enhanced by genetic and immunologic factors.*

Third, *the contention that AD is caused by some entity other than physiologic, nutritional and medical disturbances prevalent in our society ought to be challenged. Stated differently, these contributory factors are probably common, readily definable, and susceptible to avoidance or modification.*

Fourth, *reactors who experience severe confusion and memory loss after consuming products containing aspartame offer a reversible human model for studying "early" Alzheimer's disease.*

Fifth, *amyloid plaques contain both phenylalanine and aspartic acid – as do the peptide sequences of the amyloid precursor.*

Sixth, *this unique "experiment of Nature" provides fertile clues to preventing AD over the 20-30 years (!) between the initial deposition of "senile plaques" or neurofibrillary tangles and the onset of clinical dementia.*

The Tragedy of Alzheimer's Disease

Millions of Americans currently suffer from dementia due to AD. The number is expected to increase dramatically, perhaps to 14 million, within the next half century. Victims evidence severe loss of attention, memory and judgment, coupled with disorientation, increased irritability, and marked personality changes.

The strain imposed upon the spouses and families of such persons constitutes a national catastrophe. AD is an incurable physical, medical, economic and social disaster – aptly referred to as "the funeral that never ends."

- AD cost the economy $100 billion in 1995.
- The averaged annual cost of nursing home care for AD patients ranges between $25,000 and $30,000.
- About 80 percent of the care for AD patients is provided directly by family members.
- An estimated one-third of families that admit a loved one into a skilled" nursing facility become bankrupt within one year.
- Most nursing homes find it impossible to cope adequately andhumanely with the confusion, wandering, incontinence and combativeness of AD patients.

II. CLINICAL OBSERVATIONS AND PERSPECTIVES

Basic Tenets

Persons who develop otherwise-unexplained confusion and memory loss, regardless of age, should be queried about the use of aspartame products. These symptoms were reported by 28.5 percent of the first 551 aspartame reactors (Roberts 1988e, 1989a, 1991a, 1992b, 1995b).

Patients who consume them should be observed at least one month after avoiding such products before being subjected to extensive neurologic testing. Ensuing dramatic improvement could spare them the onus of being misdiagnosed as "probable Alzheimer's disease."

Similar considerations apply to the intake of phenylalanine products and other amino acid preparations. Most no longer can be purchased over the counter in Canada, which instituted this policy after it recognized the profound brain effects of these products.

Two aspects convincingly demonstrate the causative role of aspartame in thesereactions. First, there was marked improvement or disappearance of confusion and memory loss after abstaining from aspartame products. Second, they promptly and predictably recurred on rechallenge.

The Matter of Dosage

Most persons afflicted with aspartame disease consumed modest to large amounts of aspartame in many commercially-available forms, especially "diet" beverages and gum. Even relatively small amounts of aspartame could induce confusion and memory impairment, particularly diet sodas stored for many months or after adding it to hot beverages.

- A 31-year-old nurse with a prior aspartame-induced convulsion became confused and "very incoherent" the morning after drinking three sips of an aspartame beverage initially thought to be "regular" soda.
- A 61-year-old executive bought coffee at a fast food outlet before playing golf, and added an aspartame tabletop sweetener because it did not stock his saccharin sweetener. He became confused and behaved erratically on the golf course. When his memory cleared after two hours, he could not recall this episode. There had been two comparable episodes after drinking aspartame-sweetened coffee at the home of friends. None recurred with total aspartame avoidance.

Other Clinical Findings

The 3:1 female preponderance of aspartame disease is consistent with the apparent higher incidence of AD among women in many studies.

The familial incidence of aspartame disease (Roberts 1988e, 1989a, 1989b, 1955b), averaging 22 percent, was impressive. Furthermore, multiple family members often evidenced similar neurologic reactions (Chapter XVI).

575

Many patients volunteered their <u>fear of having "early Alzheimer's disease"</u> before aspartame disease was diagnosed. Most felt reassured when their confusion, memory loss and other neuropsychiatric features subsided after avoiding aspartame.

The foregoing observations have been independently encountered by the <u>FDA</u>. Numerous consumers <u>voluntarily</u> reported comparable confusion and memory loss associated with the use of aspartame products (Tollefson 1987). Over half the complainants were between 20 and 59 years of age; about 85 percent were women.

Examples of Aspartame-Induced Reactions

Aspartame-induced confusion and memory loss ranged from subtle "forgettings" and "difficulty in concentrating" to gross intellectual incapacitation.

- A 30-year-old female sales consultant noted, "I could not consciously remember what I had done or said."
- An engineer had trouble remembering "names and descriptive adjectives."
- Several persons confided that they occasionally couldn't remember <u>their own names</u> when using aspartame products.
- A 64-year-old building inspector volunteered, "I could not think straight."
- An 18-year-old male forgot where he was or where to turn when driving in his neighborhood while drinking two liters of aspartame soft drinks daily.
- A 47-year-old woman expressed extreme concern over the striking deterioration of her prized "photographic memory" when consuming aspartame products.
- Experienced secretaries described making many typing and computer errors while using aspartame products.
- A 34-year-old instructor of English and Spanish "began having trouble sequencing assignments" when she drank two cans of diet cola daily.
- A 52-year-old executive complained of difficulty in remembering whom he called after dialing a number, and expressed concern over incipient Alzheimer's disease. The problem disappeared when he avoided aspartame products.
- A 58-year-old man complained that his memory had become "so bad that if I am cooking something in the kitchen, I'm likely to forget about it." There was concomitant headache, dizziness, decreased vision and depression. These symptoms disappeared one week after discontinuing aspartame beverages, and did not recur over the ensuing two years.

- A young woman, who had been consuming a six-pack of aspartame sodas daily to lose weight, found herself "lost" in a food market. She searched desperately through her purse to get help, finally located her husband's office phone number. The confusion did not recur when she avoided aspartame products.

Dr. Nicholas Petkas, a medical colleague, depicted the "aging" effects of aspartame products in a cartoon (Figure XV-1).

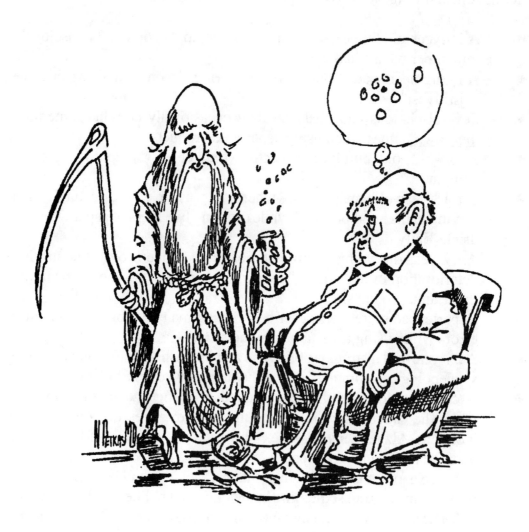

Figure XV-1

Other Clinical Associations

Individuals with both "evolving" AD and clinical dementia seem even more vulnerable. Case reports throughout this book suggest that ALL forms of dementing illness, including "small strokes," may be aggravated by aspartame disease – presumably through similar mechanisms (Chapters V, VI and VII; Section 5).

The "dry eyes" and severe memory loss/confusion in 95 aspartame reactors are germane. These observations lend further credence to the role of aspartame in the Sjögren syndrome (Chapter IV). Dr. Elaine Alexander (1986) found that as many as one-fourth of patients afflicted with this syndrome have severe cognitive dysfunction, ranging from forgetfulness to dementia.

The possibility of a specific type of optic-nerve degeneration in AD has been suggested. Widespread degeneration of nerve projections (axons) from the optic nerves were found in eight of 10 patients at autopsy (Hinton 1986). The number of ganglion cells in the retina were reduced in three. (By contrast, less than five percent of an elderly population evidence the most common types of optic neuropathy.) These observations offer other intriguing perspectives concerning the potential for memory loss and visual impairment (Chapter IV) associated with aspartame use, especially as related to chronic methanol poisoning (Chapter XXI).

III. UNDERLYING MECHANISMS

The confusion and memory loss induced by aspartame and its components probably reflect multiple mechanisms.

- Unchecked flooding of the brain by L-phenylalanine, L-aspartic acid, and their L-iso or D-stereoisomers (Chapter XXII)
- The toxic effects of free methyl alcohol (Chapter XXI)
- Metabolic breakdown products of aspartame formed during heating and prolonged storage (Chapter XX)
- Binding of excitatory amino acids to the membranes of brain cells
- Dysfunction induced by amino acid-derived neurotransmitters and related substances (Chapter XXIII)
- Induced or aggravated hypoglycemia from excess insulin secretion (Chapter XIV)
- Interference with the degradation of amyloid β-protein, which then may accumulate – perhaps involving proteolysis by insulin-degrading enzyme (Vekrellis 2000)

- A marked increase of beta endorphins (Melchior 1991)

Phenylalanine

Phenylalanine is unique in terms of brain metabolism and neurotransmitter function. It has the highest affinity for crossing the blood-brain barrier of <u>all</u> circulating amino acids. Furthermore, the exit time required for brain levels to decrease by half is longer for phenylalanine than other amino acids (Lajtha 1962).

There are other evidences for the uniqueness of phenylalanine.

- Dietary carbohydrate does not decrease its absorption, as is the case when the amino acid leucine is ingested (Krempf 1993).
- Roznoski, Huang, and Burns (1993) studied the effects of phenylalanine on the peripheral and central kinetics and metabolism of L-dopa in monkeys. Phenylalanine appears to inhibit the transport of L-dopa into cells, its metabolism within cells, or both.
- A *single* amino acid mutation in amyloid precursor protein, involving the substitution of phenylalanine for valine, appears to be the basis for at least one type of hereditary AD (Murrell 1991).

Aspartic Acid

Aspartic acid is present throughout the brain. It exerts a strong excitatory effect comparable to glutamate. These aspects of its metabolism are noteworthy.

- Aspartic acid is absorbed as a free amino acid through an active transport system, contrasting with peptides that contain aspartic acid.
- Aspartic acid is rapidly converted to aspartate and glutamate, as evidenced by the significant elevation of both aspartate and glutamate after ingesting a loading dose. It is then transported across nerve membranes and the blood-brain barrier.
- In experimental studies, insulin-induced hypoglycemia causes a sharp increase of brain aspartate concentrations, whereas glutamate and glutamine levels decline (Chapman 1987).
- The demonstration of increased concentrations of aspartate and glutamate in the cerebrospinal fluid of patients with advanced AD (Csernansky 1996) reinforces the belief that these excitatory amino acids contribute to neuronal loss.

The experiemental administration of L-aspartic acid can induce changes within the hypothalamus, especially in susceptible young animals. They later develop obesity, skeletal stunting, and reduced reproductive organ size. Both aspartic acid and its N-methyl-D-aspartate derivatives are powerful convulsants when injected into the brain (Turski 1984).

Stereoisomers (Mirror Images) and Other Metabolites of Aspartic Acid

The conversion (racemization) of amino acids tends to proceed from the biologically common L (levo) configuration to the uncommon D (dextro) configuration (Chapter XXII). D-aspartic acid and other racemate metabolites increase in aspartame products during excessive heat or prolonged storage (Boehm 1984).

The accumulation of D-aspartic acid in the brain with aging has considerable significance. Man et al (1987b) reported its considerable increase in the white matter of the human brain from infancy to about 35 years. *Increased D-aspartate levels could initiate changes in protein configuration, with associated dysfunction.*

Several related issues involving AD are germane.

- A significant amount of aspartic acid exists in the amyloid precursor protein (APP) of brain amyloid.
- Aspartate binding is reduced in the cerebral cortex of AD brains (Cross 1987).
- The uptake and binding of D-aspartic acid appears to be impaired *early* in AD brain cells.

The brain contains considerable aspartate. Dr. Andrew Procter (1986), Institute of Neurology in London, reported a striking loss of aspartate nerve endings in pyramidal cells from the cortex of AD patients (Figure XV-2). Inasmuch as phenylalanine, aspartic acid and other amino acids compete with each other for entry into the brain, this may reflect phenylalanine-aspartate competition or interference.

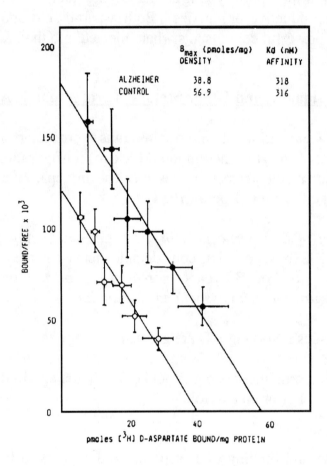

Figure XV-2

A Scatchard plot of specific sodium-dependent [³H]D-aspartate binding to human temporal cortex membranes. Each point represents the mean for nine control (●) and nine Alzheimer (o) samples. (Lines were drawn from the linear regression equations.)

Procter, A.W., et al: Glutamate/aspartate-releasing neurons in Alzheimer's disease. *New England Journal of Medicine* 1986; 314: 1711-1712.
Reprinted by permission of the *New England Journal of Medicine*

The increase of D-aspartate and beta-linked L-isoaspartate in AD neurofibrillary tangles (Shapira 1987; Payan 1992) is extraordinary. There are 1.5-2 times more total defective aspartate in AD neurofibrillary tangles, most as the beta-linked L-isoaspartate.

In a patient with late-onset AD, Peacock et al (1993) found a novel mutation in codon 655 wherein aspartate was submitted for glutamate.

Aluminum

The role of aluminum excess in AD has been reviewed elsewhere (Roberts 1955b). Aluminum increases the conversion of aspartic acid to D-aspartate in living brain protein. This is relevant to the increased amounts of D-aspartate and L-isoaspartate present in neurofibrillary tangles (see above).

Cholecystokinin

The presence of aspartic acid next to phenylalanine in cholecystokinin (CCK) poses another other remarkable coincidence. CCK is a neuropeptide that plays a significant role in learning, memory, behavior, and acetylcholine release.

- The amino acid sequence (using conventional abbreviations) of its biologically active form is ASP-TYR (SO3H)-MET-GLY-TRP-MET-*ASP-PHE*-NH2 (Brownstein 1985) (italics by author).
- CCK exists in unusually high concentrations within the cerebral cortex, the hippocampus, and related areas (Crawley 1985).
- CCK meets most of the criteria for a neurotransmitter – namely, its presence in nerve tissue, its localization in neurons, its concentration in synaptic vesicles, and its release by specific stimuli (Golterman 1985).

The amino acid sequence of cholecystokinin, and its documented biological effects could explain some of the described cerebral and metabolic reactions to products containing aspartame.

- CCK may cause or exaggerate glucose depletion in the brain. Tamminga et al (1985) reported that the peripheral administration of CCK-8 decreases glucose utilization in certain pertinent areas.
- The magnitude of weight loss has been dramatic among some persons using aspartame products (Chapter IX-B). Rogers, Keedwell and Blundell (1991) suggested that aspartame inhibits food intake in humans because it is a cholecystokinin releaser.

Nature Versus Nurture

An <u>abnormal gene</u> has been found on several chromosomes in members of families with inherited AD. These genes relate to brain amyloid, a protein that accumulates in the brains of patients having AD and mongolism.

While these observations may be pertinent to the cited familial incidence of some aspartame reactors (Chapters 11 and XVI), *the term "generational" may be more accurate than "hereditary."* Genetic studies on AD pedigrees remain inconclusive (Gusella 1988). There is as yet no evidence for the phenomenon of anticipation (or antecedence) found in other heredofamilial disorders such as Huntington's chorea and diabetes mellitus. Accordingly, even if a genetic factor exists, it may express itself only <u>after</u> exposure to some environmental neurotoxin to which the members of such families are exposed, or through cultural preferences they hold in common (Roberts 1995b).

XVI

THE FAMILIES OF ASPARTAME REACTORS

"Nature has but one judgement on wrong conduct
– if you can call that a judgement which
seemingly has no reference to conduct as such:
the judgement of death."
Oliver Wendell Holmes
(Address, 1902)

A history of known asparatame reactions existed in 211 families (17.6 percent) (Chapter II). From two to seven family members were so affected. Accordingly, *the close relatives of aspartame reactors should be regarded as being at high risk for aspartame disease.*

Pharmacogenetics refers to a relationship between inherited enzyme endowment and the metabolism of drugs and other chemicals. In this regard, the frequency with which the **same** types of reactions to aspartame products occurred – such as headache, loss of menses, difficult swallowing, or diarrhea – proved impressive (see Representative Case Histories).

- Case VI-J-5 describes severe aspartame-induced tremors in two sisters
- A woman with aspartame disease and her daughter suffered severe urinary burning ("interstitial cystitis") while consuming aspartame products.
- The suspect acceleration of familial Alzheimer's disease by aspartame was discussed in Chapter XV.
- The striking occurrence of "fibromyalgia" among family members of aspartame reactors was cited in Chapter IX-G.

Genetic variations in the gene(s) for alcohol dehydrogenase can influence the rate of alcohol metabolism appear to have clinical significance (Hines 2001). They may contribute to familial aspartame disease, and the severity of methanol effects in reactors having altered rates of oxidation.

The Emotional Impact

The emotional impact on families wherein multiple members suffered from aspartame disease was profound. Severe anguish characterized persons submitting the case reports and related correspondence. The following letters serve as examples.

"For the past ten years, I have watched in horror as my daughter's family (husband and four children) encountered one serious life-threatening condition after another. The list is too detailed and scary to go into, but suffice it to say that four members have had or continue to have seizures. Five out of six have developed chronic debilitating diseases, most of 'unknown etiology'... mysterious allergic reactions, fructose intolerance with concurrent kidney and gastrointestinal disorders, cancer, RSD (a debilitating nerve dystrophy), idiopathic angioedema, asthma, chronic migraine (even the children)... and on and on. In the month of January this year, they had 31 doctor appointments – all with specialists!

"I am convinced that the family's consumption of fat-free foods and diet sodas is at the bottom of the problem, yet my daughter discounts the information on aspartame I give her. She 'checks it out with the doctors' and is assured that there 'absolutely' could be no connection... When I think of what I see clearly happening right in front of my eyes to people I love, I could scream."

- An aspartame reactor elaborated on her reactions and those of her children. There is reference to Tourette's syndrome (Chapter VI-G). This challenging disorder begins in late childhood. Its more severe form is characterized by violent twitching, impulsive movements, and the uttering of explosive sounds and profanities.

"It has been my personal experience that headaches, dizziness, loss of memory, behavioral changes and the general feeling of 'something wrong with me' resulted from using many aspartame items. It is difficult to find things that don't contain aspartame.

"My children and several adult friends experienced similar symptoms, and avoid ingestion of this chemical as much as possible. The symptoms have disappeared. My eight-year-old exhibited signs of Tourette's syndrome."

Grandparents with aspartame disease expressed apprehension about the welfare of their grandchildren when other family members suffered reactions (Chapter XIX). They sensed that the "ghosts" of this neurotoxin reflected a genetic predisposition they had transmitted. For example, a registered nurse (Case VI-G-1) wrote her daughter about the restlessness she was experiencing. She poignantly pleaded, "Please see that none of my grandchildren are given anything containing aspartame!"

REPRESENTATIVE CASE REPORTS

Cases XVI-1 and XVI-2

A 59-year-old design engineer suggested that aspartame might be aggravating several health problems whose cause had challenged the author (his physician) for several years. They included recurrent lightheadedness, tremors, marked memory loss, depression, severe respiratory allergies, intermittent loss of hearing, intense thirst, and recurrent bronchial-sinus infections.

When the possible role of aspartame was raised, he recalled: "I do know that my discomfort in the sinuses, head and ears (in terms of pressure) were aggravated. In addition, new problems of memory loss, eye infection, apparent increased susceptibility to bronchial infection, and hearing not up to par came upon me with aspartame use."

His 23-year-old teacher-daughter had been suffering severe headache, dizziness, lightheadedness, unsteadiness of the legs, depression, "anxiety attacks," and marked frequency of urination while drinking three to four cans of diet cola daily. She also complained of decreased vision and pain in both eyes. None of these severe symptoms had occurred while taking saccharin. There was a prior history of migraine. She challenged herself four times before becoming convinced that products containing aspartame provoked her symptoms. She stated, "I find that when I have aspartame, usually in soft drinks, I feel unusual: lightheaded, headache, queasy, nauseous. My vision also becomes somewhat distorted, and my balance goes. It's kind of a tunnel vision feeling."

Case XVI-3

A concerned woman wrote about perceived aspartame addiction (Chapter VII-G) in members of her family.

"My daughter feels that she is addicted to aspartame sodas. She has half of the symptoms ascribed to it. One of my sisters has increased thirst and panic attacks that they say is caused by it. Her refrigerator is full of diet sodas, even when she is low on food. My other sister has a 21-year-old who has recently developed epilepsy. Their refrigerator is never without diet drinks. Maybe it's just a family 'allergy' which keeps us addicted and susceptible."

XVII

PATIENTS WITH PHENYLKETONURIA (PKU)

Phenylketonuria is an inherited disease. Affected individuals cannot normally metabolize phenylalanine to tyrosine because the enzyme phenylalanine hydroxylase is deficient. As a result, high concentrations of potentially neurotoxic metabolites accumulate, especially phenylacetic acid (Figure XVII-1).

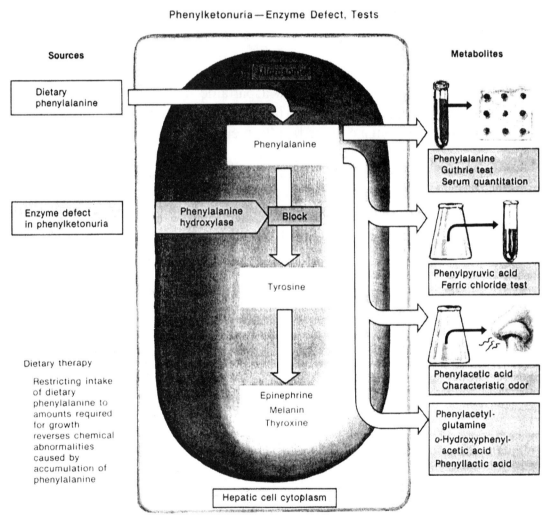

Figure XVII-1

PKU was among the first disorders identified as fulfilling the basic metabolic postulates for an inherited disease. Early investigators found that PKU patients accumulated large amounts of phenylalanine, and excreted considerable phenylpyruvic acid in the urine. The latter can be readily detected by adding ferric chloride, causing a striking green color when phenylpyruvic acid is present (Figure XVII-1).

As noted, the inability to oxidize phenylalanine to tyrosine is fundamental. In normal persons, the serum tyrosine concentration increases within 10 minutes after an oral phenylalanine load, and reaches a maximum concentration at two hours. In PKU patients, even children receiving treatment early, tyrosine levels progressively decline (Güttler 1978).

Advice from PKU Patients

PKU patients have astutely suspected aspartame disease in friends experiencing unexplained neuropsychiatric symptoms. This fortuitous situation is illustrated by the following correspondence from a college faculty member.

> "I decided to lose weight by substituting diet soda for regular soda, and began consuming up to 4 cans of diet soda each day. At first I noticed nothing wrong, but then I started getting more stupid. I lost focus and had difficulty remembering things. I started to feel very irritable and felt a loss of control over my emotions, even crying on occasion for absolutely no reason. I felt like I was losing my mind. I was lucky that a colleague, who had PKU, told me about similar problems from phenylalanine buildup. This clued me to what might be happening, and I stopped drinking diet soda. My recovery was immediate. I am thankful to be away from the stuff."

ASPARTAME AND PKU

Inasmuch as half of the aspartame molecule consists of phenylalanine, it is hazardous for persons with PKU. One liter of most aspartame soft drinks contains about 275 mg phenylalanine.

There were previous mandated warnings on labels, such as "Phenylpyruvics: contains phenylalanine." In its June 28, 1996 authorization of aspartame as a general purpose synthetic tabletop sweetener, however, the FDA removed this requirement.

The potential for severe brain dysfunction also exists among PKU heterozygotes (see below) who consume aspartame products (Elsas 1987).

There is limited information about the incidence of PKU heterozygotes in families with aspartame disease based on phenylalanine load testing (Chapter XXII). A related deficiency of short-term studies is the failure to encompass PKU heterozygotes who chronically use aspartame products.

Representative Family Case Histories

Case XVII-1

A man developed severe gastrointestinal problems and a presumed "immune deficiency problem." The latter was evidenced by alterations of his red blood cells, white blood cells and platelets. He and the following relatives had consumed large amounts of aspartame products.

His <u>wife</u> experienced decreased vision on both eyes, severe headache, extreme dryness of the mouth, and intense thirst.

Their 28-year-old <u>granddaughter</u> had PKU at birth, and subsequently evidenced learning problems. She suffered multiple grand mal convulsions while using aspartame – along with severe headaches, marked mental confusion and memory loss, recurrent depression with suicidal thoughts, a bleeding peptic ulcer, anorexia and a 15-pound weight loss.

Case XVII-2

A 34-year-old woman expressed understandable concern over the effect of aspartame on PKU carriers. She had documented PKU since childhood, but was taken off her diet at the age of ten. Aware of the potential serious nature of aspartame reactions, however, she studiously avoided any products containing it.

She added, "I also have become concerned because many carriers in my family drink beverages with aspartame." (PKU involved only her maternal relatives.) She became appalled by the large consumption of diet beverages at a recent family wedding.

Further discussion revealed the resistance by most of her extended family to avoiding aspartame products.

590

- Each of her parents consumed aspartame products to lose weight.
- A cousin with PKU, also 34, habitually drank aspartame beverages.
- Another cousin/aspartame consumer recently delivered a child with spina bifida.

Case XVII-3

A 36-year-old woman was a "learning-disabled" worker employed by Goodwill Industries. She had been diagnosed as having phenylketonuria at birth.

Her social worker reported that the patient had consumed aspartame diet sodas for three years. She wrote:

> "Aspartame is like a poison to her, but it is very difficult to avoid since she cannot go out to eat. It is everywhere in diet colas, diet root beer, and sugar-free soft drinks and gelatin. She can't sleep so she is unable to go to work. It takes five days of avoidance before her system is back to her normal."

The complaints attributed to aspartame included severe headache, dizziness, unsteadiness on the feet, mental confusion, memory loss, marked hyperactivity, intense insomnia, slurred speech, attacks of shortness of breath, palpitations, rapid heart action, abdominal pain, severe nausea, diarrhea with blood stools, and abdominal bloat. As a result, the social worker had to check all labels.

> "Her reaction is so severe that I have stayed up with her two nights for fear she might pass out, or her heart would give out. "All we could do for months was to restrict foods that made her sick as each one showed itself. (She was living on junk food and lived in the manner of a street bag lady before this.) She was tested at a medical center for allergies. Three trays of 18 extracts (each) were tried on her. The doctor says her problems were caused by the PKU factor.
>
> "I am going to continue charting and experimenting with her diet. My reward comes when she comes in from work at Goodwill and gives me that bone-crushing hug around the shoulders and says, 'Boy, do I feel good!'"

Such commendable interest by this supervisor, herself an insulin-dependent diabetic, heightened awareness of her own multiple reactions to aspartame products. Furthermore, she had two grandchildren who consumed considerable aspartame, and were being treated for hearing problems.

THE SURVEY QUESTIONNAIRE

The subject of PKU was incorporated in the survey questionnaire (Section 4). Of the first 397 aspartame reactors completing it, 224 (56.4 percent) indicated they had heard of the condition, and 108 (27.2 percent) thought they knew what it was. Four individuals were actually aware of PKU in their families (see above).

AN OVERVIEW OF PHENYLKETONURIA (PKU)

A brief review of PKU is appropriate in view of the fact that at least two-thirds of the adult population, and about 40 percent of children younger than 9 years, currently consume aspartame products.

The disease PKU is transmitted by two seemingly-normal parents who carry this autosomal recessive single gene. They are referred to as PKU heterozygotes or carriers.

The importance of making a diagnosis of PKU is indicated by the mandatory screening for PKU before newborns are discharged from a hospital. A drop of blood is collected from the heel, and placed on filter paper at least 24 hours (preferably 72 hours) after the infant has been fed with the customary amount of protein (Figure XVII-1).

Incidence

The following estimates are reasonable.

- One in 17,000 persons born in the United States has PKU.
- There is a higher incidence of PKU in some populations...as in Ireland and among the Arab populations of Israel. This probably reflects some selective genetic "pressure." It might be linked to an insulin-like growth factor, the gene of which exists on the adjacent long arm of chromosome 12 (Ledley 1987).
- One in every 50 persons (at least four million) is a carrier of the PKU gene.
- About one percent of babies delivered in the United States are born to mothers having the PKU gene.
- The incidence of PKU is much higher among inmates of mental institutions.

These figures concerning PKU heterozygotes are <u>conservative</u> owing to the increased survival of PKU infants because of required testing and the institution of a low-phenylalanine diet early in life when PKU is found.

Levy and Waisbren (1983)) estimated that as many as **20 million** persons in the United States have phenylalanine intolerance. Markedly elevated blood phenylalanine concentrations in these individuals could readily saturate the neutral amino acid transport sites at the blood-brain barrier.

Dr. Martin Banschbach, a university health educator, offered this pertinent perspective in replying to a query on the Internet.

> "One per 17,000 live births is not trivial. But the real kicker is that some PKU kids get missed for several reasons. The blood test is only reliable if blood is taken three to four days after birth. Additionally, HMOs are kicking the babies out after one day. If the pediatrician does not follow with another PKU test, there is a fall through the cracks.

> "Then there are carriers who also react badly to aspartame intake, but very few know that they are carriers of PKU. The estimated incidence is believed to be one per 11,000 live births – rather than the one per 17,000. We therefore have a lot of people with a genetic defect that prevents them from safely handling dietary phenylalanine. Until aspartame came along, the carriers were able to cope with 50% of normal phenylalanine hydroxylase activity. Now they can't if they have significant amounts of aspartame in their diet."

The Disease

When PKU is detected in infancy before severe brain damage has occurred, a low-phenylalanine diet is therapeutic. If untreated, mental retardation, seizures and other neurologic abnormalities usually become evident after six months of age. The signs and symptoms of PKU are illustrated in Figure XVII-2.

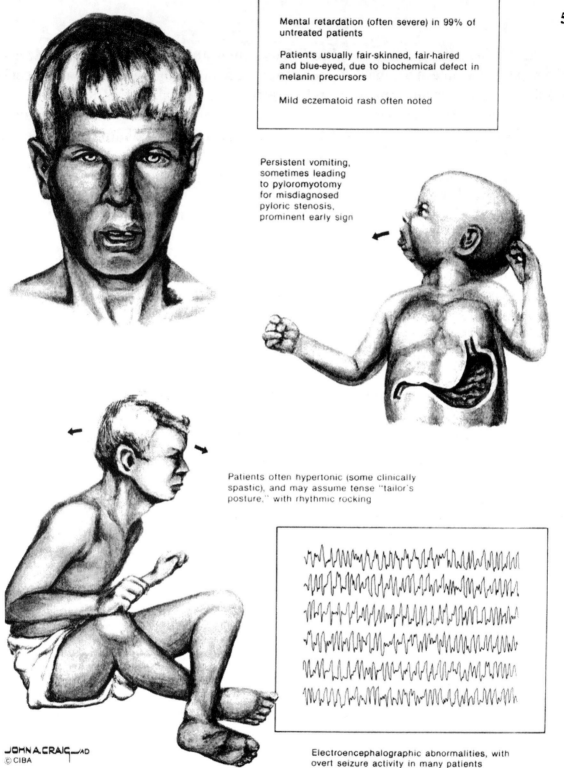

Mental retardation (often severe) in 99% of untreated patients

Patients usually fair-skinned, fair-haired and blue-eyed, due to biochemical defect in melanin precursors

Mild eczematoid rash often noted

Persistent vomiting, sometimes leading to pyloromyotomy for misdiagnosed pyloric stenosis, prominent early sign

Patients often hypertonic (some clinically spastic), and may assume tense "tailor's posture," with rhythmic rocking

Electroencephalographic abnormalities, with overt seizure activity in many patients

JOHN A. CRAIG AD
© CIBA

Figure XVII-2

An international collaborative PKU study demonstrated that even modest elevations of blood phenylalanine in pregnant women can cause fetal damage, especially microcephaly with subsequent intellectual impairment (Drogarri 1987). The Maternal PKU Collaborative Study (Waisbren 2000) convincingly demonstrated that inadequate maternal metabolic control of PKU (plasma phenylalanine levels more than 10 mg/dL) prior to or early in pregnancy increases risk for developmental problems in the offspring.

The harmful influence of phenylalanine in PKU was summarized in *Nutrition Reviews* (Volume 44: 331-333, October 1986). An excess of phenylalanine by itself tends to interfere with the brain's metabolism of amino acids, especially in infants and children.

The hypoglycemic effect of aspartame (Chapter XIV) can summate upon that of elevated phenylpyruvic acid in PKU, and thereby aggravate mental retardation (Ben-Shlomo 1999).

Presumed Dietary Control

The need to avoid aspartame products, as well as maintaining a low-phenylalanine diet, by persons treated for PKU during childhood requires emphasis. Most of the estimated 3,000 young American women of childbearing age who had been treated for PKU tend to discontinue the diet by the age of six years because their physicians believe it can be omitted with impunity after adolescence.

- Krause et al (1987) studied older PKU subjects in whom treatment was instituted early. When these investigators raised plasma phenylalanine concentrations from a mean of 6 mg percent to a mean of 23 mg percent by increasing dietary phenylalanine for one week, the following occurred: (a) prolongation of performance time on a computerized choice reaction test; (b) decreased neurotransmitter concentrations in plasma and urine; and (c) decreased EEG mean power frequency (a probable indicator of brain dopamine activity).
- Thompson et al (1991) evaluated 26 PKU patients who had been treated by diet early, and achieved phenylalanine concentrations within the desired therapeutic range during their first eight years. Even though none evidenced gross neurologic changes, abnormalities were found in 23 by magnetic resonance imaging. Results in the other three patients were equivocal. *Accordingly, such individuals remain at risk for neurological damage despite early treatment.*
- Michals and Matalon (1985) found that large quantities of phenylalanine metabolites were present in the urine during pregnancy

in PKU patients despite only modest elevations of the serum phenylalanine – even among those considered to have good phenylalanine control.

A panel of experts convened by the National Institutes of Health on October 19, 2000 concluded that patients with PKU should stay on a diet free of phenylalanine throughout **life**. It also recommended that blood tests be done monthly on affected adults, especially women planning to have children.

A suggested method for depleting phenylalanine in PKU entails the extracorporeal administration of multitubular enzyme reactors with immobilized enzymes. Ambrus et al (1987) reported a dramatic decrease of circulating phenylalanine within 5.5 hours of treatment in a patient using immobilized L-phenylalanine ammonia-lyase. (It metabolizes phenylalanine to <u>trans</u>-cinnamic acid and ammonia without requiring a coenzyme.) This treatment might reduce elevated fetal phenylalanine levels in pregnant PKU women.

Neurotransmitter Studies

Elevated phenylalanine can increase or alter neurotransmitter production, particularly the synthesis of dopamine and serotonin (Section 5).

Dr. Hans Lou (1987) (The John F. Kennedy Institute, Glostrup, Denmark) studied the effects of both a free diet and a phenylalanine-restricted diet in nine patients with classic PKU. (Vigilance was judged by the continuous visual reaction time.) Neurotransmitter synthesis was determined by cerebrospinal fluid homovanillic acid (VA) and 5-hydroxyindoleacetic acid (5HIAA) concentrations in the cerebrospinal fluid. On a free diet, HVA and 5-HIAA levels decreased significantly as the plasma phenylalanine concentration increased. On a phenylalanine-restricted diet, vigilance improved in six of seven patients found to have abnormally long reaction times.

Another observation was the addition of tyrosine as a potential therapeutic alternative. When 160 mg/kg/day were added (as three daily doses) to the free diet, the HVA/5-HIAA ratio increased in the cerebrospinal fluid of six patients, with concomitantly improved vigilance. These studies provide further evidence for the importance of dopamine synthesis in regulating attention and initiating motor activity.

Other Disorders Aggravated by Phenylalanine

Hereditary progressive dystonia, a neurologic disorder usually affecting children, is exquisitely responsive to levodopa. These patients can be adversely affected by ingesting phenylalanine because liver phenylalanine hydroxylase activity is decreased (Hyland 1997).

Rarer forms of malignant hyperphenylalaninemia (Chapter XXII) exist. One is due to tetrahydrobiopterin (BH_4) deficiency (Niederwiser 1985).

RELATED PROBLEMS OF HETEROZYGOTES

Heterozygotes are generally not aware of being carriers prior to the birth of a child afflicted with PKU. Those who are able to maintain about 15-30 percent of phenylalanine hydroxylase activity appear normal clinically (Matalon 1987). Even so, they accumulate higher and more prolonged concentrations when given a standard challenge dose of phenylalanine.

The intake of 885 mg phenylalanine by a person weighing 60 kg who also consumes the recommended daily allowance of protein (900 mg per kg) might increase the phenylalanine load by as much as 37 percent.

Another problem is introduced by the failure of some pediatricians and geneticists to warn the parents or siblings of PKU patients about limiting their phenylalanine intake. In this regard, the FDA does not require labels on aspartame products for the estimated 10 million American women who may be PKU carriers.

Data are needed relative to another important issue: frequency of the PKU heterozygote state among persons suffering aspartame disease.

Unrecognized Pregnant Carriers

High phenylalanine levels in pregnant carriers are conducive to intrauterine growth abnormalities and subsequent mental retardation (Frankenburg 1968, Mabry 1966, Farquhar 1971, Brown 1971). Most children born to mothers with plasma phenylalanine concentrations above 10 mg percent suffer mental retardation, microcephaly, retardation of intrauterine growth, and major congenital abnormalities (including congenital heart disease).

Blood phenylalanine concentrations could increase fourfold during pregnancy when PKU heterozygotes ingest aspartame products. The fetal concentrations during this critical period of brain development are even higher.

- Dr. Reuben Matalon, Professor of Pediatrics and Genetics at the University of Illinois Medical School, reported that one in 50 women are "particularly sensitive to high phenylalanine consumption. Their ingestion of aspartame during pregnancy might result in birth defects and mental retardation.

- Dr. N. V. Bhagavan (1975) warned of the potential dangers from aspartame use by women of childbearing age who are either homozygous or heterozygous for PKU. He stated, "Aspartame is a potential hazard to these women and to the fetuses that they carry."

SECTION 4

THE SURVEY QUESTIONNAIRE FOR ASPARTAME DISEASE

"That man can interrogate as well as observe nature, was a lesson slowly learned in his evolution."
Sir William Osler

"If the clinician, as observer, wishes to see things as they really are, he must make a tabula rasa of his mind and proceed without any preconceived notions whatsoever."
J. M. Charcot
(famous neurologist)

In tabulating information from the first 100 aspartame reactors in this series, dozens of issues emerged that clearly required more data. Dr. Robert H. Moser (1969), former Medical Director of the NutraSweet Company, stated in the Preface to *Diseases Of Medical Progress*, "Only painstaking retrospective analysis of many cases is required to uncover a suspect denominator." *

Having devised questionnaires for previous studies, such as the evaluation and followup of drivers involved in traffic accidents (Roberts 1971b) and of vasectomized men (Roberts 1979, 1993d), I formulated and revised one for patients and correspondents having diagnosed or suspect aspartame disease that also lent itself to computer analysis. The more recent version is reproduced.

---

* From Moser, R.J.: *Diseases of Medical Progress; A Study of Iatrogenic Disease.* 3rd edition, 1969. Courtesy of Charles C Thomas, Publisher, Springfield, Illinois.

SURVEY QUESTIONNAIRE FOR PERSONS WITH SUSPECTED REACTIONS TO PRODUCTS CONTAINING ASPARTAME

PALM BEACH INSTITUTE FOR MEDICAL RESEARCH, INC.
P.O. BOX 17799
WEST PALM BEACH, FLORIDA 33416

H. J. Roberts, M.D., F.A.C.P., F.C.C.P.
Medical Director

I. GENERAL INFORMATION

Name (optional) _____

Address (optional) _____

TELEPHONE NUMBER (optional) AREA CODE (_____) _____-_____

SEX (Circle)   Male   Female

RACE (Circle)   White   Black

PRESENT AGE (years) _____

OCCUPATION _____

II. INFORMATION ABOUT PRIOR USE OF ASPARTAME PRODUCTS
(including NutraSweet® and Equal®)

When did your first suspected reaction occur? (age) _____ years

How long had you been eating or drinking aspartame products before then?
(Aspartame was first available as a powdered tabletop sweetener in July 1981, and as soft drinks in July 1983)

_____Days   _____Weeks   _____ Months   _____ Years

Had you greatly increased such use before your symptoms began?
(Circle) Yes   No

If "Yes," how long before they occurred?

_____ Days   _____ Weeks   _____ Months   _____ Years

© 2001 H.J. Roberts, M.D.

600

Why did you use aspartame products? (Circle)

Preferred their taste
Marked thirst in hot weather
Wanted to avoid sugar because of (circle)
  Diabetes
  Hypoglycemia ("low blood sugar attacks")
  Overweight
  Other reasons _____

Did you use aspartame products under these conditions? (Circle and state how long)

While <u>pregnant</u> for   _____ Weeks   _____ Months
While <u>breast-feeding</u> for   _____ Weeks   _____ Months

How much were you eating or drinking <u>daily</u> when your symptoms began?

<u>Some examples</u>: diet colas, diet soft drinks, chocolate mixes, gelatins, puddings, pre-sweetened cereals, iced tea mixes, powdered soft drinks.

_____ cans (12 ounces) of (name of product) _____
_____ small bottles (6 ounces) of (name) _____
_____ large bottles (liter or 33 ounces) of (name) _____
_____ very large bottles (2 liters or 67 ounces) of (name) _____
_____ packets of tabletop sweetener (name) _____
_____ regular glasses of iced tea (name) _____
_____ regular glasses of soft drinks mixes (name) _____
_____ bowls of cereal (name) _____
_____ servings of puddings or gelatins (name) _____
_____ sticks of gum (name) _____
_____ (envelopes) or (teaspoons) of other products (name) _____

Were you on a <u>strict</u> diet to lose weight when your problem began?
    (Circle) Yes   No

If "Yes," for how long? _____Weeks _____ Months

Were your <u>exercising</u> to lose weight when your problem began?
    (Circle) Yes   No

III. SUSPICIONS ABOUT ASPARTAME

Who or what made you <u>first</u> think that aspartame products might be causing or aggravating your symptoms? (Circle)

Myself
A relative
A friend
My doctor
A nurse
A newspaper article
A TV program
A medical specialist (name specialty) _____
Other (state) _____

Did you then <u>completely</u> stop using aspartame? (Circle) Yes   No

If you stopped, <u>did your condition improve</u>?   (Circle) Yes   No

How soon <u>after</u> you stopped did your symptoms <u>begin</u> to improve?

_____ Days   _____ Weeks   _____ Months

Did <u>all</u> of your symptoms <u>disappear</u> after stopping? (Circle)   Yes   No

If "Yes," how soon?   _____ Days   _____ Weeks   _____ Months

If you felt better, what problems persisted?

_____

_____

If you felt better, did your symptoms <u>recur</u> when you ate or drank aspartame products <u>again</u>? (Circle)

Yes   No

If "Yes," <u>how soon</u> did the symptoms return?
_____ Days   _____ Weeks   _____ Months

How many times did you <u>retest</u> yourself until you became <u>convinced</u> that aspartame <u>really</u> caused your symptoms? (Circle)

0   1   2   3   4   More

Did the symptoms return after eating or drinking something <u>you didn't know</u> contained aspartame?

(Circle)   Yes   No

If "Yes," what was the product? _____

Did your symptoms <u>significantly</u> harm your business or personal life?

(Circle) Yes   No

If "Yes," how much? (Circle)

> A little
> Severely (loss of job; stopped school; divorce; etc.)
> I was incapacitated
> I lost my license (Circle)   driver   pilot

Please amplify _____

IV. REACTIONS ATTRIBUTED TO ASPARTAME PRODUCTS

Please **circle** any of the following complaints that you or your doctors thought might be caused or aggravated by aspartame. (You can elaborate later.)

Eyes

Marked decrease of vision in	One eye	Both eyes
Loss of vision in	One eye	Both eyes
Pain in	One eye	Both eyes
"Dry eyes"	One eye	Both eyes
Trouble wearing contacts	Yes	No
Drooping of eyelid	Yes	No

Ears

Ringing or "cracking" in	One ear Both ears
Loss of hearing in	One ear Both ears
Severe sensitivity to noise in	One ear Both ears

Brain and Head

Severe headache

Severe dizziness or lightheadedness

Severe unsteadiness of legs

Convulsions (also called seizures and epilepsy)

> How many attacks?   (Circle) 1   2   3   4   More_____

Was your brain wave test (EEG) abnormal?   (Circle) Yes   No

Epilepsy-like "fits" without convulsions

> (also called petit mal and psychomotor attacks)

Severe drowsiness and falling asleep without other reasons

Severe shaking (tremors)

Severe insomnia   (Circle) Trouble falling asleep   Awakening in night

Severe mental confusion

Marked memory loss

Severe hyperactivity (including jumping of the arms, and "restless" legs)

Severe tingling, "pins and needles," or numbness of the arms and legs

Unexplained pain in or around the face

Slurring of speech

Severe depression

> Did you actually think about suicide?   (Circle) Yes   No

Extreme irritability
Severe "anxiety attacks"
Noticeable "personality changes"
Aggravation of phobias (such as fear of crowds or heights)

<u>Chest</u>
Unexplained shortness of breath
Palpitations (heart fluttering or skipping)
Rapid heart and pulse attacks
Unexplained chest pains
High blood pressure   (Circle)   Recent   Aggravated

<u>Abdomen</u>
Pain
Severe nausea
Diarrhea
Blood in the stools   (Circle)   Red   Black
Severe abdominal bloat or swelling

<u>Skin and Allergies</u>
Severe unexplained itching
Hives (water blisters)
Other rashes   (Circle)   body   groin   vaginal area
A marked loss or thinning of your hair
Mouth reactions
Swollen lips
Swollen tongue
Pain in the mouth
Painful swallowing
Marked dental decay
Dry mouth

<u>Unintended Marked Change of Weight</u>

Gain of _____ pounds Loss of _____ pounds

<u>Other Problems</u>
Severe thirst
Increased frequency of urinating   Day   Night   Both
Gross changes of the menstrual periods
More frequent   Less frequent   They stopped
Severe muscle pains or "fibromyalgia"
Marked swelling of the legs
"Low blood sugar" (hypoglycemia) attacks
Poor control of my diabetes even while on
Diet   Oral drugs   Insulin   Combination

604

Other Suspected Reactions   (Please list)

_____

_____

V. YOUR CONSULTATIONS AND TESTS BEFORE STOPPING ASPARTAME

How many <u>physicians and consultants</u> were seen <u>in your own community</u>?
        (Circle) 1   2   3   4   _____ More

How many <u>consultants or clinics</u> were seen <u>outside of your community</u>?
        (Circle) 1   2   3   4   _____ More

Were you referred to
                A <u>psychiatrist</u>   Yes   No
                A <u>psychologist</u>   Yes   No
                Other "<u>therapist</u>"   Yes   No

<u>How many times were you hospitalized BEFORE aspartame was suspected as the cause?</u>
        (Circle) 1   2   3   4   5

<u>Which of the following tests were done BEFORE aspartame disease was suspected?</u>
        If yes, circle how many.

X-rays of the head	0	1	2	3
CT scan of the brain	0	1	2	3
MRI (magnetic resonance) of the brain	0	1	2	3
Angiograms (X-rays of brain and blood vessels)	0	1	2	3
Lumbar puncture ("spinal tap")	0	1	2	3
Electroencephalogram (EEG)	0	1	2	3
Stress test of the heart	0	1	2	3
Heart rhythm monitor (12 or 24 hrs)	0	1	2	3
Upper GI series (X-rays of stomach)	0	1	2	3
Barium enema (X-rays of the lower bowel)	0	1	2	3
Allergy tests (skin; others)	0	1	2	3
Special eye tests	0	1	2	3
Special ear tests	0	1	2	3

<u>How much did these consultations and tests cost (estimate)</u>?

        Out of <u>your</u> own pocket? $ _____
        Your insurance carrier(s) $ _____

<u>Did you report your suspected reaction(s) to aspartame</u>? (Circle)   Yes   No

        If "Yes," to whom?   (Circle)

My doctor
A consultant
My family
Manufacturer of the product
The Food and Drug Administration (FDA)
The Centers for Disease Control
Public health department
Consumer organization (name) _____
H. J. Roberts, M.D.
Other interested doctors /researchers I heard or read about (name)

_____

If "Yes," how did you report? (Circle)
      Letter   Phone call(s)   e-mail Other (state) _____

VII. REACTIONS IN MEMBERS OF YOUR FAMILY

Have other relatives had problems attributed to aspartame?   (Circle) Yes   No

If "Yes," how are they related, and how many?   (Circle or number)
Husband
Wife
Daughter(s) _____
Son(s)_____
Others _____

What kind of reaction did they have?

_____
_____

VIII. YOUR MEDICAL BACKGROUND

Did any of the following exist BEFORE taking aspartame? If so, how long before? (Circle and write
      number of months or years after each condition)

Migraine
Other headaches
Depression (feeling blue)
Severe "anxiety"
Poor vision
Ear problems
Heart problems
High blood pressure

Stomach problem
Bowel problem
Kidney problem
Hives
Other rashes   Psoriasis   Acne   Lupus   Other_____
Parkinsonism (shaking palsy)
Myasthenia gravis
Allergies
      Hay fever
      Asthma
      To medicines (such as aspirin, penicillin)   (List)

_____

_____

"Low blood sugar" (hypoglycemia) attacks
Diabetes
      Treated with   Diet   Pills   Insulin
Thyroid problem
      Goiter
      Underactive thyroid (hypothyroidism)
      Overactive thyroid (hyperthyroidism)
"Arthritis"
A marked weight problem (20 pounds or more)   Gain   Loss
Alcohol problem   (Circle) Long ago   Current
Drug abuse problem   (Circle) Long ago   Current

      What drug(s)? _____

Other conditions not listed above

_____

_____

Did you consider yourself "addicted" to aspartame?   Yes   No
      If "Yes," please explain _____

_____

Do you smoke <u>cigarettes</u>?   (Circle) Yes   No
      If "Yes," how many <u>daily</u>?   (Circle)
            Less than ½ pack   ½-1 Pack   More than 1 pack

Did you get severe symptoms after drinking alcohol while taking aspartame?
      (Circle) Yes   No

      If "Yes," how much? (Circle)   Very little   Moderate   A lot
      If "Yes," what kind of drink? (Circle)   Wine   Beer   Liquor

IX. OTHER RELATED INFORMATION

Describe any <u>impressive or unusual aspects of your reaction(s) to aspartame products</u>

_____

_____

Have <u>any friends</u> had problems with aspartame? (Circle) Yes   No

    How many?   (Circle) 1   2   3   4
    If "Yes," what kind of problems?

    _____

    _____

Do you <u>still</u> use products containing aspartame?   (Circle) Yes   No

    If "Yes," names and how much? _____

    _____

    If "No," are you using the following?
        Sugar   Yes   No
        Saccharin (as Sweet N' Low®)   Yes   No
        Stevia   Yes   No

Have you ever heard of <u>phenylketonuria</u> (PKU)?
    (Circle) Yes   No

    If "Yes," do you know what it is?   (Circle) Yes   No
    If "Yes," has anyone in your family had it? (Circle) Yes   No

Do you believe that there should be a law labeling aspartame content?
    (Circle) Yes   No

Do you think that <u>Congress</u> should attempt to regulate aspartame and its newer versions? (Circle)
    Yes   No

    If "Yes," how?

    _____

    _____

**CONTINUE ON THE REVERSE SIDE IF YOU WISH TO GIVE FURTHER DETAILS OR
COMMENTS**

XVIII

A COMMENTARY ON THE SURVEY QUESTIONNAIRE

"Multiplied testimony, multiplied views will be necessary to give solid establishment to truth. Much is known to one which is not known to another, and no one knows everything. It is the sum of individual knowledge which is to make up the whole truth, and to give its correct current through future time."

Thomas Jefferson (1823)

GENERAL COMMENTS

The questionnaire was devised to obtain more information from persons who felt they had adverse reactions to aspartame products. A frequent sequence included the onset or aggravation of complaints after consuming such products, their improvement or disappearance after avoiding them, and recurrence following subsequent challenge... deliberate or unexpected.

Most persons completing the questionnaire appreciated the need for compiling this corporate-neutral data base. A prominent engineer with severe aspartame disease asserted, "First, build up a firm mass of evidence proving your case. Then, act!"

Many reactors stated that they had gained considerable insight about aspartame disease from studying the questionnaire. One wrote, "I never expected that so many of my health problems could be related to the use of aspartame."

As in other types of chemical dependency, denial was encountered in the form of distortion or omission by aspartame abusers. This proved most impressive for aspartame addicts (Chapter VII-G). Many spouses and parents attempted to enhance the accuracy of questionnaires completed by reactors with supplementary comments. Several appear in the case histories.

A number of respondents expressed interest in learning about the final results, especially details concerning "risk factors" (see Section 3). One aspartame reactor perceptively inquired, "I wonder if you might ask in your questionnaire if there is anything unusual about each person. Maybe something will show up as a common denominator in people with reactions."

A "Handle" On The General Population

The questionnaire provided an intriguing handle for estimating the magnitude of aspartame disease in the general population. The author was predictably inundated with requests for it after radio and television inverviews. To illustrate, this topic was discussed with Miami talk-show host Neil Rogers in September 1986. The barrage of calls amazed this seasoned interviewer.

Several pregnant women had never head or read about the desirability of limiting or avoiding aspartame products during gestation. Over the ensuing weeks, my mail was swamped with requests for the questionnaire, accompanied by self-addressed, stamped envelopes. One listener asked for four questionnaires – one for herself, one for her husband, and two for friends with probable aspartame disease.

Kudos to the Public

The public deserves much credit for its willingness to assist independent research requiring input from the general population, as was the case here.

Gilbert and Wysocki (1987) expressed a similar view in their international study concerning the sense of smell. Only one person could fill out each questionnaire that appeared in the September 1986 issue of *National Geographic Magazine*. Nevertheless, many families and classrooms participated by photocopying the survey form, and then sharing the samples of six odors.

EXPRESSIONS OF APPRECIATION

Scores of letters were received expressing gratitude for this research tool and effort. A few examples are offered.

- An aspartame reactor with severe nausea wrote on top of the questionnaire, "Thank you for recognizing there is a problem. Most people tell me I imagine it." Her granddaughter also suffered adverse reactions to aspartame products.

- A 27-year-old ophthalmic assistant with intense headache, multiple other symptoms, and a strong family history of aspartame disease wrote, "Many people are still in disbelief when they hear of my reaction to aspartame. It is most reassuring to see doctors finally getting involved with this problem. It is also rewarding to be heard as a victim."

- A 52-year old businesswoman with multiple aspartame reactions stated, "Thank you for your concern. As you can see, I have been to many doctors."

- A 25-year-old hotel manager with severe aspartame disease noted, "Thank you. It's about time someone paid attention to these reactions!"

- A 61-year-old Canadian executive with aspartame-induced convulsions, confusion, and blood changes stated, "I am most grateful there is an interest in this problem."

- A 48-year-old teacher had severe migraine and other aspartame-related complaints. Her daughter suffered similar reactions and intellectual deterioration. She wrote, "Thank you for your interest in people who are exhibiting reactions to aspartame! So few doctors know the hazards of aspartame. They are unable to give victims the guidance they desperately need. As I speak with people in my community, I am finding that reactions to aspartame are quite common. You have uncovered the tip of this iceberg."

- A 43-year-old woman stated, "I'm grateful I know what caused my problems. Thank you for the information." She had experienced visual changes, lightheadedness, tremors, mental confusion, memory loss, slurred speech, irritability, and intense anxiety attacks. Her symptoms disappeared within two weeks after stopping aspartame.

- A woman with severe reactions observed, "It was true then, and is true now, that conscientious people who are 'whistle blowers' are not appreciated."

- A 51-year-old woman with multiple and incapacitating reactions to aspartame products attached the following letter to her completed questionnaire.

"I feel like you have given me back my credibility. I really didn't imagine all the things I was experiencing. My husband was very supportive throughout my illness, but I was aware that there was a certain amount of disbelief. The look on his face when I read him your questionnaire was worth a million dollars. He just kept saying, 'My God, that's you!'"

- A 38-year-old homemaker had suffered intense headache, marked weight loss, and a major decrease of vision in both eyes during recent months. She improved greatly after avoiding aspartame products. She concluded the questionnaire:

"I would like to thank you for researching this product. I feel the public needs to be warned that severe side effects can occur from the use of aspartame. I would not like to see anyone suffer through the months of pain and emotional trauma which I, as well as my family, encountered!"

- The mother of a 13-year-old boy expressed appreciation for a letter I had sent to *The Palm Beach Post* (September 25, 1987, p. E-2) defending the legitimacy of aspartame-induced seizures. Her son had also experienced severe abdominal and chest pains for nine months before she suspected their relationship to aspartame.

"I would encourage you, since you are in a position of credibility, to continue to speak out against this drug. Your letter helped me a great deal. We are not psychologically unbalanced."

This questionnaire ultimately stimulated the interest of physicians when it was handed them by their patients. One ophthalmologist promptly found seven patients having eye complaints and associated severe headache in whom there was striking improvement after abstinence from aspartame. He called to express his appreciation.

612

LIMITATIONS AND RESERVATIONS

The limitations of questionnaire surveys are recognized. In the case of drugs, Dr. Edward A. Mortimer, Jr. (1987) emphasized that "... we are dependent upon complex, carefully conducted epidemiologic studies for recognition of uncommon untoward events." The same applies to food additives suspected of causing health problems.

My ongoing observations on aspartame disease, coupled with perceptive insights from reactors, indicate limitations of even the revised questionnaire, notwithstanding its length. For example, I failed to inquire about several major symptoms or disorders that surfaced after the first version.

- Failure to ask about drooping of the eyelids (ptosis) might have uncovered more patients with myasthenia gravis (Chapters IV and VI).
- Some respondents inserted <u>unlisted</u> aspartame-associated complaints (e.g., "asthma;" "dryness of the mouth") under the appropriate systems.

The Issue of "Controls"

The confirmatory data concerning reactions to aspartame products seem convincing. Anticipating criticism about the absence of age- and sex-matched "controls," these comments are warranted.

- Most persons who carefully described the recurrence of their complaints following rechallenge with aspartame in effect served as <u>their own</u> controls. This was impressive when such exposure was inadvertent (Chapter I).
- Governmental agencies and investigators have been urged to replicate my data. They were given permission to utilize <u>the same</u> questionnaire for suspect aspartame reactors and control groups (that is, persons who never used aspartame products).
- It has been argued that one can "always" find appreciable numbers of individuals with an idiosyncrasy to foods and other substances in population surveys. This must be regarded with skepticism in the present context. The case of strawberries, an analogy often used by representatives of the industry, provides a point of reference. I attended a course given by an internationally known allergist and editor of a leading allergy journal. He repeated his longstanding offer – never yet claimed – of $100 for anyone who could produce a person truly allergic to strawberries.

- Given the extraordinary consumption of aspartame (see Overview), one may encounter several difficulties relative to a "control" study in which persons within the mainstream of society presumably had never used such products. This issue assumes added significance if there is an allergic "priming" effect (Chapter VIII).

Another matter that surfaced from my questioning of patients and acquaintances pertains to the phenomenon of denial (Roberts 1971b). A number were convinced that aspartame posed "no problem" – and therefore presumed themselves to be "controls." When asked about specific symptoms, however, it became evident in some instances that this was not the case.

Representative Case Report

Case XVIII-2

A 63-year-old friend, an experienced counsellor, was consuming large amounts of diet beverages because "they are free of sugar, like you advise your patients." He vehemently denied having difficulty with aspartame products. When asked if he suffered headaches, he paused, thought, and replied in the affirmative. Not only was he taking considerable amounts of an analgesic daily, but he had scheduled a neurology consultation the following week.

He was next asked about vision. Momentarily speechless, he admitted that his sight had deteriorated significantly in recent months. Moreover, he went out of his way to avoid heavy traffic at night because of increasingly severe intolerance to glare.

I received an elated call from this self-described "professional skeptic" four days later. He stated that the headaches had subsided, and his vision already improved significantly since avoiding aspartame. He canceled the neurology consultation. His improvement over the ensuing six months was gratifying.

Other Reservations

The term "frequent," relative to projected aspartame disease in the general population, is used by the author cautiously. Physicians and other health professionals have been justifiably criticized over the casual manner in which this and other expressions – such as "likely," "infrequent," and "almost never" – are invoked (Kong 1986).

The lack of dependability of recall poses another consideration. It had been encountered even with cooperative respondents in other areas wherein investigators sought quantitative information from survey questions (Bradburn 1987). Errors in this realm were probably <u>under</u>estimated here. For example, many details that had not been elicited during extended office visits were added by patients while completing the questionnaire at their leisure.

XIX

RESPONSES AND COMMENTARY TO THE QUESTIONNAIRE

"When you can measure what you are speaking about, and express it in numbers, you know something about it."

Lord Kalvin

The survey questionnaire was initially completed by 397 aspartame reactors (Roberts 1990). An additional 149 persons with aspartame disease subsequently submitted it – totaling 546 (45.5 percent) of the 1,200 in this series. Inasmuch as data from this latter group were virtually superimposable upon the earlier results, the first 397 replies are reviewed.

The respondents included patients and correspondents of the author, and persons referred by Mission Possible, Aspartame Victims and their friends, The Community Nutrition Institute, and Woodrow Monte, Ph.D.

More Details About the Data Base

Some respondents failed to answer or clarify certain questions. This explains the "not specified" category, and several that total less than 397.

Analysis of the data also entailed cross-indexing (see Sections 2 and 3). Results of the most pertinent correlates are listed. Some examples:

- The positive correlation between a past history of migraine or other headaches and aspartame-induced headaches, convulsions, or both.
- The importance of aspartame-induced "dry eyes" in other clinical areas.
- The lack of correlation between decreased consumption of cigarettes or alcohol and decreased vision (toxic amblyopia).

Acronym Legend

ACB	-	aspartame cola beverage
ASD	-	aspartame soft drink
ATS	-	aspartame tabletop sweetener

GENERAL INFORMATION ABOUT INITIAL 397 RESPONDENTS

Sex	-	men 94 (24%); women 300 (76%)
Race	-	white 364 (92%); black (1%); not specified 29 (7%)
Average Present Age	-	45 years
Occupation	-	Housewife 72 (18%); business 133 (34%); Professional 98 (25%); Retired 50 (12%); not specified 44 (11%)

INFORMATION ABOUT PRIOR USE OF ASPARTAME

Average age when first reaction occurred   - 43 years

1-9 years	8	(2%)
10-19 years	9	(2%)
20-29 years	68	(17%)
30-39 years	83	(21%)
40-49 years	80	(20%)
50-59 years	73	(19%)
60-69 years	48	(12%)
70-79 years	22	(6%)
80-99 years	3	(1%)

Duration of aspartame consumption prior to first reaction in these categories:

days - 2;   weeks - 3;   months - 4;   years - 1.

A great increase in aspartame consumption before symptoms began

"Yes"   182 (51%).

Reasons for using aspartame products

Preference for taste	-	15%
Great thirst in hot weather	-	9%
Desire to avoid sugar	-	76%

On a strict diet for weight loss at onset of aspartame disease

"Yes"   -   68 (17%)

Exercising to lose weight when aspartame disease began

        "Yes"   -   66 (16.6%)

Women using aspartame during pregnancy

        "Yes"   -   5

Average daily consumption of aspartame products when symptoms began

Two 12-ounce cans of soda	242	(61%)
Two 6-ounce bottles of soda	18	(5%)
One-liter bottle of soda	36	(9%)
One two-liter bottle of soda	19	(5%)
Three packets of ATS	171	(43%)
Two glasses aspartame- presweetened tea	61	(15%)
Three glasses aspartame- presweetened drink mix	102	(26%)
One glass aspartame-pre- sweetened hot chocolate	52	(13%)
One bowl presweetened cereal	26	(6.6%)
One serving presweetened pudding or gelatin	61	(15%)
Four sticks aspartame gum	47	(12%)

Comparison with FDA Data

The FDA data on aspartame consumer complaints by associated product type(s) (Tollefson 1987) are reproduced. Diet soft drinks and a tabletop sweetener again dominate.

Product Type	Total Complaints	Percentage (rounded)
Diet soft drinks	1697	41%
Tabletop sweetener	911	22%
Puddings & gelatins	290	7%
Lemonade	245	6%
Kool Aid®	239	6%
Hot chocolate	212	5%
Iced tea	194	5%

Other	156	4%
Chewing gum	115	3%
Cereal	56	1%
Punch mix	37	1%
Sugar substitute tablets	31	1%
Non-dairy toppings	4	-
Chewable multi-vitamins	3	-

SUSPICIONS ABOUT ASPARTAME CAUSING OR AGGRAVATING THE CONDITION

Who or what made you first think that aspartame might be causing or aggravating your symptoms?

Myself	195	(49%)
A newspaper article	104	(26%)
A TV program	60	(15%)
A relative	47	(12%)
A friend	36	(9%)
My own doctor	27	(7%)
A medical specialist	17	(4%)
A nurse	5	(1%)
Other	33	(8%)

Representative Case Report (also see Section 1)

Case XIX-1

A 24-year-old housewife consumed up to three liters of an ACB daily. She experienced increasingly severe headaches, but did not relate them to this product. Her initial awareness came while watching a television program.

"If it wasn't for the *Consumer's Report Special*, I might have never associated my everyday severe headaches with aspartame. Only God knows what would be wrong with me now. The night I saw the show, I immediately stopped drinking diet drinks. The next night the headaches were gone."

Did you then completely stop using aspartame?

"Yes"　346　(87%)

Symptoms improved when stopped

"Yes"   331   (83%)

Beginning of improvement after aspartame stopped (average interval)

2 days	59%
1 week	28%
2 months	13%

Disappearance of symptoms after stopping aspartame

"Yes"   256   (64%)

Average interval

2 days	57%
2 weeks	25%
2 months	17%

RECHALLENGE

The subject of rechallenge with aspartame products was considered in Chapters I and II. Some aspartame reactors, especially weight-conscious young women, purposefully tested themselves many times "to be certain" these products were the culprit.

Did your symptoms recur when you ate or drank these products again?

"Yes"   214   (54%)

Average interval

Within 1 day	90%
Within 1 week	9%
Within 1 month	1%

How many times did you retest yourself until you became convinced that aspartame really caused your symptoms?

1   41   (10%)

620

2	66	(17%)
3	59	(15%)
4 or more	40	(10%)

Did the symptoms return after eating or drinking something you didn't know contained aspartame?

"Yes"   120 of 214   (56%)

Representative Case Reports

Case XIX-2

A 23-year-old teacher suffered severe headaches, dizziness, lightheadedness, unsteadiness of the legs, depression and "anxiety attacks" the day after drinking 3 to 4 cans of an ACB. She also had decreased vision and pain in both eyes, and marked frequency of urination. These symptoms did not occur with beverages containing saccharin. There was a longstanding history of migraine. Her father had severe reactions to aspartame, especially the aggravation of respiratory allergies. She challenged herself <u>four</u> times before becoming convinced that aspartame-containing products caused her symptoms.

> "I find that when I have aspartame, usually in soft drinks, I feel unusual lightheadedness, headache, queasy, funny, nauseous. My vision also becomes somewhat distorted, and my balance goes. It's kind of a tunnel vision feeling."

Refusal to Rechallenge

The fear of suffering recurrent aspartame reactions was evidenced by the fact that 171 persons (47 percent) refused to attempt even a single rechallenge.

Representative Case Report

A 36-year-old secretary attributed visual problems, headache, dizziness, mental confusion with memory loss, slurring of speech, depression, palpitations, bloody stools, and severe itching to aspartame products. Her daughter and mother also were aspartame reactors. She expressed much apprehension about rechallenge, especially if unknowingly served aspartame in restaurants, because of "possible danger in aggravating the problems."

CONTINUED USE OF ASPARTAME-CONTAINING PRODUCTS

Forty-five aspartame reactors (12 percent) <u>still</u> used these products notwithstanding headaches, visual problems, and other complaints that were clearly aspartame-associated. These encounters recalled unsuccessful efforts in getting some patients with severe lung or cardiovascular disease to stop smoking.

Several reasons – perhaps in concert – may explain the continued consumption of aspartame under these circumstances.

- The overriding desire to taste something sweet other than sugar.
- The belief that amounts of aspartame less than those producing overt symptoms would do no harm.
- The occurrence of withdrawal symptoms among aspartame addicts (Chapter VII G), comparable to going "cold turkey" on attempted cessation of cigarettes or alcohol.

THE PERSONAL TOLL

The majority of respondents elaborated on how aspartame reactions adversely affected their lives (also see Section 1). They estimated the impact as follows:

None	72	(18%)
"A bit"	165	(42%)
"Severely" (loss of job, school, divorce, etc.)	62	(14%)
"I was incapacitated"	38	(8%)
"I lost my driver's license"	5	(1%)

Most aspartame reactors had to cope with intense "fatigue," sleepiness, headache, convulsions, and other serious health problems in their personal and business careers. An appropriate term encompassing the combined toll of aspartame disease was used in connection with chronic benign pain: the Biopsychosocioeconomic Syndrome (*Medical Tribune* July 8, 1987, p. 16).

- A 33-year-old teacher stated, "it greatly affected my family relationship, and general ability to cope and maintain control."
- A legal secretary indicated that she "was incapacitated" by the severe flu-like reaction – consisting of dizziness, lightheadedness, nausea and diarrhea – after drinking four glasses of aspartame-sweetened iced tea.

- A 35-year-old housewife experienced numerous reactions to aspartame products, especially severe depression, irritability, anxiety attacks, and a change in personality.

  > "During the four months I used aspartame, I was afraid I was losing my mind. I never had this problem before, and have not had it since stopping aspartame. Thank God I have a very patient husband or I would be circling 'divorce' in the questionnaire. I wish it had never been invented!"

- A 30-year-old elementary school teacher with many reactions to aspartame beverages and a tabletop sweetener noted,"I couldn't concentrate, and did not write down any school lesson plans from March 1985 through the end of the school year after having taught seven years."

- A 40-year-old artist was incapacitated by seizures and other complaints attributed to aspartame disease. She lost her driver's license for three months. The cost of medical consultation was $4,800, for which she received no insurance reimbursement.

  > "I could not attend graduate school. The reactions stressed my marriage because of finances and personal problems, and made me feel unsure of life. I lost my job because of the drugs prescribed to stop seizures. I feel 'doped' up all the time. I'm depressed."

- A 55-year-old priest found his career to be in jeopardy while consuming three cans of ASD and three packets of an ATS daily. He clarified his "significant" disability in these terms: "Hard to read. Double vision off and on. Loss of memory." He also suffered ringing in both ears, slurred speech, headaches, severe itching, joint pains, and a recent elevation of blood pressure. These features disappeared four days after stopping aspartame products, only to return within three days after resuming them.

- A 57-year-old woman wrote of her aspartame reaction

    "I was afraid to participate in, and avoided whenever possible, social gatherings. I always carried a plastic bag in case I had to vomit, and kept one in my car."

- A 28-year-old housewife suffered from a number of symptoms during the five months she consumed and ACB and an ATS. She was seen by more than five physicians and consultants. The impact on her personal life was poignantly described in these terms:

    "I had a five-month-old baby at the time. She's a year old now. I was so sick that I couldn't take care of her right. I feel I missed something in the months I was sick as far as her growing and learning."

Impaired Sexuality

Several persons specifically attributed their problems with sexuality to aspartame disease. The occurrence of male impotence was discussed in Chapters IXV-E and XV.

    Both spouses in one marriage had severe aspartame disease. The wife stated, "I was so sick from headache that my mate and I had no love life at all."

REACTIONS ATTRIBUTED TO ASPARTAME PRODUCTS

The many symptoms and signs noted by aspartame reactors in the questionnaire, and their relationship to aspartame abstinence and rechallenge, were comparable to those cited for the 1,200 persons with aspartame disease in Sections 2 and 3. Only the computerized data are listed below.

Several clinical and epidemiologic associations came to light in the process of collating this information. They included a history of prior or subsequent allergies (Chapter VIII), and an underactive thyroid (hypothyroidism) (Chapter IX-E).

The clinical data on 3,326 consumers who complained to the FDA about alleged aspartame reactions appear in Table II-3.

624

Frequency of Medical Complaints in 397 Respondents

Eyes

A marked decrease of vision in	one eye	20	(5%)
	both eyes	94	(24%)
Loss of vision in	one eye	12	(3%)
	both eyes	7	(2%)

Continued use of aspartame by persons with persistent decrease or loss of vision — 14

Pain in	one eye	13	(3%)
	both eyes	38	(10%)
Recent "dry eyes"	"Yes"	39	(10%)

Recent aspartame-associated "dry eyes" and severe depression — 20

Recent aspartame-associated "dry eyes" and severe mental confusion — 11

Recent aspartame-associated "dry eyes" and marked memory loss — 22

Recent aspartame-associated "dry eyes" and severe thirst — 15

Recent trouble wearing contact lens "Yes" — 16

Ears

Ringing or "cracking" in	one ear	11	(3%)
	both ears	64	(16%)
Loss of hearing in	one ear	11	(3%)
	both ears	12	(3%)
Severe sensitivity to noise in	one ear	4	(1%)
	both ears	45	(11%)

Brain and Head

Severe headaches	190	(48%)
Continued use of aspartame by persons with aspartame-induced headache	24	
Severe dizziness or feeling lightheaded	176	(44%)
Severe unsteadiness of the legs	61	(15%)

Convulsions (grand mal seizures; epilepsy)	56	(14%)
Number of attacks - 1	15	
- 2	18	
- 3	6	
- 4 or more	17	
Continued use of aspartame by persons		
with aspartame-induced convulsions	5	
History of prior strict diet by persons		
with aspartame-induced convulsions	7	
Epilepsy-like "fits" without convulsions		
(petit mal; psychomotor attacks)	32	(8%)
Severe drowsiness and falling asleep	69	(17%)
Severe shaking (tremors)	48	(12%)
Severe insomnia (trouble sleeping)	76	(19%)
Severe mental confusion	75	(19%)
Marked memory loss	102	(26%)
10-19 years	4	
20-29 years	14	
30-39 years	26	
40-49 years	23	
50-59 years	18	
60-69 years	17	
Severe hyperactivity (jumping of		
the arms; "restless legs")	45	(11%)
Severe tingling, pins and needles, or		
numbness of the arms and legs	76	(19%)
Unexplained pains in or around the face	35	(9%)
Slurring of speech	63	(16%)
Severe depression	114	(29%)
Suicidal thoughts	39	
Continued use of aspartame by		
persons with severe depression	10	

History of prior strict diet by persons with aspartame-induced depression	22	
Extreme irritability	121	(25%)
Severe "anxiety attacks"	99	(21%)
Marked "personality changes"	83	(21%)
Severe aggravation of phobias (such as a fear of crowds or heights)	47	(12%)

Chest

Attacks of shortness of breath	55	(14%)
Palpitations	87	(22%)
Rapid heart beat attacks	43	(11%)
Unexplained chest pains	47	(12%)
Recent high blood pressure	32	(8%)

Abdomen

Pain in the belly	64	(16%)
Severe nausea	66	(17%)
Diarrhea	67	(17%)
Blood in the stools		
Severe bloat (swelling)	56	(14%)
Women	51	
Men	5	

Skin and Allergies

Severe itching without a rash	38	(10%)
Hives (water blisters)	19	(5%)
Other rashes	34	(9%)
Marked loss or thinning of the hair	31	(8%)
Mouth reactions		
Lips become swollen	6	(2%)
Tongue became swollen	13	(3%)
Pain in the mouth	14	(4%)
Painful or difficult swallowing	25	(6%)

Marked Change of Weight (Unintended)

Gain	34	(9%)
Average increase - 19 pounds		
Loss	27	(7%)
Average loss - 22 pounds		

Other Problems

Severe thirst		62	(16%)
Marked frequency of urination	68		(17%)
Day	13		
Night	10		
Both	45		
Severe changes in menstrual periods		37	(12%)
More frequent	15		
Less frequent	8		
Stopped	14		
Severe joint pains		54	(14%)
Marked swelling of the legs (all were women)		19	(5%)
"Low blood sugar" (hypoglycemia) attacks		25	(6%)
Poorer control of diabetes		12	(3%)
On diet	6		
On oral drugs	3		
On insulin	3		

CONSULTATIONS AND TESTS BEFORE STOPPING ASPARTAME

Physicians and consultants seen in own community

1	86	(22%)
2	67	(17%)
3	32	(8%)
4	13	(3%)
More	16	(4%)

Number of consultants or clinics visited outside of own community

1	39	(10%)
2	13	(2%)
3	6	(2%)
4	4	(1%)
More	3	(1%)

Times hospitalized BEFORE aspartame was suspected as the cause

1	26	(7%)
2	11	(3%)
3	6	(2%)
4	1	-
More	1	-

Tests done BEFORE aspartame was suspected as the cause

X-rays of the head		45	(11%)
1	26		
2	18		
3	1		
CT of the brain		77	(19%)
1	54		
2	20		
3	2		
4	1		
MRI (magnetic resonance) of brain		22	(6%)
1	18		
2	2		
3	1		
Cerebral angiograms (X-rays of blood vessels in the brain)		18	(5%)
Lumbar puncture (spinal tap)		21	(5%)
Electroencephalograms (EEG, brain wave test)		66	(18%)
1	41		
2	15		
3	8		
4	2		
Stress test of the heart		33	(8%)

Heart monitor (12 or 24 hours)	24	(6%)
1	16	
2	7	
Upper GI series with barium	28	(7%)
1	25	
2	3	
Barium enema	23	(6%)
1	21	
2	2	
Allergy tests (skin, others)	22	(6%)
Special eye tests	50	(13%)
Special ear tests	25	(6%)

AVERAGE ESTIMATED MEDICAL COSTS (prior to 1989)

Paid by the person	-	$ 1,717
Paid by an insurance carrier	-	$ 4,544

SUSPECTED REACTIONS REPORTED TO

Own doctor	212	(53%)
Family	185	(46%)
Aspartame Victims and Their Friends	183	(46%)
The Food and Drug Administration (FDA)	95	(24%)
Another interested researcher	74	(19%)
Manufacturer of the product	59	(15%)
H.J. Roberts, M.D.	55	(14%)
Another consumer organization	51	(13%)
A consultant	33	(8%)
A public health department	26	(7%)
The Centers for Disease Control (CDC)	18	(5%)

Method of reporting

By letter	212	(53%)
By phone call	48	(12%)
Other	21	(5%)

ASPARTAME REACTIONS IN FAMILY MEMBERS

"Yes"	117	(29%)
Relationship		
Husband	20	
Wife	12	
Daughter(s)	29	
Son(s)	17	
Other relatives	54	

MEDICAL BACKGROUND AND HABITS

Migraine	40	(10%)
Other headaches	58	(15%)
History of migraine with aspartame-associated headache	27	
History of other headaches with aspartame-associated headache	31	
History of migraine or other headache with aspartame-associated headache and convulsions	30	
Depression	34	(9%)
History of depression and aspartame-associated depression	22	
Severe "anxiety"	13	(3%)
Poor vision	42	(11%)
Ear problems	17	(4%)
Heart disease	16	(4%)
High blood pressure	35	(9%)
Stomach trouble	19	(5%)
Bowel trouble	20	(5%)
Kidney trouble	4	(1%)

Hives	8	(2%)
Other rashes (such as psoriasis, acne, lupus)	12	(3%)
Allergies	126	(32%)

Hay fever	51
Asthma	20
Medicines	55
Reactors with at least one past history of allergy and at least one aspartame-induced allergic or skin reaction	27

"Low blood sugar" (hypoglycemia) attacks	31	(8%)
Diabetes	28	(7%)

A thyroid problem	26	(6%)

Goiter	1
Underactive (hypothyroidism)	21
Overactive (hyperthyroidism)	4

"Arthritis"	46	(11%)
A marked weight problem (20 pounds or more)	93	(23%)
An alcohol problem	6	(2%)
A drug abuse problem	1	-

Cigarette smoker

Yes	65	(16%)

Less than ½ pack	8
½ - 1 pack	35
More than 1 pack	18
Smokers with aspartame-associated decrease or loss of vision	29

Severe attack after drinking alcohol while taking aspartame

Yes	25	(6%)

Very little	6
Moderate	12
A lot	7

OTHER INFORMATION

Reactors still using products containing aspartame

Yes	50	(13%)

The resumption or continuation of aspartame products by reactors was motivated most often by a modest gain in weight after discontinuing "diet" soft drinks. Another factor was aspartame addiction (Chapter VII-G)

Representative Case Report

Case XIX-3

A 59-year-old secretary suffered headache, depression, palpitations, unexplained chest and joint pains, and "a recurrent weak feeling inside – like I could go down at any time."

During the summer, she consumed up to five cans of an ACB daily. There was dramatic improvement within several days after stopping it; her symptoms disappeared within one week. Two daughters and a sister also experienced striking reactions to aspartame. These subsided promptly when they avoided such products.

This person indicated, however, that she was still using 24 ounces of the diet cola daily. She explained, "I quit aspartame for six months, and gained ten pounds in a regular cola beverage. So I drink half-diet and half-regular now until the pains in the chest come on, and then cut back on the diet drink for a while."

Friends with known or suspected aspartame reactions

Yes		157	(40%)
1 person	53		
2 persons	51		
3 persons	19		
4 persons	34		

Have you ever heard of the condition known as phenylketonuria (PKU)?

Yes	224

Do you <u>really</u> know what it is?
                Yes   108   (27%)
                No   126   (32%)

Has anyone in your family had it?
                Yes   4   (1%)
                No   175   (44%)

<u>Do you believe that aspartame content labeling should be mandated by law?</u>

Yes   375   (94%)
         Would <u>you</u> study them?
                Yes   340

<u>Do you think that Congress should do anything about regulating aspartame?</u>

Yes   312   (79%)

THE OCCUPATIONAL TOLL

Aspartame reactors provided numerous accounts of occupational problems – including loss of job – from incapacitation attributed to aspartame disease.

<u>Impaired Performance At Work</u>

- A 31-year-old teacher indicated, "It is difficult to perform your professional duties to your fullest when you have a headache."
- A 42-year-old female photographer noticed marked blurring of vision in both eyes within one day after drinking a diet cola or using up to three packets of an ATS daily. This symptom subsided within one day of abstinence, but recurred during <u>four</u> separate rechallenges. She neither smoked nor drank alcohol. All aspartame products were avoided thereafter because "I'm a photographer. It was all very scary."
- A 33-year-old office manager developed severe headache, memory loss, depression, irritability, anxiety attacks with aggravated phobias, "personality changes", palpitations, frequent menses, and severe low blood sugar attacks. She stated, "I was extremely depressed on and off, and it was hard to work."
- A 52-year-old antiques dealer suffered extreme fatigue, severe eye pain, decreased vision, dizziness, drowsiness, facial pains, depression with suicidal thoughts, a change in personality, recent high blood

634

pressure, palpitations, diarrhea, and intense discomfort over the neck, shoulders and hips. She had been consuming six cans of ACB daily. Her problems culminated in both divorce and business losses. Her daughter also developed dizziness from aspartame. She wrote

> "There was a loss of work from this. I had doctors' appointments scheduled as often as 5 times a week. The extreme fatigue and intolerant pain reached the point where I didn't want anyone around me."

- A 57-year-old secretary numerous reactions to an ATS. She described the toll in these terms:

> "I continued working, but under adversity due to headaches and fatigue. I started to lose my skill and usual confidence in driving ability: sought less-trafficked routes to work, etc. I was able to continue working through sheer determination despite acute fatigue, headaches, 5 attacks of gastroenteritis, strong urine, an earache, incoordination, eyes hurting, leg pain. I avoided depression by sheer will power and determination to discover the root of this."

Loss of Work - General

- A 48-year-old teacher was incapacitated while consuming aspartame because "I became ill and couldn't perform my job." She indicated that her extreme irritability and severe nausea would return "immediately" after eating or drinking products containing aspartame.
- A 39-year-old saleswoman with a severe aspartame-associated polyneuropathy bitterly complained of the resulting incapacitation. She wrote, "I am a commission sales representative. If I don't work, I make no money. I'm broke. This isn't fair."
- A 48-year-old professor of business management was placed on permanent disability due to severe aspartame disease after filing for bankruptcy because of her inability to work.

Loss of Work - Medical Personnel

Several physicians and nurses with serious aspartame reactions – particularly seizures, visual problems and confusion – encountered extraordinary difficulty in their attempts to resume work and obtain malpractice insurance.

- A 35-year-old male nurse anesthetist consumed six cans of an ACB daily for several months. He developed hives, a striking decrease of vision in both eyes, severe headache, marked memory loss and three grand mal convulsions. He was seen by multiple specialists, both in and out of his community, and hospitalized twice. Two sets of skull x-rays, two CT scans and two MRI studies of the brain, cerebral angiograms, lumbar puncture, three electroencephalograms, and several heart studies were normal. His hives did not respond to antihistamine therapy. Phenytoin failed to abolish the seizures.

  After learning that these problems might be reactions to aspartame, he stopped the ACB. His symptoms disappeared within several weeks.

  Unfortunately, this nurse was unable to administer anesthesia because of his inability to obtain malpractice insurance due to a history of seizures. He told the Senate hearing held on November 3, 1987

  > "My problems are now re-obtaining my malpractice insurance and getting my privileges back. I have only one small hospital where I could practice and one plastic surgeon's office. As of yet, I have not been reinstated with malpractice insurance."

- A 34-year old registered nurse stated, "I felt so bad all the time that I quit a job I had for 11 years." She had been consuming up to eight 12-ounce cans of a diet cola and ten sticks of aspartame gum daily. Her symptoms included severe headache, dizziness, "fits" without convulsions, marked memory loss, slurring of speech, "anxiety attacks," palpitations, diarrhea, severe bloat, less frequent menstrual periods, recent trouble wearing contact lens, marked sensitivity to noise in both ears, and joint pains. These complaints improved within one week after avoiding aspartame, and were gone by six weeks.

636

Loss of Driver or Pilot Licenses

Aspartame reactors lost their driver or pilot licenses because of convulsions, impaired vision, or accidents ascribed to aspartame-induced confusion or sleepiness. (See case reports in Chapters III, IV, VI and XXVII). The following persons illustrate such occupational and financial distress.

- A 48-year-old clerical worker suffered severe dizziness, convulsions, shortness of breath and rapid heart action after ingesting aspartame products. She qualified the impact upon her life: "I lost my driver's license."
- A 45-year-old air traffic control specialist suffered intense pain and blurred vision in one eye within three days after drinking two 10-ounce bottles of a diet cola. He awakened to find his vision transiently clouded by a "road mad of black blood vessels." Severe thirst and an intensification of "low blood sugar attacks" ensued. His symptoms disappeared within two days after abstaining from aspartame products.

This theme has surfaced elsewhere. For example, an Air Force fighter pilot told the Senate hearing held on November 3, 1987 that he experienced a grand mal seizure several years previously while consuming up to one gallon a day of aspartame. Even though there had been no recurrence after avoiding aspartame, he was permanently grounded with a diagnosis of an "idiopathic partial seizure disorder"... at considerable reduction of pay.

Alleged Deaths

The most severe toll attributed to aspartame disease by relatives or lawyers involved fatal medical complications, accidents or sudden death ("the sweet hereafter".) (See Chapter IX-C).

Case XXVII-7 a 23-year-old male, died in an auto accident after losing consciousness while apparently convulsing at the wheel. He had been consuming two to four gallons of an ACB daily. Many of his other symptoms were consistent with aspartame disease. Furthermore, his sister experienced headaches and mood swings whenever she drank the same beverage.

FINANCIAL COSTS

Considerable monies were often spent for testing, consultation and medical care before the diagnosis of aspartame disease was entertained. The amounts – averaging $1,717 paid by the person, and $4,545 paid by the insurance carriers – appear in the representative case reports (Section 1, 2 and 3). The figures do <u>not</u> include loss of wages or other income, and related expenditures.

Additional examples underscore this financial burden.

- The mother of a child with recurrent blood changes diagnosed as histiocytic leukemia (Case IX-J-1) estimated the medical costs at $750,000 !

- A 28-year-old ballet dancer and teacher suffered repeat grand mal convulsions and other neurologic-psychiatric symptoms. She estimated the medical costs over a three-year period at $75,000. The psychiatrist's fee –two or three visits a week for one year, at $90 per hour – had to be paid out of pocket (her insurance policy covered only hospitalization.)

- A 42-year-old homemaker attributed her severe depression and convulsions to aspartame use. She estimated her personal costs at "more than $2,000," and those of her insurance at "more than $50,000."

- A 38-year-old office manager suffered nine convulsions after consuming three cans of an ACB and an aspartame soft drink for one year. Other complaints included pain in both eyes, sensitivity to noise in the ears, severe drowsiness, tremors, marked confusion and memory loss, tingling of the extremities, intense depression, anxiety attacks, personality changes, the aggravation of phobias, shortness of breath, attacks of rapid heart action, abdominal pain with nausea and diarrhea, swelling of the tongue, a gain of 15 pounds, and intensified attacks of apparent hypoglycemia. He saw three consultants in his community, and four consultants elsewhere. Two sets of x-rays, two CT scans and one MRI study of the brain, cerebral angiograms, two upper GI series, two barium enemas, and multiple studies failed to reveal another cause. He deduced "the aspartame connection" himself when the attacks recurred within two days on rechallenge. He estimated the medical costs at $10,000 out of his own pocket, and "twice that amount" for the insurance carrier.

- The author received this communication from a male aspartame reactor.

"Dr. Roberts, it was one of your articles that got me off aspartame. I wish I would have had such information about two months before date as I could have saved myself about $3,000 in tests."

- <u>Case IX-C-16</u>, a 35-year-old woman with aspartame-induced shortness of breath and other symptoms "spent a small fortune on tests that included asthma studies, gastrointestinal x-rays, ultrasound, blood work, and heart, lung and gynecologic testing" before the causative role of aspartame gum was determined.

<u>Commentary</u>

Health care costs exceeded 12 percent of the gross national product when the initial survey questionnaire was completed. As of 1990, more than half was paid by patients' private funds – specifically, 59 percent ($27 billion) of the total expenditures for health care. There have been profound changes since.

<u>Any</u> superimposed major public health problem severely exacerbates the problem for all, especially <u>futile diagnostic efforts</u>. Moreover, many aspartame reactors and their relatives stressed their enormous outlays for <u>unsuccessful treatments</u> before the crucial role of aspartame use was recognized. Some submitted long lists of previously prescribed drugs, which in turn had also caused problems.

A female administrator with severe aspartame reactions wrote

"The population certainly seems to be largely uninformed about this product. I can easily understand how many could spend a great amount of time and dollars on doctors and tests trying to find out 'what's wrong' with them !!"

"<u>Allergy testing</u>" for suspected food or inhalant offenders and auto immune reactions was costly and minimally beneficial for the large majority of aspartame reactors so tested.

<u>Needless or premature surgery</u> for complaints due to unrecognized aspartame disease proved even more costly. Examples include <u>cataract removal</u> (Chapter IV), <u>transurethral resection of the prostate</u> (Chapter IX) and <u>uterine scraping (D&C) or hysterectomy</u> in women with frequent and severe menstrual bleeding (Chapter IX-E).

Patients with aspartame disease who depend on "<u>managed care</u>" for their health needs are at a unique disadvantage. Furthermore, third-party-payors are likely not to insure such individuals with considerable prior doctoring. Another problem involves the limitation of office visits by HMO physicians or nurse practitioners who cannot obtain an adequate history in 5 -7 minutes.

EXPRESSIONS OF ANGER AND FRUSTRATION

The completed questionnaires and accompanying letters from persons afflicted with aspartame disease and their relatives or friends often contained expressions of intense anger and frustration. They lashed out at governmental regulators, physicians, dietitians, Congress, and the scientific community over the outrage to which they – as consumer victims – had been subjected. Scores enclosed copies of complaints previously submitted to the FDA, elected officials, the media, and consumer groups. In effect, this survey form provided them a vehicle for verbalizing "righteous indignation."

The following statements by such individuals constitute information volunteered for this research study. References to them do not reflect intent of malice by the author or publisher .

"Do you think that Congress should do anything about regulating aspartame?"

This question frequently evoked succinct replies with exclamation marks from aspartame reactors.

> "Ban it!"
> "Outlaw it!"
> "Take it off the market!"
> "Prohibit it!"
> "Terminate it!"
> "Stop its sale!"
> "Discontinue it altogether!"
> "Aspartame should be banned from use in all products by and act of
>   Congress!"
> "Remove it from the market until they can prove it harmless!"
> "It should be outlawed!"
> "To put it in children's vitamins is unforgivable!"
> "Congress must forbid it on the market!"

The intensity of related responses was evidenced by pleas urging further investigation and discretion in marketing.

- A 24-year-old housewife stated, "All these products should be further tested before marketing."

- A 34-year-old receptionist asked

    "What happens to the future children of America? Will they have to go through the symptoms of what I'm <u>still</u> going through? To sell the product to make money fast, is that really it? FDA, TAKE THIS OFF THE MARKET, PLEASE!"

- A 43-year-old lawyer with severe aspartame-induced depression recommended

    "Take it off the market. Please research as many suicides as you can regarding <u>quantity consumed</u> prior to the act. Also child abuse. Watch in particular the teen suicide situation!"

- The grandmother of a 7-½ year old boy who experienced two convulsions after consuming an aspartame soft drink wrote

    "Take it off the market completely!!! We will not be satisfied until this horrible menace is eliminated from the market once and for all. We feel so sorry for the unsuspecting public, and they are getting so brainwashed by being told it is natural — just harmless amino acids. An understatement if ever there was one."

- A 36-year-old Ph.D. with multiple aspartame reactions asserted, "Prohibit it! It is very dangerous. I've read the animal and human research."

- A 28-year-old woman suffered violent attacks of abdominal pain after drinking minimal amounts of aspartame cola drinks. She wrote

"Warn people. It's time to admit that this stuff is dangerous! I would rather die twenty years from now from saccharin use. The scary thing about aspartame is the immediate effect it can have. Let's get it off the market. "

- A banking executive with severe aspartame reactions had a son with aspartame-associated complaints and enlarged lymph nodes. He suggested

"I firmly believe the product should be totally removed from all products at once, and that a minimum of five years be spent restudying its effects."

- An "aspartame victim" opined

"I think they should get rid of it completely. It's no good. I hate to think that kids are eating and drinking it every day, and nobody knows the long-term effects."

- A 60-year-old woman developed dramatic reactions to aspartame shortly after she began using such products. She suggested, "It's harming many. Congress must forbid it on the market."

Related Expressions

Aspartame reactors vented their anger in other terms.

- A 31-year-old bookkeeper with multiple reactions, asserted "I feel aspartame almost killed me."
- A teacher with severe reactions attributed to aspartame products, including tea, imparted the suggestion: "What we need is another Boston Tea Party."
- A 50-year-old social worker developed mental confusion and a change in personality every time she ingested aspartame. She noted

"I can't imagine what they (Congress) can do. I have lost all confidence in the FDA. They were 'used' and we are paying the consequences. Now, economically, I don't think we can get rid of it."

642

Aspartame reactors even vented their distrust and hostility to the author!

- A 30-year-old sales consultant with neuropsychiatric reactions to aspartame inquired

    "I would like to know what took so long for me to be contacted by anyone re: aspartame. Please notify me concerning the results of questionnaires."

- A 59-year-old author wanted a reply to this request before she would complete the questionnaire: "I would like to be advised if you receive any funding from profit-making corporations using aspartame in their

    products." She was promptly assured that the author had not received one cent from such sources.

Representative Case Reports

Case XIX-4

A 60-year-old secretary supplemented her detailed responses to the questionnaire with this letter.

>"I find it odious to relate the incidences concerning my use of an aspartame tabletop sweetener. In spite of the time to answer questionnaires, I FEEL IT IS NECESSARY in the hope something can be provided as clues to bring this problem before the FDA and Congress, etc...
>
>"For some time now, I have been relatively 'trouble-free' and would like to think that things will go well from now on. I cannot stress enough the frustration which occurs during and after an incident involving aspartame usage, and never knowing whether there has been permanent damage and if, or when, problems might again develop."

She had begun to use the ATS after collecting coupons toward the purchase of this product, especially since "there was no warning printed." She consumed an estimated 3,500 packets in coffee, cereal and chocolate from January 1983 until February 1984! During this time, she suffered numerous complaints for which seven physicians (including two neurologists) were consulted. The causative role of aspartame, however, was first entertained because of "a fleeting mention of aspartame reactions on my car radio (January 23, 1984) while returning from seeing a specialist out of state. All of a sudden, it seemed to make sense."

She expressed her feelings in these terms:

> "While I basically espouse the 'free enterprise' philosophy, the potential for unwitting and unknowing damage to take place by using aspartame is, I believe, so great for some people that it SHOULD BE at least labeled as potentially harmful. I RESENT THAT THIS ASPARTAME PRODUCT WAS MARKETED, COUPONS PRINTED, AND PROMOTED WITHOUT ANY WARNING. I was trying to lose weight. It tasted good, seemed great, and I trusted THEM... I FEEL THAT ABOUT A YEAR OF MY LIFE WAS WASTED WHEN I FELT SO TERRIBLE, HAVING TO DOCTOR, AND HAVING MY LIFE UPSET."

OTHER FRUSTRATIONS

"Cornering the Market"

Dozens of consumers resented the packing of shelves in their grocery and drug stores with products containing aspartame, especially when its presence could not be easily detected on labels. This aspartame-is-everywhere lament was discussed in Chapter I.

- A 52-year-old administrator wrote

  > "I really have become resentful of having to read all labels <u>and</u> frequently not finding the aspartame content revealed. Even medications use it, as well as over-the-counter products. It seems to be everywhere, and my choices are greatly limited and restricted."

- A 34-year-old secretary lamented, "I would like to be able to purchase canned diet soda <u>without</u> aspartame."

- A 28-year-old hairdresser attributed two convulsions and numerous other complaints to aspartame. She stated

"I'd like to say that aspartame has taken over everything in your supermarkets, and that people with diabetic problems haven't got a chance anymore between aspartame and saccharin products to choose from. I'm terrified of the problem with aspartame in our country's kids. Sure, aspartame tastes better than saccharin products, but if any person on this earth went thru what I've been thru, and still am, they would never use the product. I think the Food and Drug Administration owes all of us an answer, including the manufacturer of aspartame! I'm sure they are making a mint. I wish to God I had never heard of aspartame!"

Fears Concerning Eating Outside The Home

As noted earlier under rechallenge, many aspartame reactors expressed apprehension about dining away from home – with good reason after nasty experiences. Several assumed the food they ordered at "good" restaurants did not contain aspartame... only to suffer "that same old feeling" within minutes or hours. Specific inquiry revealed that aspartame **had** been used.

Such anxiety on the part of aspartame reactors is enhanced by reports that chefs in outstanding "health conscious" restaurants began using aspartame when it allegedly became less expensive than corn syrup.

Fears Concerning Aspartame-Saccharin Combinations

A featured article in *The Miami Herald* (January 25, 1984) pointed out that many major producers of soft drinks began mixing aspartame with saccharin. This change caught aspartame reactors off guard.

Representative Case Report

Case XIX-5

A 63-year-old saleswomen repeatedly suffered severe headache, slurred speech, unexplained chest pains and shortness of breath within one hour after ingesting aspartame in soft drinks, hot chocolate or pudding. The complaints predicably subsided within 24 hours after avoiding these products. She experienced the same symptoms shortly after drinking pre-sweetened ice tea in a "health food restaurant." On learning that it had been sweetened with aspartame, she suggested, "If restaurants use it, they should have to let it be known."

A Letter to the FDA

A correspondent from Kentucky sent the author a copy of her letter to the FDA, dated February 16, 1987. The following excerpts indicated the intensity of her feelings concerning this agency's alleged "defense of aspartame."

> "Two members of my family were affected terribly from an 'over-dose' of a 'harmless' aspartame sweetener. My brother-in-law suffered from clinical depression, regression and a complete personality change. His wife (my sister) who put an aspartame sweetener in their coffee, vegetables, and almost everything they ate, suffered for three years from hyperthyroidism. Only by the grace of God did their health return after a neighbor told them that aspartame might be the cause of their problem. It was."

> "There's no need for aspartame to be on the market except for the profit the manufacturer brings in. This problem is too serious to go on any longer."

CRITICISM OF PHYSICIAN APATHY AND ATTITUDES

Many aspartame reactors stressed that physicians and consultants they had seen would not believe these products might be causing or aggravating their medical problems. Such frustration became compounded by disinterest in pursuing this subject and the discovery that consumer groups already had identified hundreds of "aspartame victims."

Numerous references to this vexation are cited in prior chapters. For example, the wife of an aspartame victim who suffered convulsions after unknowingly ingesting aspartame on three different occasions, wrote

> "I have asked doctors to report his convulsions to the FDA, and they have all refused. They all say the American Medical Association says that aspartame is harmless."

There was a notable exception in attitude when patients were being treated by physicians who had experienced aspartame disease <u>themselves</u> (Chapter I).

> A 34-year-old receptionist developed violent headaches and other symptoms while consuming large amounts to aspartame products. She wrote on the questionnaire, "The doctor I went to told me he had the <u>same</u> symptoms as I did."

Representative Case Reports

Case XIX-6

A 65-year-old accountant stated

> "My doctor didn't seem to take much interest in my belief that aspartame caused my dizzy spells, but he didn't know what caused them. I only know that I had 3 separate occasions with the dizzy spells, all beginning during the middle of the night. Since I've completely eliminated aspartame from my diet, I no longer have the dizziness. I <u>firmly</u> believe aspartame caused my problems, but this is only <u>my</u> belief and not a doctor's."

Case XIX-7

A businesswoman with severe visual, neurologic and psychiatric symptoms attributable to aspartame disease commented

> "I have come to the conclusion that none of the doctors are going to put anything in writing. Two of them have come right out and told me, 'You know, we can't put this in writing as it hasn't been proven yet. We could have a lawsuit against us.' My condition was know as "Multiple Migrating Ailments' for a while... My conclusion is that the doctors here do not want to get involved in the situation."

Case XIX-8

A 51-year-old woman with violent aspartame reactions recalled a physician encounter.

> "My doctor (an internist) here in Arizona was not at all interested when I told him I had discovered what was making me ill. He was very arrogant about the whole thing. I certainly didn't hold it against him because he didn't know what was wrong, but his attitude and lack of interest when I told him made me furious. His comment was, 'Well, if you feel better not using it, don't use it.' Needless to say, I have changed doctors."

Case XIX-9

A 23-year-old businesswoman (commercial banking) experienced many aspartame-induced complaints. They included mouth pain, difficulty in swallowing, decreased vision, ringing in the ears, severe dizziness, tremors, impaired memory, marked anxiety with aggravated phobias, attacks of shortness of breath and rapid heart action, bloody stools, a rash, and severe joint pains. She first became aware of aspartame after hearing about my discussion on a radio interview. These complaints improved within four days after stopping aspartame.. She wrote

> "The worst thing about this was that I went undiagnosed for so long. People told me it was 'all in my head' and that I needed to 'think positively' because the medical tests all came up normal. My doctor began to lose patience with me and implied that I was a hypochondriac! I was told I might have MS, but that it couldn't be diagnosed for certain.
>
> "My symptoms came and went, so that one day I would feel fine and think it was going away, and then they would be back worse that ever. There were so many symptoms and they were so varied that I felt like my body was falling apart. I was very frightened and felt very alone and depressed. I was irritable and paranoid. I had the symptoms every day for 4 ½ months.

"As soon as my friend told me she had heard about aspartame reactions on a talk show, I <u>knew</u> that was what it was. She listed symptoms that I had not described to her, and it was like hearing myself talk. I stopped immediately and the symptom began to improve. This was ten days ago. I now feel like my old self."

Neurologists

Specialists in neurology came under heavy criticism from aspartame reactors, especially those who had presented with recurrent convulsions. A vicious cycle of hostility to such professional disbelief or indifference was generated when these individuals deduced a valid relationship between the seizures and aspartame intake <u>by themselves</u> (Chapter III). Their frustration was fanned by insistence upon more CT scans or MRI studies of the brain, and other costly tests <u>already</u> done, and the recommendation that they continue taking potent anti-epileptic medication "indefinitely" long after the seizures ceased after discontinuing aspartame products.

Representative Case Reports

Case XIX-10

A 66-year-old housewife experienced a convulsion after using three packets of an ATS daily for six weeks. There was no recurrence when she stopped this product. She wrote

"My husband and I have been astounded by the doctors with whom we have tried to discuss aspartame. Only one in perhaps six gave it any thought at all. The attitude of the others, with one exception, was tolerant disinterest. The one exception would not listen, period."

Case XIX-11

A 35-year-old male anesthetist developed visual complaints, severe headaches, and three grand mal seizures after consuming up to six diet colas daily. He told a Senate hearing on aspartame (November 3, 1987) of his neurologist's comment following the third seizure: "Wouldn't it be a shame if all that's wrong with you is NutraSweet?"

Case XIX-12

A 28-year-old woman with convulsions and many other reactions to an ACB had been given the same diagnosis by most of the physicians and consultants she saw: "It's your nerves." She was infuriated because her "doctors still will not admit that they have anything to do with aspartame."

Case XIX-13

A 29-year-old businessman (Case III-5) had been subjected to <u>five</u> CT scans and <u>three</u> MRI studies of the brain, and <u>five</u> electroencephalograms for aspartame-associated convulsions. After seeing him in consultation, the author reviewed the case at length with his neurologist. This doctor then called the patient, and ridiculed the possibility of an aspartame reaction. Moreover, he <u>demanded</u> that the patient continue taking 400 mg phenytoin and six tablets of carbamazepine daily.

There had been no further seizures when the patient was next seen in six months. But the neurologist adamantly refused to reduce the dosage of either drug, even on a trial basis.

CRITICISM OF DIETITIANS

Some patients with aspartame disease, especially diabetics, leveled fierce criticism against dietitians who had **insisted** that they add aspartame to their diet.

- An aspartame reactor asserted, "Everyone treats it (aspartame) like a sacred cow because it is the 'new' thing for diabetics."
- A 36-year-old registered nurse expressed great concern over the recommendation by professional dietitians that aspartame be given to traumatized patients in order to promote weight loss. She wrote, "It should be stopped immediately. There is no question of its (adverse) effects on such persons."
- A 33-year-old graphic artist developed severe headache, drowsiness, numbness of the limbs, nausea, bloat and frequency of urination after drinking one can of diet cola daily. She stated, "I thought immediately that I was reacting to aspartame, but due to assurance by a dietitian that it was safe, I continued to use it for a year and a half." Her sister also was an aspartame reactor.

RECOMMENDATIONS

Labeling (also see Chapter XXVII)

Respondents provided numerous suggestions about aspartame labeling. A few are listed.

"Warn people like tobacco warnings."
"List aspartame in large print."
"Make warning labels on <u>all</u> products using aspartame."
"Side effects of aspartame should be listed on products that contain it."
"There should be required notice on labels of canned fruits, vegetables, puddings, and ice cream with aspartame."
"Limit allowable amounts."
"I believe it's more dangerous than saccharin, and should AT LEAST contain a warning label."
"I do not want to prevent others from using aspartame if they wish to do so. I <u>do</u> want <u>all products</u> containing aspartame to be so labeled in <u>large</u>, easy-to-read lettering!!" (This person had experienced severe blurring of vision.)

Recommendations about Commercials

Aspartame reactors objected to many of the commercials for aspartame products appearing in print and on television. For instance, a 31-year-old female sales representative with recurrent severe frequency and pain on urinating after drinking an ACB suggested that the manufacturers "...change their TV commercials. They are very misleading."

Licensing and Regulation By Congress

Aspartame reactors provided a number of terse recommendations relative to the role of Congress in regulating aspartame products. The most forceful opinions came from concerned parents, grandparents, teachers, and others involved with young persons (Chapter XI). An engineer-patient with aspartame disease, whose daughter also had severe reactions to aspartame, offered this cynical reply concerning regulation, "Congress would do the wrong thing for the wrong reason."

The following comments and suggestions by aspartame reactors are representative of <u>their</u> opinions.

"Restrict its use until further testing and research."
"State the amounts of aspartame in products."
"Require complete information on the label in large print."
"Make people more aware of the bad reactions that can be caused by aspartame."
"I do not feel it should be used in restaurants without mentioning its presence on menu items."
"Make people aware of the danger."
"Require full disclosure."
"They should limit its use, if not do away with it completely."

Aspartame reactors offered other recommendations, such as the following.

- A 72-year-old retired boilermaker asserted, "Change the bosses of FDA."
- A 39-year-old secretary with multiple reactions to aspartame wrote, "Rule that consumers have the right to know exactly what they are buying and putting in their bodies!"
- A 32-year-old registered nurse with numerous severe reactions to aspartame stated, "I think it should be fully investigated and not passed off as an 'allergic reaction,' which is what the FDA representative told me in our interview."
- A 31-year-old female administrator experienced three convulsions while taking aspartame. She wrote

> "It is the FDA's responsibility to ensure that products which are distributed in this country need certain guidelines of safety. I seriously doubt whether this product was fully tested. I think it was the big companies with all their money that pushed this product on the market before it could be fully tested. It needs to be taken off the market. If not now, it will be done when we the people bring a class action suit to protect ourselves since the government has failed to do so."

- A 33-year-old teacher suggested

> "Find out if it's safe because so many people have had problems, and remove it until long-term

effects are studied. I especially worry about children that may be affected – like mine."

- A housewife averred, "Aspartame should not be in products normally used by children."
- The comptroller of a major corporation opined, "I believe it (aspartame) needs further testing, and proven either safe or unsafe for human consumption."
- Several respondents pleaded, "Don't remove other artificial sweeteners." One even requested "Legalize cyclamate. It is sold in Canada."
- The mother of a 2 ½ year-old girl with focal seizures attributed to aspartame wrote, "Set safe limits for children. Set a standard to ensure a safe 'shelf life'."

SECTION 5

ASPARTAME: CHEMICAL STRUCTURE, METABOLISM, AND BIOPHYSIOLOGIC CONSIDERATIONS

"Try to penetrate to the secret of their occurrence (facts), persistently search for the laws which govern them."
Ivan Pavlov (1849-1936)

"The guarantee of science is the verification of experience, direct or indirect. It distrusts the validity of prior conclusions, or of any explanation drawn solely from general ideas of Nature's order, unless those general ideas have themselves been rigorously demonstrated to be necessities of thought, or to represent the observed order."
George Henry Lewes
"Aristotle" in *The History of Science*
(Smith, Elder & Company, London 1864)

654

Aspartame disease underscores the ongoing need for pharmacovigilance of drugs and "supplements."

The Chemical: General Considerations

Aspartame consists of three components – phenylalanine (an essential amino acid); aspartic acid (a nonessential amino acid); and a methyl ester that is metabolized to free methyl alcohol (methanol). Figure 5-1 depicts its chemical structure.

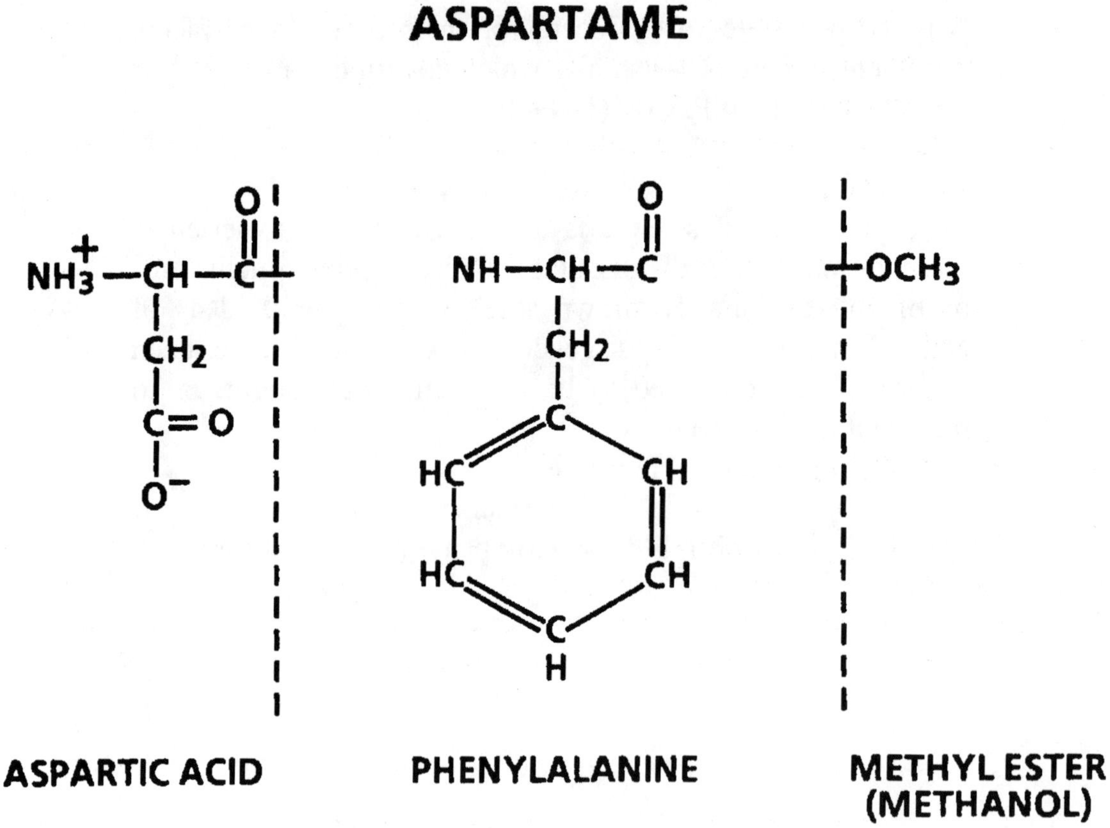

ASPARTAME

ASPARTIC ACID   PHENYLALANINE   METHYL ESTER
(METHANOL)

Figure 5-1
The chemical structure of aspartame

Consumers often infer that aspartame is a "natural" or "organic" substance. In reality, a major Japanese chemical company that pioneered this industry combined methyl alcohol and phenylalanine, which was sold to manufacturers. A former vice-president for nutrition and medical affairs of another company refused to give a definitive answer about the source of aspartic acid, but did admit that "phenylalanine might not come from soy beans and corn."

A major manufacturer provided food scientists with this information:

- There is a synergy when aspartame is used in combination with sucrose, dextrose, fructose and saccharin.
- Aspartame is adapted to use in carbonated beverages by controlling pH, time and concentration. For example, the pH ranges from 2.4 -3.1 for cola, and up to 4.8 for root beer.
- About 40 percent degradation of aspartame is required before sweetness perception is no longer acceptable.

The promoters of products containing aspartame repeatedly emphasize its two "building blocks of protein." Reference to the presence of methyl alcohol, however, is generally omitted.

The Soft Drink Industry

The National Soft Drink Association initially objected to incorporating aspartame in carbonated beverages. It referred to this chemical as "inherently unstable" in the May 7, 1985 *Congressional Record*. Moreover, it protested that the safety of aspartame had not been conclusively demonstrated because of "inadequate and unreliable" studies.

Sweetness

Multiple receptors in the tongue mediate "sweetness." The receptor site for aspartame is apparently not identical with that for sodium saccharin.

Each component of aspartame contributes to the perception of sweetness by screening out other taste bud sensations. The methyl ester is a "potent paralytic," while aspartic acid alters nerve cells in the tongue receptive to sugar. Phenylalanine serves to exaggerate the effect.

XX

ASPARTAME METABOLISM; THE EFFECTS OF HEAT AND STORAGE

"Medical science often cannot give adequate answers to questions of toxicological action, not only as regards new compositions but even in the case of substances long in use. Indeed, to the medical man unpleasant surprises are constantly being revealed, in the case of both drugs and of chemicals used in food preparations."*
Sir Edward Mellanby (1951)

When metabolized in the body, aspartame yields about 50 percent phenylalanine, 40 percent aspartic acid, and 10 percent methyl alcohol on a weight basis. Stegink and Filer (1984), along with other researchers, reviewed the physiology and biochemistry of aspartame. Information concerning its breakdown products and their pharmacologic effects (Chapter XXV), however, remains limited. For example, the absence of excessive peak plasma aspartame concentrations in normal adults given "abuse doses" (Stegink 1987) does not exclude the rise of its components in the portal vein and the brain.

There were errors concerning the decomposition products of aspartame in data originally submitted to the FDA. The *Congressional Record-Senate* (1985, p. S-5508) indicated that high pressure liquid chromotography is a superior analytical method for detecting and quantifying amino acids than the thin layer chromatography used, which may not even detect aspartic acid. Indeed, as much as 39 percent of aspartame's breakdown products could not be accounted for using these prior methods.

---

*© *British Medical Journal.* Reproduced with permission.

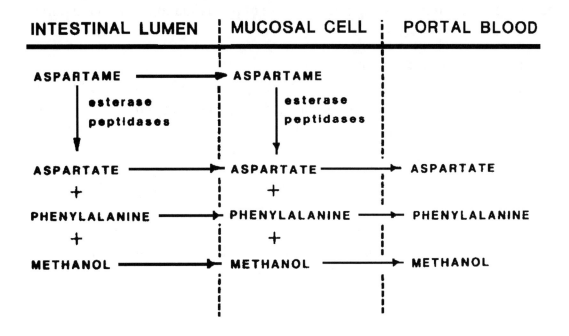

Figure XX-1
Intestinal metabolism of aspartame

Stegink, L.D., and Filer, L.J., Jr.
Aspartame: Physiology and Biochemistry. Marcel Dekker, Inc.
New York, 1984, p. 608
Reprinted by courtesy of Marcel Dekker, Inc.

The ester bond of aspartame is first broken. Aspartylphenylalanine or the individual amino acids are then absorbed and handled in a manner comparable to other dipeptides and amino acids derived from protein digestion. Tobey and Heizer (1986) reported the following:

- Three previously-reported brush border dipeptidese enzymes have very low affinity for ASP-PHE.
- A substantial portion of the dipeptide may be transported intact into the enterocytes, and hydrolyzed in the cytosol.
- All such hydrolytic activity is detected in a single additional band on starch gel, and a single peak on ion-exchange chromatography – inferring that a single enzyme within the cytosol hydrolyzes ASP-PHE.

The greater rise of plasma phenylalanine than plasma aspartate after aspartame loading may reflect more rapid metabolism of the aspartic acid than phenylalanine within the enterocyte, and the ensuing larger release of phenylalanine within the portal circulation (Surget 1984).

Possible Absorption From The Mouth

Some aspartame reactors <u>promptly</u> develop generalized symptoms and signs after taking small amounts, especially chewing gum (Chapter II-D). This suggests absorption through the mucosa of the mouth (as used therapeutically with nitroglycerin), and simple diffusion from the oropharynx directly into the brain. The latter phenomenon has been demonstrated with small molecules – as glucose, sodium chloride and ethyl alcohol (Maller 1967; editorial, *British Medical Journal* 1966; 1:184).

The flavor and sweetness of aspartame in chewing gum can last 30 minutes, compared to 5-6 minutes with sugar-sweetened gum. Accordingly, more is likely to be absorbed.

These considerations have added relevance in view of (a) the commercial availability of aspartame "flavor sprays" to induce satiety, (b) the widespread use of aspartame mints, wafers and mouth washes to control bad breath, and (c) the severe neurologic reactions induced by chewing aspartame gum, most dramatically as convulsions (Chapter III).

Distribution

Matsuzawa and O'Hara (1984) followed the distribution of aspartame labeled with a radioactive-carbon isotope in adult rats. They detected prompt and significant uptake in the pancreas, gastrointestinal tract, salivary glands and liver – with less in the eye and brain.

Metabolic Pathways

The metabolic pathways of aspartame, illustrated by Ranney et al (1976), appear in Figure XX-2.

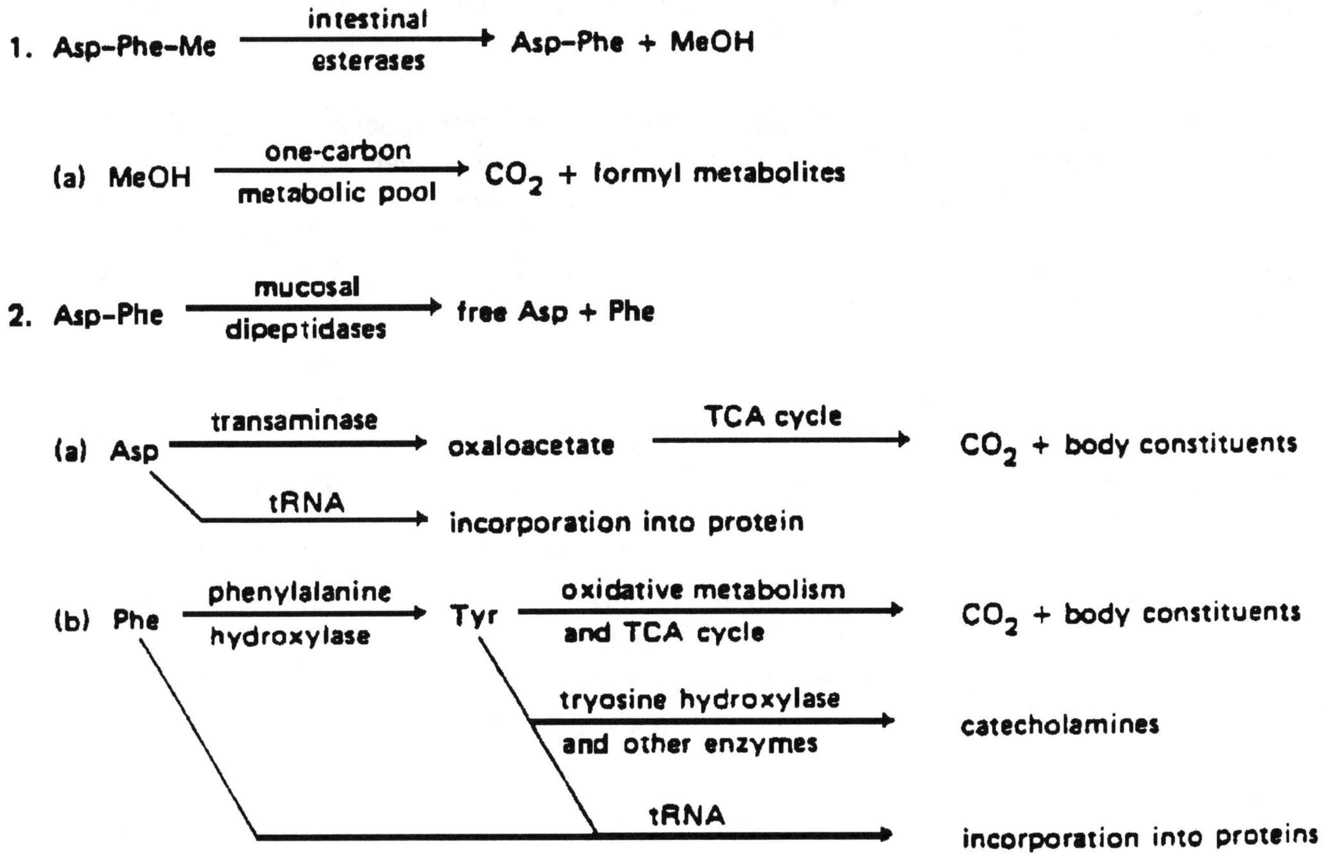

1. Asp-Phe-Me $\xrightarrow[\text{esterases}]{\text{intestinal}}$ Asp-Phe + MeOH

   (a) MeOH $\xrightarrow[\text{metabolic pool}]{\text{one-carbon}}$ CO_2 + formyl metabolites

2. Asp-Phe $\xrightarrow[\text{dipeptidases}]{\text{mucosal}}$ free Asp + Phe

   (a) Asp $\xrightarrow{\text{transaminase}}$ oxaloacetate $\xrightarrow{\text{TCA cycle}}$ CO_2 + body constituents

        $\xrightarrow{\text{tRNA}}$ incorporation into protein

   (b) Phe $\xrightarrow[\text{hydroxylase}]{\text{phenylalanine}}$ Tyr $\xrightarrow[\text{and TCA cycle}]{\text{oxidative metabolism}}$ CO_2 + body constituents

        $\xrightarrow[\text{and other enzymes}]{\text{tryosine hydroxylase}}$ catecholamines

        $\xrightarrow{\text{tRNA}}$ incorporation into proteins

Figure XX-2

The metabolic pathways of aspartame. Abbreviations: Phe = phenylalanine; ME = methyl ester; MeOH = methyl alcohol; Tyr = tyrosine; tRNA = transfer ribonucleic acid; TCA = tricarboxylic acid; CO_2 = carbon dioxide.

Ranney, R.E., et al.
Comparative metabolism of aspartame in experimental
  animals and humans.
Journal of Toxicology and Environmental Health 1976;
  Volume 2:441-451.
(Reproduced with permission from Hemisphere Publishing Corporation,
  Washington, D.C. and New York)

INFLUENCE OF THE PHYSICAL STATE OF ADMINISTRATION

Stegink et al (1987) reported marked differences in plasma phenylalanine and aspartate concentrations when normal subjects were given three grams aspartame in solution and in capsule. This suggested that the pharmacokinetics of phenylalanine and aspartate are influenced by these physical states.

- The peak plasma phenylalanine levels, and the area under the four-hour plasma phenylalanine concentration-time curve were significantly higher when administered as solution than capsules.
- Administration as a solution resulted in a significantly higher ratio of plasma phenylalanine concentration to the sum of the plasma concentrations of the other large neutral amino acids.
- Peak plasma aspartate concentrations were higher when aspartame was ingested in solution.

Joachim et al (1987) demonstrated the importance of aspartame particle size in effervescent forms.

The influence of particle size and homogenization has been raised in other realms. An example is cholesterol absorption and metabolism when whole eggs or milk are homogenized (Oster 1982). Homogenization of milk appears to increase availability, perhaps due to formation of new mycellae that enhance the absorption of free cholesterol and vitamin D_3. By contrast, the serum cholesterol is not significantly increased when normal persons ingest eggs in a nonhomogenized form.

THE INFLUENCE OF HEAT

Instability of aspartame in heat occurs when aspartame soft drinks are exposed to temperatures higher than those used in company-sponsored studies. The *Federal Register* (Volume 48, No. 132, July 8, 1983) indicated that the degradation of aspartame is 38 percent at 86° F, and over 50 percent at 104° F.

Aspartame is converted to its racemate breakdown products during heating (Novick 1985). (It also occurs at room temperature by interactions with other components of food and beverages.) Bada (1987) demonstrated that boiling causes an internal rearrangement of aspartame. Stated differently, the L-isomers of phenylalanine and aspartic acid are transformed to unnatural D-isomers (or mirror images).

Boehm and Bada (1984) investigated racemization of the aspartic acid and phenylalanine in aspartame at 100° C (Figure XX-3).

- A pH 6.8, the racemization half-lives for aspartic acid and phenylalanine were 13 and 23 hours, respectively. Racemization at this pH occurred in its diketopiperazine decomposition product rather than aspartame itself.
- At pH 4 (the typical acidity of most foods and beverages sweetened with aspartame), the half-lives were 47 hours for aspartic acid and 1,200 hours for phenylalanine – with racemization occurring in the aspartame molecule.

These peptide chemists made other pertinent observations.

- The heating of aspartame-sweetened foods and beverages at a neutral pH (7.0) generates D-aspartic acid and D-phenylalanine, coupled with an associated loss of sweetness.
- Some components of foods and beverages might act as catalysts at a more acid pH wherein racemization rates tend to be slow. (The heating of chocolate products containing aspartame may pose a special problem.)

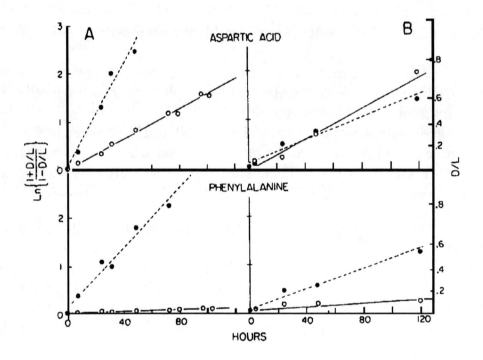

Figure XX-3

The racemization kinetics of aspartic acid and phenylalanine in solutions of pure aspartame (A) and an aspartame tabletop sweetener (B) heated at 100° C and pH 4 (●) and pH 6.8 (o). The $\underline{t}$ = 0 point represents the amount of racemization that occurs during the HCl hydrolysis step.

Boehm, M.F., and Bada J.L. Racemization of aspartic acid and phenylalanine in sweetened aspartame at 100° C. *Proceedings of the National Academy of Science USA* 1984; 81:5263-5266.

(Reproduced by courtesy of Dr. Jeffrey Bada)

THE INFLUENCE OF STORAGE

When aspartame is dissolved in liquid, it becomes unstable and begins to break down into its individual components. The rate of breakdown is largely dependent upon temperature and pH. Even refrigerated drinks are sold with an eight-week shelf life owing to their acidic pH.

According to the original stability data submitted to the FDA as part of the approval process for use of aspartame in carbonated beverages, 11-16% breaks down after eight weeks at 68°F, 38% breaks down at 86°F, and over 50% breaks down after nine weeks at 104°F.

Independent tests by Tsang (1985) demonstrate how quickly aspartame can break down in carbonated beverages stored at room temperature. The following are figures for one-liter (1.057 quart) bottles of diet cola sweetened with aspartame and stored at 71.6°F.

Substance	At Time of Bottling	6 Months after Bottling	36 Months after Bottling
Aspartame	550.0 mg	155.34 mg (28%)	19.70 mg (4%)
L-Phenylalanine methyl ester	0.0 mg	28.62 mg (9%)	13.01 mg (4%)
Diketopiperazine (DKP)	0.0 mg	135.66 mg (28%)	173.28 mg (35%)
L-Aspartylphenylalanine	0.0 mg	158.31 mg (30%)	189.05 mg (36%)
L-Phenylalanine	0.0 mg	42.22 mg (14%)	101.27 mg (33%)

Jennifer Cohen, a student at Oradell Public School (New Jersey), conducted a study titled, "The Effects of Different Storage Temperatures on the Taste and Chemical Composition of Diet Coke®." (The analysis of samples was performed by Winston Laboratories.) These results appeared on the Internet on April 13, 1997.

"The level of aspartame in a can of Diet Coke® was found to be 0.06% by a food testing laboratory. The remaining cans from one case of Diet Coke were stored under three different heat conditions for 10 weeks. Seven cans were stored in an incubator (104 degrees F); seven cans were stored at room temperature (68-70 degrees F). At the end of 70 days, samples were tested for levels of aspartame, formaldehyde and diketopiperazine (DKP). The refrigerated sample contained 0.051 percent aspartame, 0.002 percent DKP, and 231 parts per

664

billion of formaldehyde. The <u>room temperature sample</u> contained 0.051 percent aspartame, 0.002 percent DKP, and 231 parts per billion of formaldehyde. The <u>incubator sample</u> contained 0.026 percent aspartame, 0.010 percent DKP, and 76.2 parts per billion of formaldehyde.

In addition, 10 human subjects tested each soda sample plus a new can of Diet Coke, and rated each sample for taste on a 1-4 scale – 1 being the best, and 4 the worst. The new can of Diet Coke received an average rating of 2.0. The sample stored in the refrigerator received an average rating of 2.6. The sample stored at room temperature received an average rating of 2.5. The sample stored in the incubator received an average rating of 3.8."

CLINICAL SIGNIFICANCE

The effects of physical heat and storage on aspartame products must be taken into account when provocative clinical trials or double-blind testing are conducted. The limiting of such studies to intake of aspartame in dry form, or as non-heated foods or liquids prepared within one hour of solution, could be misleading.

- The father of a young patient with severe aspartame reactions ridiculed the absence of FDA recommendations about the handling, distribution, avoidance of heat, and storage of aspartame products as lacking reality. He wrote, "The Agency must know that diet colas are being transported in closed steel trucks where the inside temperature reaches more that 125° in the summer sun. At this temperature, charts indicating spoilage rates must be off the wall."
- Kreusi et al (1986) studied aggression and activity in 30 preschool boys following the ingestion of sugar or aspartame. Behavior patterns were observed both in a playroom setting and at home. The children received sucrose, glucose, aspartame and saccharin on separate challenge days, separated by five-to-seven-day washout periods. These investigators concluded neither sugar nor aspartame significantly disrupt behavior. In this study, however, the sweeteners were added as syrups kept in the refrigerator and crushed ice, and the drinks were served <u>cold</u> (personal communication, February 9, 1987).

The FDA recommended that aspartame ought to be delivered in a milk-based formula when tested (*Food Chemical News* 1999 [March 15]; Volume 41: p. 34). Aspartame taken with milk and dairy products does not break down as readily within the stomach, and therefore has longer pharmacologic activity. This was inferred from the development of epileptic seizures in Rhesus monkeys fed aspartame in milk-based formula.

"Bad Chemical Taste"

Numerous individuals stated that they intuitively avoided aspartame products because of their "bad chemical taste." Others who experienced this sensation persisted consuming them on the premises, "Oh, you'll get used to it," or "It tastes better if you drink it real cold."

Industry has attempted to counteract the "palate fatigue" of diet sodas by increasing their aspartame content, or by adding another ingredient (such as a acesulfame potassium) to enhance the "sweetness profile."

A correspondent observed that the "bizarre" taste of diet cola, which had been stored for several seasons and subjected to considerable heat, disappeared after re-chilling. Accordingly, consumers may be ingesting decomposed aspartame sodas when again chilled!

THE "NORMAL-PROTEIN-BUILDING-BLOCKS" FALLACY

Dr. Frank Young, a former FDA Commissioner, told the Senate hearing on November 3, 1987 that the amino acids of aspartame are metabolized similar to "natural" amino acids of protein. Inasmuch as this premise is crucial to aspartame disease, it requires scrutiny.

Differences Between The Digestion Of Protein And Aspartame

Proteins are complex molecules made up of numerous bonded amino acids. The chemical and physical reactions within the stomach and small intestine that break such bonding through the action of multiple enzymes are equally complex. The released amino acids are then absorbed into the portal vein, and subsequently transported to the liver and brain.

The progression of protein digestion within the gastrointestinal tract is relatively prolonged. This precludes a sudden and unbalanced increase of circulating individual amino acids.

By contrast, the absorption and metabolism of aspartame are rapid, requiring only two enzymatic actions. The first involves the methyl ester bond with phenylalanine. The ensuing rapid rises of phenylalanine and methyl alcohol in the blood and brain, and their consequences, are described in Chapters XXI and XXII.

Promotional Considerations

Ads for aspartame products have asserted that at least half the food eaten contains what is in aspartame (*Newsweek* June 30, 1987) – presumably phenylalanine and aspartic acid, two of "the building blocks of protein."

Such promotional material also infers that (a) these amino acids are "natural," and (b) the body treats them in the same way as amino acids derived "from a peach or a string bean or a glass of milk." The synthetic combination of these amino acids, however, may not be innocuous. (An analogy might be made to isolating two words from a sentence, and expecting them to function properly alone or out of context.)

The increases of L-phenylalanine, L-aspartic acid, and their D-isomers after aspartame ingestion (Chapter XXII) are biologically unique. This argues against assertions that "an amino acid is an amino acid," and "the body doesn't know aspartame from beans" (ad in *Annals of Internal Medicine* August 17, 1987, p. I-45).

A further paradox was encountered in the promotion of researches pertaining to memory loss and related areas by the pharmaceutical company then holding the trademark for aspartame. Full-page ads in major medical periodicals stated: "Excessive activity of these excitatory amino acids may produce nerve cell destruction resembling that which occurs in Alzheimer's, Huntington's chorea, and other degenerative diseases." Indeed, the firm's ongoing researches focused on antagonists capable of blocking related amino acid receptor systems that might prevent "neuronal dysfunction and disruptions."

Other Amino Acid Considerations

Young and Marchini (1990) reviewed the ability of altered intakes of amino acids, especially phenylalanine, to modulate rates of the major systems (protein synthesis; protein degradation; amino acid oxidation) responsible for maintenance of protein and amino acid homeostasis in organs and the whole body.

Concern over the widespread use and potential adverse effects of L-tryptophan (another amino acid) spawned ISTRY, an organization that monitored reactions to it. Such concern is comparable to that for phenylalanine – namely, the large consumption of an amino acid in the absence of other neutral amino acids present in protein that tend to suppress its rapid ingress into the brain.

The combining of amino acids with drugs by the pharmaceutical industry also requires careful regulatory monitoring. A case in point is <u>L-arginine</u>. Inasmuch as it is the precursor to nitric oxide (the so-called "endothelium derived relaxing factor"), this amino acid has been tried in conjunction with thiazide diuretics for managing hypertension. The stimulation of insulin by arginine, and the documented association of hypertension with hyperinsulinemia, however, ought to invite caution.

These additional observations relate to aspartame's amino acids and their stereoisomers.

- Bowie et al (1990) emphasized the considerable tolerance of proteins to amino acid substitutions, including aspartic acid and phenylalanine.
- Noren et al (1989) reported the site-specific incorporation of unnatural amino acids in proteins, with particular reference to several mutants of phenylalanine.
- Mapelli et al (1988) analyzed four stereoisomeric analogs of aspartame. They found them tasteless as either solids or aqueous solutions. (Their lack of taste is probably explained by positioning of the phenyl group.) These observations also pertain to the cited loss of taste of aspartame products with prolonged storage.

XXI

METHYL ALCOHOL (METHANOL) TOXICITY

"It is all very well to say 'Drink me,' but the wise little Alice
was not going to do that in a hurry. 'No, I'll look first,' she
said, 'and see whether it's marked *poison* or not.'... She had
never forgotten that if you drink very much from a bottle
marked 'poison' it is almost certain to disagree with you,
sooner or later."

Lewis Carroll
(Alice in Wonderland)

The toxic effects of methyl alcohol (methanol) are paramount in aspartame disease, especially severe visual impairment (Chapter IV). They have been recognized since wood was dry distilled in French provinces during the 19th century to obtain "wood alcohol." Methanol imparts the sweet taste to aspartame. (The ancient Aztecs used another toxic substance as a flavor enhancer: arsenic.)

This metabolic poison is rarely found in nature as the "free" form. Six years before FDA approval of aspartame, Dr. Herbert S. Posner (1975), National Institute of Environmental Health Sciences, wrote a review titled, "Biohazards of Methanol in Proposed New Uses." He stressed the failure to recognize "delayed and irreversible effects on the nervous system" of methanol... at widely varying levels of exposure and at rather low levels." Furthermore, he suggested that "when a safer compound is available, methanol should not be utilized."

In their pharmacology text, Goodman and Gilman (1980) assert that methanol is "purely of toxicological interest." Analyzing 323 cases of methyl alcohol poisoning, Bennett et al (1952) found that as little as three teaspoons of 40 percent methanol could be fatal.

The public is more familiar with methanol as an ingredient of fuels (such as Sterno®), antifreeze, solvents (see below), and fluids used in duplicating machines.

- The husband of a patient expressed alarm on learning that methanol is an ingredient of aspartame because he had worked in a chemical plant manufacturing it. Three pipefitters who savored methyl alcohol, notwithstanding warnings against doing so, died.
- The toxicity of methanol made headlines when 25 persons in Italy died after consuming table wine tainted with "only" 5.7 percent methanol (*The Philadelphia Inquirer* March 25, 1986, p. C-26).
- Methyl alcohol is one of many solvents to which persons are exposed at work and in the home. They can remain in some tissues for prolonged periods. A number of studies implicated solvents as causative or contributory to major diseases – including rheumatoid arthritis, lupus erythematosus, scleroderma, birth defects, and cancer of the breast and other tissues.
- Hundreds of persons in Kenya recently died or became blind after drinking a cheap home brew that had been laced with methanol to enhance its potency (*The Lancet* 2000; 356:1911).

Quantitation in Aspartame

The digestion of aspartame yields approximately ten percent methanol by weight. The FDA calculated its presence in the aspartame molecule as 32/394, or 10.9 percent (*Federal Register* February 22, 1984, pp. 6672-6682).

These approximations are listed for reference.

- 19 mg aspartame (the equivalent of one teaspoon sugar) yields 1.9 mg methanol.
- One liter of an aspartame soft drink averages 555 mg aspartame, which yields about 55 mg methanol.
- Methanol concentrations rise with both the heating and prolonged storage of aspartame (Chapter XX).
- Case III-1 consumed two liters of an aspartame soft drink (110 mg methanol) prior to the onset of her first convulsion.

METABOLIC CONSIDERATIONS

Methyl alcohol, probably the first component of aspartame released within the small intestine, is rapidly absorbed. The enzyme chymotrypsin releases free (that is unbound to protein) methanol from aspartame. The correlation between aspartame intake and blood methanol concentrations appears in Figure XXI-1

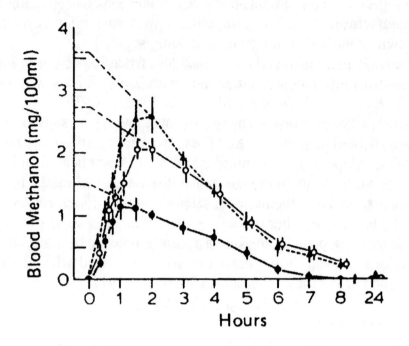

Figure XXI-1

The mean blood methanol concentrations in normal adults administered aspartame at 100 (●...●), 150 (○–○), or 200 mg/kg body weight (△---△). Standard deviations are included.

Reproduced from Stegink, L.D. and Filer, L.J., Jr.
Aspartame: Physiology and Biochemistry Marcel Dekker, Inc.,
 New York, 1984, p. 543.
Reprinted by courtesy of Marcel Dekker, Inc.

Blood Levels

Techniques for measuring plasma methanol that are sensitive to 0.012 mg/liter have been devised (Davoli 1986b). (Earlier statements about levels of methanol not being detectable in the blood after aspartame ingestion were erroneous. They derived from an outmoded test for measuring plasma methanol that was limited to 4 mg/liter.) Davoli et al (1986a) reported that ingesting 8.7 mg/kg of aspartame instead of 6 mg/kg significantly increases plasma methanol concentrations, nearly doubling in some instances.

"Abuse doses" of aspartame (100 mg/kg or more) ingested by normal subjects markedly elevate blood methanol concentrations, which remain detectable <u>eight or more hours later</u> (Steginik 1984).

Elevated "blood alcohol" levels have been detected in persons consuming diet sodas who appeared drunk. Methyl alcohol also can be detected by breath alcohol analyzers.

- A famous long-distance swimmer was found in her car, 55 yards from home, wearing pajamas. Her blood alcohol reading was 0.12. She had been drinking only diet colas.
- Washington State addictionologist personally informed the author about a female patient who consumed from 6-12 cans of diet sodas daily, and became comatose. Her blood alcohol level was 0.5. She adamantly denied drinking any alcoholic beverages.

METHANOL TOXICITY

Humans are more vulnerable to the toxic effects of methanol than laboratory animals. Two or more enzymes required to metabolize it have been lost in evolution (Roe 1982). Whether the rhesus monkey serves as an acceptable experimental model for methyl alcohol poisoning in man (Cooper 1961) remains debatable.

The effects of formaldehyde and formic acid, breakdown products of methanol, are amplified below.

Rate of Oxidation

The toxicity of methanol is enhanced by its <u>slow rate of oxidation</u>, only one-seventh that of ethyl alcohol (ethanol).

Robert Forney and Francis Hughes (1968), Professors of Pharmacology at Indiana University School of Medicine, noted that <u>the elimination of methanol by man takes five times longer than an equivalent amount of ethyl alcohol</u>. Furthermore, the daily ingestion of "individually innocuous amounts of methyl alcohol" could result in "eventual poisonous effects."

The oxidation of methanol occurs chiefly within the liver and kidneys. Even though its half life in human volunteers ingesting small amounts (1-5 ml) is about three hours, complete oxidation to carbon dioxide usually requires several days.

672

Metabolic Demands

Many of the reactions to aspartame could be interpreted as resulting from either decreased substrate for energy or greater metabolic demands within vital tissues. Increased energy demand has been documented in chronic alcoholics (Chapter XII), presumably from microsomal induction (Jhangian 1986). It is also likely to exist in persons who constantly ingest methyl alcohol in aspartame products.

Methanol in small amounts may exaggerate hypoglycemia by delaying the release of epinephrine as a protective counterregulatory mechanism, as has been shown with non-intoxicating doses of ethanol (Sood 2001).

A severe metabolic acidosis might be induced clinically after the ingestion of a large amount of aspartame, especially by children. A London physician wrote about his nine-year-old daughter who had been given an aspartame cola.

> "In all, she probably drank about 1.5 litres over a 24-hour period together with eating a few slices of toast in the same 24 hours. The following morning she was found semi-conscious and confused. She had a metabolic ketoacidosis, but a normal blood sugar on admission to hospital. Tests for metabolic poisons such as aspirin were negative. Fortunately, re-hydration restored her to normal biochemically within 4-5 hours together with restoration to normal levels of con-sciousness. I thought at the time that the diet cola could be responsible, but could not find any evidence to support this. The company in the UK was very defensive about the effects of aspartame, and denied any knowledge of the adverse effects of aspartame."

Toxic Concentrations

Certain FDA requirements are intended to provide an adequate margin of safety for heavy consumers of products, and for persons who may be uniquely sensitive to compounds in foods that can cause adverse effects. Section 170.22 of Title 21 of the Code of Federal Regulations decreed that this margin of safety should be 100 times below the "highest no-effect" level.

It has been averred that 200 12-ounce cans of an aspartame soft drink would be required to yield a fatal amount of methanol – about six grams (6,000 mg). The fatal dose

---

of methyl alcohol, however, varies considerably. In terms of the foregoing FDA guidelines, Monte (1984) calculated that one-hundredth the fatal level translates into **two cans**! The one-hundredth projection of the dose preceding the convulsion in Case III-1 would have been 11 grams (11,000 mg).

Exposure in Infancy

The hazards of methanol exposure to an infant from the breast milk of a mother drinking diet sodas or other products containing aspartame can be inferred from several studies. The level of alcohol dehydrogenase activity during the first year of life is less than 50 percent the adult level (Pikkarainen 1967). Another observation is the impaired neurologic development in children who had been exposed to alcohol through breast milk (Little 1989).

FORMALDEHYDE AND FORMATE

The body attempts to detoxify methyl alcohol by oxidizing it to formaldehyde, and then to formic acid or formate. The pathways in mammals (particularly man and monkey) involve an alcohol dehydrogenase system, formaldehyde dehydrogenase, and catalase peroxidation. Formic acid appears to be largely responsible for the clinical effects of methanol poisoning (Brent 2001).

The oxidation of methanol to formate occurs within minutes. Filer and Stegink (1989) reported significantly increased urinary formate excretion for eight hours after the ingestion of 200 mg aspartame/kg body weight – indicating conversion of methanol to formate. The measurement of formate in urine, however, is not an appropriate test for low-level formaldehyde poisoning.

Folacin catalyzes the elimination of formic acid (Reitbrock 1971). The rate of formate oxidation is markedly diminished by folate deficiency (Tephly 1984). Aspartame-associated depletion of folic acid therefore could have important clinical and pathologic implications, including anemia and neoplastic transformation in blood-forming tissues (Chapter IX-J). Additionally, the decline in neural-tube defects attributed to fortifying grain products with folic acid might be negated among pregnant women who consume aspartame products that deplete tissue folate levels.

USDA #13, published in 1908, reported that formaldehyde is poisonous even in small amounts, and should be prohibited for use in food.

Allergists also recognize that sensitivity to formaldehyde can be clinically significant.

The mutagenic and carcinogenic properties of formaldehyde are considered in Section 6. An early evidence for the mutagenicity of formaldehyde in humans exposed to it occupationally is the demonstration of DNA-protein crosslinks and sister chromatid exchanges in their circulating lymphocytes (Shaham 1997). These related considerations are noteworthy.

- The emission of formaldehyde from vehicles using methanol as an auto fuel has raised concerns about its potential carcinogenic effects (*The Wall Street Journal* September 4, 1987, p. 38).
- Some vaccines for children contain formaldehyde. (Triple antigen DPT also contains mercury and aluminum phosphate.)

Mechanisms of Toxicity

Alcohol dehydrogenase and formaldehyde dehydrogenase are the enzymes chiefly involved in methanol metabolism. The retina, cornea and liver have the greatest alcohol dehydrogenase activity.

The highly reactive formaldehyde molecule becomes bound to proteins and nucleic acids, forming adducts. (These are little groupings of formaldehyde molecules that grow as more molecules become placed on top of existing ones.) They are difficult to eliminate through the usual metabolic pathways.

Trocho et al (1998) convincingly demonstrated that *formaldehyde derived from dietary aspartame binds to tissue components in vivo*. These findings were observed in adult male rats given oral aspartame ^{14}C-labeled in the methanol carbon. Most of the radioactivity was bound to protein in plasma and liver, but it also could be detected in fat, muscle, brain and eye (both cornea and retina). The half life was long.

Progressive accumulation of even more label occurred when non-labeled aspartame was administered over ten days... suggesting that the amount of formaldehyde adducts coming from aspartame in tissue proteins and nucleic acids is cumulative. The presence of large amounts of label in DNA proved impressive. These investigators commented: "The cumulative effects derived from the incorporation of label in the chronic administration model suggests that regular intake of aspartame may result in the progressive accumulation of formaldehyde adducts. It may be further speculated that the formation of adducts can help to explain the chronic effects aspartame consumption may induce on sensitive tissues such as brain."

Formaldehyde may also contribute to toxicity and nervous system/immune dysfunction through its <u>conjugation with human serum albumin (F-HSA) to form a new antigenic determinant</u>. Patients with multiple health complaints who had been exposed chronically to formaldehyde develop anti-F-HSA antibodies and elevated Tal cells (antigen memory cells), consistent with sustained antigenic stimulation of the immune system (Thrasher 1988).

Another insight derives from the behavioral (limbic system) <u>cross-sensitization</u> to cocaine after repeated low-level exposure to formaldehyde. Sorg et al (1998) asserted that this phenomenon is relevant to multiple chemical sensitivity in humans who manifest fatigue, irritability, problems with memory and concentration, depression, headache, muscle/joint pain, and gastrointestinal problems.

"Pre-Embalming"

Inferences by funeral directors about the "pre-embalming" of persons who had been heavy aspartame consumers initially evoked considerable skepticism.

But this theme kept surfacing. One experienced undertaker literally warned his family against using diet sodas after repeatedly detecting the deposition of formaldehyde crystals deposited in the organs of such individuals. Some funeral directors even insisted on closing the caskets of persons who had consumed large amounts of aspartame because formaldehyde seeped through the skin.

This issue has religious ramifications. Jewish law forbids embalming because it considers prompt burial a sign of respect for the deceased.

THE METHYL ALCOHOL SYNDROME

Dr. Woodrow Monte (1984), Director of the Food Science and Nutrition Laboratory at Arizona State University, described methanol toxicity in man as the methyl alcohol syndrome. It may **not** have a direct correlation with blood methanol concentrations.

<u>Eye damage (retinopathy</u> (Chapter IV)

Methanol causes blindness, largely due to the toxic effects of formaldehyde and formic acid on the retina. Indeed, suspicion of "wood alcohol poisoning" was raised by ophthalmologists in several patients with aspartame disease.

Formate, a metabolite of formaldehyde, probably induces retinal damage through energy depletion because it inhibits adenosine triphosphate (ATP).

Edema of the optic disc (Hayreh 1977) and retinal ganglion cell degeneration (Baumbach 1977) occur in monkeys poisoned with methanol.

Involvement of the peripheral nerves (neuropathy) (Chapter VI).

The symptoms include numbness, "pins and needles" sensations (paresthesias), and shooting pains. They are most likely to occur after chronic exposure. Marked improvement of carpal tunnel syndrome has occurred among patients with aspartame disease after they avoided aspartame products (Chapter VI-E).

Inflammation of the pancreas (pancreatitis)

Pancreatitis was the probable basis for severe abdominal pain in some aspartame reactors (Bennett 1952) (Chapter IX-D).

Inflammation of the heart muscle (cardiomyopathy).

A number of patients with aspartame disease complained of palpitations, rapid heart action, and atypical chest pain (Chapter IX-C). Persons who smoke heavily and ingest much aspartame are probably at greater cardiovascular risk. (Cigarette smoke also may contain methyl alcohol.)

Monte (1984) alluded to the case of a 21-year-old man who worked as a material handler in the aspartame area of a plant that packaged this product. He was exposed to a fine dust of aspartame daily for seven months. The patient developed a dilated heart, and ventricular ectopy requiring quinidine. Other complaints included visual disturbances, headache, dizziness and severe depression. At autopsy, an enlarged and dilated heart due to cardiomyopathy was found.

The author has received reports of other persons working in a similar environment whose illnesses were attributed to inhaled aspartame (Chapter XXVII-G).

Central Nervous System Involvement

The cerebral effects of methanol contribute to the magnitude of neurologic and psychiatric manifestations in aspartame disease (Chapters III, V, VI and VII).

Imaging studies of the brain in patients with methyl alcohol toxicity have revealed areas of <u>presumed infarction</u> (McLean 1980; Shwartz 1981). Methanol intoxication causes symmetrical necrosis and hemorrhage of the putamen.

Marked <u>reductions of both cerebral blood flow and cerebral oxygen consumption</u> have been documented during methanol poisoning.

Observations concerning <u>brain edema and vascular stasis</u> after methanol exposure are also relevant to the neuropsychiatric reactions in aspartame disease.

- Edema of the brain in methanol poisoning has been found in humans and animals (Menne 1938; Bennet 1953; Erlanson 1965; Rao 1977).
- Rao et al (1977) noted significant alterations in brain water, sodium and potassium when methanol was administered to male rabbits and monkeys. Concomitant vascular stasis was evidenced by colloidal carbon studies. These changes occurred in both acute and chronic studies. (With chronic administration, the concentration of blood methanol progressively increased after the third week, suggesting partial inhibition of methanol degradation.)

Methanol-induced <u>parkinsonism</u> has been attributed to postsynaptic dysfunction, perhaps by interference with dopamine reuptake at nerve terminals. McLean et al (1980) reported two survivors of acute severe methanol intoxication who developed parkinsonism, dementia, other neurologic abnormalities (including bilateral Babinski responses), and blindness due to optic atrophy.

The National Institute for Occupational Safety and Health (NIOSH) includes methyl alcohol in *Organic Solvent Neurotoxicity* (*Current Intelligence Bulletin* Volume 48, March 31, 1987). The neuropsychiatric features of chronic toxicity from organic solvents range from a mild "organic affective syndrome" (characterized by fatigue, impaired memory, irritability, mild mood disturbances and difficulty in concentrating) to severe toxic encephalopathy with profound and generally irreversible dementia.

A Dissenting Corporate Viewpoint

Some of the foregoing assertions were criticized by Frank M. Sturtevant, Ph.D. (1985), a member of the Research and Development Division of G. D. Searle & Co. He regarded reference to methanol as a "cumulative poison" as misleading. Furthermore, he stated that the <u>instantaneous</u> consumption of 50 cans of an aspartame diet beverage would not result in a detectable increase of blood formate. (The carcinogenic and teratogenic potential of formaldehyde resulting from the degradation of aspartame to methyl alcohol also was challenged).

Fomepizole Treatment

Fomepizole (4-methylpyrazole) given intravenously appears to be a safe and effective treatment for methanol poisoning (Brent 2001). This inhibitor of alcohol dehydrogenase should be considered in patients presenting with severe metabolic acidosis, cardiovascular instability, or acute blindness following the ingestion of considerable asparatame. The decline of formic acid concentrations, the resolution of metabolic abnormalities, and improvement of vision have been dramatic in methanol poisoning caused by other agents (windshield-wiper fluid; antifreeze), especially as suicidal attempts.

Representative Case Reports

Case XXI-1

A 53-year-old man developed blindness in both eyes – first on the left, and then on the right. He neither drank alcohol nor used tobacco. There was numbness and tingling in all limbs, confusion, memory loss, headache and irritability. Having recently been diagnosed as a diabetic, he eliminated sugar and began using large amounts of aspartame products. When he presented with bilateral visual loss, a physician stated that he had "the symptoms of a person who consumes wood alcohol."

Case XXI-2 (FDA Project #5307; Courtesy, Dr. Linda Tollefson)

A 31-year-old woman wished to lose "a few pounds" after childbirth. She was 5 foot 8 inches, and weighed 125 pounds. She consumed diet colas and soft drinks, and an aspartame tabletop sweetener. Symptoms attributable to aspartame disease occurred shortly thereafter. They included memory loss, severe dizziness, blurred vision, headache, numbness, shooting pains, a rash involving the arms and eyes, nausea, slurred speech, anxiety attacks, depression, palpitations, frequent urination, and two blackout attacks. These features subsided following the avoidance of aspartame products. A major university clinic had previously diagnosed her as being "allergic to formaldehyde." She then inquired as to whether her severe reaction to aspartame could be related to such an allergy.

THE ISSUE OF METHANOL IN "NATURAL" AND SUSPECTED SOURCES

There are limited data from the FDA about the "free" methanol content of fruits, fruit juices, alcoholic beverages and other products, based on current sensitive assays. The author repeatedly requested this information because the FDA and the Council on Scientific Affairs of the American Medical Association (1985) continued to maintain that "fruits and vegetables are also sources of dietary methanol," and "dietary methanol also arises from fresh fruits and vegetables" (*Federal Register* Volume 48, No. 132, July 8, 1983, p. 31380). Similarly, the *FDA Talk Paper* (January 24, 1984) asserted, "FDA said that no safety issues appeared to be involved, there being more methanol in many fruit juices than in long-stored aspartame products, including carbonated beverages."

Dr. David G. Hattan (Chief of the Regulatory Affairs Staff, Office of Nutrition and Food Sciences, Center for Food Safety and Applied Nutrition, FDA) told the author that he was not aware of recent data concerning the methanol content of fruit juices, wines and other beverages (personal communication, June 8, 1987). His principle references were assays that had been performed many years earlier. The one used to indicate that "average fruit juice" contains more methanol than aspartame was published three decades before (Francot 1956).

I have studied translations of the three major reference articles on this subject originally published in German (Sommer 1962), Russian (Ivanitskiy 1973), and French (Le Moan 1956). The emphasis upon methanol in pectin-containing fruit and fruit products, some vegetables, wines and other alcoholic beverages appears to have little relevance to aspartame products. Indeed, Ivanitskiy (1973) concluded: "From the standpoint of health, it is not correct to apply the standards of the methanol content of alcoholic beverages arbitrarily to fruit juices, as has been done by several authors."

A related issue concerns repeated reference by the aspartame industry to the methanol content of tomatoes. While they may contain five times or more methanol than oranges, tomatoes and various fruits contain protective factors (see below) that are not provided by aspartame.

Monte (1984) suggested that the daily intake of methyl alcohol from natural sources averages less than 10 mg. He compared the available methyl alcohol in nonalcoholic and alcoholic beverages in Table XXI-1.

	METHANOL mg/liter	CALORIC DENSITY Calories/Liter	METHANOL (mg.) Consumed per 1,000 Calories	RATIO Ethanol (wt.) Methanol (wt.)	*Methanol (mg.) Consumption per day	
Juices						
*Orange, fresh	1	470	2	475	1	
*Orange, fresh	33	470	70	20	6 mg	
*Orange, fresh	34	470	72	16	6 mg	
*Orange, canned	31	470	66	15	6 mg	
*Grapefruit, fresh	1	400	1	2000	1 mg	
*Grapefruit	43	400	108	5	7 mg	
*Grapefruit, Canned	27	400	68	9	5 mg	
Grape	12	660	18	—	—	
Alcoholic Beverages						
Beer (4.5%)	0	400	—	—	—	
Grain Alcohol	1	2950	1	500000	—	
Bourbon, 100 proof	55	2950	19	9090	—	
Rum, 80 proof	73	2300	32	5000	—	
Wines (French)						
White	32	800	44	2500	—	
Rose	78	800	98	1000	—	
Red	128	800	160	667	—	
Pear	188	1370	137	250	—	
Cherry	276	1370	201	294	—	
Wines (American)						
Low	50	800	62	2500	—	
High	325	800	406	385	—	
Aspartame Sweetened Beverages					2 liters	5 liters
Uncarbonated Drinks	55	8	6875	0	110 mg	275 mg
Cola (Carbonated)	56	8	7000	0	112 mg	280 mg
Orange (Carbonated)	91	8	11375	0	182 mg	455 mg
Aspartame, pure			25000			

*17.6% of U.S. Population consume an average of 185.5 gm. of Orange Juice a day
*1.1% of the U.S. Population consume an average of 173.9 gm. of Grapefruit Juice a day

Table XXI-1
Available methanol in various beverages.

Monte, W.C.
Aspartame: Methanol and the public health.
Journal of Applied Nutrition 1984; 36:43-54.
Reproduced with permission of *Journal of Applied Nutrition*
and Dr. Woodrow Monte.

Monte also stressed that none of the foods to which aspartame was added could be considered as significant dietary sources of methyl alcohol prior to their sweetening with this chemical.

These points are relevant to aspartame disease.

- The methanol consumed in aspartame beverages could readily exceed 250 mg daily, especially in hot weather or after exercise. This is 32 times the consumption limit for methanol recommended by the Environmental Protection Agency (EPA).
- Methanol concentrations are likely to be higher when aspartame products have decomposed during exposure to heat or prolonged storage (Chapter XX).

The small amount of methanol in fruit juices is countered by the accompanying ethanol which tends to minimize or reduce its toxicity (see below) (Gilger 1959)... contrasting with absent ethanol in diet drinks. Ethanol is also present in some vegetables and fruits.

Using gas chromatographic methods, Lund et al (1981) and Nisperos-Carriedo and Shaw (1987) clarified the methanol, ethanol and acetylaldehyde concentrations of citrus products.

- Orange juice and grapefruit juice average as much as ten times more ethanol than methanol, and from two to ten times more acetylaldehyde.
- The concentration of methanol is higher in fresh-squeezed orange juice compared to the small amounts in pasteurized orange juice (22 mg/liter), frozen concentrate (3.4 mg/liter), reconstituted juice from concentrate (trace/one glass), and orange juice in tin cans (trace). The former probably reflects persistence of the pectinmethylesterase enzyme in unpasteurized juice. (It demethylates some pectin, and liberates methanol in the process.)

Unsuspected sources of methanol exposure could summate upon its effects from aspartame. Examples are flavors and food colors in which the methanol used as an extraction solvent was not completely removed, and styrofoam containers.

682

OFFICIAL POSITION OF THE FDA

A statement by the FDA concerning the methyl alcohol component of aspartame is found in the following excerpt of a letter (dated September 8, 1986) written by Hugh C. Cannon, Associate Commissioner for Legislative Affairs of the FDA.

"The Agency does not believe that methanol exposure equivalent to 10 percent of the aspartame dose is of sufficient quantity to be of toxicological concern under acute or chronic use conditions. A study submitted by Searle in support of its petition for the dry use of aspartame showed no detectable levels of methanol in the blood of human subjects following the ingestion of aspartame at 34 milligrams per kilogram (mg/kg) body weight. Assuming complete hydrolysis after ingestion, this 34 mg/kg dose of aspartame is equivalent to a dose of 3.4 mg/kg body weight of methanol. Even following administration of an abuse dose of aspartame of 200 mg/kg body weight (equivalent to 20 mg/kg body weight of methanol or drinking more than 13 quarts of aspartame-sweetened orange soda) in a clinical study conducted by Searle, the mean peak blood methanol concentration reached only 26 mg per liter.

"The Agency has recently become aware, however, of clinical data that indicate that the toxic effects of methanol are due to formate accumulation and not to formaldehyde or methanol itself. Formate is the oxidation product of formaldehyde which is itself formed from the metabolism of methanol. In the Searle clinical study using abuse doses of aspartame, equivalent to 20 mg/kg body weight of methanol, no significant increases were observed in plasma concentration of formate, suggesting that the rate of formate production does not exceed its rate of urinary excretion. In fact, studies in human subjects given oral dosages of methanol of 71 to 84 mg/kg body weight showed no toxic effects with blood levels of methanol reaching 47 to 76 mg per liter 2 to 3 hours afterwards. More recently, four adult males were give 550 mg of aspartame in a single dose (equivalent to aspartame in 2½ diet sodas); the resulting methanol level was found to be within the range of basal levels found initially within these individuals (Fd. Chem. Toxic. 24; 187-9, 1986).

"From estimates based on blood levels in methanol poisonings, it appears that the ingestion of methanol on the order of 200 to 500 mg/kg body weight is required to produce a significant accumulation of formate in the blood which may produce visual and central nervous system toxicity.

"The toxic doses of methanol (200 to 500 mg/kg body weight) are approximately one hundred times that ingested when aspartame is consumed at 34 mg/kg body weight. Moreover, orange soda, which may contain the highest concentration of aspartame in carbonated beverages (335 mg aspartame per 12 fluid ounces or 930 mg per liter), results in a lower methanol level (93 mg per liter) than that found in certain fruit juices (140 mg per liter). Under the most conservative assumption, the complete hydrolysis of aspartame to methanol, consumption of aspartame would not result in toxicologically significant methanol and formate levels.

"Finally, it is well known that many foods contain significant quantities of methanol. In fruit juices, content of methanol is as much as 140 mg per liter and grain alcohols (such as gin and whiskey) contain as much as 1000 mg per liter. Moreover, fresh fruits and vegetables also contain compounds that are metabolized in the body to methanol. Normal metabolic processes such as purine and pyrimidine biosynthesis and amino acid metabolism require methyl groups from compounds like methanol. It also appears that either methanol or formaldehyde may serve as precursors for the methyl groups in choline synthesis.

"Thus, the intake of methanol derived from aspartame consumption is far below the level which would provide toxicological concern from humans. In addition, methanol is widely distributed in commonly ingested foods and is required as a component of normal metabolic processes."

The basis for multiple criticisms by the author was reviewed above.

ETHYL ALCOHOL INTERACTIONS

Clinically significant interactions between methanol and ethanol-related compounds can occur. They include the hypoglycemic sulfonylureas, metronidazole (an antibacterial agent), and allopurinol (a drug used for treating gout).

Ethyl alcohol has been used as an antidote for methyl alcohol poisoning because it slows the rate of conversion to formaldehyde.

> Martensson et al (1988) demonstrated the persistence of high methanol blood levels in chronic alcoholics who drank a cleansing solution containing 90 percent ethanol and five percent methanol. This was attributed to the lower rate of methanol elimination. Paradoxically, such dual ethanol-methanol consumption minimized both the acidosis and other features of classic methanol poisoning.

The familial ramifications of aspartame disease (Chapter II-1) suggest genetic influences comparable to those with alcohol abuse/dependence. There is a three-to-fourfold higher prevalence of alcoholism among first-degree relatives of alcoholics (Schuckit 1999). Moreover, the rate increases another twofold in identical twins of alcoholic parents.

Possible Enhancement of Methanol Toxicity by Disulfiram Therapy

The intake of considerable methyl alcohol in aspartame products might prove harmful to alcoholic patients being maintained on disulfiram (Antabuse®). The following data are pertinent.

- An estimated six percent of the adult population is trying to cope with alcoholism at any given time.
- Disulfiram has been prescribed to cause an aversion for alcohol – both as Antabuse® and less expensive generic products.

The risk of increased methanol concentrations in persons taking disulfiram who abuse aspartame is heightened owing to further slowing of methanol degradation.

- Koivusalo (1958) demonstrated that the rate of methanol elimination in rabbits is considerably retarded by disulfiram treatment. Methanol was still detectable in the blood 100 hours after the smallest dose administered.

685

- Way and Hausman (1950) found the toxicity of oral methanol in rats and rabbits to be more rapid after prior disulfiram administration. Furthermore, it was more severe and protracted than among control animals receiving only methanol.
- Linden et al (1983) reported a 36-year-old man with severe metabolic acidosis who had ingested both methanol and ethylene glycol while taking disulfiram for chronic alcoholism.

Others have reflected on this issue. MacDougall and MacAulay (1956) did not administer disulfiram to patients with methanol toxicity because they were concerned about the accumulation of an excessively toxic metabolite (presumably formaldehyde).

FORMALDEHYDE: ECONOMIC AND POLITICAL CONSIDERATIONS

There have been formidable economic and political apologists for formaldehyde. Their activities could extend to aspartame consumption.

- Industries generating products containing formaldehyde successfully staved off attempts to regulate this chemical. One method involved funding scientists to give "independent" testimony aimed at minimizing the risks.
- Several scientists expressed considerable concern in letters to *Science* (1983; 224:550-551) over a feature dealing with federal policy concerning regulation of formaldehyde that downplayed any "significant risk."

XXII

PHENYLALANINE; ASPARTIC ACID;
STEREOISOMERS; AMINO ACID IMBALANCES

"It has often been held that the method a physician uses to acquire facts is that of observation, while that used by the scientist is experiment, and that there is a fundamental difference between them. This, I think is to misunderstand the nature of experiment. Experiment is no more than planned observation."

Sir George Pickering
(Harveian Oration, Royal College of
Physicians, London, October 19, 1964)

The two amino acids in the aspartame molecule (Figure 5-1) are discussed in this chapter, which consolidates and amplifies material mentioned in other sections.

Author's Note

It may surprise the reader that the author, as a practicing physician, chose to focus much attention in this biochemical realm. An explanation seems appropriate.

The high concentrations of phenylalanine and aspartic acid in aspartame provided an important, albeit unintended, "experiment of nature." Serendipitously, observations on aspartame disease offered plausible clues to the pathogenesis of major disorders.

These controversial corporate-neutral insights prodded me to research them because of their profound ramifications in both the basic sciences and medical practice.

The Phenylalanine – Aspartame Acid Juxtaposition

The frequency with which these two amino acids occur adjacent to each other in important endogenous peptides underscores the foregoing assertion. Some examples:

- <u>Cholecystokinin</u> (CCK) ... Tyr-Met-Gly-Trp-Met- Aspartame-Phe-NH$_2$
- <u>Human growth hormone</u>... Leu-Ser-Arg-Leu-Phe- Aspartame-Asn-Ala
- <u>Human gastrin 1</u>... Glp-Gly-Pro-Trp-Leu-Glu-Glu-Glu-Glu-Glu-Ala-Try-Gly-Trp-Met-Asp-Phe-NH$_2$

Aspartame has been referred to as "a drug masquerading as an additive." The gastrin configuration probably influenced conceptualization of aspartame as a drug for treating peptic ulcer.

A. PHENYLALANINE
GENERAL CONSIDERATIONS

Phenylalanine is classified as an "essential" amino acid by virtue of being nutritionally indispensable to mammals.

Healthy adults require 1-2 grams (gm), or 1,000-2,000 mg, of phenylalanine daily. This can be derived from about 50 gm of quality protein. High protein foods (such as milk or eggs) provide 5 gm phenylalanine per 100 gm protein.

The so-called "hamburger argument" avers that there is more phenylalanine in hamburger and other protein foods than aspartame. For perspective, dietary proteins generally contain about <u>5 percent</u> phenylalanine by weight (Brimboecombe 1961), a concentration that does not approach the <u>50 percent</u> present in aspartame. (Estimates of its phenylalanine content range from 40 to 56 percent [Jobe 1987]).

The enormity of aspartame consumption appears in the Overview. More than a decade ago, Pardridge (1987, p.206) calculated that 3.6 million kg (eight million pounds) phenylalanine were being introduced annually into the food supply as aspartame.

Metabolism

Phenylalanine is readily converted to tyrosine by the action of phenylalanine hydroxylase (see below). Tyrosine then serves as a precursor for synthesis of the brain catecholamines that regulate food intake, and influence mood and arousal.

Dihydroxphenylalanine (DOPA) can cross sympathetic neuronal membranes and reach the general circulation. It then becomes a source for the synthesis of tissue catecholamines (dopamine; epinephrine; norepinephrine), even in the absence of tyrosine hydroxylase (Goldstein 1987).

688

The greater increase of phenylalanine than aspartate in plasma after aspartame loading is impressive. This may reflect the more rapid metabolism of aspartate than phenylalanine within intestinal cells, thereby releasing of more phenylalanine within the portal circulation (Burget 1984).

Another evidence for the uniqueness of phenylalanine is failure of dietary carbohydrate to decrease its absorption, as occurs when leucine (a branched-chain amino acid) is ingested (Krempf 1993).

Non-Aspartame Phenylalanine Consumption

Large amounts of L- and DL-phenylalanine are consumed by the public in products other than aspartame. About one-third of ingested D-phenylalanine is rapidly excreted in the urine; another third is converted to the L-isomer. One author cautioned that amino acids should be taken as far as possible from meals so "they don't get shouted down by other amino acids" (Kilmer 1987).

- A "holistic" physician suggested during a nationwide talk show that taking 4-5 gm (4,000-5,000 mg) phenylalanine in the morning can relieve pain.
- An ardent promoter of bee pollen for weight control attributed its appetite-suppressing effect to the high phenylalanine content. The release of cholecystokinin (a hormone that can reduce food intake) by phenylalanine was noted in Chapter IX-B.
- A popular "nutritional beverage mix" alleged to increase energy contains 600 mg L-phenylalanine per tablespoon. The label indicates that up to four tablespoons – containing 2,400 mg phenylalanine – could be consumed daily.

Pravda, the Russian paper, reported a warning from the Novosibirsk State Medical Academy that substitution of phenylalanine for sugar in bubble gum may be hazardous for children and pregnant women (January 30, 2001). Retardation, delayed growth and nervous system disorders might result. Blond and blue-eyed persons were regarded at higher risk because of deficient enzyme activity involving the metabolism of phenylalanine.

The extensive promotion of D-phenylalanine and DL-phenylalanine by "wellness" periodicals and businesses as over-the-counter remedies for the relief of arthritis, migraine and whiplash, and for treating depression, dyslexia, alcoholism and obesity warrants concern. The severe reactions of Case I-1 to both aspartame and this individual amino acid are germane.

<u>Stress and Depression</u>. Relatively large amounts of phenylalanine have beenadvocated for managing "chronic stress," presumably based on a reduction of excess serotonin. (It was suggested that phenylalanine be taken in the morning to avoid inhibiting sleep-promoting serotonin at the end of the day.) Another explanation for the purported usefulness of phenylalanine in chronic stress and depression derives from being the dietary precursor of phenylethylamine, a natural analog of amphetamines.

<u>Pain</u>. The alleged scientific basis for phenylalanine's analgesia involves the brain's "natural pain relievers" known as endorphins. The brochure of one product purported "good to excellent pain relief" in every patient. It emphasized not only the absence of adverse side effects, but also that "a toxic dose is almost impossible."

These claims have not held up under critical scrutiny by clinicians. Dr. Neil J. Nathan (1987) reported a randomized crossover study lasting from 2-26 years to the American Pain Society. Thirty "enthusiastic" volunteers with back pain took D-phenylalanine 250 mg four times daily, which failed to relieve their pain or increase function. Furthermore, four patients reported "significant" side effects (including dizziness, nausea and muscular cramps) that necessitated termination of the study in two.

<u>Adverse Effects</u>. Aspartame reactors have made other pertinent observations.

- A 44-year-old man expressed surprise that he could tolerate L-phenylalanine. He speculated "L-phenylalanine and DL-phenylalanine are probably not made from the same synthetic ingredients as aspartame." This point is appropriate because the phenylalanine in aspartame is combined with a methyl ester (methanol) (Chapter XXI).
- In addition to consuming considerable diet soda, presweetened tea and diet cranberry juice, a young woman with headache, impairment of memory, anxiety and gastrointestinal complaints had been taking phenylalanine, arginine and ornithine to lose weight – even though she weighed only 135 pounds.
- A California woman inquired about the side effects of phenylalanine and tyrosine. She had previously enjoyed "excellent health," and "<u>never</u> experienced any losses in my life." On the advice of a "health food clerk," she took 2 gm phenylalanine and tyrosine daily for six months. She suffered progressive "memory loss, dizziness, inability to concentrate, shooting pains in the left arm and leg, marked sensitivity of the eyes to light, and extreme cold in the left limbs" until discontinuing these amino acids.

Phenylalanine-Induced Pathology

Excessive phenylalanine can interfere with the ability of the brain and other tissues to metabolize amino acids, especially infants and children having phenylketonuria (Chapter XVII). The brain and nerve changes induced by phenylalanine are amplified below.

The experimental administration of considerable phenylalanine causes tissue damage. After four weeks, rats develop marked pancreatic and liver changes, hyperkeratosis, inhibition of spermatogenesis, and a loss of body weight (Klavins 1967). The mortality increased when given conjunction with tyrosine.

BIOPHYSIOLOGICAL CONSIDERATIONS

Figure XXII-1 indicates the relationship between dosages of ingested aspartame and plasma phenylalanine concentrations in normal subjects.

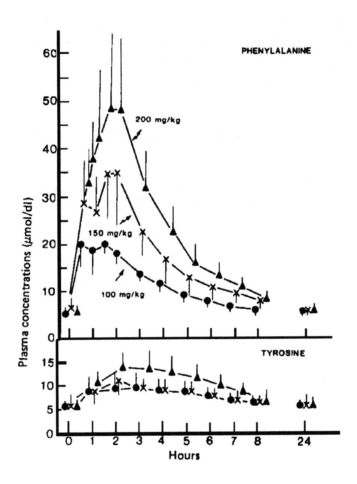

Figure XXII-1

The mean plasma phenylalanine concentrations (μmol/dl) in normal adults ingesting aspartame in amounts of 100 (●), 150 (X), or 200 mg/kg body weight (△), including standard deviations.

Stegink, L.D., and Filer, L.J., Jr.
Aspartame: Physiology and Biochemistry, Marcel Dekker, Inc.,
  New York, 1984, p.519.
Reproduced by courtesy of Marcel Dekker, Inc.

Aspartame administration to rats by gastric feeding (gavage) greatly increases the plasma and brain concentrations of both phenylalanine and tyrosine (Yokogoshi 1984). Moreover, whole body autoradiographs of rats given either radioactive-labeled aspartame or radioactive-labeled phenylalanine indicate appearance of the radiolabel in the brain and spinal cord within 30 minutes.

Phenylalanine Hydroxylase

Most dietary phenylalanine is hydroxylated to tyrosine by phenylalanine hydroxylase (PH). This enzyme exists only in the liver and catecholamine-synthesizing neurons. Its deficiency in phenylketonuria (PKU) was discussed in Chapter XVII. Over 95 percent of phenylalanine reaching the liver via the portal vein is hydroxylated to tyrosine.

Several reports indicate that high dietary intake of phenylalanine depresses the conversion of phenylalanine to tyrosine (Harper 1970). This phenomenon has clinical relevance when considerable phenylalanine is ingested, whether as aspartame or the single amino acid.

Information concerning the homeostatic mechanisms regulating plasma concentrations of phenylalanine is limited. Furthermore, one must bear in mind when analyzing experimental data that there are marked species differences in phenylalanine hydroxylation, the process being much slower in man than rodents. Indeed, the rat liver metabolizes phenylalanine five times faster than human liver.

Plasma Levels and Ratios

Matalon et al (1987) reported that plasma phenylalanine concentrations rose ten times higher than normal when adult controls and PKU carriers were given 100-200 mg aspartame/kg.

Using 6 mg percent phenylalanine as the plasma level probably harmful to pregnancy outcome, Matalon et al (1987) found that up to 14 percent of normals and 35 percent of PKU carriers exceeded this concentration. Concentrations above 10 mg percent were detected in 5 percent of normal persons and 12 percent of carriers.

The ingestion of aspartame causes an increase in the phenylalanine/large neutral amino acid ratio. (This contrasts with its decline after a high-protein meal.) The ratio increases disproportionately when larger amounts of aspartame are ingested by normal persons and those with the PKU gene. It is estimated from rat studies that the phenylalanine brain concentration doubles for every 0.1 change in the plasma phenylalanine ratio (Caballero 1987).

Plasma phenylalanine levels tend to be higher in a number of medical disorders – notably iron deficiency, liver disease, diabetes and obesity (Introduction to Section 3).

- Patients with liver failure are particularly prone to deterioration of brain function from increased concentrations of phenylalanine and other amino acids (Fischer 1971).
- Significantly higher fasting plasma phenylalanine concentrations occur in obese persons (Caballero 1987). This finding – and the blunted response to carbohydrate intake – presumably evidence resistance to insulin action on plasma amino acid levels (Felig 1969).
- The splanchnic uptake of phenylalanine is greater in diabetic patients 24 hours after the withdrawal of insulin, compared to healthy controls (Wahren 1972).

Other Factors Affecting Plasma Concentrations

Plasma phenylalanine concentrations peak earlier when aspartame is given in solution than in capsule form (Steginic 1987) because it is relatively insoluble (Introduction to Section 5). Filer and Stegink (1897) indicated that some clinical studies may have been "compromised" when aspartame was administered as a slurry or in capsules with minimum quantities of fluid. (Distinct variations in both the rapidity and levels of plasma phenylalanine occur when aspartame is given in slurry form.)

The metabolism of phenylalanine in the peripheral tissues is influenced by hormone action (Chapter XXIV). As a case in point, the secretion of insulin following meals facilitates its uptake into skeletal muscle, thereby reducing plasma phenylalanine concentrations (Caballero 1987).

The levels of plasma and brain phenylalanine and tyrosine are significantly increased, both in man and animals, when aspartame is taken with a high-carbohydrate meal. The administration of glucose by gavage also elevates brain phenylalanine and tyrosine concentrations, and enhances their increments from aspartame (Yokogoshi 1984). (Brain phenylalanine is nearly doubled.) Concomitantly, the aspartame-glucose combination reduces brain concentrations of leucine, isoleucine and valine much more than when aspartame or glucose are given alone.

Such rapid increases in the concentration of critical neutral amino acids within the brain undoubtedly influence the synthesis of major neurotransmitters and their clinical expressions. For example, the ensuing increases of norepinephrine and dopamine may elevate blood pressure (Chapter IX-C). Conversely, the decrease of other neurotransmitters resulting from amino acid competition could alter sleep or satiety, leading to severe insomnia or a marked loss or gain of weight, respectively.

Lawrence and Iyengar (1987) determined the beta-aspartame content in diet soft drinks and other products. They noted an increase of beta-aspartame with decreased pH, and nearly double the amount in diet gingerale than in diet cola.

PHENYLALANINE LOADING

Güttler et al (1978) investigated the effects of an oral phenylalanine load on plasma glucagon, insulin, amino acid and glucose concentrations in six healthy men of normal weight. They ingested a load of 0.6 mmol L-phenylalanine/kg body weight after an overnight fast. Their observations support these concepts: (a) insulin facilitates the transport of both glucose and amino acids from the extracellular to the intracellular space; and (b) increased glucagon release decreases the extracellular concentrations of amino acids.

- Serum phenylalanine increased within 10 minutes after the load, reaching a maximum concentration at 30 minutes.
- Serum tyrosine increased within 10 minutes after the load, reaching a maximum concentration at two hours. (By contrast, it progressively declined in 58 children with early-treated PKU.)
- Plasma glucagon and insulin increased during the first 10 minutes after the load, reaching a peak of twice the fasting levels at 30 minutes (Figure XXII-2).
- The molar insulin/glucagon ratio remained unchanged during the first 20 minutes after this load. It then declined by 50 percent at two hours.
- The plasma concentrations of amino acids other than phenylalanine and tyrosine decreased about 15 percent – especially isoleucine, leucine, methionine and valine. It is known that the hypoaminoacidemic effect of insulin and glucagon is greatest for these four amino acids.

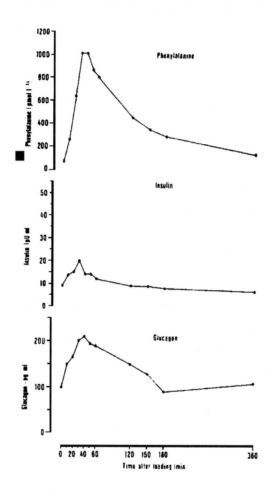

Figure XXII-2

The response of plasma insulin and glucagon concentrations to an oral phenylalanine load given six normal adult men.

Güttler, F., Kühl, c., Pedersen, L., Påby, P.
Effects of oral phenylalanine load on plasma glucagon, insulin,
   amino acid and glucose concentrations in man.
   Scandinavian Journal of Clinical and Laboratory Investigation 1978;
   38: 255-260, 1978.
Reproduced with permission of Blackwell Scientific Publications Limited.

PHENYLALANINE TOLERANCE TESTING

Phenylalanine tolerance testing can demonstrate a reduced capacity to metabolize phenylalanine. Subjects ingest a single dose of this amino acid, such as 100 mg/kg body weight (Koch 1982). The results are illustrated in Figure XXII-3.

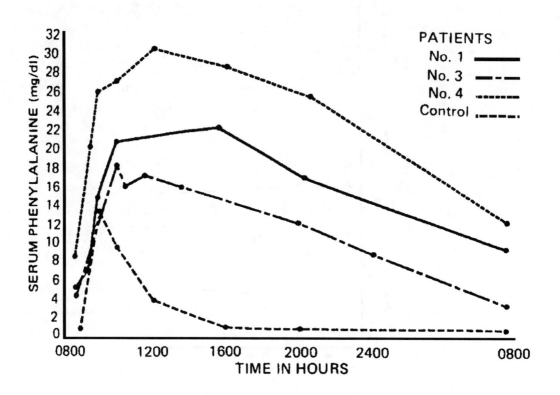

Phenylalanine Metabolism

Figure XXII-3

The serum phenylalanine concentrations of normal control and hyperphenylalaninemic subjects given a single dose of 100 mg/kg body weight of phenylalanine. They ingested regular meals after 12:00.

Stegink, L.D., Filer, L.J., Jr.
Aspartame: Physiology and Biochemistry.
Marcel Dekker, Inc., New York, 1984, p. 93.
Reproduced by courtesy of Marcel Dekker, Inc.

Increased fasting phenylalanine-tyrosine ratios and postload phenylalanine-tyrosine ratios characterize <u>phenylketonuria</u> (PKU) (Chapter XVII). PKU carriers handle phenylalanine at only about half the rate of normal individuals.

Persons with <u>acquired iron deficiency</u> show similarly elevated ratios (Lehmann 1986). The existence of an iron molecule in phenylalanine hydroxylase might account for the elevated phenylalanine concentrations noted during phenylalanine loading in persons with iron deficiency.

Elevated ratios have been found in a number of <u>other states and medical disorders</u>. They include pregnancy (Yakymyshyn 1982), oral contraceptive drug therapy (Landau 1967; Rose 1970; Craft 1971), cirrhosis of the liver (Jagenberg 1977; Heberer 1980; Dhont 1982), malnutrition (Antener 1981), obesity (Brown 1973), renal disease (Pickford 1973; Jones 1978; Stonier 1984), infection (Wannemacher 1976), and leukemia (Wang 1961). *Such individuals therefore risk being classified as PKU heterozygotes.*

PHENYLALANINE-INDUCED BRAIN AND NERVE CHANGES

The consequences of flooding the brain with phenylalanine are profound. Phenylalanine serves as a precursor of two major neurotransmitters, dopamine and norepinephrine (Chapter XXIII). Altered amino acid ratios also can modify tryptophan concentrations... and therefore cerebral serotonin.

There are clinical and experimental manifestations of increased phenylalanine conentrations in the central nervous system – for example, prolongation of the reaction time. Aspartame-associated headaches, convulsions, confusion, erratic behavior and other neuropsychiatric features were detailed in Section 2. The neurotoxicity of excessive phenylalanine for the fetus and during infancy was discussed in Chapter XI.

Excessive phenylalanine "handicaps the nutritional flow of amino acids to the brain" (Christensen 1987). Elsas and Trotter (1987) reported that increased blood phenylalanine decreases plasma L-DOPA, slows brain electrical discharge, and prolongs performance of certain neuropsychologic tests reflecting higher brain function. Furthermore, phenylalanine concentrations inducing such changes could be attained by the chronic ingestion of 34 mg aspartame/kg/day in both adult PKU heterozygotes and normal controls.

The increase of phenylalanine in the brain lesions of Alzheimer's disease is reviewed in Chapter XV. Shoji et al (1992) detected phenylalanine at positions 4, 19 and 20 in amyloid β protein.

698

Murrell et al (1991) provided further evidence that a single amino acid mutation may be important in the pathogenesis of Alzheimer's disease. They studied a family with the classic early-onset disease (autopsy proven) in which there appeared to be an autosomal-dominant inheritance pattern. Direct sequencing of DNA revealed only the substitution of phenylalanine for valine in the transmembrane domain of the amyloid precursor protein. These investigators hypothesized that this "missense mutation" could cause both amyloid fibril formation and dementia.

> Protein engineers are impressed by the dramatic effects on the stability of protein folding when single amino acids are substituted. In this regard, Professor Gregory A. Petsko (1988), Massachusetts Institute of Technology, stressed that the foremost revelations encountered in attempts to manipulate gene coding for protein by using recombinant DNA technology have been "surprise" and "horror." As an example, he noted that the introduction of the dextro forms of amino acids is usually toxic for E. coli.

Blood and Brain Levels

The consumption of phenylalanine as a constituent of dietary protein does not significantly elevate brain phenylalanine concentrations. By contrast, ingesting an aspartame soft drink with dessert food that is rich in carbohydrate and poor in protein can double brain phenylalanine (Yokogoshi 1984).

There is a very high affinity (low Km) transport system for ^{3}H-phenylalanine into isolated brain capillaries. In fact, *phenylalanine has the highest affinity for transport across the blood-brain barrier among the circulating neutral amino acids.* Pardridge (1981) demonstrated this high affinity transport system in both man and the rat.

Induced selective hyperphenylalaninemia also alters the brain concentrations of amino acid-derived neurotransmitters (Choi 1986). These effects are reviewed in Chapter XXIII. Lajtha (1962) reported that the exit time for brain levels of several amino acids to decrease by half was longer for phenylalanine than leucine and proline.

The apparent paradox of decreased phenylalanine concentrations after protein consumption represents a disproportionate greater increase of other neutral amino acid plasma concentrations (viz., valine, leucine, isoleucine, tyrosine and tryptophan). In turn, these compete with phenylalanine for brain uptake. They are transported into the brain by a common facilitated diffusion system. Studies using brain scanning or positron emission tomography (PET) confirm the inhibited uptake of other neutral amino acids (e.g., methionine) by the brain when blood phenylalanine concentrations are increased.

Such competition with other neutral amino acids probably occurs within the capillary endothelial cells that comprise the blood-brain barrier. Inasmuch as phenylalanine has a greater affinity for these transport binding sites, its intake in pure form or as aspartame disproportionately increases brain phenylalanine (Caballero 1987), and reduces other amino acid concentrations.

Neurotoxicity In Infancy

Elevated phenylalanine concentrations are undesirable in pregnant women and in infants. They may incur considerable damage at a period of maximum brain growth during the third trimester and the first year of life. Infants with PKU (Chapter XVII) offer convincing proof that increased phenylalanine concentrations severely impair brain function.

High concentrations of phenylalanine inhibit specific ATP-sulfurylase activity within the central nervous system. (ATP-sulfurylase, the first enzyme of sulfate activation, is most active within those areas of the brain that tend to be more severely affected in PKU.) This leads to decreased synthesis of sulfatides. Hommes and Matsuo (1987) hypothesized that such changes effect an increased turnover of central nervous system myelin unaccompanied by increased synthesis, and the regression of synaptic contacts found in PKU patients.

These observations are uniquely important for pregnant women and infants who consume aspartame because sulfatides are actively synthesized and incorporated into the myelin sheath. The smallest increase of phenylalanine concentrations capable of damaging the brain and myelin sheath requires study, especially in view of the simulation of multiple sclerosis by aspartame disease (Chapter VI-D).

Dr. William M. Pardridge (1986) considers phenylalanine the major neurotoxic amino acid of aspartame. He challenged the Council on Scientific Affairs of the American Medical Association over the following issues.

- There is little scientific basis for postulating a threshold relationship between increased blood phenylalanine concentrations and neurotoxicity, notwithstanding the Council's belief concerning a toxic threshold (1 mmol/L plasma phenylalanine) below which no adverse central nervous system effects occur.

- A linear relationship exists between increased blood phenylalanine concentrations and adverse brain effects. As a case in point, the IQ of babies born to mothers with 225 µmol/L increments in plasma phenylalanine concentration declines (Levy 1983; Kirkman 1984). Similarly, the choice reaction time in adults decreases approximately 10 percent with a 250 µmol/L increase in plasma phenylalanine concentration (Krause 1985). Accordingly, a fivefold increase in plasma phenylalanine concentration (e.g., from 50 to 250 µmol/L) could cause distinct impairment of brain function in children, adults, and a developing fetus. Such an increase could occur if the estimated 20 million persons having impaired phenylalanine metabolism (Levy 1983) were to consume 50 mg/kg aspartame daily.

- The Council's assumption that only one percent of the population consumes more than 34 mg/kg aspartame daily is probably incorrect, especially for children.

Phenylalanine given intravenously to sick infants with immature livers can result in high, and potentially neurotoxic, plasma phenylalanine concentrations (Walker 1986).

- Puntis et al (1986) emphasized the risk of neurotoxic hyperphenylalaninemia when intravenous solutions of amino acids are infused into newborns. It may be exacerbated by breast milk. Such a child evidenced cerebral atrophy and delayed motor development at one year of age.

- Evans et al (1986) noted that the commercial solutions used for total parenteral nutrition in newborns have different phenylalanine contents. Accordingly, they recommended monitoring phenylalanine concentrations during such therapy.

B. ASPARTIC ACID
GENERAL CONSIDERATIONS

Aspartic acid constitutes 40 percent of the aspartame molecule. While not classified as an essential amino acid, aspartic acid participates in major metabolic processes. This is evidenced by the fact that aspartate and glutamate account for up to 30 percent of the total free amino acid content in the brain.

Metabolism and Distribution

The Federation of American Societies for Experimental Biology summarized many aspects of the absorption and metabolism of aspartic acid for the FDA in its July 1992 monograph, *Safety of Amino Acids Used as Dietary Supplements*.

The free form of aspartic acid (that is, not bound to protein) from aspartame is promptly absorbed into the blood stream. By contrast, an immediate and considerable increase of the aspartic acid blood concentration infrequently occurs after ingesting natural foods, contrary to assertions by some representatives of this industry.

Aspartic acid is absorbed as a free amino acid via an active transport system. By contrast, peptides containing aspartic acid must be hydrolyzed by specific intracellular peptidases.

The rise of circulating aspartic acid is decreased when consumed with carbohydrate or protein. Conversely, the ingestion of considerable aspartic acid as aspartame beverages results in greater levels of this amino acid.

Aspartic acid crosses the blood-brain barrier, albeit less readily than phenylalanine. It is transported across the blood-brain barrier and the neuronal membrane in association with two sodium ions per molecule of aspartic acid.

Aspartic acid is importantly involved in brain metabolism, being linked to pyridoxyl phosphate by an aspartate transaminase. It is present throughout the mammalian brain.

Aspartic acid has a strong excitatory effect, as does glutamate (see below). There are least three receptor subtypes for excitatory amino acids, the majority of L-aspartate effects being mediated through NMDA receptors.

Aspartate is converted by the liver into glumatic acid, the toxic component of monosodium glutamate (MSG) (Chapter VIII-G). Accordingly, blood glutamate levels following the ingestion of both aspartame and MSG may exceed those after taking only MSG.

Aspartic acid is also involved in other major metabolic processes, both normal and abnormal. Craik et al (1987) demonstrated its crucial role in the function of serine proteases for the hydrolysis of specific polypeptide bonds within many biologic systems.

Aspartame Ingestion

Plasma aspartate concentrations increase significantly when normal subjects ingest 47 mg aspartame/kg of body weight (Stegink 1987).

Dr. Jon B. Pangborn (personal communication, 1992) noted a rise of plasma aspartic acid in persons drinking one or more aspartame colas during the postprandial state. Heavy users of aspartame were found to have elevated plasma levels in an overnight fasting sample. In view of the "aspartame-phenylalanine peak," he requested client-doctors to have their patients avoid aspartame products before and during the blood/urine sampling for amino acid analysis.

Aspartic Acid (Aspartate) and Glutamic Acid (Glutamate)

Aspartic acid is closely related to glutamic acid (glutamate), another amino acid. They not only have similar chemical structures and transport systems, but also comparable toxicity in animals. The toxicity of monosodium glutamate (MSG) may be enhanced by aspartame (Chapter VIII-E).

Ingested aspartic acid is rapidly converted to aspartate and glutamate, as indicated by the significant elevation of <u>both</u> aspartate and glutamate after a bolus of aspartic acid.

The high-affinity glutamate transport system apparently cannot distinguish between aspartate and glutamate. Subtoxic doses of aspartate (and glutamate) can be cumulative to the point of toxicity.

The extracellular fluid concentrations of glutamate and aspartate play an important role in the pathogenesis of hypoxemic and epileptic brain injury (Tendler 1991).

The demonstration of increased concentrations of aspartate and glutamate in the cerebrospinal fluid of some patients with advanced Alzheimer's disease (Csernansky 1996) reinforces the belief that these excitatory amino acids contribute to neuronal loss. The markedly diminished aspartate binding found in the brain cells of patients with Alzheimer's disease (Procter 1986) is also germane (Chapter XV).

There has been considerable interest in *N*-acetylaspartylglutamate (NAHE) concerning neurotransmission and the mediation of hormonal effects. The concentration of NAHE is exceptionally high in the brain and spinal cord. It is also concentrated in retinal ganglion cells and other neurons of the visual system (Tieman 1988).

Neurotoxicity

Aspartate toxicity has been demonstrated in every experimental species studied, including primates. Some evidences for the neurotoxicity of excess aspartic acid are cited.

- Neurotoxicity occurs in the young of certain animal species (Olney 1980; Finkelstein 1983; Steginik 1984) when plasma concentrations of aspartate and glutamate are markedly increased.

- Large amounts of aspartate and glutamate can destroy nerve cells in the hypothalamus of neonatal rodents (Olney 1970, 1979; Steginik 1984). There is subsequent obesity, skeletal stunting, and reduced reproductive organ size.

- The neurotoxic effects of aspartate and glutamate are additive. Insulin, carbohydrate, or both, reduce such damage (Takasaki 1979, 1980), presumably by increasingly intracellular glucose.

- Dr. John Olney, a Washington University neuropathologist, raised the possibility that aspartic acid may interact with monosodium glutamate (MSG), and potentiate its neurotoxic effects, especially in children (*The Argus* [Rock Island, Illinois], May 6, 1986.)

The selective toxic effects of aspartame and monosodium glutamate, relative to neuronal degeneration of the arcuate nucleus of the hypothalamus, have been attributed to capillary permeability (*Environmental Health Perspectives* 1978; Volume 26: 107-116). (The inefficient blood-brain barrier and blood-cerebrospinal fluid barrier in the hypothalamus presumably allow substances to diffuse into the local tissue spaces, especially among susceptible young animals.) Rapid exchange of a plasma filtrate can occur through slits or fenestrations in the brain capillaries.

The issue of reactions to aspartame preparations was repeatedly raised by correspondents. Several aspartame reactors whose symptoms persisted after the avoidance of such products (notably ringing in the ears or tinnitus) found as a result of considerable personal research that various preparations chelated with aspartic acid caused or exacerbated their problems. Examples are vitamins, minerals (most notably magnesium, potassium and calcium), "enzyme therapies," and "fitness" powders/supplements.

Endocrine Effects

The free aspartate liberated after digestion can adversely affect the brain and endocrine system when it enters the circumventricular structures that control hormonal output from the pituitary, adrenal and other glands.

The effects of excessive aspartic acid on endocrine functions may be significant. It increases pituitary prolactin and gonadotropin hormones in the adult female rhesus monkey (Wilson 1982). These observations explain in part the severe menstrual disturbances among women consuming aspartame products (Chapter IX-E).

The substitution of aspartic acid in the B chain of human insulin can increase its absorption (Kang 1991), causing an earlier and greater decline of the blood glucose concentration. A high frequency of aspartic acid at position 57 of the HLA-DQ β-chain has been reported in Japanese patients with insulin-dependent diabetes mellitus (Awata 1990).

Excessive aspartic acid intake influences the subsequent accumulation and metabolism of <u>N</u>-acetylaspartic acid. Its concentration in the brain is uniquely high (Tallan 1957), being localized chiefly within neurons.

- <u>N</u>-acetylaspartate appears to have unique significance during myelinization, perhaps serving as a transporter of acetyl groups from mitochondria to the cytosol for lipogenesis (D'Adamo 1966). It is synthesized from aspartate and acetyl-CoA by an enzyme, and efficiently kept within neurons.
- The accumulation of <u>N</u>-acetylaspartate due to aspartoacylase deficiency could be directly toxic to the central nervous system (Hagenfeldt 1987).

Canavan's Disease

Other clues suggest the profound effects on brain function of altered aspartic acid metabolism. There is derangement of this amino acid in Canavan's disease, also referred to as spongy degeneration of the nervous system.

This leukodystrophy ranks second in frequency to Tay-Sachs disease among Jews in the New York area having Ashkenazi ancestors (Dr. Anne B. Johnson, personal communication, February 13, 1988). Children with Canavan's disease lack a gene that regulates the production of the enzyme aspartocylcase, which controls the amount of <u>N</u>-acetylaspartic acid.

C. AMINO ACID STEREOISOMERS

Repeated reference is made in other chapters to the stereoisomers or mirror images of phenylalanine and aspartic acid. They are of sufficient significance in aspartame disease to warrant further discussion. In view of the profound metabolic ramifications of these stereoisomers, the classic words of Lewis Carroll assume even greater meaning: "Perhaps, looking-glass milk isn't good to drink."

The aspartame molecule and its amino acid components can open as either the natural L (levo) isomers or the aberrant D (dextro) isomers. <u>Racemization</u> refers to conversion of amino acids from the biologically common L form to the uncommon D configuration.

The author also has emphasized the potential harm of uncommon stereoisomers in amino acid supplements and "fake fat" (Roberts 1989c), and the potential adverse effects of tocopherol (vitamin E) racemates (Roberts 1994c).

Only the L-form of amino acids is found in the numerous enzymes of the human body. Moreover, they are promptly absorbed by L-enzymes within the digestive tract, whereas D- or DL- form amino acids require up to four times longer for absorption.

Small dipeptides or tripeptides containing D-forms of amino acids can diffuse through membranes. Once in the tissues, however, they are not readily metabolized by either oxidases or proteases (Dr. J. Bada, personal communication, March 2, 1988). D-amino acid oxidases in liver that can decompose dietary amino acids chiefly affect free amino acids, not those incorporated in proteins or amino acid chains.

While the D and L stereoisomers of amino acids have nearly identical physical and chemical properties (other than for opposite effects on rotating plane polarized light), it is primarily the L-forms in living organism proteins that are physiologically active. The D stereoisomers of the essential amino acids tend to be poorly utilized, and are excreted mainly in the highly acidic urine by mammals (Neuberger 1948; Man 1987).

There is evidence for a deficiency of D-amino acid oxidase activity in mammals (Koono 1988). Accordingly, the D-forms of amino acids probably qualify as harmful "metabolic garbage" that can damage nucleic acids, proteins and other vital cellular building blocks. The potential toxic effects of ingesting large quantities of D-amino acids in the form of marine bivalves have been raised (Felbeck 1987).

The unexpected complications associated with use of synthetic amino acids caused the FDA to drop DL-amino acids from the Generally Recognized As Safe (GRAS) listing. Some manufacturers, however, continue to use DL-forms to fortify processed foods and supplements for animal feed.

Phenylalanine

Evaluations of the phenylalanine component of aspartame generally focus on the L form of this molecule. Yet, the biological consequences of its D stereoisomer, especially after heating or prolonged storage, ought to be cause for concern (Chapters XX and XXV).

- As noted earlier, persons taking D-phenylalanine for its alleged relief of pain have experienced dizziness, nausea and muscular cramps (Nathan 1987).

- The author received correspondence from a woman who sold a product promoted as a neurotransmitter precursor for "brain food." Up to six capsules daily on an empty stomach were recommended, each capsule containing 300 mg DL-phenylalanine. She wrote, "I consumed it for three days and constantly had a severe headache (which I rarely have), and felt on edge and easily irritated."

Dr. Jeffrey Bada (personal communication, January 1987) provided the following information relative to D-phenylalanine and the D stereoisomers of other amino acids.

- Being tightly bound as peptides, such peptides tend to be more resistant to hydrolysis, and therefore absorbed in this form.
- These stereoisomers are excreted more rapidly by the intestinal tract. There may be adverse nutritional consequences, such as considerable loss of protein and weight.
- The ability of D-phenylalanine to inhibit enzymes metabolizing endorphins could account for the prolonged duration of morphine when given in conjunction with phenylalanine.

D-phenylalanine tastes sweet to man, and is preferred to water by some mammalian species (Ninomiya 1987). By contrast, there are decided strain differences, suggesting that D-phenylalanine probably tastes sweet to C57BL mice, but not to BALD and C3H mice (Ninomiya 1987). Moreover, the chorda tympani fibers of sucrose tasters who evidenced high sensitivities to sucrose also responded to D-phenylalanine, whereas those of non-sucrose tasters did not. Ninomiya et al (1987) suggested that the site of action of the possible gene (*dpa*) is in the taste cell membrane.

Aspartic Acid

Historically, Pasteur found in 1852 that aspartic acid derived from vetch plants was optically active, whereas its synthetic production by heating ammonium fumarate was optically inactive.

Bada and his colleagues documented the faster racemization of aspartic acid than other amino acids (Poinar 1996). The rate at which the L amino acids undergo racemization to produce D amino acids, and then establish an equilibrium, depends on several factors. Aspartic acid has activation energy and rate constants over a wide temperature range (at neutral pH).

The Life Science Research Office of the Federation of American Societies for Experimental Biology prepared a review for the FDA titled, *Safety of Amino Acids Used As Dietary Supplements* (July 1992). The author could find no reference to the D form of aspartic acid (pp. 131-139) in this review. It concluded that "the use of aspartic acid as a supplement in doses up to 8.6 g/day has not been associated with documented detrimental effects in adult humans." In view of the aforementioned observations, this assertion must be regarded with reservation.

There is a progressive accumulation of the D-aspartic acid isomer in the white matter of the brain with aging (Man 1983). This is underscored by the intake of D-aspartic acid in aspartame beverages resulting from heating and prolonged storage.

- D-aspartic acid may accelerate aging and possibly contribute to memory loss (Chapter VI-C).
- Postmortem studies of both the uptake and binding of radiolabeled D-aspartic acid have demonstrated the loss of terminals of cortical neurons in Alzheimer's disease (Procter 1988). Such loss seems to occur relatively early, especially as reduced pyramidal cell counts in temporal lobe biopsies.

Anderson et al (1990) demonstrated that aluminum catalyzes the racemization of aspartic acid in living brain protein. The feeding of rats with supplementary aluminum salts for ten weeks resulted in the accumulation of between 65-182 percent excess aluminum in their brains, compared to controls. There was a concomitant increase in the level of D-aspartate in brain tissue. Such increased amino acid racemization to the abnormal D-enantomer is highly significant because of the increased amounts of D-aspartate and L-isoaspartate in the neurofibrillary tangles of Alzheimer's disease (Roberts 1995b). These changes can lead to functional or structural alterations of myelin in the brain.

Other Considerations

Mapelli et al (1988) analyzed four stereoisomeric analogs of aspartame. They were tasteless as solids or aqueous solutions. Their lack of taste is explained by the rigid positioning of the phenyl group. These observations are also relevant to the loss of taste of aspartame products following prolonged storage.

The following facts about stereoisomers are also noteworthy.

- Lajtha (1962) found that the rate of exit of the D isomers of amino acids from the brain was more prolonged than for the L isomers.

- The microwaving of milk results in the isomerization of amino acids (Luber 1990).
- Lubec (1990) noted that the replacement of a single amino acid moiety in a protein can induce immunological and functional changes.
- The D-glutamate in processed food also appears to cause or enhance adverse reactions to MSG (Chapter VIII), and is increased by cooking.
- The biologic importance of stereoisomers has been further demonstrated by PET scanning relative to the stereoselectivity of monoamine oxidase types A and B for so-called suicide enzyme inactivators of L-deprenyl (an inhibitor of monoamine oxidase type B) and clorgyline (Fowler 1987).

D. AMINO ACID IMBALANCES

After their ingestion in meat and other proteins, the neutral amino acids tend to "neutralize" one another within the gastrointestinal tract. As noted earlier, this does **not** apply to the intake of large amounts of individual amino acids. Dr. C. Wayne Callaway (1986) stressed the failure of many physicians to appreciate "the potentially harmful effects of supplementation with megadoses of single amino acids or other nutrients." He questioned the long-term safety of oral tryptophan (see below) that was previously used for its alleged soporific and neuropharmacologic properties.

The pathologic processes induced by amino acids have been described as "amino acid imbalances," "amino acid antagonism," and "amino acid toxicity" (Brown 1967). The latter refers to adverse effects that cannot be overcome by various supplementations.

Another therapeutic consideration is germane. Amino acids from dietary protein are known to cause crippling fluctuations in the motor performance of patients with parkinsonism, even while receiving levodopa (Pincus 1986). One suggested mechanism is interference with the transport of levodopa from serum across the blood-brain barrier. This may occur with aspartame products (Chapter VI-J).

The chemical configuration of amino acids also is pertinent (see above). Differences exist in the toxicity of the L, D or "DL" forms of phenylalanine (Klavins 1967) and other amino acids (Chapters XXII and XXV).

In its solicitation of studies on the project, "Dietary Amino Acid and Brain Function" (No. 223-86-2095, dated August 6, 1986), the FDA asserted

"Whether consumed as peptides or amino acids, these compounds are metabolically indistinguishable from other dietary amino acids, yet any change in the balance of amino acids, especially when large doses are consumed, has the potential to affect neuro-chemical processes... Hence, a fundamental question has arisen as to whether dietary exposure to such amino acids can modulate central neurotransmitter systems and, if so, could this result in significant changes in brain function and behavior?... At this time, there is insufficient knowledge regarding diet, neurotransmitters, and brain function."

Age-Related Consideration

Amino acid requirements decline sharply with age (Stegink 1984). Accordingly, the ingestion of large amounts by older patients, already a high-risk group (Chapter XV), might lead to problems.

Avoidance of Single or Combined Amino Acids

Mention was made of the considerable promotion of various amino acids as potential curative nutrients for dozens of medical disorders. They include the aromatic amino acids, sulfur amino acids, urea cycle amino acids, glutamate amino acids, threonine amino acids, branched chain amino acids, and amino acids having important metabolites. Further considerations pertain to which stereoisomers (i.e., the L-form, D-form or DL-form) should be utilized. For example, all the essential amino acids have been recommended for Alzheimer's disease, and phenylethylamine, tyrosine, tryptophan, methionine and L-dopa for Parkinson's disease.

Insights from the Eosinophilia-Myalgia Syndrome (EMS)

The hazards of ingesting single amino acids, with or without neurotoxic contaminants, is underscored by the eosinophilia-myalgia syndrome following the use of L-tryptophan. Its clinical manifestations include severe muscle pain, fatigue, rash, marked joint pain, peripheral edema, polyneuropathy, and striking elevation of the eosinophil count in the absence of an infectious or neoplastic disease. The long-term follow-up of such patients, predominantly women, is pertinent.

Sack and Criswell (1992) followed 22 patients with EMS. Marked fatigue, weakness and myalgia remained in all. Only mild gliosis was found by brain biopsy following a grand mal seizure. They commented

"What of the future? Could a situation similar to EMS occur with even more devastating consequences? We say yes, for the following reasons. First, the general public, and probably many physicians, regard food constituents as 'natural' and hence safer than synthetic compounds. This was clearly the case with L-tryptophan, because in 1989 an estimated 2% of American adults were using this agent. Second, the FDA, though long concerned with the safety of substances, has not been successful in controlling their use. In the 1970s, the FDA removed amino acids (including L-tryptophan) from the 'generally regarded as safe' category, and classified them as 'food additives.' As such, amino acids can 'be used to significantly improve the biological quality of the total protein in a food containing naturally occurring primarily intake protein,' but it is illegal to use such supplements to 'treat or prevent' an illness. Yet this is precisely how consumers were using L-tryptophan before the recognition of EMS. Third, the FDA has not introduced new regulations to prevent similar events from occurring again."*

XXIII

ALTERED NEUROTRANSMITTER FUNCTION (INCLUDING SEROTONIN AND CHOLECYSTOKININ)

"Each science confines itself to a fragment of the evidence and weaves its theories in terms of notions suggested by the fragment. Such a procedure is necessary by reason of the limitations of human ability."

Alfred North Whitehead
Nature of Life (University of Chicago Press, 1934)

More than 40 neurotransmitters control or modify brain, nerve and endocrine function. Some are nitrogenous compounds consisting of, or related to, essential and nonessential amino acids – including aspartate, glutamate, glycine and gamma aminobutyric acid. The major neurotransmitters derived from them are norepinephrine, epinephrine, serotonin, acetylcholine, histamine, dopamine and cholecystokinin.

Much literature exists on this subject. The present discussion is limited to the effects of aspartame and amino acids on proteins. The author previously reviewed (a) norepinephrine-serotonin-cholinergic interrelationships, (b) their influence on sleep, arousal, hunger, thirst and drug action, and (c) alterations in narcolepsy, diabetes mellitus and hypoglycemia (Roberts 1971b). Additional comments appear throughout this book.

The blood-brain barrier prevents most peptides from entering the central nervous system because of their hydrophilic character, and the presence of peptidolytic enzymes in this lipoidal barrier. The ability of water-soluble molecules (e.g., glucose; essential amino acids; glutamate) to enter the brain occurs almost exclusively through carrier-mediated transport.

There is concern by scientists and regulatory agencies in the United States and Canada about over-the-counter availability of aspartame and pure phenylalanine because of their potential to alter neurotransmitter physiology and brain function.

712

AN OVERVIEW

Aspartame induces "functional" changes in the central nervous system involving neurotransmitters independent of proneness to phenylketonuria.

Dietary Precursors

Dietary proteins serve as neurotransmitter precursors. Lovenberg (1986) diagrammed their role in Figure XXIII-1.

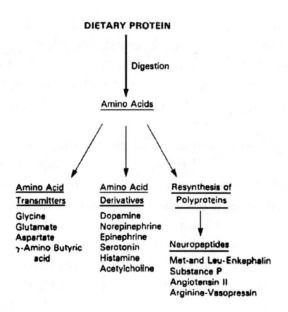

Figure XXIII-1

Lovenberg, W.M.
Biochemical regulation of brain function. *Nutrition Reviews*
    May, 1986, pp. 6-11.
Reproduced with permission of International Life Sciences
Institute - Nutrition Foundation and Dr. Walter Lovenberg

Sequential Synthesis of Neurotransmitters

Lovenberg (1986) also depicted the points at which diet could influence the synthesis of biogenic-amine neurotransmitters (Figure XXIII-2).

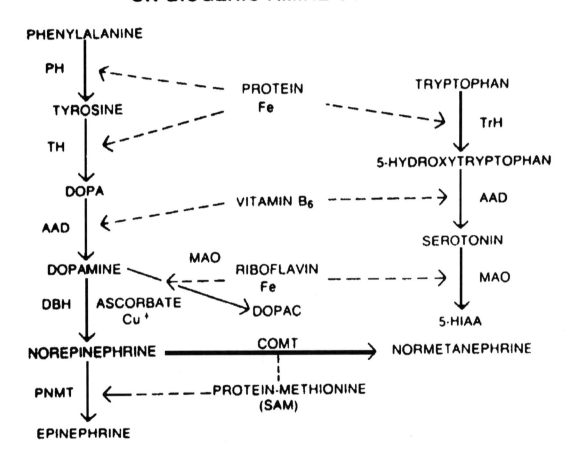

POSSIBLE POINTS OF DIETARY INFLUENCE ON BIOGENIC AMINE SYNTHESIS

Figure XXIII-2

Lovenberg, W.M.
Biochemical regulation of brain function. *Nutrition Reviews*
  May, 1986, pp. 6-11
Reproduced with permission of International Life Sciences
Institute - Nutrition Foundation and Dr. Walter Lovenberg)

714

Tyrosine (Chapter XXII) is converted to dihydroxyphenylalanine (DOPA) through a series of enzymatic processes. The reaction continues with creation of dopamine, and then norepinephrine. The sequence by which these catecholamine neurotransmitters evolve appears in Figure XXIII-3.

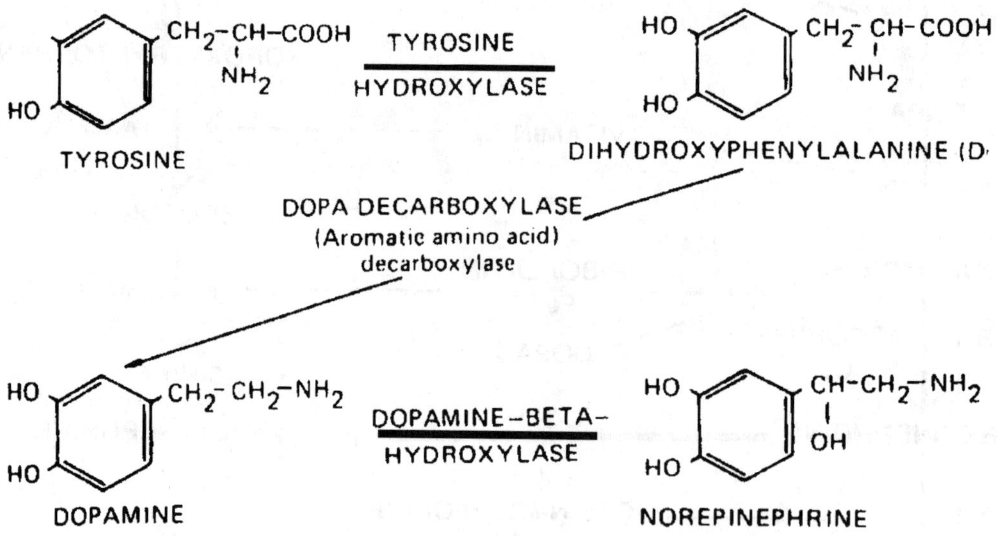

Figure XXIII-3

The pathways of synthesis of catecholamine neurotransmitters from tyrosine after its metabolism from phenylalanine.
Stegink, L.D. and Filler, L.J., Jr. *Aspartame: Physiology and Biochemistry*
Marcel Dekker, Inc., New York, 1984, p. 95.
Reprinted courtesy of Marcel Dekker, Inc.

Reservations Concerning Animal Studies

There is great variation in the brain concentrations of neurotransmitters among animals. This necessitates caution in interpreting studies such as the ability of aspartame to block a carbohydrate-induced rise of brain tryptophan (Wurtman 1987).

Another inherent fallacy involves animal studies used to project the margin of safety in man – namely, some multiple of the acceptable daily intake (ADI). The rate of conversion of phenylalanine to tyrosine, for instance, is considerably slower in humans than rodents.

AMINO ACID INTERACTIONS AND
NEUROTRANSMITTER DYSFUNCTION

Derangement of the major neurotransmitters, whether by dietary or other influences, can alter memory, behavior and divers aspects of brain function. One may conceptualize the complexity of this matter by recalling that its cortical surface alone contains more than <u>100 trillion</u> interconnections.

The long-term consequences of altering amino acid-releasing neurons could be profound. The loss of glutamate/aspartate nerve endings in the brain cortex of patients with Alzheimer's disease (Proctor 1986) provides an example.

- The blockade of N-methyl-D-aspartate (NMDA) glutamate receptors by drugs during late pregnancy is known to cause neurodevelopmental disorders (*The Lancet* 1999; 353:126).
- N–acetylaspartylglutamate (NAHE) affects neurotransmission and the mediation of hormonal effects. Its concentration is exceptionally high in the brain and spinal cord. NAHE is also concentrated in retinal ganglion cells and other neurons of the visual system (Tieman 1988). Its receptors have been implicated in learning, seizures and other forms of neurotoxicity.

Most of the large neutral amino acids within the brain have specific transport systems (Stegink 1984). As noted earlier, phenylalanine, tyrosine, tryptophan, leucine, isoleucine and valine tend to compete with each other for ingress into neurons across the blood-brain barrier. Rats fed a high phenylalanine diet develop marked elevations of cerebral phenylalanine and tyrosine, coupled with reductions of leucine, isoleucine, valine, methionine and histidine (Peng 1973). Their feeding behavior is altered even though blood concentrations of these amino acids remain normal.

716

Patient experiences in other areas suggest comparable amino acid interactions. A tyramine-restricted diet, such as recommended in migraine management, appeared to benefit a 60-year-old woman with severe headaches and petit mal episodes induced by aspartame.

Krassner (1986) listed the following ways in which chemicals naturally present in foods and food additives can affect brain activity.

- Interference with neurohumoral transmission by altered synthesis of neurotransmitters within the neuronal cell body.
- Interference with neurotransmitter release (as by thickened presynaptic membranes) or by blocking release into the synapses.
- Increased release and depletion of neurotransmitters.
- Altered structure of neurotransmitters.
- Effects on enzymes regulating the concentrations of neurotransmitters.
- Blocking neurotransmitters through competitive inhibition at postsynaptic receptor sites.

Altered DOPA and Dopamine Metabolism

Considerable information exists concerning dopamine-serotonin balance, and the marked neuropsychologic changes that can occur when this balance is upset. These neurotransmitters work in concert to modulate activities of the nervous system... analogous to the peripheral sympathetic and parasympathetic systems. Alterations of dopamine metabolism have extraordinary clinical implications (Chapter VI).

Dihydroxyphenylalanine (DOPA) can cross sympathetic neuronal membranes to reach the general circulation, where it becomes a source for the tissue synthesis of catecholamines (dopamine; epinephrine; norepinephrine), even in the absence of tyrosine hydroxylase (Goldstein 1987).

> Roznoski, Huang, and Burns (1993) studied the effects of phenylalanine on the peripheral/central kinetics and metabolism of L-DOPA in monkeys. Their findings suggest that phenylalanine inhibits the transport of L-DOPA into cells or its metabolism within cells.

These observations amplify the subject.

- Walter et al (1987) reported that two dopamine receptor subtypes (D1 and D2) exert synergistic effects on the firing rates of basal ganglia neurons and stereotyped behavior in rats.

- There is evidence that neurotransmitters regulate developing or regenerating nerve cells through an influence on specialized structures called growth cones. Investigators at Northwestern University found that dopamine inhibits the outgrowth of certain vertebrate neurons (Klein 1986).

- Dr. Hans Lou (1987) studied the effects of elevated phenylalanine on the synthesis of dopamine and serotonin in patients with classic PKU. He followed the concentrations of homovanillic acid (HVA) and 5-hydroxyindoleacetic acid (5-HIAA) in the cerebrospinal fluid, both on a free diet and a phenylalanine-restricted diet. The details appear in Chapter XVII.

EFFECTS ON SEROTONIN

Aspartame decreases the availability of L-tryptophan (a precursor of serotonin) and alters its balance with norepinephrine, another important neurotransmitter. Its effects have been likened to a lesion in the lateral hypothalamus that causes neuropsychiatric problems and eating disorders.

The ability of aspartame and its components to inhibit glucose-induced release of serotonin can have profound effects involving satiety, food choice, sleep, and emotional behavior.

- Aspartame-induced decrease of serotonin is pertinent to psychiatric/psychological disorders, especially among weight-conscious women who restrict their carbohydrate intake. A rapid lowering of brain serotonin has been shown to precipitate depression in untreated susceptible individuals when well (Smith 1997).

- Aspartame appears to uncouple the sensory dimension of foods from their calorific properties by distorting regulatory mechanisms concerned with hunger and satiety (Blundell 1986). Persons of normal weight placed on severe diets are vulnerable to such distortion (Chapter IX).

- Unusual alterations of neurotransmitter responses to precursor amino acids have been found in obese persons (Anderson 1986).

- The striking rise of brain phenylalanine concentrations following aspartame ingestion, with ensuing alterations of catecholamine and serotonin synthesis, have been ascribed to a reduction of other neutral amino acids (Wurtman 1985).

- A decrease of brain monoamine levels could lower the seizure threshold of susceptible (albeit previously asymptomatic) individuals. Although Fernstrom et al (1986) felt that the ingestion of large amounts of aspartame would be clinically insignificant, the experience of aspartame reactors (Chapter III) suggests otherwise.

- The large intake of aspartame within a relatively short time suppresses the rise in brain tryptophan levels – and ensuing synthesis of serotonin – that accompany a carbohydrate meal (Fernstrom 1986). Under normal circumstances, tryptophan gains a competitive advantage for such transport over the other large neutral amino acids because their concentrations are lowered by the insulin secreted after a carbohydrate meal. Serotonin synthesis then increases through the action of tryptophan hydroxylase.

Persons with enzyme deficiencies that affect the metabolism of neurotransmitters could manifest unique responses to aspartame. A case in point is congenital dopamine beta-hydroxylase deficiency (In 'T Veld 1987) (see introduction to Section 3). Four percent of the population have minimal amounts of dopamine beta-hydroxylase, presumably indicating an inherited autosomal recessive trait.

CHOLECYSTOKININ

Another remarkable "coincidence" concerning aspartame is the presence of aspartic acid next to phenylalanine in cholecystokinin (CCK). This substance plays a role in memory and acetylcholine release. The amino acid sequence (using conventional abbreviations) of its biologically active form is ASP-TYR (SO3H)-MET-GLY-TRP-MET-*ASP*-*PHE*-NH2 (Brownstein 1985). CCK was reviewed in a symposium edited by Jean-Jacques Vanderhaegagn and Jacqulinen Crawley (1985). (Vanderhaegagn discovered this gastrin-like immunoreactive peptide within the rat brain in 1975.)

There are a number of additional perspectives concerning neuronal cholecystokinin.

- CCK exists in unusually high concentrations in the central cortex, amygdala, septum and olfactory tubercles. Indeed, the concentration of CCK (expressed as mean picomoles per gram of protein) is greater than 4 nmol/gm protein in the rat cerebral cortex – representing at least one order of magnitude above the concentration of norepinephrine or dopamine!

- CCK also is found in relatively high concentrations in the hypothalamus, where it likely plays an important role in regulating the release of pituitary hormones.
- The presence of CCK in both brain and gut suggests evolutionary significance for separate pools of this peptide in two discrete biological systems... including the influence of dietary protein and amino acids.
- CCK is heterogenous in all regions of the mammalian brain with the exception of the cerebellum and pineal body (Goltermann 1985).
- CCK meets most of the criteria for a neurotransmitter – namely, its presence in nerve tissue, its localization in neurons, its concentration in synaptic vesicles, and its release by specific stimuli (Goltermann 1985).
- The enzymatic degradation of cholecystokinin in the central nervous system has been reviewed by Deschodt-Lanckman (1985). The peptidic bonds are cleaved by both an exopeptidase and an endopeptidase. In addition, "enkephalinase" cleaves CCK-8, primarily at the Asp 32-Phe 33 bond.
- Cholecystokinin-dopamine receptor interactions in the central nervous system suggest that CCK-8 may increase striatal dopamine transmission (Agnati 1985).

The amino acid sequence of cholecystokinin and its documented biological effects appear to explain in part some reactions encountered in aspartame disease.

- Possible alteration of the high concentration of CCK in the hypothalamus by a high influx of phenylalanine, aspartic acid, or both, might alter adrenal, gonadal and insulin metabolism. It could be manifest by loss of menses, excessive uterine bleeding, severe hypoglycemia, impaired diabetes control, and obesity (Roberts 1989.)
- Another feature in some persons reacting to aspartame products is marked weight loss (Chapter IX-B). The satiety effect of cholecystokinin, evidenced by reduced intake of both liquid and solid food, has been repeatedly documented (Stacher 1985).
- CCK may cause or exaggerate cerebral glucopenia and its clinical manifestations. Tamminga et al (1985) demonstrated that acute peripheral administration of CCK-8 tended to decrease cortical glucose utilization in certain areas of the brain, particularly the entorhinal cortex and the medial prefrontal cortex.

- Perry et al (1981) reported decreased CCK in Alzheimer's disease.
- Others have noted that memory improved after the experimental administration of CCK, presumably due to enhanced release of acetylcholine from the cerebral cortex (Urakami 1991).

XXIV

EFFECTS ON HORMONES AND METABOLISM

"Whatever can happen to one man can happen to every man."
Seneca

A number of clinical reactions in aspartame disease can be ascribed largely to hormonal and metabolic effects. They are collated here to supplement material in other chapters.

EFFECTS ON INSULIN AND GROWTH HORMONE

Glucose ("body sugar") is the chief fuel for brain under ordinary circumstances. Its supply may be drastically reduced by the release of excessive insulin in response to ingesting table sugar (sucrose), and the administration of insulin or oral drugs for diabetes.

The problem becomes compounded when carbohydrate intake is replaced to a significant degree by noncaloric/hypocaloric aspartame foods and beverages in persons having diabetes mellitus and hypoglycemia. (An analogy could be made to pumping water into a vehicle gas tank.) Melchior et al (1991) demonstrated that the rise of insulin after ingesting aspartame drinks equalled that of sucrose stimulation (Figure XIV-1).

Phenylalanine

Phenylalanine, alone or as the component of aspartame, can increase insulin release and intensify its metabolic consequences. Some of the mechanisms by which these effects aggravate diabetes and hypoglycemia in aspartame disease were described in Chapters XIII and XIV.

It has been known for three decades that phenylalanine, with or without arginine, increases the release of insulin, growth hormone and glucagon. This is depicted in Figures XXIV-1 and 2.

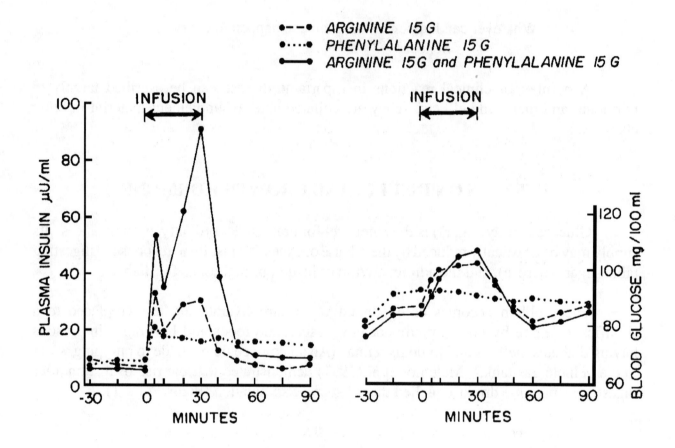

Figure XXIV-1

Plasma insulin and blood glucose concentrations following the infusion of phenylalanine, arginine, and a mixture of arginine and phenylalanine in seven healthy subjects.

Floyd, J.C., Jr., et al
Synergistic effect of certain amino acid pairs upon insulin secretion in man.
   Diabetes 1970; 19: 102-108.
Reproduced with permission of the American Diabetes Association, Inc.,
   and Dr. John C. Floyd.

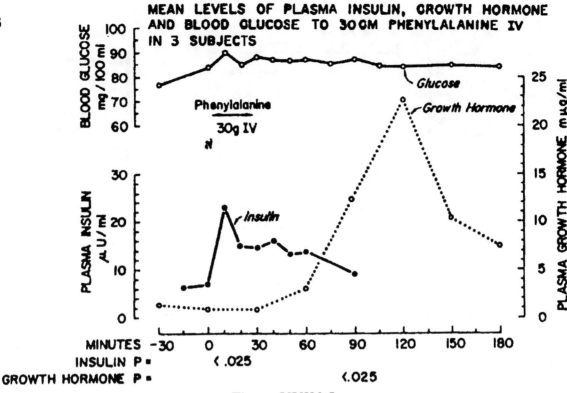

Figure XXIV-2

The plasma insulin, plasma growth hormone, and blood glucose
responses to 30 gm infusion of phenylalanine in three healthy subjects.
Knopf, R.F., et al.
The normal endocrine response to ingestion of protein and infusion of amino
 acids. Sequential secretion of insulin and growth hormone.
Transactions of the Association of American Physicians 1966; 79: 312-320.
Reproduced with permission.

Güttler et al (1978) administered L-phenylalanine to healthy nondiabetic men with no
known family history of phenylketonuria. An oral dose of 0.6 mmol/kg body weight, given
after an overnight fast, caused the serum phenylalanine concentration to reach peak values
of 100 μmol/dl. The plasma insulin and glucagon concentrations increased during the first
10 minutes, doubling the fasting levels at 30 minutes (Figure XXII-2).

Phenylalanine and its analogs also influence glucose and insulin metabolism through
the binding and activation of glucose-dependent insulinotropic polypeptide (GIP) receptors
(Yip 1999). GIP receptors regulate insulin release, increase the binding affinity of the insulin
receptors, and enhance the effects of insulin on target tissues.

Similarly, amino acid combinations can elevate these hormones. Reitano et al (1978)
demonstrated the effects of priming premature infants with a mixture of amino acids relative
to blood glucose, serum insulin, growth hormone and plasma amino nitrogen concentrations
(Figure XXIV-3).

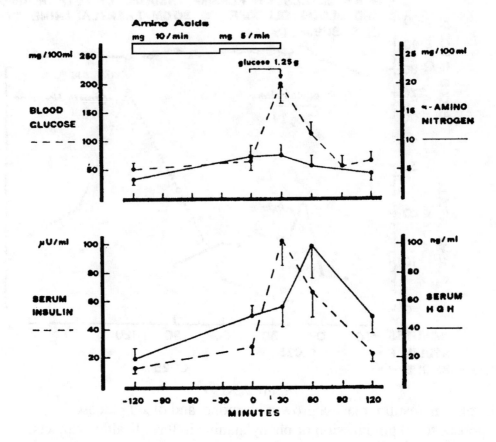

Figure XXIV-3

The effect of priming with a mixture of amino acids on blood glucose, plasma a-amino nitrogen, serum insulin, and human growth hormone (HGH) in the preterm infant.

Reitano, G., et al
Effect of priming of amino acids on insulin and growth hormone response
  in the premature infant.
  Diabetes 1978; 27: 3343-337.
Reproduced with permission of the American Diabetes Association, Inc.

Schmid et al (1989) reported a 3.6-fold greater insulin response among obese subjects given an infusion of amino acids (including phenylalanine and aspartic acid) than lean subjects.

The marked increase of plasma insulin after ingestion of phenylalanine drinks by healthy men is further elevated when the amino acid is ingested with carbohydrates (van Loon 2000).

Cholecystokinin-Insulin Relationships

The ingestion of protein and amino acids is a more potent stimulant of cholecystokinin (CCK) release than glucose. CCK (Chapter XXIII) is one of several compounds termed incretins that modulate insulin output from the pancreatic beta cells. They play an important role in the enteroinsular axis – specifically, the regulation of postprandial plasma insulin and glucagon concentrations after protein ingestion (Rossetti 1987).

In turn, aspartame-associated stimulation of cholecystokinin can enhance amino acid-induced insulin release. Rushakoff et al (1987) found a striking increase of insulin secretion when arginine was infused along with CCK (Figure XXIV-4). A similar response occurred with a mixture of amino acids.

726

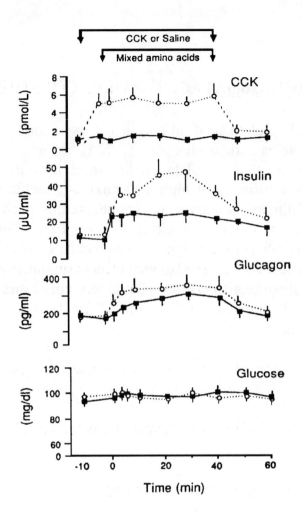

Figure XXIV-4

Mean (±SEM) plasma cholecystokinin (CCK), insulin, glucagon, and glucose responses to the intravenous infusions of mixed amino acids and CCK in four men who were studied on two separate occasions. After drawing baseline plasma samples, a 50-min infusion of either saline (■) or 24 pmol/kg.h CCK (0) was started. An infusion of mixed amino acids (15 g in 40 min) was started ten minutes later. Note the significantly elevated insulin and glucagon levels during infusions (P<0.005).

Rushakoff, R.J. et al
Physiological concentrations of cholecystokinin stimulate amino acid-
  induced insulin release in humans
Journal of Clinical Endocrinology and Metabolism 1987;
  65:395-401.
Reproduced with permission of the *Journal of Clinical Endocrinology
  and Metabolism*, and Dr. Roger A. Liddle.

RELATED HORMONAL/METABOLIC CONSIDERATIONS

Carbohydrate Intake

The experimental evidence that high aspartame <u>and</u> carbohydrate intake induces major neurochemical changes was reviewed in the preceding chapter. The apparent interaction of aspartame and dietary carbohydrate (Council on Scientific Affairs 1985; Ferguson 1987) assumes added clinical significance. For example, Case III-1 experienced her first convulsion 12 hours after consuming two liters of an aspartame-containing orange soft drink. She stressed that she also had been eating more fruit that day.

Reflex Hyperinsulinemia

Aspartame may potentiate the cephalic phase of insulin secretion (Chapter XIV). The methyl ester is required for aspartame's taste since aspartyl-phenylalanine is tasteless.

This phenomenon also has been demonstrated with the artificial sweetener acesulfame K (Liang 1986).

Decreased Substrate; Increased Energy Demands

Reactions following considerable intake of aspartame products might reflect the body's inability to meet habitual energy requirements.

- Porikos and Van Itallie (1984) noted that healthy adults who were given food in a controlled laboratory setting reduced their energy intake at 85 percent of baseline when aspartame was substituted for sucrose.
- In rat studies conducted by these investigators over a period of 15-30 days, neither normal-weight control rats nor obese rats increased their intake sufficiently to maintain energy intake at baseline levels when sucrose was replaced by aspartame.

Methyl alcohol (Chapter XXI) may increase energy demands. As a point of reference, chronic alcoholics use more energy, even at rest. This is attributable in part to the stimulation of microsomal enzymes involved in alcohol oxidation (Jhangian 1986).

The Role of Severe Dieting

Individuals who are overweight – or so perceive themselves – often curtail caloric intake while satisfying their "sweet tooth" with aspartame products. They could suffer serious complications if the reduction becomes drastic (Chapter IX). These include potentially fatal disturbances of the heart rhythm (notably ventricular tachycardia) associated with potassium loss (Roberts 1964a, 1965b, 1967a, 1971b, 1985). Other factors may be operative.

- The ingestion of amino acids or "liquid protein" products by such persons can release considerable insulin, perhaps exceeding that of a glucose stimulus. Lantigua et al (1981) found significantly decreased plasma glucose concentrations among patients receiving a commercially available amino acid mixture as their sole protein source. Similarly, Dr. John E. Potts (personal communication) demonstrated equivalent glycemic and hyperinsulinemic responses to beefsteak and dextrose among overweight non-insulin-dependent diabetics).
- The D-forms of phenylalanine and aspartic acid may be poorly absorbed (Chapter XXII and XXV).

EFFECTS ON PROLACTIN AND FEMALE HORMONES

The striking menstrual, breast and sexual changes in aspartame disease were detailed in Chapter IX-E.

Representative Case Report

Case XXIV-1

A 33-year-old woman experienced more frequent menses, marked breast tenderness, and more prolonged features of the premenstrual syndrome (PMS) while consuming considerable aspartame colas. These features disappeared within one week of abstinence... only to recur within two days after retrial.

Prolactin

Prolactin stimulation contributes to the reduction or loss of menses in aspartame disease.

Carlson, Hyman and Blitzer (1990) demonstrated that phenylalanine (given orally or intravenously) stimulates prolactin secretion, even in males. This effect could not be completely abolished by the concurrent infusion of valine.

Observations by a number of investigators implicate prolactin as a tumor-promoting substance in various tissues (Chapter XXVII). They include the pituitary (Oliveira 1999), endometrium (Brosens 1999), and human breast (Maus 1999).

Yano et al (1997) demonstrated that phenylalanine[576] plays an important role in the secondary structure and intracellular signaling of the human luteinizing hormone/chorionic gonadotropin receptor.

DIURESIS FROM COLD-INDUCED INHIBITION OF VASOPRESSIN

The diuresis in many aspartame reactors consuming cold aspartame beverages has been impressive (Chapter IX-F). This may be partly to stimulation of oropharyngeal receptors by cold water, with subsequent inhibition of vasopressin (antidiuretic hormone) release (Salata 1987).

XXV

OTHER HAZARDOUS METABOLITES

"Right up there with the fluoride and mercury-
in-your fillings scandals is the aspartame mass
poisoning of the world."
Dr. William Campbell Douglass
(Second Opinion, July 1999)

Aspartame reactions may be caused by the aspartame molecule or its metabolic products. The biological effects of its amino-acid stereoisomers (Chapter XXII) and other metabolites remain incompletely studied. The FDA suggested its inability to account for 30 percent of aspartame decomposition products was largely attributable to analyses performed at 104°F (40°C) rather than lower temperatures (*Federal Register* February 22, 1984, p. 6675).

STUDIES OF DR. BADA

Jeffrey Bada, Ph.D., Professor of Chemistry at the University of California (San Diego) and researcher at the Amino Acid Dating Laboratory of the Scripps Institution of Oceanography, has made significant contributions in this field. He detected up to ten different breakdown products of aspartame (personal communication, November, 1986), the diketopiperazine derivatives constituting about half.

Using reversed phase high performance liquid chromatography to separate the dipeptides and diketopiperazines generated from the decomposition and epimerization of aspartame, Gaines and Bada (1987) identified six such diastereomeric products. The proposed decomposition scheme is shown in Figure XXV-1.

730

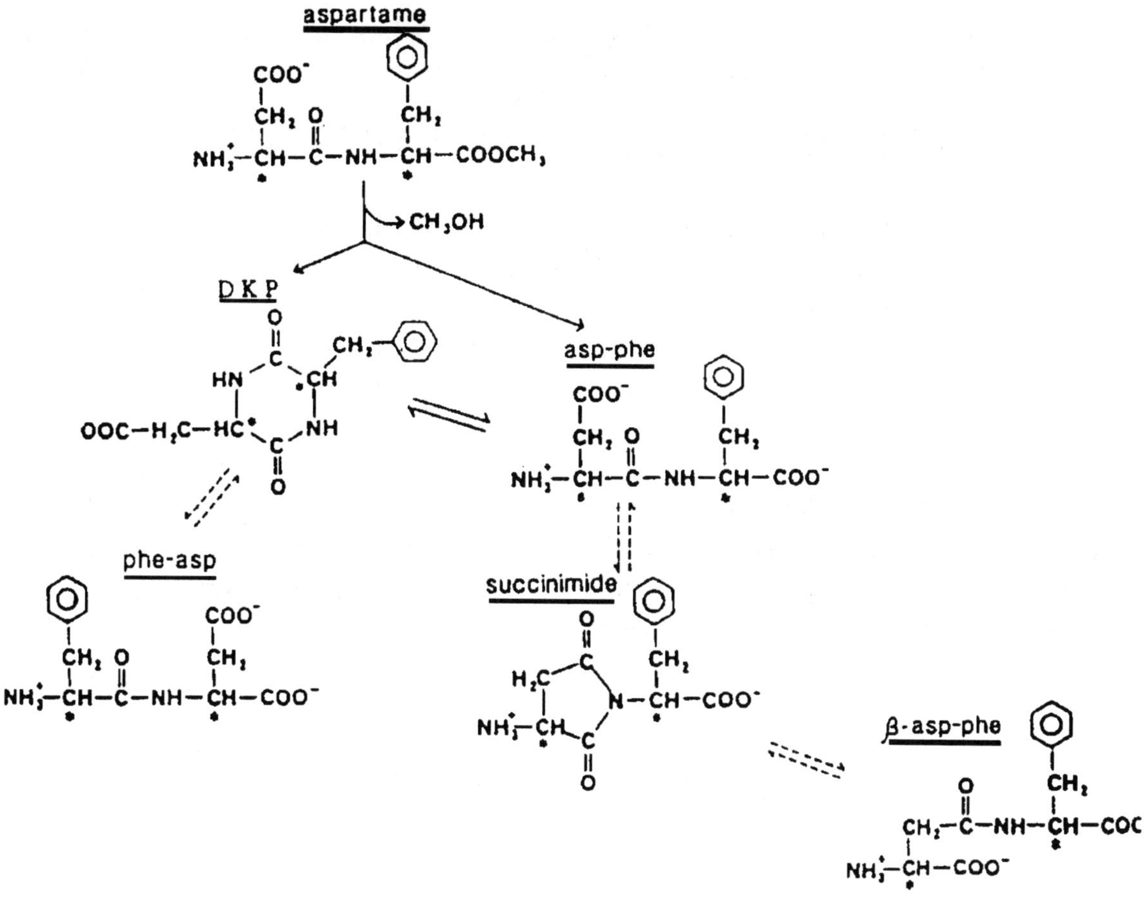

Figure XXV-1

A proposed scheme of aspartame decomposition showing the various possible products. The symbol * indicates chiral centers. Each of these products may undergo epimerization producing four stereoisomers. Solid and dashed arrows represent the possible dipeptide and diketopiperazine (DKP) pathways that may occur during aspartame decomposition.

Gaines, S.M., and Bada, J.L.
Reversed phase high performance of aspartame diastereomeric liquid separation decomposition products.
Journal of Chromatography 1987; 389:219.
Reproduced with permission of Elsevier Science Publishers, B.V., Amsterdam.

732

DIKETOPIPERAZINE

A diketopiperazine (DKP) derivative (3-benzyl-2,5-piperazinedione-6-acetic acid) is formed in solution and in storage, especially at higher temperatures (Boehm 1984). Its conversion from aspartame is depicted in Figure XXV-2.

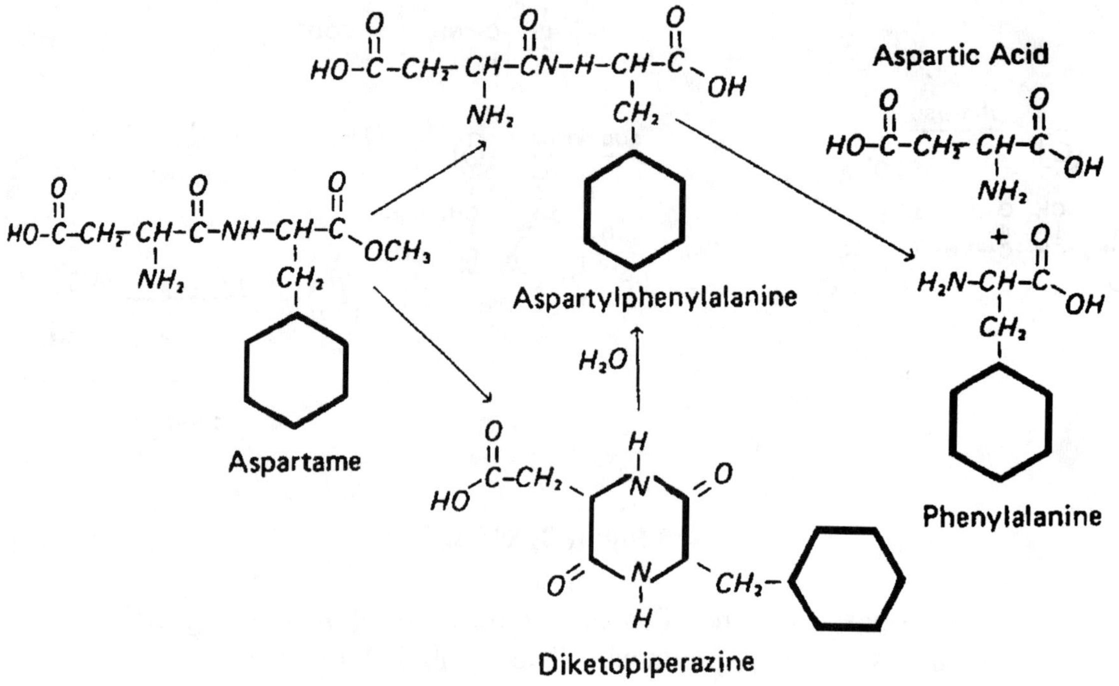

Figure XXV-2

The conversion of aspartame to diketopiperazine and its components.

Stegink, L.D. and Filer, L.J., Jr.
Aspartame; Physiology and Biochemistry
Marcel Dekker, Inc., New York, 1984, p. 249.
Reprinted by courtesy of Marcel Dekker, Inc.

Sophisticated analytic technics (as differential scanning calorimetry) confirm the dramatic increase of DPK after heating of solid-state aspartame hemihydrate.

This toxic metabolite is not usually present in the human diet. Kulczycki (1986, 1987) suggested that DKP might act as an antigenic haptene-like intermediary in allergic reactions (Chapter VIII). Its potential for carcinogenicity is also suspected (Chapter XXVII).

REACTIONS WITH ALDEHYDES

Aspartame can react with certain aldehydes, another class of flavor compounds. Using gas chromatographic analysis, Hussein et al (1984) demonstrated such reactivity with several aldehydes in ethanol. The degree of reactivity differed with each of the model aldehydes – namely, benzaldehyde, cinnamaldehyde, citral, *n*decanal, and vanillin. They also found that (a) the presence of water in the model system slowed the reaction, and (b) citric acid could counteract the effects of water.

These observations explain in part the dramatic reactions experienced by patients after ingesting aspartame fruit juices and flavored soft drinks.

Dr. Bada also noted that a popular aspartame tabletop sweetener reacted differently than pure aspartame after being heated. Its increased aldehyde content might account for the severity of such reactions.

THE BROWNING REACTION

A brown coloration develops when solutions of an aspartame tabletop sweetener at pH 6.8 are heated. This is due to the formation of melanoidins, condensation products of amino acids and peptides with carbohydrates.

Such nonenzymatic browning involves the Maillard reaction, a reaction of dipeptides with reducing sugars in the presence of water. Stamp and Labuza (1983) demonstrated that this reaction increases with rising temperatures. A related finding has considerable significance: the shelf life of aspartame in an aqueous system at 45° C is 60 days (Chapter XX).

The brown substances resulting from cooking amino acids and sugars may be highly mutagenic and even carcinogenic because of the DNA-damaging agents so produced (Abelson 1983).

SECTION 6

THE IMMINENT PUBLIC HEALTH THREAT ISSUE

"As soon as questions of will or decision or reason or choice arise, human science is at a loss."
Noam Chomsky

"Few subjects cause greater controversy than the assessment of the potential health hazard of a chemical. The more widely the chemical is used, the greater will be the potential impact on public health and the subsequent scatter opinions and attitudes. Often, these opinions are impossible to equate."
D. D. Bryson (1981)*

"No new chemical or no chemical that is subject to any question as to safety should be employed until its possible injurious effect, both on an acute and on a long-time chronic basis, has been shown to be nonexistent. In other words, any chemical that is proposed for use ought to be proved in advance of distribution in a food product to be utterly and completely without the possibility of human injury."
Dr. Paul B. Dunbar (1950)
(former FDA Commissioner)

GENERAL CONSIDERATIONS

Joseph D. Douglass, Jr. and Neil C. Livingstone (1987) wrote *America The Vulnerable: The Threat Of Chemical And Biological Warfare* (D. C. Heath & Company, Lexington, Massachusetts). This title is relevant because the public is being increasingly exposed to chemicals in its food and water that can have serious adverse effects, especially in the long term.

Citizens of the United States properly take pride in a judicial system wherein an accused individual is presumed innocent until proven guilty by a jury of peers. To demand "ultimate proof" of adverse reactions to products being consumed by over half the population, and in the face of thousands of such volunteered reports, is a different matter. In the absence of legislative or executive restraint, "battles of the experts" supported by self-serving interests having almost unlimited funds for legal defense can drag on for decades, during which more millions could be affected. This scenario appears to be the case with aspartame disease.

In the author's opinion, based on five decades as a practicing physician and corporate-neutral researcher, aspartame disease can be considered a contemporary "thirteenth plague" in the wake of biological and chemical warfare, and the AIDS epidemic. Others support this conviction. Dr. William Campbell Douglass stated in *Second Opinion* (April 1999): "Right up there with the fluoride and mercury-in-your fillings scandals is the aspartame mass poisoning of the world."

The issue of aspartame's safety ought not be whitewashed by reassuring pronouncements, pseudoscientific arguments based on limited or flawed double-blind tests from corporate-sponsored researchers, disinformation rebuttals to valid "anecdotal" reports, or media campaigns waged by vested interests. Senator Howard Metzenbaum stated during the November 3, 1987 Senate hearing on aspartame: "We need new, independent tests of safety. We don't need the company, or non-profit institutes fronting for the company, telling us this product is safe."

- A case in point is the administration of dry aspartame placed in cool solutions, or as capsules, for double-blind studies. Some of the problems associated with aspartame and its breakdown products stem from the effects of heat and prolonged storage (Chapter XX).
- When boiled, the two amino acids undergo structural changes wherein they rotate to the right (rather than the left), a process known as *racemization* (Chapter XXII). The presence of other chemicals in

various substances (such as coffee, chocolate and flavorings) also may alter the molecular structure of this chemical (Chapter XXV).

- Camfield et al (1982) obtained an aspartame product from a grocery store in conducting an independent double-blind study of epileptic children. They reported an increase in the frequency of spiked-wave discharges by electroencephalography, contrasting with the results of other studies using aspartame capsules or freshly-prepared cool drinks.

Commentary: "The Principle of Precautionary Action"

Aspartame disease reinforces the need for regulators to adopt "the principle of precautionary action" when dealing with potentially toxic dietary and environmental hazards. The permissive "prove harm" philosophy heretofore used is no longer acceptable. The author has repeatedly urged such a policy relative to other harmful substances. They include the pesticide pentachlorophenol (Roberts 1990b, 1997d), mercury (Roberts 1995b), lead (Roberts 1995b), and the fluoridation of water supplies (Roberts 1992f, 1998h).

A definition of the precautionary principle, cited by *The Lancet* (2000; 356: 265), avers: "When an activity raises threats of harm to the environment or human health, precautionary measures should be taken even if some cause and effect relationships are not established scientifically."

The appropriateness of this attitude as a condition of public health surveillance is bolstered by considerable clinical observation and scientific input. Alarmed consumers concur that these must not be disregarded because corporate and other interests demand "certainty." It is folly to tamper with human biology and our ecosystems in the face of unequivocal brain damage, multiple types of cancer, and disorders of the immune system legitimately attributable to contamination of food, water and air by the foregoing substances.

The importance of aspartame disease within this realm is underscored by its magnitude and potential long-term ramifications. The many years that regulators previously required in order to "line up the bodies" for satisfying prove-harm apologists can be justifiably criticized as unreasonable foot-dragging. It is unrealistic to expect the body to ward off, detoxify and excrete poisons once the toxic load becomes excessive.

The old joke, "It must be something in the water or the air," assumes considerable significance in the context of aspartame sodas. The coordinator of special programs for high school students with disability from emotional/behavioral disorders (E/BD) in

Minnesota became increasingly convinced about a relationship between the phenomenal rise of E/BD disability over the previous decade and aspartame consumption.

A. IMPLICATIONS OF ASPARTAME CONSUMPTION: AN OVERVIEW

"If we do not pay proper attention to the nutritional problems association with food technology, we run the risk of eventually producing an abundance of palatable, convenient staple foods that are not capable of meeting man's nutrients needs. We run the risk of undermining the nutritional well-being of our nation."

O. Stewart (1964)

The escalation of aspartame consumption (see Overview) justifies re-evaluation <u>all</u> evidences for suspect adverse effects to products containing it. This is emphasized because companies producing or selling food "additives" and "supplements" need not prove they are effective or curative. Moreover, there are no standing committees to evaluate the safety of new food additives that demand long-term pre-marketing studies on humans.

Many clinical observations and experimental studies that pertain to the public health have been detailed in preceding chapters. There is special concern over its use by pregnant women, lactating mothers, children and the elderly. Related sentiments by consumers appear in Chapter XIX.

Others issued warnings concerning potential hazards of aspartame after its approval.

- In an early publication suggesting the toxic potential of the aspartylphenylalanine methyl ester as a low-calorie sweetener, Cloninger and Baldwin (1970) suggested that "by maintaining low concentrations of sweetening agents, problems of toxicity are less likely."
- The initial reservations concerning aspartame by the National Soft Drink Association (1985) appeared in the *Congressional Record*.
- One analyst estimated that 85 percent of all aspartame consumed in the United States during 1996 was as soft drinks.
- Two decades ago, Uribe (1982) criticized the FDA for not having carefully investigated its possible toxicity in patients with liver disease.

738

- In its January 8, 1982 edition reporting the availability of aspartame, *The Medical Letter* concluded "...its long-term safety remains to be determined." The editors expressed concern over each potentially toxic component.

- Dr. Jacqueline Verrett, a former FDA biochemist and toxicologist, told the Senate hearing held on November 3, 1987 that she had found serious departures from standards while examining the original crude studies performed by the manufacturer in the early 1970s. Verrett used terms such as "woefully inadequate" and "uninterpretable." She also deplored discarding the findings of uterine polyps and other abnormalities because they were considered too minor.

Estimated Population Affected

The author is frequently asked to estimate the percentage of persons in the general population adversely affected by aspartame products. The answer obviously depends on the clinical and scientific criteria used. It is my opinion, however, that the **majority** are affected, especially when aspartame is taken large amounts over prolonged periods.

A comparable attitude has been expressed by afflicted scientists on the basis of their personal experiences.

A 29-year-old research chemist at the University of Cambridge (England) began experiencing severe migraine, joint pain, a flushed sore face, extreme fatigue, confusion, and other symptoms on returning to England after having lived three years in Switzerland. He was told that his symptoms represented "the stress of moving," depression, and "chemical exposure at work." He found a link to aspartame during an Internet search for triggers of migraine. After one week of abstinence, his symptoms disappeared or had markedly improved. He commented: "Being a chemist, I am truly horrified that this chemical is so widely used in so many foods and drinks. I have worked with hundreds of different chemicals for years without consequences. Yet, I was quite ignorantly poisoning myself everyday with diet colas from the drinks machine down the corridor."

Even if only one-tenth of one percent of persons currently using aspartame products in the United States were to suffer reactions, the total number – over 140,000 – remains impressive.

The severity and magnitude of allergic reactions to aspartame products were considered in Chapter VIII. Potential victims in this category probably exceed persons with peanut allergy, for whom the Department of Transportation proposed an accommodation in the form of a "peanut-free zone" by ten major United States airlines. Yet, the Centers for Disease Control estimate that less than one percent of the population is allergic to peanuts (*The Wall Street Journal* September 2, 1998, p. A-1).

Accordingly, the public ought to heed the classic advice of *caveat emptor* ("let the buyer beware") – or the dictum of Senator Howell Heflin, "If in doubt, don't."

Senator Howard Metzenbaum

A concerned Senator Howard Metzenbaum (1985) pointed out the absence of human studies on aspartame prior to its licensing. He further asserted, "The Government does not have that burden of proof. The manufacturer must prove that... aspartame is safe, and that there is reasonable certainty that no harm will result from its use."

In introducing The Aspartame Safety Act of 1985, Metzenbaum criticized the FDA as "more of a handmaiden of the food and chemical industry than it is a defender of the health and safety of American consumers." His defeated bill would have mandated independent studies conducted under the auspices of the National Institutes of Health, and appropriate informative labeling.

Concern of the Author

The author's position relative to safety represents professional concern as a physician, consultant and researcher. It does NOT reflect bias against the manufacturers or representatives of this industry. He certainly did not choose to become a "majority of one" in the face of an impressive list of organizations that "unanimously" approved aspartame (see Overview) and issued statements such as the following:

- "Few compounds have withstood such detailed testing and repeated, close scrutiny, and the process through which aspartame has gone should provide the public with additional confidence of its safety." (Statement by the FDA Commissioner approving aspartame for use as a food additive, July 1981, 46 FR 38285)

- "The Committee... has previously reviewed all the toxicological data available for aspartame on several occasions. As a result of these reviews, the Committee has been satisfied that aspartame is safe for use in food and drink." (The Committee on Toxicity of Chemicals in Food, Consumer Products and the Environment of the Ministry of Agriculture, Fisheries and Foods in the U.K., 1983)
- "The data on the safety of aspartame is the most comprehensive ever received by the Health Protection Branch in support of a food additive." (Canadian Health Protection Branch)
- "We have been disturbed by recent reports in the news media that suggested that aspartame... is harmful to the fetus and therefore should be avoided by pregnant women. These articles have been so incomplete they have seriously misled and unnecessarily frightened the public." (American Council on Science and Health, *News and View* November/December 1985)
- "Recent publicity on aspartame and seizures have prompted calls from concerned patients. As an organization devoted to people suffering from seizure-related problems, we at the Epilepsy Institute investigated this allegation and found aspartame to be safe for people with epilepsy." (Richard Reuben, M.D., Chairman, Professional Advisory Board, Epilepsy Institute)
- "Dr. Harold Rifkin, President of the American Diabetes Association, reaffirmed that aspartame has been found to be an effective artificial sweetener." (An American Diabetes Association news release, June 24, 1985)

The author's observations and expressed concern went unheeded by official agencies charged with protecting health. (Serious majority-of-one researchers involved in public health problems have been likened to an orchestra conductor who must turn his back on the crowd.) This dilemma was compounded by many of the obstacles described in Section 7.

Several factors have enhanced the risks.

- The FDA approved the use of aspartame in juice drinks, frozen novelties, tea beverages and breath mints during November 1986.
- The FDA approved the sale of aspartame in bulk, even though reactors already were worried about products incorporating "100 per cent" aspartame. For example, a 31-year-old secretary wrote, "When they switched aspartame from the blend to full strength, I passed out after three days of consumption."

- The government's review of the process by which the FDA approved aspartame failed to come to an assertive conclusion. The United States General Accounting Office (1987) offered this disclaimer: "We did not evaluate the scientific issues raised concerning the study used for aspartame's approval or FDA resolution of these issues, nor did we determine Aspartame's safety. We do not have such scientific expertise." On the other hand, 12 of 69 scientists who responded to a GAO questionnaire had serious reservations about the safety of aspartame.

- *The FDA approved aspartame as a general-purpose sweetener in June 1996.* This meant that the chemical could be used as a sweetener in **ALL** foods and beverages for which prior approval had not been obtained. Even baked goods were included, provided the aspartame content did not exceed 0.5 percent.

Concern of the Public: The "Imminent Public Health Hazard" Issue

The imminent public health hazard of aspartame will be discussed below. Phenformin (DBI®), a drug that had been used successfully for years by many physicians to treat patients with diabetes mellitus, was declared an imminent public health hazard – and removed from the market – because a rare complication (lactic acidosis) occurred in a few who should have
been receiving insulin or another drug. (Its analog, metformin, was subsequently approved, and remains in wide use even though occasional reports of lactic acidosis are published.)

In the present context, aspartame is classed as a food additive, not a drug. The father of a young aspartame reactor who had been misdiagnosed as having multiple sclerosis wrote, "I believe we are on the brink of a national tragedy, not unlike that due to thalidomide and other drugs that were prematurely sanctioned as safe."

Scores of aspartame reactors have complained that "aspartame is everywhere" (Chapter I). Their attempts to avoid aspartame often proved difficult and frustrating.

A 43-year-old teacher had frequent and excessive menstrual periods while consuming up to four cans of an aspartame soft drink daily. Her daughter suffered aspartame-induced headaches. She wrote

> "It is becoming increasingly difficult to avoid aspartame. I am constantly irritated by people <u>not informing me</u> when a product containing aspartame is served. This has happened time and again at church suppers and friends' homes. I do not want it foisted on me!"

Paul B. Ruggles, a member of Aspartame Victims and Their Friends, wrote this letter to a disbelieving journalist on August 14, 1987.

> "What we are seeing is ironically reminiscent of the posture that the NASA assumed prior to the 1967 Apollo fire and the Challenger accident... As the Rogers Commission points out, there was also a dangerous shift in policy at the NASA which changed the contractor's burden to prove that all was safe to that of proving that is was unsafe. This subtlety was essentially the difference between success and tragic failure. The analogy with aspartame is also clear: the FDA has certified it to be safe based on assumed safety, and now it's up to the <u>individual</u> consumer to prove that aspartame is unsafe. Lots of luck." (Reproduced with permission.)

Jane E. Brody (1987), a nutrition journalist, expressed concern over the statement that aspartame is the most extensively tested food additive in view of the probability that it may be consumed for a lifetime. Accordingly, this assertion could not be equated with having been "adequately tested."

B. THE CONCEPT OF FOOD ADDITIVE SAFETY

The United States General Accounting Office (1987) defined a food additive as "a substance intentionally used that becomes or may become a component of food or otherwise affect its characteristics."

The food additive amendment approved by the Congress in 1958 was intended to offer the public the same degree of protection against unsafe food additives as unsafe drugs. According to *Congressional and Administrative News: Legislative History of Food Additives Amendment of 1958* (p.5302), "Safety requires proof of reasonable certainty that no harm will result from the proposed use of an additive." It also clarified the "Concept of Safety" for food additives in these terms.

"The concept of safety used in this legislation involves the question of whether a substance is hazardous to the health of man or animal. Safety requires proof of a reasonable certainty that no harm will result from the proposed use of an additive. It does not and cannot require proof beyond any possible doubt that no harm will result under any conceivable circumstances.

"This was emphasized particularly by the scientific panel which testified before the subcommittee. The scientists pointed out that it is impossible in the present state of scientific knowledge to establish with complete certainty the absolute harmlessness of any chemical substance.

"In determining the 'safety' of an additive, scientists must take into consideration the cumulative effect of such additive in the diet of man or animals over their respective life spans together with any chemically or pharmacologically related substances in such diet. Thus, the safety of an additive in such diet. Thus, the safety of a given additive involves informed judgements based on educated estimates by scientists and experts of the anticipated ingestion of an additive by man and animals under likely patterns of use.

"Reasonable certainty determined in this fashion that an additive will be safe, will protect the public health from harm and will permit sound progress in food technology.

"The legislation adopts this concepts of safety by requiring the Secretary to consider in addition to information with regard to the specific additive in question, among others, the following relevant factors (1) the probable consumption of the additive and of any substance formed in or on food because of the use of such additive; (2) the cumulative effect of such additive in the diet of man or animals, taking into account any chemically or pharmacologically related substances in such diet; and (3) safety factors which qualified experts consider appropriate for the use of animal experimentation data.

"In determining the safety of an additive, the Secretary would have to consider not only the food to which the additive is directly added, but also other foods derived from such foods.

For example, in evaluating the safety of an additive for poultry feed, the Secretary would have to consider any residues that might appear in eggs produced by the poultry. Similarly, in determining the safety of additive-treated cattle feed, account would have to be taken of residues of the additive in the milk or edible flesh of the animal.

"Since the scientific investigation and the other relevant data to be taken into consideration by the Secretary include information with respect to possible cancer causing characteristics of a proposed additive, the public will be protected from possible harm on this count."

Dr. David C. Hattan (1987) (Chief, Regulatory Affairs Staff of the Office of Nutrition and Food Sciences Center, FDA) focused upon the standard of "reasonable certainty of no of no harm" in discussing the regulation of food additives with neurotoxic potential. In order to resolve the regulatory dilemmas involved, he asserted that "the law must change or evolve, and science must provide us additional insight concerning the mechanisms of neurotoxicity so that the FDA can confidently justify permitting the presence of the minute quantities of neurotoxins in food."

The Bureau of Drugs has indicated that it did not fully agree with the criteria used by the Bureau of Foods for the safety of additives.

C. THE IMMINENT HAZARD REGULATION

A House of Representatives report on the Food Additives Amendment stated, "Safety requires proof of a reasonable certainty that no harm will result from the proposed use of the additive" (H.R. Report No. 2284, 85th Congress, 2nd Session, 1958).

A Legal Overview

The pertinent FDA regulation (21 CFR 2.5) concerning imminent public health hazards reads

"(a)   Within the meaning of the Federal Food, Drug and Cosmetic Act an imminent hazard to the public health is considered to exist when the evidence is sufficient to show that a product or practice, posing a significant threat of danger to health, creates a public health situation (1) that should be corrected immediately to prevent injury and (2) that should not be permitted to continue while a hearing or other formal proceeding is being held. The imminent hazard may be declared at any point in the chain of events which may ultimately result in harm to the public health. The occurrence of the final anticipated injury is not essential to establish that an 'imminent hazard' of such occurrence exists.

"(b) In exercising his judgment on whether an 'imminent hazard' exists, the Commissioner will consider the number of injuries anticipated and the nature, severity, and duration of the anticipated injury."

Provision for the "Amendment or Repeal of Regulations" was set forth in Section 409(h) of the Food, Drug and Cosmetic Act.

"(h) The Secretary shall by regulation prescribe the procedure by which regulations under the foregoing provisions of this section may be amended or repealed, and such procedure shall conform to the procedure provided in this section for the promulgation of such regulations."

Historical Perspective

The FDA has been successfully challenged on a number of occasions after its concurrence with the alleged safety of a particular drug, additive or device. The tragic birth defects attributed to use of thalidomide by pregnant women for sedation, and of doxylamine succinate for nausea in pregnancy, provide examples.

Such instances not only reflect insufficient testing prior to marketing, but also the considerable time needed to obtain ironclad proof that a drug or chemical is indeed the offender. As an illustration, the author maintained an international registry of aplastic anemia attributed in pentachlorophenol, a pesticide, for four decades (Roberts 1961, 1983).

Dr. Robert H. Moser (1969), prior Medical Director of the NutraSweet Company, asserted in *Diseases of Medical Progress*

746

"Often it takes years before the full spectrum of efficacy or toxicity of a drug becomes evident... and it may take almost twenty years to appreciate the complete spectrum of drug efficacy and toxicity".*

"Imminent Public Health Hazard" Precedents

The FDA and the Environmental Protection Agency (EPA) have removed a number of products and drugs in the face of mounting evidence they posed an imminent public health hazard. Such pressure of consumer complaints, for instance, caused the FDA to ban the use of sulfite preservatives on fresh fruits and vegetables in August 1986.

The removal of phenformin was mentioned earlier. Even though it had been successfully used for more than two decades in managing numerous diabetics, this action was taken on the basis of little more than a score of reported cases... a number that pales in comparison to the thousands of consumers who developed aspartame disease (Chapter XXVI). The United States District Court for the District of Columbia, in upholding reliance on Imminent Hazard in the case of phenformin, asserted

"As recited in the Order, the criteria used by the Secretary to determine the imminence of the hazard included:

"1. The severity of the harm that could be caused by the drug during the completion of customary administrative proceedings to withdraw the drug from the general market.

"2. The likelihood that the drug will cause such harm to users while the administrative process is being completed.

"3. The risk to patients currently taking the drug that might be occasioned by the immediate removal of the drug from the market taking into account the availability of other therapies and the steps necessary for patients to adjust to these other therapies.

---

* From Moser, R.H.: *Diseases of Medical Progress: A Study of Iatrogenic Disease.* 3rd edition, 1969, p.xx. Courtesy of Charles C Thomas, Publisher, Springfield, Illinois

"4. The likelihood that after the customary administrative process is completed, the drug will be withdrawn from the general marketing.

"5. The availability of other approaches to protect the public health. (Secretary's order of suspension July 25, 1977, at 34.)

"...Further, we are not inclined to adopt plaintiff's 'crisis' interpretation of imminent hazard. Rather we are more persuaded by defendant's suggested analogy to cases interpreting the imminent hazard provisions of the Federal Insecticide, Fungicide and Rodenticide Act which caution 'against any approach' to the term imminent hazard...that restricts it to a concept of crisis, and adopt the view that 'It is enough that there is substantial likelihood that serious harm will be experienced during...any realistic projection of the administrative process.' See *Environmental Defense Fund v. Environmental Protection Agency*, 167 U.S. Apparent. D.C. 71, 76, 510 F.2d 1292, (1975) (E.D.F. II); *Environmental Defense Fund v. Environmental Protection Agency*. 150 U.S. App. D.C. 348, 360, 465 F.2d 528, 540 (1972) (E.D.F.I.).

"We decide accordingly that the Secretary's criteria for evaluating the existence of an imminent hazard were not improper. *Forsham v. Califano*. 442 F. Supp. 203 at 208 (1977)."

Relevance to Aspartame

It is clear that laws passed since the "thalidomide revolution" have been inadequate for assessing the safety of newer food additives. The preceding sections that contain many documented adverse reactions to aspartame products serve as proof. Other misgivings exist. For example, no extensive public hearings were held (to the author's knowledge) prior to permitting the incorporation of aspartame in soft drinks.

In his review of nutrition for the *Journal of the American Medical Association*, Dr. C. Wayne Callaway (1986) stressed that "food supplements" are not subject to as rigorous regulatory restraints as drugs. Furthermore, manufacturers need not provide evidence for safety and efficacy if specific therapeutic claims do not appear on the package label.

Entire realms of plausible concern about additives are still downplayed or ignored. A case in point is the absence of reference to brain tumors in animals given N-[N-(3,3-dimethylbutyl)-L-*a*-aspartyl]-L-phenylalanine 1-methyl ester (Neotame) in its Environmental Assessment as a high intensity sweetener, dated December 17, 1998. (The petition for this analog of aspartame was published in the February 8, 1999 issue of the *Federal Register*.) Yet, the suspected role of aspartame in brain tumors remains (see below and Chapter XXVII-G).

By contrast, the *Reinheitsgebot*, Germany's purity law (codified in 1516), aims to protect beer drinkers against "adulterant" additives by mandating that beer sold in Germany be made with only four ingredients – malt, hops, yeast and water. While additives are present in exported German beers, they have been forbidden heretofore in domestic brews, which are considered nourishment for the population. (The annual consumption of local beer in Bavaria averages 60 <u>gallons</u> for every man, woman and child.)

Many other observations challenge the classification of aspartame products as "Generally Recognized As Safe" (GRAS).

- Spiers et al (1987) reported on aspartame and human behavior. In terms of safety, they noted that "the absence of proof cannot be taken as proof of absence," and "aspartame may have more widespread and diverse effects on human behavior than has heretofore been contemplated."
- Higher incidence rates of brain tumors in rats (especially males) were found after aspartame administration by Dr. Innes (a neuropathological consultant), and by the Universities Associated for Research and Education in Pathology (UAREP) (Cornell 1984). This subject is considered in Chapter XXVII.
- <u>Small doses</u> of aspartame have been associated with severe reactions (Chapter II-D). A 42-year-old dentist so afflicted wrote, "I suspect that all humans are affected by aspartame, some more than others."
- The hypertensive effect of aspartame (Chapter IX) might summate upon that of other drugs (both prescription and over-the-counter) that elevate blood pressure, such as phenylpropanolamine which has been incriminated in hemorrhagic stroke.

The alarm of citizens is further evidenced by statements volunteered in replies to my survey questionnaire (Section 4) and letters to the media. Some parents and grandparents have expressed extreme concern (Chapter XI).

- An aspartame reactor with severe hives and menstrual bleeding stated

  "I thought of writing to the company or the FDA, but figured it would do no good. These people have some conviction that their product is safe beyond a reasonable doubt. I am willing to testify that for me it was very unsafe. I am frightened about the growing use of this product in children's foods and so many of our foods. Just think about how much aspartame kids drink during the summer. You can liken this to my drinking lots of iced tea and diet sodas, and what it did to my body. I believe there's a national tragedy in the making."

- An insulin-dependent diabetic who developed seizures after consuming several products containing aspartame sued the manufacturer for breach of an "implied warranty" that these sweeteners were "fit for ordinary use" (*The Grand Rapids Press* March 6, 1986, p. C-6). He believed that a product liability statute had been violated.

Other observations suggest the inherent toxicity of aspartame. For example, several correspondents described the apparent effectiveness of aspartame packets in eradicating carpenter ants.

The National Soft Drink Association actually lobbied **against** the incorporation of aspartame in soft drinks during 1983. It detailed its objections, including marked deficiencies in the stability studies using aqueous media (*Congressional Record* (S507-S5511).

Other Nations

India illustrates the concern of other governments about aspartame soft drinks. It approved such use in May 1999. Within a week, however, the Indian Health Ministry announced that any carbonated drink should contain at least five percent sucrose. (This would add 99 calories per can.) Such action pertained to the stipulation that anything classified as food must have some nutritional value (*The Wall Street Journal* July 21, 1999, p. B-1). Moreover, the Ministry ordered that every can and bottle must carry the label warning: "Not recommended for children."

The absence of official concern invites expansion of aspartame disease abroad. A major Chinese chemical company began promoting "high quality and cheap" aspartame in

August 2000. Its consumption, both in China and internationally, will undoubtedly increase dramatically.

D. BROADER PUBLIC HEALTH PERSPECTIVES

"Food additives are big business. The chemical and drug industries have joined the food industry in a food-industrial complex that the FDA is supposed to regulate. The result is a proliferation of food chemicals that are unnecessary, an unknown number that are unsafe, many of them untested, and most of them poorly monitored, at best."
Senator Gaylord Nelson (1972)

The magnitude of aspartame consumption and the serious nature of aspartame disease (Sections 2, 3 and 4) should be considered in a broader context – namely, prevailing habits of the general population and other conditions that affect our society. They may trigger vicious cycles.

When questioned about the safety of aspartame being added to their products, producers have stated that this substance has been "tested up, tested down, and tested sideways." But one cannot rely on laboratory studies to detect the effects of neurotoxin exposure on humans, especially when of a prolonged and low-level nature. Indeed, the literature on neurotoxins is largely useless for clinicians in dealing with suspected neurotoxic illness. This becomes a special problem when corporate-funded testing is tantamount to "kill and count them."

The emphasis upon happiness and personal satisfaction derived from consuming products featured on television that may be harmful, including "diet" drinks and foods, should bother those concerned with the future of our society. This state of affairs has been allowed to develop through the influence wielded by corporate giants on officials having regulatory functions with but one aim: profit. Such emphasis has intensified with the merging of large companies in the food, drug and chemical industries.

Wealthy corporations have bought their way to the top of both government and the media. Mintz and Cohen (1971) focused on the protection the FDA affords giant drug companies against small competitors through extensive regulatory requirements. While Chairman of the Federal Trade Commission, Casper W. Weinberger told the Senate Subcommittee on Antitrust and Monopoly (February 1970, p. 4815), "The disappearance of healthy, medium, middle-sized firms is a matter of concern not only for competition but for social and political institutions."

The unrestrained ingenuity of aspartame-product producers in expanding their markets for faux sugars is remarkable. But the potential hazards of drinking excessive "liquid candy" must be considered in these money-making ventures.

- Manufacturers of new "sports drinks" target athletes and "fitness enthusiasts." One product contains sugar, aspartame <u>and</u> acesulfame-K.
- Some cash-strapped school systems encourage the sale of soft drinks in vending machines at high schools as a way to pay for football uniforms, computers and other expenses.
- The industry anticipates increased consumption in hot weather by utilizing vending machines equipped with a temperature sensor and computer chip that can automatically raise prices (*The Palm Beach Post* October 28, 1999, p. A-1), and that respond to credit cards.

The Limited Adaptability of Human Metabolism

Man has limited ability to cope with the high consumption of sugar and of aspartame. Dr. Rene Dubos, a renowned physician-scientist, expressed these relevant fears to the 22nd World Health Assembly concerning human adaptation.

> "The evolution of biological mechanisms is far too slow to keep up with the accelerated pace of the technological and social upheaval of the modern world.
>
> "Today, everything changes so quickly that the processes of adaptation do not have time to come into play. The cost is likely to be an increase in degenerative disabilities.
>
> "It will require extreme alertness and greater social responsibility on the part of physicians and public health experts to protect mankind from great health disasters."

Dr. Robert H. Moser (1969), former Medical Director of the NutraSweet Company, provided another generic overview. He prefaced *Diseases of Medical Progress* with the following commentary on unprecedented pharmacologic manipulations.

> "We have designed molecules unique to human physiology and have intruded them into blood and tissue by techniques that are

also unique in physiologic experience... and you begin to appreciate the magnitude and genius of man's conspiracy to bypass the conventional avenues for introducing new environmental factors to the physiology of man... The implications of these ingenious tactics of assault, these strange manmade chemicals and emanations upon the beleaguered human mechanism, are fascinating to contemplate."*

Pathophysiologic Changes Induced By Aspartame

Aspartame reactions may reflect responses to the chemical itself, each of its three components (phenylalanine; aspartic acid; methyl alcohol), and stereoisomers or other toxic breakdown products. Many in the latter category are not known or have been incompletely studied.

Roak-Foltz and Leveille (1984) estimated that the mean daily consumption of aspartame per person would be 867 mg if aspartame were to replace all sugar and other sweeteners in the United States. In this scenario, the mean daily intake of its components would increase as follows: phenylalanine – 433 mg (12 percent); aspartic acid – 347 mg (five percent); and methanol – 87 mg.

The scientific evidences were reviewed in Section 5. A few examples are germane.

- Sustained levels of methyl alcohol in heavy aspartame consumers may damage the retina, optic nerves, and many tissues. Humans cannot promptly and adequately detoxify methanol, especially its breakdown products: formaldehyde and formic acid.
- Adverse cerebral effects may reflect flooding of the central nervous system with high concentrations of phenylalanine, which in turn alter the function of major neurotransmitters and hormones.
- Other metabolic actions and interactions must be considered. For instance, the combined effects of voluntary severe caloric restriction, amino-acid induced secretion of excess insulin, and vigorous exercise could deprive vital organs (especially the brain, retina and inner ear) of

---

*From Moser, R. H.: *Diseases of Medical Progress; A Study of Iatrogenic Disease*. Third edition, 1969, p. xix. Courtesy of Charles C Thomas, Publisher, Springfield, Illinois.

energy needed for proper function. The increase of plasma insulin after ingestion of phenylalanine drinks by healthy men is exaggerated when the amino acid is ingested with carbohydrates (van Loon 2000).

- Selective amino acid imbalances within the brain created by an excess phenylalanine and aspartic acid might accelerate or aggravate intellectual impairment, behavioral disorders, parkinsonism and Alzheimer's disease.

ASPARTAME DISEASE AS A NATIONAL HEALTH PROBLEM

Over half the population in the United States currently consumes aspartame, and is largely oblivious to its potential adverse effects. In view of the author's data, those of the FDA, and other information to be detailed, shortcomings involving prior aspartame research and its licensure require reevaluation. The regulatory agencies involved ought to alter their benign attitudes to aspartame, which some consumer advocates have captioned "a recipe for disaster."

The United States Accounting Office (1987) indicated that 12 of the 69 scientists who responded to a GAO questionnaire expressed major concerns about the safety of aspartame. It even extends to persons in this industry.

> The health ramifications of adding aspartame to soft drinks, coupled with potential prolonged lawsuits, were major factors in the sale of his company by a famous private soda bottler. He "did not wish to leave that kind of an inheritance to my children." Another crucial aspect of this decision was the alleged report of "toxic gases evident" in tests on aspartame that had been stored in a hot desert area.

Shortcomings Concerning Aspartame Safety

A chronological outline of some details about this bittersweet story appears at the beginning of Section 6. The National Research Council (1991) warned, "Anecdotal reports of neurotoxicity in humans need to be pursued vigorously with clinical surveillance and follow-up."

The following deficiencies pertaining to the licensing, use and surveillance of aspartame ought to be challenged.

- The neglect or casual interpretation of clinical complaints submitted by consumers.

- The failure to make such complaints available to interested professionals.
- The inadequate testing for aspartame-induced tumors in experimental animals, especially within the brain and the urinary bladder of male rats.
- The arbitrarily high maximum allowable daily intake (ADI) of aspartame approved by the FDA.
- The resistance by Congress to legislating adequate labeling or products containing aspartame, including justified precautions concerning heating and prolonged storage (two months or longer).
- The virtually unchallenged emphasis upon the safety of aspartame (exclusive of persons afflicted with phenylketonuria) in advertising campaigns.

Challenging "Authoritative" Approval

The approving comments by regulatory agencies outside the United States, mentioned earlier, must be regarded with reservation.

- Many researchers presented by the manufacturer were accepted without insisting upon additional corporate-neutral clinical trials.
- Although aspartame products are licensed in Europe and elsewhere, their inhabitants tend to shun them because of reflexive health concerns, as well as cost.

Physicians have learned from experience that thoughtful challenges to the alleged safety of drugs and additives after their approval by the FDA **must** be encouraged. The tragic birth defects from thalidomide and from doxylamine succinate taken during pregnancy were largely attributable to insufficient testing prior to marketing. They also reflect the considerable time needed to prove that a given drug or chemical is harmful. Another example is bone marrow toxicity (aplastic anemia) caused by the pesticide pentachlorophenol (Roberts 1963, 1983b).

Needless Radiation

Many aspartame reactors in this series had been subjected to considerable diagnostic radiation, especially studies of the brain and gastrointestinal tract, before the nature of their problem was suspected. X-rays of the stomach, small intestine and large bowel for possible peptic ulcer, Crohn's disease or ulcerative colitis were commonly performed in young persons.

Hazards For the Weight-Conscious

An estimated six out of every ten Americans currently watch their weight in an attempt to become Jack Sprats. Their use of diet soft drinks probably exceeds that of other beverages. Such excessive use of aspartame could be tantamount to "the slender trap."

Drs. Jerome P. Kassirer and Marcia Angell (1998), editors of the *New England Journal of Medicine*, warned physicians about the public's excessive infatuation with thinness. They editorialized: "Countless numbers of our daughters and increasingly many of our sons are suffering immeasurable torment in fruitless weight-loss scams, and some are losing their lives. Doctors can help the public regain a sense of proportion."

The arbitrary and severe dieting by weight-conscious young women deserves condemnation. Such nutritional neglect has assumed epidemic proportions on the college campus. In a survey of 364 female college freshmen by Frank et al (1991), nearly 60 percent were currently on a diet to lose or maintain weight. Furthermore, 29 percent had resorted to crash dieting or fasting since entering college, 20 percent had used diet pills at some time, and 13 percent resorted to purgatives or diuretics.

In this pervasive cult of thinness, the United States public is spending more than $20 billion a year on diets, dietary supplements, and other products purported to facilitate weight loss. The promotion of aspartame products to weight-conscious persons, especially young women, obviously has been successful. There is also the problem of "affluent malnutrition" among persons who perceive themselves as overweight.

An important caveat exists: *there is as yet no convincing evidence for the long-term effectiveness and safety of most crash reducing programs.* The enormous consumption of non-nutritive sweeteners has had only a minimum effect on the frequency and degree of obesity (Stark 1987). Women using aspartame products paradoxically may gain weight because of altered satiety and the tendency to consume extra calories (Chapter IX). Another explanation, applicable both to humans and experimental animals, is the body's metabolic response in the anticipation of calories after perceiving sweetness.

Our culture has spawned a related epidemic problem, "the fear of fat." In its wake, children, teenagers and adults frequently curtail calories coupled with using considerable amounts of foods and beverages containing aspartame. By so masking or ignoring hunger in the pursuit of ill-advised and unattainable goals dictated by the high priests of fashion, they defy "the wisdom of the body." (Coco Chanel, the famous designer, once observed that fashion is generated by men who basically hate women.) The developmental, medical and psychologic consequences may become evident thereafter as stunted growth, anorexia nervosa, bulimia, and a host of other disorders. Some have not been considered in this context, such as "desk rage" in the workplace.

These statements may seem heretical to some. Yet, they are based on the author's longstanding interest in the potential hazards of indiscriminate caloric restriction (see below). The ability to lay down fat reserves (e.g., the "thunderous thighs" that many women find so objectionable) represents an evolutionary survival trait in the face of severe food deprivation – especially when metabolic demands are increased, as in pregnancy.

Serious complications have been provoked or aggravated by inappropriate caloric restriction due to an unrealistic obsession with modest "obesity." They include severe headache (Roberts 1967d), angina pectoris and cardiac arrhythmias (Roberts 1965b, 1967a), nonthrombotic stroke, leg cramps (Roberts 1965, 1973), multiple sclerosis (Roberts 1966b), and hyperthyroidism or thyroiditis (Roberts 1969a). (One consumer activist characterized sudden death provoked by a severe aspartame reactions as "the sweet hereafter.")

The combination of phenylpropanolamine and aspartame in a number of "appetite suppressant' products – including "maximum-strength" appetite control formulas and diet gums – may induce or aggravate hypertension and its complications.

The author also has reported the apparent greater susceptibility to thrombophlebitis (inflammation of the veins with possible blood clot formation) in the lower limbs, and subsequent pulmonary embolism (clots to the lungs) among persons using liquid protein diets (Roberts 1978, 1985), or vigorously exercising against machine resistance (Roberts 1986b).

Another long-term consequence of "fear of fat" among young women is the choice of nonparenthood. Several childless women having aspartame disease boldly asserted that "pregnancy will make me fat."

Diabetes Mellitus

A striking 33 percent rise in the incidence of diabetes nationally between 1990 and 1998 was reported by the Centers for Disease Control and Prevention. Various explanations were offered (e.g., overweight, stress, fast foods and less exercise), but not the possible contributory role of aspartame products.

Aggravated Hypoglycemia

So-called reactive hypoglycemia ("low blood sugar attacks") is <u>common</u> in our society, notwithstanding reflexive denial of its prevalence by some physicians. An estimated <u>one-third</u> of the general population harbors this trait.

The condition reflects interactions of a genetic tendency to produce excess insulin ("the thrifty gene"), contemporary eating habits (overeating and so-called forced feeding), enhancement of insulin release by aspartame (Chapter XIV), and other factors. The striking increased mitogenicity of insulin glargine and other insulin analogs over human insulin (Berger 2000) assumes considerable relevance relative to brain, prostate and other tumors.

A partial list of the author's researches and reviews of <u>diabetogenic hyperinsulinism</u> (Roberts 1962a-d, 1968) appears in the bibliography. This term implies that the repeated and prolonged secretion of excessive insulin could culminate in diabetes mellitus.

Recurrent hunger and a craving for sweets are two hallmarks of reactive hypoglycemia. If unrecognized and untreated, the associated extreme weakness, sleepiness, and other symptoms invite overindulgence in sugar, sugar substitutes, caffeine, nicotine, alcohol, amphetamines, and other stimulants (Roberts 1970, 1971a,b). These influences may then compound the ravages of hypoglycemia on the brain and other organs.

Birth Defects

The subject of aspartame-associated birth defects was considered in Chapter X. It is known that a fetus may suffer serious injury from pesticides and other chemicals at levels of exposure considerably lower than the concentrations affecting adults.

This issue requires clarification. The author's belief that pregnant women should avoid aspartame products (Appendix C) has been criticized by industry. In this context, corporate funding was withdrawn from Dr. Diana Dow-Edwards when her study suggested this problem. She then had to pay personally for further research.

Fractures; Osteoporosis

Increased brittleness of bones has been identified among girls who consume considerable carbonated beverages, especially colas. The risk of broken bones was <u>five times higher</u> for active cola-drinking girls in a study of 460 ninth- and tenth-grade girls at a Boston-area high school (Wyshak 2000). It probably results from deficient calcium intake and the effects of phosphoric acid.

Altered Sex Ratio

The possible altered sex ratio among offspring of aspartame users requires clarification. Males before and during puberty appear to be at greatest risk, even with exposures to only parts per <u>trillion</u>.

Hints about this phenomenon exist in other areas. For example, the male/female sex ratio is lower in the offspring of men exposed to a dioxin (TCDD). Indeed, this effect may persist years after such exposure (Mocarelli 2000).

Aspartame Addiction

The term "substance abuse" justifiably can be invoked relative to clinical aspartame addiction. This serious problem was described in Chapter VII-G.

Unnecessary Surgery and Interventions

Many aspartame reactors were subjected to needless operations and major interventions. They included hysterectomy, prostate surgery, cataract removal, laser treatment for presumed symptomatic diabetic retinopathy, and coronary arteriography. Removal of the gallbladder had been performed in Case IX-D-15 for recurring nausea and abdominal pain. These symptoms persisted postoperatively until she realized that she was an aspartame victim.

Disinformation For the Medical Profession and the Public

Education of both physicians and the public about aspartame disease has been curtailed. The specifics appear in Section 7.

<u>High-risk groups</u> (Section 3) ought to be warned. They include pregnant women, nursing mothers, young children, older persons, families with members who are aspartame reactors, and persons having a genetic tendency to phenylketonuria (PKU). Individuals with histories of migraine, hypoglycemia, diabetes mellitus, alcoholism and drug abuse also should be so informed.

It is incumbent upon doctors to question patients presenting with <u>any</u> of the complaints listed in Sections 1 and 2 about aspartame use. If encountered, a brief trial of abstinence should be recommended <u>before</u> embarking upon expensive tests and consultations. Unfortunately, conveying such awareness has been a challenge.

- The *Journal of the American Medical Association* repeatedly refused its forum for reports on aspartame disease even though the A.M.A. Council on Scientific Affairs (1985) published its approval of aspartame therein. (This periodical contained expensive full-page multicolor advertisements for popular aspartame products nearly every week in the 1980s.)

- A short letter written by the author to the *New England Journal of Medicine*, commenting on three recent articles about aspartame it had published, was not accepted. The editors stated "this subject has been sufficiently covered and needs no further discussion in the *Journal*."

- An abstract submitted for the 1987 annual scientific session of the American Diabetes Association was titled, "Complications Associated with Aspartame in Diabetics." It summarized my experience with 58 diabetic patients. The Committee on Medical and Scientific Programs not only rejected it for presentation, but refused to print the abstract in the program supplement.

E. RELATED CONSIDERATIONS

"Congress has shown little interest in protecting consumers from the hazards of dietary supplements."
　　　　Dr. David Kessler (2000)
　　　　(former FDA Commissioner)

It is prudent to recall an adage when regulatory agencies and consumers make premature decisions about novel foods and additives: "Nature does not play favorites, it plays tricks." Proposals for new chemical sweeteners and synthetic food substitutes **must** be carefully analyzed **before** approval. This is particularly true if large long-term pre-marketing studies on humans were not performed, as was the case with aspartame.

The author has repeatedly emphasized the shortcomings of animal studies in this realm for various reasons, including differences in metabolism and life span. (The life cycle of rats or mice is only four years.) Persons interested in the multiple deficiencies of animal studies involving aspartame should read the 1977 Bressler Report, which is available on the Internet.

The Need For Careful Scrutiny of New Sweeteners

A major lesson to be learned from the aspartame experience is the need for extreme vigilance by regulatory agencies when considering proposed high-potency sweeteners, particularly derivatives of L-aspartic acid. Owing to industrial support and leverage in the daunting task of obtaining approval for any "breakthrough," research technologists receive considerable encouragement.

- A compound being studied at French Universite Claude Bernard is 7000 times sweeter than sucrose.
- A major beverage company is experimenting with a series of L-aspartyl-D-*a*-aminoalkanoyl-S) - *a*-alkylbenzylamines.

The Evaluation and Regulation of "Fake Foods"

The hard-earned insights about aspartame disease should be extended to the barrage of applications for low-calorie, low-fat, low-cholesterol and sugar-free food or food substitutes. Such products ought NOT be released without confirmation of long-term safety by extensive pre-marketing trials on humans. Risk may be introduced by homogenization, reduced particle size, malabsorption, and combinations with aspartame or other additives.

Attempts by the food industry to stay ahead of successful promotional campaigns that increase demand are illustrated by breakfast cereals. Computerized automation has enabled the continuous production and more sophisticated manipulation of cereal grains. The cooking extruder, for example, can create highly palatable cornflakes and other cereals sweetened with sugar or other sweeteners.

Physicians and dietitians continue to find themselves outpaced by these imaginative innovators of "guilt-free" low-calorie, sugar-free foods or food substitutes that can fool the taste buds. Similarly, governmental regulators are confronted by producers for the approval of faux sugars and "fake foods" without extensive pre-marketing trials on humans. They contend that these products are made from substances classed "generally recognized as safe" (GRAS). In the case of Simplesse®, it was asserted that this fat simulator derived from proteins in milk and egg whites is "simply cooked, chopped egg white" (Berger 1988).

In the light of researches on aspartame, issues such as the following require clarification by corporate-neutral scientists before approval of comparable "new all-natural fat substitutes."

- Does decreased particle size and homogenization influence the absorption and metabolism of its component amino acids? As a case in point, alteration of milk and whole eggs increases the absorption of free cholesterol (Oster 1982). Particle size also significantly alters the physical characteristics of aspartame (Joachim 1987; Stegink 1987).

- Could the product induce malabsorption and other nutritional deficiencies?
- Can the rapid influx of phenylalanine and other "egg white" amino acids into the brain cause neurologic, psychiatric or behavioral reactions?

Regulation of Non-Aspartame Phenylalanine

Concerned investigators believe that the use of pure amino acids, especially phenylalanine, must be carefully monitored in view of many reported suggestive alterations affecting brain and neurotransmitter function (Chapter XXII). Editorializing on the eosinophilia-myalgia syndrome precipitated by use of L-tryptophan, Duffy (1992) stressed that physicians should be better informed about the potential hazards of such consumer products – including the health and welfare of future generations.

Many popular books and periodicals in "health" stores in the United States extol the value of phenylalanine for restoring energy, minimizing stress, combating depression, improving memory, and aiding weight loss. Similar claims are made for other amino acids. A feature writer for *The Evening Times* of West Palm Beach (April 14, 1987, p. A-14) wrote an article titled, "Mainlining Amino Acids Can Work." She reported the "miraculous" regression of depression after taking tyrosine, DL-phenylalanine, tryptophan and arginine. Other dramatic responses to specific amino acids were alleged by dyslexics, patients with chronic pain, drug addicts, obese persons, and alcoholics – the "trick" being to ingest them as far as possible from meals so "they don't get shouted down by the other amino acids."

- Part of the rationale for using L-phenylalanine as an antidepressant is its conversion to tyrosine, and then to dopamine and norepinephrine. This amino acid also can be decarboxylated to phenylethylamine, a compound having chemical and behavioral effects similar to amphetamine.
- Another explanation for the use of D-phenylalanine in treating pain is the inhibition of metenkephalin degradation(Young 1987).

The general failure of L-phenylalanine and D-phenylalanine to ameliorate depression and pain (Chapter XX) led to prohibition of their sale in Canada (Young 1987). Moreover, Health and Welfare of Canada designated single amino acids, or mixtures of amino acids demonstrating pharmacologic effects, as "drugs" in 1985. They include the D, L or DL forms of phenylalanine, tryptophan, tyrosine and lysine. Such regulation was passed to minimize any toxic effects of these products in the long term, particularly with curtailed protein intake.

XXVI

EPIDEMIOLOGY

"As physicians, we are not here to do battle with the
government for our self-interests... Patient advocacy
 means putting forth intensive efforts to eradicate
threats to public health."
> Dr. William S. Hotchkiss (1987)
> Former President, American Medical Association

Epidemiology encompasses those factors that influence the development, frequency and distribution of disease. The magnitude of aspartame disease, coupled with the enormous consumption of aspartame, warrants epidemiologic consideration. Unfortunately, epidemiologists are regarded with suspicion by some scientists who joke that they are good at discovering a health problem only when it has become epidemic... as in the present context.

Aspartame products have been available commercially since 1981. Physicians and public health professionals ought to consider their possible role in major problems that developed or intensified thereafter. Examples include migraine, epilepsy, visual problems, allergies, attention-deficit/hyperactivity, multiple sclerosis, parkinsonism, and Alzheimer's disease. Similarly, birth defects, impaired intelligence, sex ratio changes, and behavioral abnormalities among children whose mothers consumed aspartame during pregnancy require scrutiny. Aspartame reactors and their relatives have repeatedly stressed these apparent associations in correspondence.

Several caveats are appropriate.

- While the science of epidemiology may enable determining the incidence of a particular disease in the population, it does not establish the causation of that disease in a given individual.
- Dr. Ephraim Kahn (1987), a specialist in environmental epidemiology, asserted

762

"But reports by patients or parents in response to
a pre-designed questionnaire and as part of a
study design, although subjective, are not
anecdotal. Their validity would depend on the
quality of the study design and the care with
which the study was performed.*

REPORTED ASPARTAME REACTIONS

Many thousands of complaints about aspartame consumption – exclusive of those in the author's data base – have been submitted by letter, phone or e-mail to the following:

- The Food and Drug Administration (FDA)
- Centers for Disease Control (CDC)
- G. D. Searle & Company
- The NutraSweet Company
- The Community Nutrition Institute
- Aspartame Victims And Their Friends
- The Aspartame Consumer Network
- Mission Possible
- Dr. W. C. Monte (Arizona State University)
- Dr. R. J. Wurtman (Massachusetts Institute of Technology) – more than 100 persons with seizures attributed to aspartame, and "well over 1,000" letters and "related communications" reported in the *Congressional Record – Senate* (May 7, 1985)

The projections are staggering. For example, Dr. Anthony Kulczycki, Jr. (1987) estimated a minimum of six thousand (!) individuals with aspartame allergy in the United States over a decade ago.

The CDC Analysis - 1984

The Centers for Disease Control (1984) reported its "passive surveillance" of 517 complainants who were interviewed during 1984. Two-thirds experienced neurologic or behavioral symptoms such as headache, dizziness and mood alteration. Other problems included gastrointestinal complaints (24%), allergic skin reactions (15%), and menstrual disorders (6%).

---

*©1987 *The Journal of Pesticide Reform*. Reproduced with permission.

This analysis of 231 selected complainants analyzed by the CDC is pertinent: "13% reported that symptoms recurred after rechallenge with more than one product, and another 15% reported that symptoms recurred on second use of the same product."

The FDA Analysis - 1995

The major side effects reported to the FDA by 6583 aspartame complainants as of April 20, 1995 are summarized in the following table. It is noteworthy that this agency arbitrarily chose to exclude 649 of the initial reactors because of "differences in the adverse reaction information collected."

MOST FREQUENT SYMPTOMS BY 6583 ASPARTAME COMPLAINANTS*

Symptom	Count	Percent
Headache	1647	28.1%
Dizziness/Poor equilibrium	735	11.2%
Change in Mood	656	10.0%
Vomiting or Nausea	647	9.8%
Abdominal Pain and Cramps	453	6.9%
Change in Vision	362	5.5%
Diarrhea	330	5.0%
Seizures and Convulsions	290	4.4%
Memory Loss	255	3.9%
Fatigue-Weakness	242	3.7%
Other Neurological	230	3.5%
Rash	226	3.4%
Sleep Problems	201	3.1%
Hives	191	2.9%
Change in Heart Rate	185	2.8%
Itching	175	2.7%
Grand Mal	174	2.6%
Change in Sensation (numbness, tingling)	172	2.6%
Local Swelling	114	1.7%
Change in Activity Level	113	1.7%
Difficulty Breathing	112	1.7%
Oral Sensory Changes	108	1.6%
Change in Menstrual Pattern	107	1.6%
Symptoms reported by less than 100 complainants	1812	-----

*Some consumers described more than one symptom attributed to aspartame products

Additional Comments

On August 7, 1986, the author requested copies of FDA data on aspartame reactors. An FDA representative replied that there had been "approximately 2,800 consumer complaints describing adverse reactions allegedly due to the ingestion of aspartame" <u>since</u> the earlier CDC report cited above. Several important points are noteworthy.

- Those aspartame reactors who concluded that aspartame caused their problems, and then made the effort to contact this agency or other interested groups, represent a **small** fraction of persons so affected.
- Suspected aspartame reactions remain underreported because physicians are **not** required to report complaints about food additives, as mandated in the case of drug reactions.
- The number of regional FDA investigators who handled these complaints (and numerous additional ones about other products) have been limited. The author was told that each of the estimated eleven FDA investigators in South Florida forwards only about five alleged aspartame-related problems to Washington.

Statistics published in *Morbidity And Mortality Weekly Report* (December 19, 1986 Supplement) serve as a "silent footnote." They emphasize that the Years of Potential Life Lost (YPLL) through premature mortality had increased only for diabetes mellitus and chronic obstructive pulmonary disease. The widespread use of aspartame products by diabetics is germane.

PERSONAL ENCOUNTERS

The author's data on 1,200 aspartame reactors, and results collated from the detailed survey questionnaire, appear in Sections 2 and 4, respectively.

The extensive annotations and supplementary letters from persons with aspartame disease who completed the questionnaire proved remarkable. Such a concentrated barrage of product-related complaints had never been encountered by the author during five decades of medical practice and research. Intelligent consumers railed bitterly against manufacturers, the medical profession, and governmental bureaus charged with the responsibility for monitoring the challenged foods and additives.

Appearances on talk shows also evoked a deluge of calls... including scores of requests for the questionnaire. This experience offered added proof for the existence of **many** aspartame reactors in the general community.

- The day after my interview on local TV Channel 5 (November 3, 1986), <u>28</u> calls for the questionnaire were received from persons who felt they had aspartame disease.

- The office manager of a major local law firm called that same day and requested 90 (!) forms. When asked about this unusual request, she mentioned having observed profound changes (especially depression and erratic behavior) and poor work performance in many employees. Furthermore, several young secretaries had expressed concern over the unexplained loss of their menstrual periods. Being in charge of the beverage machines, this manager <u>already</u> had correlated such complaints with their large consumption of diet cola beverages.

- More than 100 letters, cards and phone calls were received after my one-hour interview on the Irv Homer talk show, featured by WWBD (Philadelphia).

XXVII

SAFETY CONSIDERATIONS

"One really can't tell from animal testing how safe an additive will be in man. So the prudent thing to do, on the basis of the experimental data, is to lean over backward not to greatly increase risks."

Dr. Paul E. Johnson (1970)

"Long-delayed effects are frequently difficult to relate to their specific causes. Thus, it is conceivable that injuries due to unrecognized causes have been produced by common materials that have long been produced by common materials that have long been considered safe as foods or for use in foods. In this regard we are concerned with cancer, genetic damage and birth defects, premature old age, cardiovascular, endocrine and mental disorders, and other human ills of unexplained etiology."*

Dr. Julius M. Coon (1970)

The severe reactions to aspartame products detailed in preceding sections, – coupled with increasing numbers of persons diagnosed as having unexplained "chronic fatigue syndrome," fibromyalgia" and other evolving public health problems – validate reference to an "aspartame Armageddon." A concerned European Union banned the addition of aspartame to any food consumed by infants (Directive 96/83/EC).

Governmental agencies and scientific organizations charged with evaluating alleged reactions to aspartame products reported by health professionals and consumers, however, continue to ignore the long-term ramifications. These attitudes recall the assertion of famed psychologist, B. F. Skinner (1986): "The people who control the condition in which we live have no reason to think beyond more than five or ten years."

---

*©1970 *Modern Medicine*. Reproduced with permission.

- Experience in many fields, including medicine, agriculture and politics, indicates how the failure of a single system can synergize other system failures. Accordingly, concerned scientists recognize the need for a new multivariate measure of "possibility" monitoring, to project future threats, and to institute earlier intervention – whether in technologic, social or public health realms.

- In her book, *Living Downstream: An Ecologist Looks at Cancer And The Environment*, Sandra Stingraber (1997) urged the principle of the least toxic alternative for all activities having potential public health consequences. This guide presumes that toxic substances would not be used when there is another way of accomplishing the task.

About half the reactors in this series used aspartame products because of the conviction they would help them lose or "control" weight (Section 1). Moreover, patients with diabetes, hypoglycemia, heart disease, and a host of other disorders felt that substituting aspartame for sugar was both desirable and risk-free. These perceptions usually derived from focused advertising. On other hand, Section 101.9 of the Federal Food, Drug and Cosmetic Act (FDCA) asserts

> "A food labeled under the provisions of this section shall be deemed to be misbranded... if its labeling represents, suggests or implies that the food because of the presence or absence of certain dietary properties is adequate or effective in the prevention, cure, mitigation or treatment of any disease or symptom."

Cumulative Toxicity

The adverse effects of aspartame products, and other chemicals or activities having potential neurotoxic and carcinogenic effects can be cumulative. This is illustrated by persons who travel frequently by air at altitudes above 30,000 feet, and are thereby subject to increased radiation. Other examples are pesticides (Roberts 1990b), megadoses of vitamin E (Roberts 1994c), excessive female hormones, and arbitrary fluoridation (Roberts 1992f).

Challenged Pre-Certification Data

Some of the critical data submitted to the Food and Drug Administration (FDA) before it approved aspartame have been challenged. They include animal studies and clinical trials. The debates thereon appear in the *Congressional Record-Senate* of May 7, 1985 and August 1, 1985.

Senator Metzenbaum expressed his belief that *the burden of proof for the safety of aspartame is the responsibility of the manufacturer and producers, NOT government.* He made this statement about aspartame during the November 3, 1987 hearing of the Committee on Labor and Human Resources.

> "In the history of the FDA, has there ever been any other case in which the scientific data submitted to the FDA caused the FDA to be so concerned about the representations made to it that it was sent to a U.S. attorney for presentment to a grand jury for indictment — any other cause? ... It is my understanding — I think this occurred in 1977 — that prior to that time there had never been a case in which the submissions of a company to the FDA had provided a basis to submit their file, their record, to the U.S. Attorney for submission to a grand jury, and that since then there has certainly been none. Is that correct?"

Thomas Scarlett, Chief Counsel for the FDA, replied to the Senator on December 22, 1987: "There was at least one case referred to the FDA to the Department of Justice for the consideration of criminal charges because of irregularities in the reporting of test data. The case involved the drug MER-29, and was referred sometimes in the 1960s."

Senator William Proxmire

Senator Proxmire (cited by Honorof 1975) was one of the first pubic officials to criticize rapid attempts for licensing aspartame. He was disturbed by the allowance of only 30 days for scientific and public comment after notice in the July 26, 1974 *Federal Register*. He commented that the supporting data "took four large whiskeycase-like boxes to contain it... There is no way it could be analyzed or criticized thoroughly in such a short period of time." He demanded further scientific tests concerning potential brain damage to children, especially in combination with monosodium glutamate (MSG).

Senator Proxmire issued a press release on October 20, 1974 that became a prelude of future concern.

- He charged the then-FDA Commissioner with *"misfeasance in office by allowing a potentially brain-damaging sweetener to be manufactured and sold even before a hearing into its dangers is held."*
- *"While the general use of aspartame can bring a financial killing to the manufacturer, it may also kill the brain cells of countless children."*

Accusing the FDA of "stacking the deck in favor of the manufacturer and against the public," the Senator emphasized that 30 days is not enough to catalog the documents and evaluate these massive data. Failing this, he asserted that every box of breakfast food, bottle of soft drink, and basket of fried chicken which includes aspartame or MSG should be labelled: "<u>Danger, this product can cause brain damage</u>."

Other Considerations

Misleading information pertaining to the use of aspartame products by <u>diabetics</u> offers another case in point. My observations suggest that its consumption can be conducive to loss of control and the aggravation or simulation of diabetic complications (neuropathy, retinopathy, vasculopathy (Chapter XIII). The problem, however, is often subtle.

Aspartame reactors can be likened to canaries used in mines for the early detection of toxic exposure. To my knowledge, *there is no dependable animal model for evaluating the toxicity of aspartame in humans.* The rat liver metabolizes phenylalanine more efficiently than the human liver. Some monkeys detoxify methyl alcohol to a limited extend, but man hardly can do so (Chapter XXI). Moreover, rats and other animals apparently fail to perceive aspartame as "sweet," and therefore do not replicate changes involving the cephalic phase of insulin production triggered by the taste of sweet.

Neotame: Will History Repeat Itself?

The Monsanto Company petitioned the FDA on January 23, 1999 to approve its high intensity sweetener, N-[N-(3,3-dimethylbutyl)-L-*a*-aspartyl]-L-phenylalanine 1- methyl ester, as an all-purpose sweetener and flavor enhancer. This analog of aspartame (on which the patent had expired), named Neotame, is 30-60 times sweeter than aspartame.

The author submitted detailed letters of professional opposition to such approval – dated March 3, 1998, February 25, 1999, and April 10, 1999 – pending additional data about the safety of this chemical in humans. He concluded with this opinion:

"I am a totally corporate-neutral physician who is concerned about the ongoing exposure of the population to aspartame and numerous other chemicals that were approved without adequate long-term studies by corporate-neutral investigators and politically-neutral regulators. Let me repeat: I anticipate a public health tragedy if the aspartame problem is allowed to be repeated in the case of Neotame without these safeguards!"

Remarkably and coincidentally, my novel projecting a public-health scenario caused by a fabricated analog of aspartame was published. It is titled, THE CACOF CONSPIRACY: LESSONS OF THE NEW MILLENNIUM (Sunshine Sentinel Press, 1999). When conceived a decade earlier, the author had no knowledge of Neotame.

A. ASPARTAME AS A "DRUG"

The impressive biophysiologic effects of aspartame (Section 2 and 5) provide justify classifying aspartame as a "drug." Indeed, this chemical was first devised as a drug for treating peptic ulcer.

Deficient Reporting of Aspartame Reactions

All practising physicians are urged by the FDA to report "serious reactions, observations of events of described in the package information insert (of drugs), and reactions to newly marketed products of particular importance." They receive copies of the relevant Form FDA-1639, along with detailed instructions, in the *FDA Medical Bulletin*. But this agency has NOT insisted upon comparable accountability about overt reactions to aspartame products, or criticism about disinformation thereon, from manufacturers and producers despite current use by a majority of the population.

According to current regulations, manufacturers, packers and distributors are required to file reports about any "serious and unexpected" adverse reactions to drugs, and "any significant increase in the frequency" of expected or serious reactions, within 15 working days.

Contrary to the "Dear Doctor" letters mailed to physicians by drug firms after reports of side effects following the release of drugs, such vigilant postmarketing surveillance is NOT required for approved GRAS additives.. The paucity of drug reports in the postmarketing experience outside of the United States – as with the "flank pain syndrome" associated with suprofen, a nonsteroidal anti-inflammatory drug (Rossi 1988) – is equally

772

disturbing. The infrequent publication of aspartame-associated problems by journals abroad, for reasons discussed in Section 7, represents a comparable phenomenon.

A food claimed to prevent disease is considered a "drug"... and therefore subject to pre-marketing verification relative to both safety and effectiveness. Realistically, the FDA has supported health claims implied for "low calorie" and "reduced calorie" products – with particular reference to weight loss or control – in the management of diabetes, heart disease and hypertension. In effect, the current consumption of aspartame constitutes a massive uncontrolled "clinical trial."

The Consequences of Delayed Warnings

The harmful side effects of new drugs and "supplements" may become evident only after being taken by several hundred thousand persons. The specific reaction patterns negate manufacturer allegations that the initial reports were "individual idiosyncratic reactions" or "coincidence." Furthermore, one cannot rely on the clinical safety of chemically-similar compounds (*The Wall Street Journal* August 10, 1990, p. A-12).

Historically, congressional investigators reported that more than half of the new drugs sold in the United States were found to have severe or fatal side effects after their approval by the FDA. These findings appear in *FDA Drug Review: Postapproval Risks 1976-85* (GAO/PEMD-90-15. The term "serious" was applied to any adverse reaction leading to hospitalization, increased length of hospital stay, severe or permanent disability, or death. Included among adverse reactions were heart failure, shock, convulsions, kidney or liver failure, blood disorders, blindness, birth defects and fetal toxicity. The GAO report also emphasized a time lapse of up to five years between recognition such problems and action by the FDA, including other side effects known to the FDA before approval!

> The serious delayed consequences of drugs and other chemicals have been numerous. One involves reproductive abnormalities in males and females from fetal exposure to diethylstilbestrol (DES) – including misshaped uterus, premature delivery, miscarriage, atopic pregnancy, infertility, and cervical/testicular cancer.

B. MISLEADING AND INADEQUATE LABELING

Three agencies are empowered to enforce federal laws governing foods and their labeling. The Food and Drug Administration is responsible for all foods except meat, poultry and egg products, which the United States Department of Agriculture (USDA) regulates. The Federal Trade Commission (FTC) oversees the advertising of foods.

Regulations for food labeling began with the Federal Food and Drug Act of 1906. It prohibited false or misleading statements on food or drug labels. A 1975 nutrition-labeling regulation developed by the FDA mandated the net content or net weight of a product, and the listing of ingredients in descending order of predominance by weight (that is, from the greatest to least amounts). Dr. Allen L. Forbes (1986), Director of the Center for Food Safety and Applied Nutrition of the FDA, appropriately wrote, "Extreme care is needed to maintain the accuracy of such information and the integrity of the food label generally."

General Considerations

The FDA had 30 percent fewer inspectors for preclearing label claims in 1986 than in 1980 (*News/Sun Sentinel of Fort Lauderdale*, November 28, 1986, p. F-6). Raymond Newberry (Chief, Labeling Enforcement for the FDA) stated, "If I were to walk into a grocery, I could find technical violations on the labels on every third or fourth product; and 50 percent of those would be substantially misleading" (*News/Sun Sentinel of Fort Lauderdale*, November 28, 1986, p. F-1).

The Nutrition Agency Committee of London's Coronary Prevention Group (1986) published a "rational approach" to the nutritional labeling of foods. It proposed that the total fat, saturated fat, total sugar, salt and fiber content be classified as "high, medium and low." This Committee averred

> "Consumers need clear, informative food labeling which is readily understood to help them in choosing a healthy diet by purchasing foods with a known nutrient content... The numerical expression of nutrient is too complex for most consumers. Consumer surveys clearly demonstrate the public's need for an additional simpler and more meaningful display of the information."

Physicians need to be constantly reminded of deficient labeling relative to other food additives.

- There have been near-fatal cases of high blood potassium concentration (hyperkalemia) from the liberal use of potassium-containing salt substitutes. Patients with severe kidney disease and diabetics taking medications that influence potassium metabolism are at high risk. But labels may not warn against the use of such products

in cooking, or indicate the safe maximum daily dose. Some even have wide-bore openings to facilitate cooking (Hoyt 1986).
- The Ad Hoc Advisory Committee on Hypersensitivity to Food Constituents of the FDA indicated that allergic reactions to foods have become a serious health problem warranting better food labeling (*Internal Medicine News* November 1, 1986, p. 3). It recommended that restaurants and fast food establishments provide **complete** ingredient information for **all** their products.
- Persons highly sensitive to manufactured monosodium glutamate (MSG) are in danger when labels fail to reveal its presence or that of related substances (Roberts 1993a).

Aspartame: A Neglected Label Ingredient

Products containing aspartame should be labeled properly.

Consumer advocates emphasize the importance of misleading labeling, with particular emphasis on confusing "buzz words." Examples include "sugar-free," "naturally," "no preservatives added," "no artificial flavors," "light," and "all natural." They also stress that the potential for abuse is not as "obvious" as it would seem, even for alcoholic beverages.

Patients who are allergic to aspartame (Chapter VIII) and other additives (such as monosodium glutamate) must pick their way through "the label mine field" to avoid the severe consequences of their inadvertent consumption. In the absence of terms that are easily readable and understood, they must resort to analyzing **all** ingredients listed on labels.

The importance of labeling aspartame products likely to be used by infants and children was emphasized in Chapter XI .

Where the FDA gave virtual blanket approval for the incorporation of aspartame, aspartame reactors were forced to be even more vigilant. For example, the National Yogurt Association petitioned the agency to allow the addition of aspartame to yogurt without labeling this ingredient. Yet, many patients with aspartame disease have singled out "light" yogurt as a cause of severe reactions.

In its June 28, 1996 authorization of aspartame as a general purpose synthetic tabletop sweetener, the FDA rescinded the requirement that labels of aspartame products state: "Phenylketonurics: Contains Phenylalanine."

Representative Case Report (Also see Case XXVII-B-3)

Case XXVII-B-1

A female attorney promptly experienced severe reactions to aspartame products on several occasions, two being inadvertent exposures. They included incapacitating headache, flashes of light, dizziness, and vomiting. She then could not work for two days. These reactions occurred even after chewing a stick of aspartame gum. One of the culprits was an aspartame-containing yogurt. She complained to the manufacturer: "Your non-fat yogurt container had absolutely no indication of the fact that it contains aspartame, nor does it have the little red label indicating aspartame is an ingredient. I acknowledge that your label does indicate a term equivalent to a warning against aspartame, but it is not commonly understood."

Many aspartame reactors have expressed the conviction when completing the questionnaire (Section 4) that products containing aspartame **must** be properly labeled. Some cited the precedent of cigarette packaging, as the label reading, "SURGEON GENERAL'S WARNING: Smoking causes lung cancer, heart disease, emphysema, and may complicate pregnancy."

The <u>actual content</u> of aspartame also should appear on labels.

- The American Diabetes Association (1987) issued a position statement wherein the food industry was encouraged "to label products with the amounts of noncaloric sweeteners present, as it should all food ingredients."
- A statement by Dr. Richard Wurtman published in the *Congressional Record-Senate* (1985, p. 5493), asserted: " I doubt that one consumer (or physician) in a thousand now realizes, for example, that a can of TAB provides less than one fourth aspartame than a can of Diet Pepsi or Diet Cola."
- More aspartame is added to certain soft drinks to compensate for alterations in sweetness caused by its breakdown products (Chapter XX).

Case III-1 illustrates the importance of adequate labeling. This registered nurse suffered a severe seizure after ingesting two liters of an orange drink containing aspartame. In her discussions with the FDA, she discovered that this brand and various "diet" orange sodas contain appreciably higher concentrations of aspartame – 335 mg per 12 fluid ounces, or 930 mg per liter – than other flavors.

The undetermined biologic effects of racemization of aspartic acid and phenylalanine after heating, or during the prolonged storage of aspartame products at high temperatures (Chapters XX and XXV), underscore the need for adequate labeling relative to exposure to heat and duration of storage. This may be even more important for products containing certain components that might act as catalysts, such as chocolate.

These labeling are mandated by other countries.

- Since 1984, labels in Israel state, "Do not consume more than three grams aspartame daily for adults" – both in English and Hebrew. In addition to an expiration date two months after production, labels advise, "Store in a cool place not over 22 Centigrade."
- The smaller cans (280 ml) of a popular diet cola in Toronto indicate the presence of aspartame.
- Some companies recognize this problem by indicating, "Best taste if used by (date)." (It also serves as a defense tactic in the event of suit.)

The issue of disinformation on labels compounds the problem.

Representative Case Report

Case XXVII-2

A 66-year-old diabetic woman had been controlled with oral medication. She developed "such severe headaches I couldn't function and was disoriented" after drinking one brand of diet cola. The same reaction recurred during three retesting trials. She had multiple allergies, including hives and drug reactions.

The patient avoided this cola beverage after hearing about aspartame reactions on a television program. She subsequently drank another diet beverage because its label indicated that saccharin was the sweetener. After drinking a few sips, she experienced an intense headache. ("I felt my brain was swelling and to be too big for my cranium.") She wrote

> "I called the bottling company and asked if they were using aspartame. They said yes! I told them the can said saccharin. They told me they were just using up the old cans, and would then change the contents as listed. I didn't get any satisfaction from them, so I called the Food and Drug Department in Gahu.

777

I told them the story and they just said, 'Yes, that's what they do.' They were very uncooperative. I felt I was hitting my head against a brick wall. They didn't care a thing about me.

"The outcome is that I eat nothing with aspartame listed as an ingredient. I find very few drinks without it. It is difficult for me, as I am not a coffee drinker."

Problems With "The Fine Print"

Even highly motivated parents have overlooked "the A word" because of small print on labels. Some were appalled that a magnifying glass was needed to read them.

Another problem encountered with ineffective "warning" labels on numerous products is that consumers become inured to them, in part because they are a source of unwanted advice. The warnings about smoking, and the fetal alcohol syndrome risk among pregnant women drinking alcoholic beverages, provide examples.

Representative Case Report

Case XXVII-B-3

A 53-year-old aspartame reactor developed depression, lethargy and fibromyalgia after consuming aspartame products. When these symptoms recurred after taking yogurt, he found that aspartame was indeed present – but with the help of a magnifying glass. He suggested

> "The government should at least make it easier to identify toxins in our food, and let us decide for ourselves. People with difficulty reading small print should be protected by the government. The FDA needs to develop an international "coding" system, such as ASP or MSG in bold red letters. Why can't the government make it easier for us to 'censor' our foods. Even movies have easily identifiable rating symbols. Heck, anyone knows that K inside a circle means that the food is kosher!"

Diagnosis By Ordeal

The problem of inadequate labeling is illustrated by the cited case reports. Another involves the following experience of a college educator who developed severe symptoms within one or two hours after ingesting aspartame. She actively attempted to avoid such products thereafter. This reactor raised the added possibility that the manufacturer may have used the same mixing equipment without thoroughly removing the aspartame when subsequently making "regular" candy.

> "I used to think that it would be enough to read the labels, but I'm becoming more and more convinced that the only way to stay completely free from consuming aspartame involuntarily is to have the product taken off the market. The other day I bought some regular candy. The package said nothing about aspartame. For two days in a row after eating a few pieces, I had terrible ringing in my ears, felt slightly dizzy, and had awful mood swings just like when I used to consume a lot of aspartame. They don't even give you a choice to avoid the substance. You stumble across it by accident."

C. THE MAXIMUM ACCEPTABLE DAILY INTAKE (ADI) ISSUE

The FDA originally set the ADI for aspartame at 20 mg/kg. (One kg is 2.2 pounds.) It then ignored its own standard safety factor for soft drinks (see below) by doubling the ADI in 1983. Accordingly, an adult weighing 130 pounds would have to drink four to five liters of aspartame soft drinks to attain the new level.

Others here and abroad disagree with this recommended ADI guideline. The State of Israel asserts that two liters of an aspartame beverage should not exceed 50 percent of the ADI for a 70 kg adult.

Other parameters for toxicity in animal studies also have severe limitations. Measurement of the acute toxicity of a drug or product by determining the LD_{50} has been incorporated in applications for licensure. This refers to "the lethal dose" in 50 percent of a population so exposed. With the availability of other methods for assessing acute toxicity since this assay was first proposed in 1927, Dayan et al (1984) challenged the wisdom of the "formal" LD_{50}.

Criticisms of the Current ADI

Quantitative information about aspartame content is lacking on the labels of such products in the United States (see below). Accordingly, even concerned parents are unable to calculate the amounts their children consume.

Dr. Frank E. Young, former FDA Commissioner, defined the ADI during the November 3, 1987 Senate hearing on aspartame as "an estimate of the amount of the food additive, expressed on a body weight basis in *animal* studies, that can be ingested daily *over a lifetime* without appreciable health risk. It focuses on continued exposure *over a lifetime*, and not on the exposure that could occur on any given day" (italics supplied).

An arbitrarily high ADI could have serious consequences.

- Elsas and Trotter (1987) expressed concern over the potential for severe brain dysfunction caused by elevated plasma phenylalanine concentrations when PKU heterozygotes ingest the amounts of aspartame approved by "several biopolitical organizations."
- Dr. M. Adrian Gross, an FDA investigator-scientist, challenged the licensing of aspartame. He noted in the *Congressional Record-Senate* of August 1, 1985: "I would view the Acceptable Daily Intake (ADI) set by the FDA for aspartame (50 mg/kg body weight/day) as totally unwarranted and extremely high in that it can be associated with completely unacceptable risks as far as the induction of such (brain) tumors is concerned." Dr. Gross concluded his discussion with this statement: "It is clear that risks of this magnitude for what the FDA regards as a 'safe' level of exposure to aspartame represent an outright calamity or disaster."
- Senator Howard Metzenbaum (see above) took the FDA to task for having increased the acceptable daily maximum intake of aspartame from 20 mg/kg body weight to 50 mg/kg. He pointed out that this action represented an exception to the usual 100-fold safety factor used for regulated food additives.

The maximum daily intake of "aspartame that is safe" remains unknown. It is the author's opinion that the current arbitrary ADI is high. For example, the cited 31-year-old nurse developed her first convulsion within 12 hours after ingesting two liters of an aspartame soft drink – calculated as 18.3 mg/kg of her weight.

Corporate representatives have asserted that a person would have to drink enormous quantities, such as one can of aspartame-containing soda every eight minutes for 24 hours, before achieving blood concentrations approaching the purported toxic threshold. I disagree. There are no practical means at present for measuring concomitant brain elevations of phenylalanine or methanol. The great variations in brain concentrations of tryptophan and neurotransmitters in experimental animals precludes projecting the ADI from such data onto man. Moreover, the conversion of phenylalanine to tyrosine is much slower in man than rodents.

Pregnant Women

The potential hazards to the fetus when a pregnant woman consumes aspartame, independent of proneness to phenylketonuria, have been discussed in Chapter X. Fetal plasma phenylalanine concentrations were nearly double those of the maternal levels when normal pregnant women took "potential abuse concentrations" (100-200 mg/kg body weight) of aspartame.

Infants and Children

The concern over aspartame ingestion by breast-feeding mothers and young children was discussed in Chapter XI. These considerations warrant repetition.

- A child weighing 30 pounds could exceed the current ADI of aspartame by drinking just three or four cans of such soft drinks, excluding the amount also consumed in other products.
- Pardridge (1987, p. 206) asserted that the 10 mg/kg aspartame intake regarded by Levy and Waisbren (1987) as "large amounts" could be consumed by a 50-pound child drinking a single can (12 ounces) of a carbonated aspartame beverage.
- Children weighing 45 pounds who drink a two-liter bottle of an aspartame cola beverage (containing over 1,100 mg aspartame and 110 mg methyl alcohol) already have exceeded the daily limit. Furthermore, they could have easily consumed 30 mg/kg aspartame before dinner in the form of cereals, chocolate milk, milk shakes, chocolate pudding, gelatins, cereals, orange drinks, chewing or bubble gum, and numerous other products so sweetened.

- The minimal potentially "toxic" amounts are suggested by reports of convulsions in infants as their breast-feeding mothers drank an aspartame beverage.

Expressing extreme concern over the large consumption of aspartame by children, Senator Metzenbaum stated, "We cannot use America's children as guinea pigs to determine the safe level of aspartame consumption" (*Philadelphia Enquirer* March 4, 1986, p. A-4).

A few pediatricians and geneticists have voiced concern about potential brain damage and other problems induced by aspartame. They expressed the belief that aspartame ought not be used by mothers who breast-feed nor by children less than six months of age. Striking rises of phenylalanine levels at these critical periods of brain development could interfere with the normal migration of brain cells, perhaps later becoming manifest as mental retardation, attention deficit, and deviant behavior.

Adverse Effects of Small Doses

Severe reactions to small amounts of aspartame, as from chewing a stick of <u>gum</u>, were described in Chapter II-E. It is obvious that such intake does not begin to approach the ADI. Two possible mechanisms for the rapid entry of aspartame are absorption from the mouth into the blood stream (akin to the placement of nitroglycerine under the tongue in treating angina pectoris), and direct entry from the oropharynx into the brain (see Preface to Section 5).

Most physicians and consumers are likely to consider the parts-per-million content of a drug or chemical in food, liquids and drinking water as "very small." This mistaken idea was compounded by the FDA, which reduced the environmental assessment requirements by manufacturers to less than one part per billion in July 1997.

I have repeatedly emphasized the potential ecologic hazards of pesticides (Roberts 1990b), fluoride (Roberts 1992f), and other toxic substances when present even in concentrations of pars per <u>trillion</u>. Other investigators have made comparable observations, such as the effects on *E. coli* and other bacteria of antibiotics in parts-per-trillion concentrations.

In submissions to the FDA concerning approval of the Neotame petition (see above) the author stated: "It is erroneous to assume that a dietary concentration of less than 10 ppb of each minor degradant is innocuous. My published work on highly toxic pesticides indicates that there are several molecules in each cell even from parts-per-TRILLION exposure."

782

Representative Case Reports

Case XXVII-C-1

A 59-year-old fashion coordinator experienced extreme "head swimming, dizziness and slight nausea" after swallowing <u>a single cup</u> of aspartame gelatin. She adamantly refused to retest herself.

Case XXVII-C-2

An 8-year-old girl complained of daily headaches. Concerned over the frequency with which she was giving her child aspirin, the mother made arrangements for a neurologic consultation. The girl then volunteered that her headaches occurred <u>exactly</u> 10 minutes after she began chewing aspartame-containing bubble gum. They disappeared when it was avoided.

Case XXVII-C-3

A young woman described her reactions in this letter sent to Aspartame Victims and Their Friends.

> "In April of 1984, I started chewing aspartame gum. I had just quit smoking. I chewed perhaps three sticks a day. In October 1984, I started to feel strange, and discovered I was reacting to the gum. I stopped chewing it. The symptoms are primarily
>
> - Headache or pressure around the skull
> - Tingling primarily in head and face, although sometimes in extremities as well
> - Occasional numbness on the left side of the face and sometimes in extremities, particularly on the left side
> - Mental confusion
> - Blurred vision
> - A general "spaced-out feeling"

The Question of Tolerance

Among the initial 397 aspartame reactors who completed the questionnaire, 50 (12.5 percent) continued taking small amounts of these products because they equated the seeming absence of some symptoms with safety. This assumption is unproved. It requires testing persons with other overt features of aspartame disease for subtle changes involving attention, perception, memory, reaction time responses, and additional parameters. The "clinical threshold dose" will be discussed below.

Individual "Biological Titration"

Several aspartame reactors offered valuable insights concerning <u>their</u> maximum allowable daily intakes. These were derived from clinical tolerance thresholds based on the <u>predictable</u> onset or recurrence of symptoms. In point of fact, these persons qualify as "experiments of Nature" for the biologic titration of active compounds. (Some classic examples in medical pharmacology include the effective doses of digitalis leaf for "the dropsy," and of colchicine for managing gout.) *The calculated intake for aspartame reactions in my patients* ranged from 10 to 18.3 mg/kg.

The key was a perceptive individual who could promptly recognize the onset of some non-gastrointestinal reaction to aspartame or phenylalanine. The most notable were itching, a rash, headache, mental confusion, visual changes and depression. These convincing "titrations" were defined in terms of the <u>maximum</u> intake of an aspartame product (variously measured as cans, glasses, bottles or servings) that could be tolerated before symptoms appeared. Their reproduction by the subsequent ingestion of phenylalanine <u>alone</u> (as in Case I-2) provided another dose-related insight.

These clearcut trial-and-error evaluations underscore the contention that the ADI for aspartame currently set by the FDA is arbitrarily high. Wurtman (1987) estimated from studies indicating the tendency to increased seizures in animals given low doses of aspartame that 12 mg/kg (about three cans of diet soda) could do so in humans.

Representative Case Reports

Case XXVII-C-4

A 35-year-old woman and two close relatives experienced diarrhea after drinking a beverage containing aspartame. She observed

> "Tolerance levels seem to vary. Only one or two cans of the
> soft drink affect my mother immediately. For me, it took more.
> If I had one glassful during the day, no problem. But at several
> throughout the day or over two days, the problem will begin."

Case XXVII-C-5

A 34-year-old woman weighing 50 kg <u>predictably</u> developed a severe itch and rash within two hours whenever she consumed four 8-ounce glasses of a diet cola in one day – her ADI approximately 11 mg/kg. Lesser amounts (as four glasses a week) did not do so.

D. OTHER POTENTIAL HAZARDS TO THE PUBLIC

Many persons with aspartame disease in this series held responsible positions – e.g., as vehicle drivers, pilots, medical technicians and nuclear facility operators. They recognized that aspartame reactions could lead to serious difficulty, as in the case of pilots with aspartame-induced convulsions (Chapter III).

A. Implications Of Altered Behavior

Extreme changes in mood, personality and behavior among aspartame reactors were described in Chapter VII. The potential ramifications of <u>severe depression with suicidal thoughts</u>, and of <u>psychopathic behavior</u> are frightening. For example, a 42-year-old registered nurse/"aspartame victim" expressed extreme concern when projecting "bizarre killings" by persons with an aspartame reaction.

<u>Businesses might be jeopardized</u> when key personnel suffer aspartame problems. The most notable are confusion, loss of memory, depression, sleepiness and aberrant behavior. "Executive stress" associated with aspartame reactions (Chapter VII) has had devastating corporate consequences.

Unexplained <u>highway violence</u> has escalated dramatically in recent years (*The Wall Street Journal* August 3, 1987, p. 1). The "Jekyll-and-Hyde" nature of this problem, including "road rage," continues to puzzle law enforcement officials when otherwise-responsible citizens engage in fist fights, shootings and other forms of mayhem after some minor encounter (e.g., the flashing of high beams by an oncoming car; failure to yield.) This phenomenon on Southern California's crowded freeways and in other areas where mass transportation is proving inadequate has been referred to as "road wars" and "copycat shootings." It necessitated the installation of more bullet-proof windows and the wearing of bullet-proof vests by highway troopers.

The author reviewed many of the factors that contribute to comparable behavior by drivers in a previous text (Roberts 1971b). The role of aspartame disease in "road rage" also requires serious study. The American Automobile Association found a 51 percent increase of motorists behaving in an overtly hostile manner since 1990 (*The New York Times* September 20, 1977).

Other aspects of traffic accidents relating to aspartame disease are considered below.

B. Malnutrition

Marked anorexia, severe weight loss, and other nutritional sequelae of "diet" products were discussed in Chapter IX. Comparable complications can be anticipated with the emergence of post-aspartame technological "miracles" that dissociate pleasure from gastronomic "sin." William Raspberry (1987) conjectured that this feat for achieving slimness could usher in a tidal wave of deficiency diseases.

C. Traffic Accidents

Severe fatigue, confusion, visual disturbances, irritability, altered behavior (see above), and seizures in persons with aspartame disease who drive motor vehicles are invitations to disaster. Aspartame reactors repeatedly emphasized the deterioration of their driving ability. Some avoided traffic by taking "the long way home." Case XXVII-D-3 illustrates the potential for fatal accidents.

Aspartame-induced brain reactions are described in Chapters VI and VII. The soporific and hypnotic effects can be exaggerated by prolonged confinement, darkness, physical fatigue, and use of nicotine commonly associated with driving occupations.

One-third of Americans have 6½ hours sleep a night during the work week. Accordingly, superimposed aspartame-related insomnia (Chapter VII-F) constitutes another public health consideration relative to poor performance at work from "fatigue" and driving accidents.

Representative Case Reports

Case XXVII-D-1

A woman who consumed diet colas and other aspartame products had been experiencing unexplained headache. She was involved in an automobile accident while driving. The front of her car slid under the rear wheels of a tractor-trailer. This incident was attributed to "some loose gravel at the base of the hill."

Several weeks later, she drove toward an intersection and suddenly could not determine the stop pedal... causing her to enter traffic. She "blacked out" but fortunately recovered in time to stop. A friend mentioned that her difficulties might be due to aspartame consumption. The headaches and "blackouts" ceased within a few days after abstinence, and did nor recur.

Case XXVII-D-2

A 71-year-old former saleswoman experienced intense drowsiness and an uncontrollable desire to fall asleep while driving after she began to consume one packet of an aspartame tabletop sweetener daily. She stated

> "My judgment was affected a number of times while driving. I would drive across the center line without being aware of it until I would notice an approaching car. I couldn't understand what was happening to me. I have always been an excellent driver. The sleepiness increased to the point where I had to lie down every day!"

After reading an article about reactions to aspartame, she eliminated the product and felt markedly improved within three days.

Case XXVII-D-3

A 23-year-old man suffered an apparent grand mal convulsion while driving. He had been consuming from two to four gallons (!) of aspartame cola daily. His complaints included depression, anxiety attacks, irritability, headaches, visual problems, slurred speech, weight loss, abdominal pain, nausea, shortness of breath, and unexplained chest pain. A sister provided the following information about his fatal accident.

> "I am writing because you are currently collecting medical data about aspartame. I have a very sad story to relate to you. On March 18, 1987, my youngest brother G___ died from massive internal injuries sustained in an auto accident. He was

unconscious at the wheel when the accident occurred. He had also been found unconscious at the wheel of his auto on December 23, 1986.

"On March 18, 1987, the night of the fatal accident, one of the first people at the scene said the upper part of G__'s body was convulsing with tremors and his legs were pinned in the wreckage. The man who stated this to me said G__ was totally unconscious and never regained consciousness. It took the paramedics and firemen an hour to cut my brother from the wreckage. They had Med-Evac waiting to fly him to a trauma unit.

"Before G___ died, he had been having numerous problems which could be attributed to aspartame. His consumption of diet cola grew by leaps and bounds. In the last year of G__'s life, he was drinking from 2 to 4 gallons of this diet cola each day.

"G__ was an extremely responsible young man. He never took time off from his employment, and he frequently worked overtime. G____'s employer chose him to go for special schooling to learn to operate a computerized tape lathe. He was an excellent machinist.

"In this last year, noticeable changes began to occur. G___ started to lose weight. He was almost 6' tall and had been pudgy a few years ago. Then he dropped to slightly below normal weight. His moods began to change radically. He became depressed and was having anxiety attacks. He knew something was wrong but was terrified of doctors and needles because of a traumatic experience in his earlier years. This was what kept him from getting these problems checked out. He also seemed to become extremely irritable and short-tempered about everything.

"Within 3 months before G__ died, he was having trouble with his eyes. He also was having pain in his stomach and side. He had moments of being nauseated. G___ had a few occasions where his speech would slur. He had shortness of breath and unexplained chest pain.

"I myself experience mood swings and headache every time I drink a cola containing aspartame.

"For a very long time, my mother kept saying G_____ was addicted to this diet cola (see Chapter VII-G). I truly believe G ___ couldn't go a day without it. I never connected the occurrences with aspartame until I happened to see a special on Channel 10 in Philadelphia about six weeks ago. That was when I realized what had happened to my brother. I can't bring my baby brother back but maybe I can help others so they don't end up dying like G___. I just wish I had known all of this information sooner. It might have made the difference and saved everyone who loved G__ a lot of pain and suffering.

"If you wish to add this information to your research, please do. I can provide witness statements from family and friends who watched what happened over the last year. I would like to see aspartame controlled or banned completely. I think it is a very dangerous substance to humans."

Driver Fatigue and Drowsiness: An Overview

The role of "driver fatigue" was underscored in my text on traffic accidents (Roberts 1971b). It encompasses lapses of attention, overlooking cues, altered depth perception, and dozing at the wheel – all conducive of a fatal "syndrome shift." The potentially disastrous nature of such "functional" disturbances was conveyed in a *British Medical Journal* editorial titled, "Natural Death at the Wheel" (1969; 1:332).

"A sudden departure from normal health might easily be sufficient to interfere with the driver's capacity enough to cause an accident to a fast-moving car, yet not be detectable clinically if he survives. Moreover, if the driver is killed, it might not be evident as a significant lesion postmortem, either because he has suffered multiple injuries which mask the disease, or because it may be of such a minor nature that the pathologist could not be sure, in the absence of a clinical history, that it would be enough to cause any symptoms."*

---

*© 1969 *British Medical Journal*. Reproduced with permission.

Intrusive drowsiness, other forms of fatigue, and the effect of alcohol or drugs can impair a driver's attention, perception, comprehension, and motor responses in dangerous situations. The following indicate the important relationships between such dysfunction and vehicular accidents.

- "But, I didn't see" accidents account for many unanticipated mishaps.
- Officials of the heavily traveled New Jersey Turnpike reported that driver lack of attention was by far the greatest cause of accidents. Of 2,272 during 1969, the leading contributory factors were inattentive driving (971), excessive speed (362), mechanical defects (279), and apparent sleep or drowsiness (137) (*U.S. News & World Report* March 30, 1970, p. 77). Accordingly, half of these accidents could be accounted for by inattentive driving while drowsy or asleep.
- Thomas (1968) discussed the phenomenon of "looking without seeing" in his investigations on eye movement.
- Lindsley (1960) commented upon lapses of attention and the overlooking of cues even in a seemingly attentive posture.
- The *Mainichi Daily News* (Tokyo, August 19, 1969) editorialized that the biggest cause of traffic accidents had shifted to "not looking where one is driving."

As a corollary, alertness and the anticipatory skills needed to cope with the "man-machine-road equation," otherwise referred to as defensive driving, may avert a potential accident. Schlesinger (1967) observed, "There's a moment of grace in any accident... if the driver can take appropriate corrective action."

- Lansing, Schwartz and Lindsley (1959) demonstrated a striking effect of alerting on the visual reaction time to a visual stimulus by interposing a brief forewarning auditory signal. The reduced reaction time was interpreted as quicker central cortical processing.
- General Motors engineers estimated that the severity of crash impacts can be reduced 80 percent if a restrained occupant can anticipate the crash, and assume a pre-crash position.

D. Plane Accidents and Near-Accidents: Pilots and Air Traffic Controllers

Pilots, emergency medical services (EMS) helicopter pilots, and air traffic controllers **must** remain alert. To this end, many consume large amounts of coffee, tea and cola beverages. Most also seek to avoid sugar because they are health-conscious ...and therefore tend to use aspartame products.

Pilots and air traffic controllers have experienced confusion, behavioral changes, and even convulsions while consuming aspartame (Chapter III). Many volunteered their relevance to the increasing number of collisions and near-collisions in the sky and at major airports.

- Wurtman (1987) reported epilepsy in a 35-year-old test pilot who consumed six liters of an aspartame beverage daily following his mid-day jog.
- A pilot experienced in acrobatics would become temporarily disoriented "every time I was drinking a diet soda or chewing gum with aspartame in it."
- Several commercial pilots made reference to peers who allegedly became incapacitated or lost their licenses because of aspartame reactions. An airline pilot offered this answer to the question in the survey questionnaire concerning other friends with aspartame-related problems: "One who was a pilot lost his job due to ruined eyesight." (See Chapter IV)

The air industry has been baffled by unexplained and sometimes totally disabling complaints of flight attendants, such as headache, dizziness, nausea and tremors. The possible role of noxious fumes and other substances relating to hydraulic fluids, air ventilation systems and ozone have been analyzed, with but little effect when upgraded. Inasmuch as flight attendants tend to be health- and weight-conscious, they are inclined to drink diet sodas, especially if available at no cost.

In the context of this experience, concerned consumer groups regard flights by pilots who consume aspartame products as a form of Russian roulette for both the passengers and crew. A seasoned pilot for a major airline offered the following insight

"I would like to see any aspartame-based drinks banned from use on airplanes, but it is an uphill battle. My airline does not provide us with crew meals. As pilots, we never seem to get a chance to eat right while on the road. We are either up too early, in too late, or just too tired to get to the restaurant during our scheduled rotation. What is always available on flights are soft drinks, peanuts and pretzels. Being very conscious of gaining weight, we opt for diet drinks that contain aspartame."

This subject is elaborated in IGNORED HEALTH HAZARDS FOR PILOTS AND DRIVERS (Roberts 1998d).

Representative Case Reports

Case XXVII-D-4

A concerned captain of large commercial planes called to inform me about his reaction to aspartame as perceptible deterioration in flying skills. He also had become depressed and experienced unaccustomed crying spells. Dramatic improvement occurred after stopping aspartame with apparent normalization of his physical and psychological health.

The senior pilot then amplified his reason for calling: the serious implications of comparable reactions he had observed in colleagues consuming large amounts of aspartame products. They were most evident during lengthy delays before departure and landing.

Case XXVII-D-5

A member of the U.S. Air Force had served from April 1992 to August 1996. He wrote

> "Late in my service time, I experienced some strange illnesses that I could not explain, nor could the military doctors. I had a major and sudden onset of hearing loss, dizziness, numbness in my hands, blurry vision, tiredness, muscle and joint aches, blood pressure variation, stress/anger, and other symptoms.

"My doctors said that it may have been due to stress Meniere's syndrome, ear infection, allergies, environment, etc. I finally got tired of their inability to do anything about it, and I quit going to see them. I was never before a sickly person, and it was a new experience for me.

"At the same time that this was happening, I was drinking a large quantity of diet cola to reduce my caloric intake. I started doing this because I had gotten married recently, and we had a new child. I was exercising less and gaining weight. I typically drank 4-8 cans of sodas per day, and tried to replace sugar with some aspartame sweetener whenever I could. Before this period, I had water/milk/juice drinks, but I rarely drank diet drinks."

Case XXVII-D-6

A pilot issued this personal warning for overweight pilots concerning the use of aspartame to lose weight.

"It was the summer of 1992. After loading my aircraft the load master told me that if I didn't lose weight, they would have to get a new pilot. I went to the aeromedical examiner who put me on a 1000-calorie diet. The instructions stated: 'You can have as much diet soda, tea or coffee you desire.' So my colas became those sweetened with aspartame. I also started using it in baking etc. to reduce the calorie content of my meals.

"Within six months I started to experience joint aches and difficulty in remembering. The symptoms were insidious in onset. They started with difficulty copying instrument clearances, so I installed a computer to do that. Then it was vertigo; time for a inner ear check. Then the joint pain. Then it was irritability, with outbursts of temper over the smallest incident. I then developed skin lesions on my scalp and arms.

"By accident, while cruising the net, I found information about aspartame, and discontinued any product that contained it. My symptoms are reversing. The ironic thing is that I did lose my job not because of my weight, but due to the fact I couldn't function at my job.

"I do feel a lot better, and my mental confusion is no longer present. My ability to remember numbers is improved, along with my ability to transfer objects to long-term memory. My skin lesions are healing, and the intestinal problems are diminishing. Even my weight loss is improved, in part because I no longer battle a craving for chocolate.

"I intend to pursue any legal remedy because I lost my ability to be employed. I fully believe it was due to aspartame poisoning."

Related Considerations

There were an estimated 2,000-3,000 near-collisions in the air annually a decade ago (*The Wall Street Journal* July 21, 1987, pp. 33.) (The FAA defines a near-collision as any event involving a plane coming within 500 feet of another.) Even these figures represent underreporting because of different interpretations as to the nature of a near-collision, and the reluctance of pilots to jeopardize the occupation of their peers.

A series of airline mishaps was termed a "breakdown in pilot professionalism and pilot vigilance" by the head of the Federal Aviation Administration (*The Wall Street Journal* August 6, 1987, p. 28).

- A notorious example of such pilot error involved the inadvertent shutting off of a large jet's engines while in flight!
- Pilot error was inferred in the nation's second-worst air disaster during August 1987 (*The Miami Herald* August 28, 1987, p. A-11). The plane's flight-data recorder indicated that the crew had not set the wing flaps to takeoff position... a routine flight procedure.
- The National Transportation Safety Board found that 17 of 26 incidents involved oversights by air traffic controllers, generally due to failure of coordination or communication. It concluded that the danger of on-the-ground collisions at airports has become a significant problem (*The Miami Herald* November 7, 1986, p. A-9).

- Increased attention is being paid to the intense drowsiness and uncontrollable sleep occurring in commercial airline pilots (*The Miami Herald* December 23, 1986, p. A-11). Some have flown on automatic pilot. It is common knowledge within the Federal Aviation Administration that pilots routinely nap on long-haul flights, at times as long as 40 minutes (*The Wall Street Journal* January 21, 1998, p. B-1). Similarly, "navigator's snooze" has resulted in planes overshooting their destinations. In a few instances, an <u>entire</u> three-member crew dozed simultaneously!

- Ninety percent of EMS helicopter accidents are currently attributable to pilot error, most often from dozing at the controls.

E. Nonaccidental Sudden Death

The author is repeatedly asked about nonaccidental deaths attributable to aspartame reactions. This possibility exists, even in FDA records. The underlying mechanisms may include changes in heart rhythm (Chapter IX-C), allergic (anaphylactic-like) shock, and severe swelling of the mouth and upper respiratory passage (Chapter VIII). For example, Case IX-C-5 experienced <u>complete heart block</u> shortly after drinking an aspartame beverage for the <u>first</u> time.

F. Potential Nuclear Reactor Accidents

The hazards of inattentiveness or sleeping by key person while on duty at nuclear reactors are obvious. This was emphasized by the mandated shutdown of Philadelphia Electric Company's Peach Bottom nuclear power station on March 31, 1987. (It is situated only 37 miles from the Three Mile Island reactor, scene of the worst commercial nuclear accident in the United States.) The executive director of operations for the Nuclear Regulatory Commission stated, "Continued operation of the facility is an immediate threat to the public health and safety" (*Sun/Sentinel* of Fort Lauderdale, April 1, 1987, p. A-3).

> The problem was most severe during the 11 PM to 7 AM shift in the control room. During this time, licensed operators, senior licensed operators and shift supervisors had been observed to doze or otherwise become inattentive to their duties. Had such behavior occurred when lightening struck electrical wires, they would have been unable to respond promptly.

A similar problem occurred at Miami's nuclear power plant (*The Palm Beach Post* April 23, 1987, p. D-5).

Comparable scenarios attributable to aspartame analogs appear in a novel, THE CACOF CONSPIRACY (Roberts 1998f).

E. TUMORS AND CANCER; THE DELANEY AMENDMENT

"By far the most mutagenic agents known to man are chemicals, not radiation. And in this regard, food additives rather than fallout at present levels may present a greater danger."
Dr. Richard Caldecott (1961)
(Atomic Energy Commission)

Heavy consumers of aspartame products appear to be at increased for developing tumors in the brain (see below) and elsewhere. The author initially considered "anecdotes" about cancer involving organs other than the brain in aspartame reactors to be coincidental. As the number increased, however, a relationship could not be ignored.

Reference was made in Chapter IX to aspartame-induced vaginal bleeding, breast tenderness, and changes involving blood cells and lymph nodes.

Admittedly, this realm remains controversial. The Bressler Report (1977) underscored the numerous shortcomings of aspartame studies in rats, especially tumor induction. Dr. M. Adrian Gross, a senior FDA pathologist-scientist, stated

"In view of all these indications that the cancer-causing potential of aspartame is a matter that had been established way beyond any reasonable doubt, one can ask: "What is the reason for the apparent refusal by the FDA to invoke for this food additive the so-called Delaney Amendment to the Food, Drug, and Cosmetic Act?" (*Congressional Record-Senate* August 1, 1985, p. S10837).

There may be a long hiatus between the introduction of a drug or chemical and awareness of its link to cancer. This is illustrated by phenolphthalein, the main ingredient of several popular laxatives. Nearly a century lapsed before documentation of its carcinogenic activity in rodents – including tumors of the ovaries, kidneys, adrenal glands and thymus (McGinley 1997).

Selected Tumors

Dr. George Schwartz (1999) suggested a connection between aspartame consumption and breast cancer and prostate cancer. Both markedly increased following the release of aspartame in 1981, based on governmental surveillance statistics.

There are suggestive anecdotal reports in this serious. For example, a diabetic male developed retinopathy and joint pain while consuming diet colas, and then cancer of the breast.

The puzzling rise of certain cancers over the past decade, especially among younger weight-conscious women, warrants consideration of the contributory role of aspartame products.

- Ductule breast carcinoma in situ rose 52 percent from 1983-1989; during this period, the use of aspartame products quadrupled. The numbers subsequently rose to 23,000 case in 1992 and 36,000 in 1998, 200 persons higher than had been projected.
- A fourfold increase of adenocarcinoma of the cervix in England's East Anglia region, most notably in the 30- to 39-year-age group was reported in 1997 by Diane Stockton of the Institute of Public health at Cambridge University.

The Delaney Amendment

Congress included the Delaney clause in the 1958 Food Additives Amendment. Its intent was to ban the ingestion of cancer-causing chemicals.

> The circumstances surrounding the adoption of this Federal law may be of interest to "Trivia" buffs. Representative James Delaney of New York unsuccessfully tried to obtain its passage for five years. Delaney's staff then briefed actress Gloria Swanson, a health food advocate, in 1956. She enlisted sympathetic wives of congressmen, who in turn encouraged their husbands to support the bill.

Unfortunately, the Delaney clause was emasculated by the Senate's Comprehensive Regulatory Reform Act of July 19, 1995. Without defining the terms "negligible" or "insignificant," it stated that a substance or product shall not be prohibited or refused approval when it "presents a negligible or insignificant foreseeable risk to human health."

The Author's Perspective

Having monitored the controversy about saccharin and urinary bladder tumors (see below), the following revelations proved troublesome.: (a) deficiencies involving <u>comparable</u> testing with aspartame; (b) ignored reports of brain tumors in mice given aspartame; and (c) reluctance of governmental agencies to invoke the Delaney Amendment.

In prior publications, the author reported increased tumor rates attributable to divers influenced to which the population is exposed. They include

- The ability of insulin to enhance the action of male hormone (testosterone) on prostatic growth (Sirek 1953; Calame 1964; Roberts 1966a, 1967c).
- Diaz-Sanchez et al (1999) demonstrated enhancement of insulin biosynthesis and secretion by testosterone, consistent with the hyperinsulinemia encountered in hyperandrogenic syndromes.
- A variety of tumors caused by exposure to the pesticide pentachlorophenol – especially lymphoma, sarcoma, leukemia and other blood disorders (Roberts 1990b, 1997d).
- Breast enlargement/tumors in persons taking megadoses of vitamin E (Roberts 1994c).
- Prostate cancer after vasectomy (Roberts 1993d).

Aspartame As a Co-Carcinogen

A potentiated carcinogenic effect by aspartame in our increasingly complex environment demands study. Others share a similar orientation.

- Dr. Samuel S. Epstein (1999) (Professor of Environmental and Occupational Medicine, University of Illinois) stated, "Much cancer is avoidable and due to past exposure to chemical and physical carcinogens in the air, water and food and the workplace."
- Huff, Haseman and Rall (1991) offered this summary concerning chemical carcinogens.

"We believe our scientific and public responsibility must continue to be directed toward identifying those chemicals, mixtures of chemicals, and exposure circumstances that present potentially the most predictable carcinogenic (and other toxicologic) hazards to humans... The important issue is not whether we are undeniably correct in extrapolating carcinogenic responses in laboratory animals up the evolutionary trail to humans, but rather to concentrate our vigilance to assure and improve the entrusted public health."

Possible Carcinogenic Mechanisms

Several of the potential cancer-inducing properties of aspartame, its three components (phenylalanine; aspartic acid; and a methyl ester that promptly becomes free methanol after ingestion), and the many breakdown products on exposure to heat and storage are cited here and in the ensuing discussion of brain tumors.

- Many constituents in the human diet are nitrosated within the gastrointestinal tract to form potentially carcinogenic nitroso compounds. Shephard et al (1993) reported mutagenic activity by aspartame after nitrosation, using *Salmonella typhimurium* as the test organism.

- The diketopiperazine derivative of aspartame (Chapter XXV) has been incriminated as a tumor-causing chemical.

- Formaldehyde released from the breakdown of methyl alcohol (Chapter XXI) is known to be carcinogenic.

- The potential carcinogenic effects of chronic hyperinsulinemia (Chapter XIV) has been discussed in prior publications, with special reference to the prostate (Roberts 1967d). Others have implicated hyperinsulinemia in the pathogenesis of breast cancer (Diamanti-Kandarakis 1999).

- Alteration of glucose transport is a characteristic of experimental tumors. Reporting on this phenomenon, and the dramatic increase in total cellular glucose transporter protein, Birenbaum et al (1987) emphasized the induction of such transformation when fibroblasts are starved for glucose.

- <u>Increased phenylalanine may play a role</u>. Animal and human studies indicate that restricting dietary phenylalanine decreases tumor growth and metastases (Norris 1990).

- Several investigators have implicated <u>prolactin</u> (Chapter XXIV) as a tumor-promoting substance in various organs – including the pituitary (Oliveira 1999), endometrium (Brosens 1999), and human breast (Maus 1999).

- The brown substances created by <u>the heating of amino acids</u> during cooking may be mutagenic and carcinogenic (Abelson 1983). They include a number of DNA-damaging agents.

- The causation or enhancement of brain and other tumors in persons consuming aspartame products may summate upon a <u>hyperimmune state</u> induced by early and multiple immunizations with vaccines whose long-term safety is being increasingly challenged (Section 6-D). A number contain formaldehyde (Chapter XXI) and mercury as preservatives.

The mutagenic and carcinogenic potential of other chemicals might intensify under the influence of aspartame and its breakdown products. The ability of aspartame to induce or aggravate the multiple chemical sensitivity syndrome, including pesticide reactions, was discussed in Chapter VIII-E.

The Issue of Gender

The agencies responsible for approving aspartame apparently overlooked an important gender-related detail in experimental studies. The assessment for potential urinary bladder cancer following administration of aspartame and its diketopiperazine derivative was studies <u>only</u> in female mice. Professor George T. Brian (1984) noted that <u>female</u> Swiss albino mice were used for "all" such studies.

The author expressed reservations about limiting the testing to female animals at the First International Meeting On Dietary Phenylalanine and Brain Function held on May 10, 1987 in Washington, D.C. Information to the contrary from those present – including at least five professionals and scientific consultants for the manufacturer – was <u>specifically</u> solicited. No verbal or written response, then or since, has been received.

The subject of urinary bladder tumors induced by saccharin will be discussed below. There is little doubt, however, that it is largely a phenomenon of <u>male</u> rats. Miller and Howe (1977) asserted, "For bladder cancer, the distinction between males and females seems to us to be fundamental."

F. BRAIN TUMORS

Pre-Approval Perspectives

On September 60, 1980, a Public Broad Of Inquiry (PBI) unequivocally advised against the approval of aspartame owing to the high incidence of brain tumors among animals receiving this chemical. It did not mince words: "The Board has not been presented with proof of a reasonable certainty that aspartame (NutraSweet) is safe for use as a food additive under its intended conditions of use."

The observations of Dr. John Olney concerning aspartame-related brain tumors are detailed below. Other investigators also reported increased rates of brain tumors (gliomas) in rats given aspartame (*Congressional Record-Senate* 1985a, b). Cornell, Wolfe and Sanders (1984) reviewed the data. Dr. M. Adrian Gross stated, "At least one of those studies has established beyond any reasonable doubt that aspartame is capable of inducing brain tumors in experimental animals" (*Congressional Record-Senate* 1985b).

Professor Walle Nauta (Massachusetts Institute of Technology) chaired the Public Board of Inquiry (PBOI) convened by the FDA in 1980 to evaluate the issue of aspartame-related brain tumors. This Board recommended that aspartame NOT be approved. It concluded that the evidence from the Lifetime Rat Study and the Two Year Rat Study "...appeared to suggest the possibility that aspartame, at least when administered in the huge quantities employed in the studies, may contribute to the development of brain tumors" (United States General Accounting Office 1987). The carcinogenic potential of aspartame was further suggested by early occurrence of tumors in dosed animals.

The Board's recommendation was overruled, however, by the FDA Commissioner. Nauta emphasized that he had been under the clear impression aspartame would be <u>excluded</u> from soft drinks! He asserted that the inquiry would have been conducted differently had he known otherwise (*Congressional Record-Senate* 1985, p. S5503).

Dr. Douglas L. Park (Staff Science Advisor, Office of Health Affairs of the Department of Health & Human Services) submitted his analysis of the hearing by this PBOI in 1981. He pointed out that <u>his</u> interpretation of the term "authentic," as used by the Universities Associated for Research and Education in Pathology (URAEP), was primarily that the experiments "had indeed been done." Park then explained his concerns about the occurrence of brain tumors in the treated rats. *"I believe that aspartame has not been shown to be safe for the proposed food additive uses.* Along with the Board of Inquiry, I must recommend, therefore, that aspartame *not* be approved until additional studies are carried out using proper experimental designs." (Italics supplied)

The FDA was influenced by the Ishii (1981) report. These investigators administered aspartame and its diketopiperazine to SLC Wister rats for 104 weeks at the Ajinomoto Company's research laboratories. Although two astrocytomas, two oligodendrogliomas and one ependymoma were found among the four test groups, it was concluded that neither agent caused brain tumors.

The same gender difference noted above for urinary bladder tumors is again suggested by a higher incidence of brain tumors among <u>male</u> rats given aspartame. (The incidence rates in female rats and controls were the same.)

Does Aspartame Cause Human Brain Cancer?

The author's initial report on this topic (Roberts 1991a) was published a decade ago. Since then, more than a score of reports have been personally received about patients who developed brain tumors after consuming considerable aspartame. They included astrocytoma, oligodendroglioma, other gliomas, meningioma, and hypothalamic tumors.

Examples of the prodigious consumption of aspartame are cited.

- A 19-year-old woman developed an acoustic neuroma after prolonged use of five to six cans diet soda daily.
- The husband of a woman who died of a brain tumor at the age of 37, leaving an 8-year-old daughter, wrote this poignant note:

> "She was a heavy user of aspartame. On a typical day, she would consume 6-12 cans of diet cola. I used to joke to her about drinking so much diet cola that she could cut out the middleman by having them deliver the stuff right to our house. She also consumed it in many products everyday because, like most women, she was obsessed with watching her weight."

- The wife of a man who died of a glioblastoma wrote of his addiction to a diet cola. "He drank gallons of this soda each week. I personally saw our 20-gallon trash cans filled each week to the brim with his empty large diet cola bottles. He was obsessed with intense thirst for the diet cola."

- A man who developed an astrocytoma had been putting 20 aspartame tablets in each cup of coffee, along with consuming from two to three 2-liter bottles of diet soda daily.

- A 49-year-old woman attempted drastic reduction of weight. She developed a large glioblastoma in the posteror fossa within several months after "ingesting massive quantities of aspartame." In addition to various diet sodas, ice cream and puddings, she drank "tons of coffee," adding six packets of a tabletop sweetener to each cup.

- A 43-year-old woman developed severe depression, a 60-pound weight gain, and a subsequent brain tumor after consuming diet colas for many years. On learning about aspartame disease, she commented, "This supposed miracle sweetener of the century turns out to be the silent killer of my life."

Dr. Lennart Hardell (2000) (Department of Oncology, Orebro Medical Center, Orebro, Sweden) found an odds ratio of 1.24 patients with malignant brain tumors who consumed low-calorie drinks, compared to controls. Furthermore, this risk increased among persons exposed to radiation.

Representative Case Reports

Case XXVII-F-1

A 41-year-old woman had consumed at least two to three cans of aspartame soft drinks more than 11 years. She developed a grand mal seizure. A brain tumor (oligodendroglioma) was found. Surgery was followed by radiation therapy. Her previous non-neurologic complaints included palpitations, abdominal pain, blood in the stools, severe itching without a rash, a gain of ten pounds, and unexplained discomfort in the knees and elbows.

Case XXVII-F-2

A 62-year-old manager switched to aspartame products in the wake of publicity about the tumor-causing effects of saccharin. He averaged six packets of an aspartame tabletop sweetener in his coffee daily, and also added it to iced tea.

The patient experienced decreased vision in both eyes, partial loss of hearing, headaches, mild confusion, slurring of speech and leg cramps. His granddaughter developed hives from aspartame sodas.

A diagnosis of primary brain lymphoma was later made by biopsy. There was no evidence for immunosuppression or overt exposure to environmental carcinogens. As with other aspartame consumers who developed brain tumors, this patient had difficulty in determining whether his neurological manifestations were primarily due to a brain tumor evolving over several years, or aspartame disease which was then complicated by the tumor.

Case XXVII-F-3

A diabetic man was advised to drink a minimum of one gallon liquid daily because of concomitant high uric acid levels. He did so by using aspartame sodas.

Within several months, he experienced persistent headaches, "zoning out", and a striking decline in his body temperature to 95.6 degrees. An MRI of the brain ten years before was normal. He consulted an endocrinologist. A repeat study revealed a large tumor (hamartoma) in the hypothalamus.

The Rising Incidence Of Primary Brain Cancer

The incidence rates for primary malignant brain tumors have increased by 2.5 percent annually since 1980 according to a National Cancer Institute registry, particularly among older persons. This phenomenon cannot be attributed solely to better diagnostic technology.

The National Cancer Institute's Surveillance Epidemiology and End Results (SEER) statistics (*Cancer Statistics Review* 1973-87, NIH Publication No. 89-2789) indicate an impressive increase in the age-adjusted incidence rates of primary brain cancer since 1985 – possibly as early as 1984. This phenomenon was documented in the categories "All Races, Males and Females," "All Races, Males," and "All Races, Females," "All Races, Males," and "All Races, Females."

Statistically significant rises in brain cancer also were found in the Estimated Annual Percent Change (EAPC) over the 1983-1987 period. SEER Table II-34, containing the five-year trends for all races, indicated that the annual percent change rose from 2.1 in 1975-1979 to 8.7 in 1983-1987 for males; for females, it increased from 2.1 in 1975-1979 to 11.7 in 1983-1987.

It has been argued that such increases reflect more accurate diagnosis by recent scanning and other procedures. In rebuttal, these considerations are germane.

- Adequate brain scanning devices had been widely available for at least one decade previously.
- The rise of primary brain tumors was quantitative.
- The incidence rates for cancer involving most other systems either remaining stable or declined during the 1983-1987 period.

Recent data continue to confirm that the incidence rates for brain cancer in the United States have increased in both adults (Devesa 1995) and children (Gurney 1996). In fact, the increased reporting of brain tumors among young persons causes children with headache to worry about a tumor as the cause!

The Rising Incidence Of Primary Brain Lymphoma

The subset of primary brain lymphoma is of unique interest.

- Eby et al (1988) reported a nearly threefold rise in incidence of this previously-rare tumor among immunologically normal persons in the 1982-1984 SEER data. Specifically, the rate increased from 2.7 cases per ten million population in 1973-1975 to 7.5 cases per ten million in 1982 through 1984 ($P=0.001$). The age-adjusted rise was more striking among women – from 4.9 per ten million in 1979-1981 to 8.9 per ten million in 1982-1984. This could not "be explained completely by confounding effects."
- Yau et al (1996) reported a steep rise in the incidence of primary lymphoma of central nervous system in non-immunocompromised patients between 1981 and 1991 in southeast Scotland. Primary brain lymphoma accounted for 7.6 percent of all gliomas managed by the Edinburgh Department of Clinical Neurosciences, compared to a median of 1.5 percent for the previous decade. These investigators noted similar increases of primary brain lymphoma in other European centers.

The foregoing phenomenon assumes considerable pertinence in light of these facts: (a) the formal approval of aspartame in July 1981, and (b) the 3:1 preponderance of women with reactions to aspartame (Section 1). Eby and al (1988) commented: "A possible explanation of the increased incidence might be other noninfectious environmental exposures. One could conjecture that primary brain lymphomas may have a long latency period and are the result of occupational or other chemical exposures. However, the similar increases in incidence in both men and women, particularly in older persons, make occupational exposures an unlikely cause."

Experimental Aspartame-Associated Brain Tumors

Prior experimental evidence corroborates this association. An unexpected high incidence of primary brain tumors was found experimentally in rats during the 1970s. Although FDA scientists and others expressed considerable concern, the statutes of limitations on two such studies were allowed to expire before the Delaney Amendment (XXVII-E) could be invoked. The details appear in the *Congressional Record-Senate* hearings of May 7, 1985 and August 1, 1985, and in prior text (Roberts 1989a).

Even though aspartame continues to be touted as "the most thoroughly tested additive in history," there remains a paucity of corporate-neutral studies aimed at proving or disproving carcinogenesis in rats and other species.

Related Criticisms Of The FDA

A. Dr. M. Adrian Gross

Dr. Gross, a senior FDA pathologist, told the Senate hearing held on August 1, 1985 (pp. S108220-10847)

> "In view of all these indications that the cancer-causing potential of aspartame is a matter that has been established way beyond any reasonable doubt, one can ask: *'What is the reason for the apparent refusal by the FDA to invoke for this food additive the Delaney Amendment to the Food, Drug, and Cosmetic Act?'"* (Italics supplied)

In a subsequent stinging rebuke of the FDA, Dr. Gross stated in his sworn analysis of corporate experimental studies (November 3, 1987)

> "At least one of those studies had revealed a highly significantly dose-related increase in the incidence of brain tumors as a result of exposure to aspartame. The full incidence of those brain tumors was not disclosed by G. D. Searle & Co. to the FDA prior to the initial approval for the marketing of aspartame in 1974; moreover, as a review of that study in the FDA was so

flawed, the Agency apparently did not even realize it at the time that only a portion of the observations on brain tumors had in fact been submitted by G. D. Searle & Co. in their petition for that approval."

B. Dr. John Olney

Dr. Olney (Professor of Psychiatry and Neuropathology, Washington University School of Medicine) wrote the following statement to Senator Howard Metzenbaum, dated December 8, 1987 concerning aspartame-related brain tumors.

"This is an exceedingly complex topic which, unfortunately, has a history riddled with appearances of fraudulent practices by the manufacturer of NutraSweet and ineptitude and/or malfeasance on the part of the FDA officials. In the mid 1970's, when I reviewed the NutraSweet record in preparation for the hearing I had been promised, I came upon a peculiar study which the manufacturer had submitted to the FDA and which FDA had unquestioningly accepted as evidence for the safety of NutraSweet. The study showed that in 320 NutraSweet-fed rats there were 12 brain tumors, whereas in a group of concurrent control rats which were not exposed to NutraSweet there were no brain tumors. Being a neuropathologist, I know that spontaneous brain tumors in laboratory rats are extremely rare. The archival literature documents an incidence not exceeding 0.6%. Since the above incidence in NutraSweet-fed is 3.75%, this suggests that NutraSweet may cause brain tumors and certainly suggests the need for additional in-depth research to rule out that possibility...

"I seriously doubt whether this method of data analysis would stand the scrutiny of competent disinterested statisticians. Even more seriously I wonder why FDA allows microscopic slides to disappear (while supposedly impounded) and why they do not question the de novo emergence of a brain tumor among the controls when the slides reappear.

"The PBOI panel member who was primarily responsible for reviewing the brain tumor issue was Peter Lampert, M.D.,

Neuropathologist and chairman of the pathology department at Univ. of Calif. San Diego. *Dr. Lampert personally examined the microscopic slides pertaining to the brain tumor studies, and told me a year or so after the PBOI report was completed that he had been surprised at the large size of the brain tumors in the NutraSweet-fed rats.*" (Italics supplied)

C. Senator Howard Metzenbaum

Senator Metzenbaum offered this commentary at the May 7, 1985 Senate hearing.

"I do not claim children will develop brain tumors. I do not know that. I do know that the FDA was worried about it. I do know that three of the six FDA scientists advising the FDA Commissioner on final approval were sufficiently worried about it that they were not willing to approve the product. The FDA's own scientists were split on the issue." (P.S5492)

D. The Community Nutrition Institute

The Community Nutrition Institute and others filed a petition on August 8, 1983 seeking (a) a public hearing by the FDA concerning its approval of aspartame in liquids ("wet use") because one had not been held, and (b) a stay of such approval pending the hearing due to concern over neurotoxicity. The United States Court of Appeals for the District of Columbia Circuit (9) denied both requests (No. 84-1153 and No. 84-5253 [D.C. Civil Action No. 83-03846, decided September 24, 1985].)

This court was aware of prior misgivings by scientists and the Public Board of Inquiry convened in January 1980, including the Board's plea for "further study to establish whether or not a relationship existed between the ingestion of aspartame and brain tumors." (In the three years since the Board's recommendation, G. D. Searle & Co. "chose not to conduct cancer studies on aspartame... and the FDA failed to require such studies.") The Court made the following pertinent comment (p.14):

"Our scope of review, the exactitude of the fit that we require between the agency's conclusions and the germane facts is investigated, is necessarily deferential. *The judiciary is ill-equipped to conduct investigations and analyze facts of the type involved in this case. Because of the agency's expertise and broad discretion in ensuring the safety of food additives, we cannot substitute our judgment for the agency's. The Commission's finding that there were no material issues of fact can be overturned only if an examination of the record discloses that material issues of fact are apparent to any reasonable examiner."* (Italics supplied)

Brain Cancer in Females

The apparent rise of these tumors in women is noteworthy. The threefold higher incidence of severe reactions to aspartame products in females (Section 1) is germane.

Malignant brain tumors in adults previously occurred more often among men (Salcman 1985, Cole 1989). Older male rats also develop more spontaneous brain tumors (chiefly granular-cell meningiomas) than females (Krinke 1985).

The increase of fatal brain cancer among women is illustrated by the following death rates (per 100,000 population) among females of all ages (kindly supplied by Mr. Edwin Silverberg, Department of Epidemiology & statistics, American Cancer Society): 1979 - 3.4; 1980 - 3.5; 1981 - 3.5; 1982 - 4.0. These increases were more striking among white women than non-white women. (Socioeconomic and cultural factors pertaining to the consumption of "diet" drinks during the early 1980s in part explains these discrepancies.)

Pathogenetic Insights

The following newer concepts concerning the etiology and pathogenesis of primary brain tumors are pertinent.

- Aspartame and its components or metabolites might activate some proto-oncogene, such as the epidermal growth factor-receptor (EGF-R) gene (Hoy Sang 1989) – either directly or indirectly (e.g., by tissue glucopenia or the influence of uncommon amino acid dextroisomers.)
- The substitution of no-calorie or low-calorie products for conventional foods and beverages, whether as meals or snacks, can have serious sequelae in the brain (Chapter IV). Under usual circumstances, this organ is almost totally dependent upon glucose for optimal function. This point is emphasized relative to the pathogenesis of multiple sclerosis (Roberts 1966).

- The initial rise of primary brain lymphoma in 1982 – when the consumption of aspartame was much less than after its approval of "wet" use during 1983 – might be explained by the need for a less intense biophysiologic or toxic stimulus than the more common types of brain tumor.
- The unchecked hyperinsulinized state (Chapter XIV) may be critical.

The author is impressed by the prolonged use of <u>aspartame gum</u> in some of these patients. The ability of small molecules to enter the brain directly from the opharynx was described in Chapter II-E.

Primary Tumors

Pituitary tumors occurred in patients who had consumed considerable aspartame for years, and evidenced other clinical features of aspartame disease. For example, one female aspartame reactor developed a pituitary tumor in 1992, which recurred in 1995. She had continued consuming six diet colas, and aspartame yogurt and hot chocolate daily.

Attention is directed to several <u>prolactin-secreting pituitary tumors</u> encountered (see Chapter XXVII-F-5). The stimulation of prolactin by phenylalanine was discussed in Chapters IX-E and XXIV.

Animal studies validate this association. Multiple instances of pituitary tumors were cited in the Bressler Report – e.g., the following female rats:

No. M15CF - pituitary adenoma
No. H18HF - pituitary adenoma
No. K18HF - pituitary adenoma
No. M17LF - marked enlargement of pituitary <u>and</u> both adrenal glands
No. J30HM - marked enlargement of pituitary

Representative Case Reports

Case XXVII-F-4

A 35-year-old man with longstanding diabetes had been consuming considerable diet cola since its availability. In recent years, he suffered severe unexplained headaches, numbness of the hands, and intermittent diarrhea. He felt "my mind was in a fog," and gained 80 pounds. A pituitary tumor enveloping the optic nerve was found and removed. Continuing to drink diet cola, his blood glucose did "some weird things." He then learned about aspartame disease, and improved after stopping the diet soda.

Case XXVII-F-5

A female aspartame reactor repeatedly developed "horrible headaches whenever I knowingly or unknowingly consume aspartame." As a teenager, she "literally existed on diet sodas and a low caloric intake because I was so very body conscious." She then developed a prolactin-secreting pituitary tumor. This caused her to focus on aspartame disease because "I come from an incredibly healthy stock, and live a healthy life style in a reasonably uncontaminated environment."

G. OCCUPATIONAL EXPOSURE THROUGH INHALATION

The author initially regarded reports of aspartame disease caused by exposure in the manufacturing environment with skepticism. As more were received from perceptive professionals, the association seemed more plausible.

These findings are relevant.

- The Material Safety Data Sheet on aspartame lists its potential adverse effects on the eyes, skin and respiratory tract, along with required personnel protective equipment (including an approved air purifying or mist respirator) and first aid measures
- Visitors to an aspartame manufacturing plant are advised to wear protective clothing in order to avoid hazardous exposure.
- There have been related instances of non-occupational exposure. One woman reported "I am allergic to aspartame. If I break open a packet containing it, and inhale the powder, I instantly develop a headache."

Representative Case Reports

Case XXVII-13

The head of an engineering firm wrote the author after reading about aspartame disease. He described the problem of a friend, the installation engineer of more than a dozen automatic centrifuges used in the manufacture of aspartame. After exposure to the dry aspartame powder as these machines were started up, he suffered multiple symptoms – "hot flashes," marked weakness and insomnia. They slowly disappeared after completion of the installations, and without further exposure.

Case XXVII-14

A 21-year-old man was exposed over one year to a fine dust of aspartame at the packaging plant where he worked. He complained of blurred vision, headache, dizziness and depression. An autopsy following his sudden death revealed degenerative changes in the liver, kidneys, heart and lungs. The cardiac abnormalities suggested alcoholic cardiomyopathy, but he did not consume alcoholic beverages.

Case XXVII-15

A 33-year-old worker at a plant manufacturing aspartame developed progressive dizziness, palpitations, a rapid heart rate, intermittent "fuzzy vision" with a "sparkly light," "needles" over the right face, and leg weakness. He blended aspartame with citric acid, with or without a acidulent containing phosphoric acid. (He would cut the bags, and slowly pour the chemical in 140-degree water.) Any exposed skin was covered with a fine talc. He could detect the sweetness through his mask.

The author saw him in consultation because prior neurologic and psychiatric evaluations failed to uncover another cause. One neurologist began his report by indicating the patient's concern over occupational exposure to aspartame, but made no further reference to it in his three-page analysis.

Commentary

Sensational but premature exposes of diseases in workers and their communities have been attributed to chemicals used in industry.

This apparently was the case with problems affecting residents in Hinkley (California), a desert town. They were ascribed to the chromium-6 used in a Pacific Gas & Electric plant manufacturing a rust inhibitor. On the other hand, this scenario may apply to exposed personnel through the manufacture of aspartame.

This story formed the basis for a hit movie *Erin Brockovich*. A huge settlement was made <u>before</u> the publication of scientific

812

information indicating that this substance is a toxin and carcinogen **only** when inhaled during production (*The Wall Street Journal* March 28, 2000, p. A-30).

H. THE SILICONE BREAST IMPLANT ISSUE

"Why has the hypothesis that breast implants cause these diseases been so readily accepted with so little evidence to support it?"*
Dr. Marcia Angell (1994)
Executive Editor, *New England Journal of Medicine*

The author did not anticipate a marked interest in the silicone breast implant controversy. It evolved from the striking overlap of systemic symptoms in patients with severe reactions to aspartame products and those experienced by women with breast implants. The magnitude of this issue was suggested by the fact that breast augmentation had become the second most popular cosmetic surgery.

The frustration of being unable to obtain a forum for these observations over five years became compounded by the huge punitive damages – a proposed $3.2 billion settlement filed on November 9, 1998 – against a major manufacturer of these implants on the basis of unwarranted inferences. Rosenberg (1996) termed them "the neuromythology of silicone breast implants."

The enormity of silicone breast implant litigation (Associated Press 1995; Bandow 1998) is briefly summaried.

- At least 170,000 women filed claims against Dow Corning. (This firm stopped producing silicone breast implants in 1992.)
- Thousands of additional plaintiffs sued other manufacturers, notably Bristol-Myers Squibb Company and Minnesota Mining & Manufacturing Company.
- Juries awarded as much as $25 million in silicone breast implant cases (Burton 1998).
- Dow Corning Corporation filed for Chapter 11 bankruptcy court protection in 1995 as a result of these suits.

---

*©1994 *New England Journal of Medicine*. Reproduced with permission.

The perceived medicolegal travesty is unparalleled in the annals of forensic medicine. It culminated in writing the book, BREAST IMPLANTS OR ASPARTAME (NUTRASWEET®)DISEASE? (Roberts 1999).

Two additional points serve to preamble this discussion. First, the author continues to remain corporate-neutral... meaning that no grants or contracts from any party were received. Second, he has not testified in related litigation.

The Inference

A number of women with silicone breast implants experienced perplexing and disabling **systemic** symptoms. In addition to joint pain (arthralgia) and muscle pain (myalgia), their complaints frequently focused on chronic fatigue, headache, dizziness, mental confusion, insomnia, peripheral neuropathy, rashes, the dry eye-dry mouth (Sjögren) syndrome, and atypical chest pain (Germain 1991; Bridges 1993, Gabriel 1994; Lu 1994; Sanchez-Guerrero 1995).

These features were reflexively attributed to immunologic reactions involving connective tissue. They presumably occurred when silicone debris came in contact with the immune system after the polymer (technically known as polydimethylsiloxane) leached from the implants. Some thought these molecules combined with proteins to form so-called haptenes, thereby initiating an inflammatory reaction.

Lack of Convincing Proof

Most investigators have **NOT** been able to find convincing clinical or investigational proof for the foregoing explanation of systemic complaints (Germain 1991; Bridges 1993; Gabriel 1994; Sanchez-Guerrero 1995). Negative reports also were issued by a British government scientific panel (the Independent Review Group), and the European Committee on Quality Assurance and Medical Devices in Plastic Surgery (Bandow 1998).

The inability to find an association between silicone breast implants and connective-tissue diseases or other disorders is illustrated by the report of Gabriel et al (1994). They followed 749 women in Olmsted County (Minnesota) who had received a breast implant for various reasons over a mean period of 7.8 years, and 1498 community controls over a mean period of 8.3 years. They only significant increase found among the breast implant group was morning stiffness.

U.S. District Judge Sam C. Pointer, Jr., who oversaw thousands of breast implant cases, appointed an independent scientific panel to help evaluate systemic illness allegedly caused by these devices. The four members had expertise in the fields of toxicology, immunology, epidemiology and rheumatology. They declared on December 1, 1988: "The main conclusion that can be drawn from existing studies is that women with silicone breast implants do not display a silicone-induced systemic abnormality in the types of functions of cells of the immune system" (Burton 1998).

The Aspartame Connection

Attention is directed in this context to aspartame-related headache, dizziness, confusion, memory loss, insomnia, chronic fatigue, dryness of the eyes and mouth, joint pain, skin eruptions, hair loss, paresthesias, atypical pain syndromes (most notably involving the face and chest), and dysuria (burning on urination) with sterile urine cultures. These complaints were detailed in the preceding sections.

The following clinical observations are germane.

- Dozens of patients in this series who had been diagnosed as having "fibromyalgia" (Chapter IX-G) experienced striking improvement after avoiding aspartame products.
- Allergic-type reactions occur in about one-fifth of aspartame reactors (Chapter VIII).
- The finding of skin eruptions, joint symptoms, other suggestive complaints, and even a high antinuclear antibody (ANA) titer had led to a diagnosis of systemic lupus erythematosus in more than a dozen patients with aspartame disease (Chapter VIII).
- The dry eye - dry mouth (Sjögren) syndrome (Chapter IV) also was reported in patient-plaintiffs with breast implants.
- The combination of aspartame disease and silicone breast implants was encountered in the author's practice.

The probable mechanisms for these reactions appear in Section 5.

It is noteworthy that the vast majority of reports concerning symptomatic women with breast implants occurred after 1982 (German 1991; Sanchez-Guerrero 1995.) For reference, aspartame was approved by the Food and Drug Administration in July 1981.

While this presentation focuses on the systemic complaints of women with breast implants, aspartame-induced damage to soft tissue may contribute to their local complications. The chronic effects of formaldehyde are noteworthy in this regard.

Inability To Obtain Epidemiologic Data

Despite many attempts by the author, specific statistical data about aspartame usage by female litigants with silicone breast implants could not be obtained.

Repeated suggestions were made to the major corporate-defendant about obtaining such information, chiefly as supplementary interrogatories – to no avail. Even though its senior officials continued to deny that silicone implants caused systemic illness, they did not pursue these leads after receiving pertinent published reports about aspartame disease! The facts sought entailed parts of the Questionnaire (Chapter XVIII) and information about the following:

- Date(s) of silicone breast implant surgery
- Medical background before implant surgery – including drugs and habits
- Symptoms that developed after implant surgery, and dates of onset
- Date(s) of breast implant removal
- Medical status (improved; worse; unchanged) after implant removal (if performed)

Additionally, attempts to obtain the cooperation of several groups involved with breast implants proved futile. The inference of finding associated aspartame disease was viewed as counterproductive by litigants. The possibility that the systemic symptoms might represent reactions to aspartame in conjunction with changes induced by the silicone polymer was raised. The court-appointed scientific panel, referred to earlier, also conjectured on "the potential for silicone breast implants to exacerbate disease." The writer's letter requesting assistance of these groups stated

> "In view of the profound medical and legal ramifications involved, I would like to suggest that you and members of your network engage in a simple study. It entails completion of a questionnaire, modified after the one printed in my books on aspartame disease (enclosed), by persons with silicone breast implants and controls. This voluntary study – with no grants from any of the legal parties involved – would establish its neutrality."

Pertinent Socioeconomic and Ethical Aspects

The prodigious consumption of products containing aspartame by weight- and-figure-conscious women provides a crucial socioeconomic common denominator. The majority of women (60 percent) with silicone prostheses elected to have breast augmentation for cosmetic reasons rather than for deformity resulting from breast cancer surgery (Cook 1995).

Most figure-conscious women in our society consume "diet" products to avoid or control weight gain. This phenomenon is striking among white women with greater household incomes... the same group that predominates in electing silicone implant surgery for cosmetic reasons (Cook 1995).

Such economic selectivity has been validated by the producer of a popular diet cola. Its researches concluded that middle-age women are not only the prime consumers of this drink, but also the chief purchaser's of best-selling novels. As a result, the firm inserted excerpts from six new books in its six-packs (*The Miami Herald* April 13, 1999, p. A-13).

It is unfortunate that this inquiry has to address ethical professional considerations, including "sciencegate." Discussing "The Code of Silence," Dr. Peter Wilmshurst (1997) wrote, "I contend that those who should uphold the ethics of medicine and medical research tolerate and help to conceal dishonesty."*

A fundamental issue involves the extent of "junk science" in mass torts of questionable validity. Judge Bernstein (1996) warned in *Blum v Merrell Dow Pharmaceuticals* (1996) that " 'scientific consensus' can be created through purchased research and the manipulation of 'scientific' literature." The demand for "evidence based" statistical validation poses a paradox. As noted, the author repeatedly attempted to obtain it, only to encounter disinterest or stiff resistance, even from the defendants being sued!

A related matter involves self-serving interests. Criticism of those disputing the systemic manifestations of silicone implants has been leveled by persons who served as consultants and "expert witnesses" in breast implant litigation on behalf of plaintiffs (Angell 1996, p. 1156). This costly quagmire reaffirms the "call for activism by scientists" issued by Rosenbaum (1997) based on "lessons from litigation over silicone breast implants."

Possible Related Unwarranted Litigation

There are pertinent counterparts to litigation involving silicone breast implants as the alleged cause of systemic symptoms in a society where over 70 percent of adults consume "diet" products.

A case in point is the business decision by American Home Products Corporation to settle injury suits over its Norplant® contraceptive device by paying $50 million (*The Wall Street Journal* August 27, 1999, p. B-5). It was made despite universal rejection by courts that the claims of attorneys representing these women with a variety of systemic complaints were attributable to inadequate disclosure. The tendency to gain weight by women on contraceptive hormones undoubtedly influenced their preference for aspartame products.

I. THE GULF WAR (DESERT SHIELD) SYNDROME

Considerable debate continues about the so-called Gulf War syndrome. Many patients in this category and their relatives incriminated aspartame as a likely factor.

Dr. Robert Haley (1999), University of Texas Southwestern Medical Center, listed a "reproducible pattern of symptoms reported by many Gulf War veterans." The following multisystem features resemble those occurring in aspartame disease (Chapter II-A).

- Memory problem
- Depression
- Fatigue (daytime sleepiness)
- Speech problems
- Insomnia
- Distractibility
- Migraine headaches
- Moodiness
- Anxiety
- Mental confusion
- Vertigo
- Sexual impotence
- Joint pains
- Muscle pains
- Tingling or numbness in the extremities

No reasonable factor identifiable among Americans, British and Canadian troops engaged in the Gulf War should be ignored in view of the magnitude of disability among nearly two-thirds of the 50,000 troops involved. Persistent fatigue, irritability, headache, insomnia and complaints of breathlessness rendered many unfit for duty. Epidemiologic studies have not convincingly identified a cause.

- Unwin et al (1999) conducted a cross-section epidemiologic survey of United Kingdom servicemen who served in the Persian Gulf area. Their findings did not support a unique Gulf War syndrome.
- Ismail et al (1999) analyzed three UK military cohorts of men serving in the Gulf War and others who had not been actively deployed to it. They could not determine a unique syndrome.

Aspartame disease was raised by a number of correspondents for several reasons.

- There were official requests that relatives and other persons not send servicemen any items containing sugar. As a result, many thousands of packets of Diet Kool Aide® arrived.
- Gulf War veterans had independently reported observing many pallets of diet colas exposed for weeks to the Arabian sun.
- The mother of a Gulf War veteran with memory problems, visual difficulty, and other unexplained disorders wrote, "The water was bad, and they drank diet colas all day." A remarkable aspect involved the recommendation of his best friend, who had worked for a manufacturer of aspartame: "Do not let your family use aspartame!"

Admittedly, exposure to pesticides and other chemicals (Chapter VIII-G) may have summated upon the effects of aspartame, resulting in confusion, dizziness and central pain. Examples included the wearing of flea collars meant for pets, and the application of insect/tick repellants containing high concentrations of DEET.

Representative Case Reports

Case XXVII-I-1

A male registered nurse on active duty in the United States Navy during the Gulf War drank a gallon of diet soda every day. He experienced increased headaches, nausea, vomiting, and shaking of the hands. There was marked improvement after avoiding aspartame products, notwithstanding "nasty withdrawal symptoms" during the initial four days of abstinence.

Case XXVII-I-2

A pilot served in a squadron during the Desert Shield operation. He brought "cases upon cases of diet sodas from package stores, which were nothing more than open, non-airconditioned warehouses." An "avid drinker of diet sodas," he developed severe complaints that were variously diagnosed as "MVP, TM, MS, migraine, hypoglycemia, tendonitis, arthritis, carpal tunnel syndrome and depression." (These initials refer to mitral valve prolapse, transverse myelitis and multiple sclerosis.) He also developed optic neuritis in the left eye.

J. OTHER AREAS REQUIRING RESEARCH

Many issues raised above and throughout this book invite extensive research to clarify the "pharmacoepidemiology" of aspartame disease. Only a few are briefly presented.

Dr. Gerald A. Faich (1986), Office of Epidemiology and Biostatistics, Center for Drugs and Biologics at the FDA, editorialized on the importance of "total drug risk" and the inherent limitations therein. (It is recalled that aspartame originally was conceived as a drug for peptic ulcer.)

"The presentation of an impressive pharmacoepidemiologic study reminds us how few such studies are carried out. To examine risks of marketed drugs, appropriate cohorts or case series and comparison populations must be located in the community. Dealing with confounding by indication and other complexities of observational studies of ill patients requires carefully designed approaches and sophisticated analyses. Who will fund and conduct such studies? Usual sources of research support find that most pharmaceutical safety issues are too mundane or are lacking in basic scientific significance. Regulatory bodies have few funds for research. The pharmaceutical industry, while not homogeneous, largely commits its post-approval research funds to clinical trials having potential for product enhancement. The result is that

there are few academic or industry based pharmacoepidemiologists in the United States or elsewhere.*" (Italics supplied)

Additionally, the "junk science" from partnership arrangements between universities and multinational chemical companies has confused both regulators and the public.

Commentary

Many jolting encounters during decades of self-motivated clinical research convinced me of two issues: (a) I could not depend on sympathy or support for my studies on aspartame disease, and (b) I would be more productive by "going it alone."

> Clinical investigators in other fields recognize this struggle in contemporary science. In his book, *And The Waters Turned to Blood: The Ultimate Biological Threat* (Simon & Schuster), Rodney Barker, describes the tribulations facing an aquatic ecologist who discovered *Pfiesteria piscicida*, the organism responsible for "red tide." This crusader had to contend with the establishment, rigged grant proposals, conniving colleagues, and deceit by health department bureaucrats and environmental officials.

Insights From Student Projects

The diligence of students – even in grammar school – who performed studies involving aspartame as a result of their interest in aspartame disease has been impressive.

- Jennifer Cohen studied the rates and percentages of aspartame breakdown products at different temperatures (Chapter XXII).
- Susi Morse of Price, Utah reported a three-year study conducted on elderly rats. She demonstrated that sucrose-fed animals could run a six-course maze 30 percent faster than aspartame-fed rats (*The Palm Beach Post* August 30, 1998, p. A-16). Her report was presented at the 15th Annual International Sweetener Symposium sponsored by the American Sugar Alliance.

Several middle school and high school students who performed science projects involving the effects of aspartame on animals described the rejection of this chemical.

> Jyoti V. Deo, a student at Glenridge Middle School in Winterpark, Florida, gave ten dogs a choice between Sprite® (containing sugar) and Diet Sprite® (containing aspartame) when they were made thirsty after walking or running. Only one dog (a mixed breed) preferred the diet soda. This student also found that the weakest detectable concentration of aspartame was 4.5 mg per 100 ml of water. Another dog was given the choice between a pile of sugar and a pile of aspartame; only the aspartame remained the next day.

I. Aggravation of Allergies (Chapter VIII)

The increase of mortality from asthma among children in recent years has been striking. It raises questions concerning the influence of food additives and other environmental agents (*The Wall Street Journal* February 18, 1987, p. 29.)

Cross-sensitization to additional additives and chemicals by aspartame products, especially manufactured monosodium glutamate (Roberts 1993a), was reviewed in Chapter VIII-E.

II. Intellectual and Behavioral Performance of Children (Chapter VII and XI)

The frequency of abnormalities in development, attention-deficit disorder, and lowered school performance among children consuming aspartame products must be clarified. This also applies to the offspring of mothers who used them during pregnancy.

The contributory role of aspartame to aberrant behavior, the rising number of suicides among teenagers, and crimes committed by children below the age of ten (*The Miami Herald* December 29, 1986, p. A-16), requires comparable study.

III. High-Risk Groups (Chapters X to XVII)

Medical disorders other than those listed in Section 3 increase the risk of consuming aspartame in large amounts. They include kidney disease, liver disease, hypothyroidism (underactive thyroid), gout, and many neurologic disorders. Examples of the latter are myasthenia gravis, narcolepsy, stroke, multiple sclerosis, parkinsonism, and evolving Alzheimer's disease.

The use of aspartame by children with the sudden infant death syndrome (SIDS) and near-miss SIDS should be investigated in view of its apparent contribution to sleep apnea (Chapter VI-K).

The subject of aspartame-accelerated Alzheimer's disease was discussed in Chapter XV. This issue evolved from my encounter of many relatively young aspartame reactors who experienced severe confusion and memory loss.

IV. Altered Behavior in Drivers and Pilots (see above)

The dramatic increase of traffic confrontations involving otherwise-responsible citizens, and the rising number of "near-misses" by pilots, should alert all to the consumption of aspartame by drivers and pilots. This issue was stressed in a separate title (Roberts 1998d).

V. Susceptibility to Infectious Diseases and Their Complications (Chapter IX-1)

The apparent increased susceptibility of some aspartame consumers to recurrent infection deserves investigation, as does possible damage to the immune system. Reasonable questions concern whether such immunologic stress is compounded by feminity (Chapter II), the high intake of phenylalanine, and administration of live virus or bacterial vaccines.

The correlation of aspartame consumption with certain infectious diseases that have become problems also deserves attention.

- Women with aspartame disease repeatedly experienced <u>fungal infections</u> while using aspartame products.
- The resurgence of <u>acute rheumatic fever</u> ("the red plague") since 1984 has puzzled researchers. Serious outbreaks occurred among the children and young adults of affluent families (*Newsweek* December 22, 1986, p. 60), contrasting with its characterization as a "slum disease" earlier in the century. Utah's outbreak of 133 confirmed cases, for example, could not be attributed to an increased incidence of

streptococcal infection (*Medical World News* March 23, 1987). The <u>chronic Epstein-Barr virus syndrome</u> (Chapter IX), possibly involving lowered immunity, has become more prevalent in recent years.

- The so-called <u>postpolio syndrome</u> surfaced among poliomyelitis victims decades after their acute paralytic illness. It presumably reflects "exhaustion" of the remaining nerve cells that innervate muscles and other organs. Current evidence suggests that progressive death of individual nerve terminals when their cell bodies cannot maintain the metabolic demands of the increased sprouts (editorial, *The Lancet* 1985; 2:1195-1196) – a realm in which aspartame metabolites can have adverse effects.

- Considerable aspartame is consumed by some victims of <u>HIV infection</u> in an attempt to avoid sugar. They consider sugar intake as conducive to fungal super-infection.

VI. <u>Unexplained Sudden Deaths</u>

Aspartame disease should be considered when an adult in apparent good health who had consumed considerable aspartame products is found dead without demonstrable cause (Chapter IX-C). For example, a 50-year-old woman unexpectedly died at home. The only pertinent history obtained from her daughter was having "a diet cola in her hand every waking minute of the day and night."

VII. <u>Carcinogen or Co-Carcinogen</u> (see above)

Aspartame may serve as a co-carcinogen, especially with viruses, in the case of cancers that have escalated. An example may be hepatocellular carcinoma associated with hepatitis B and C viruses. This tumor nearly doubled during the past decades, with a progressive shift toward younger persons (El-Serag 1999).

VIII. <u>Effects on Satiety</u> (Chapter IX)

Aspartame can play a paramount role in anorexia nervosa and bulimia. Such patients, particularly weight-conscious young women, binge on food and then attempt to rid themselves of it by vomiting or the use of laxatives. This compulsive behavior poses a dilemma for physicians, psychologists and others as eating disorders keep increasing in our society.

IX. <u>Genetic Disorders</u>

A possible adverse role of aspartame in genetic diseases must be considered in persons other than pregnant women and phenylketonuria (PKU) "carriers" (Chapter XVII). They include individuals with enzyme deficiencies, both congenital and acquired, that can affect the metabolism of neurotransmitters. Congenital dopamine beta-hydroxylase deficiency (In 'T Veld 1987) is a case in point.

"Dry eyes" (Chapter IV) and "dry mouth" (Chapter IX) can be induced by aspartame. In simulating Sjögren's syndrome, studies are needed to determine whether aspartame interferes with DNA synthesis in proliferating cells.

The possible aggravation of other glandular secretory deficiencies, including some that are genetic or familial in nature, also warrants attention. Cystic fibrosis, chronic pancreatitis, "the fragile X syndrome," and disorders causing gastrointestinal malabsorption are candidates.

X. <u>Birth Defects</u>

The number of drugs and chemical products capable of inducing birth defects increases annually. Examples are anticonvulsants, dioxins, spray adhesives, insecticides, industrial solvents, and isotretinoine (marketed for the treatment of acne). *Chemically Induced Birth Defects*, a book by James L. Schardein, Frederick J. DiCarlo and Frederick W. Oehme (Marcel Dekker, Inc., 1985), contains 879 pages.

There are ample grounds for suspecting the teratogenic effects of aspartame and its metabolites.

- Aspartame has been shown to be capable of inducing cell aging by its effects on human diploid cells in culture, with a corresponding decrease of mitochondrial activity (Kasamaki 1993).
- The increased concentration of methanol-derived formaldehyde in DNA (Chapter XXI) is relevant.

The chromosomal abnormalities and congenital deformities involving women who used aspartame at the time of conception and during pregnancy (Chapter X) requires investigation. The fetal neurotoxicity of such indulgence poses another challenge for our pay-later society.

XI. Potentiation by Other Additives, Amino Acids and Drugs

The potentiated adverse effects of aspartame by other additives, pesticides and chemicals/drugs seem fertile area for investigation. Gulf War servicemen receiving drugs to protect against poison gas exposure, who consumed considerable diet sodas (see above), suggest this scenario. Unfortunately, corporate-sponsored researchers usually investigate their effects on health individually rather than as "illness by a thousand cuts."

The adverse effects of aspartame on brain function may increase when consumed with other additives or drugs. Reference to this phenomenon was made in the case of manufactured monosodium glutamate (MSG) (Chapter VIII-E), a seasoning used in processed foods and Chinese dishes. Aspartic acid interacts with MSG to synergize its neurotoxicity, especially among children (Olney 1986).

The potentiated action of standard medications by aspartame, particularly psychotropic drugs and tranquilizers, warrants study. Some of the associated "side effects" or "withdrawal symptoms" (e.g., blurred vision, numbness, seizures) may have been caused or aggravated by concomitant aspartame use (Chapter VII-G).

XII. Additional Pharmacologic Considerations

Possible differences in the metabolism of aspartame when consumed at different times of the day require pharmacologic clarification. An example is the taking of aspartame – sweetened coffee, tea or cola products to increase alertness at night.

- Persons working swing-shift jobs tend to have a desynchronization of circadian rhythms, as manifest by disturbed sleep (Roberts 1971b).
- Physicians recognize that patients with diabetes, epilepsy, hyperthyroidism and other disorders often have exacerbations when their work schedules are shifted.
- Experimentally, certain medications and toxins given at night are known to result in higher mortality than when administered in the morning.

Phenylalanine (Chapter XXII) is a precursor of chemicals in the body that influence skin pigmentation. Accordingly, there should be clarification of whether patients with prior melanoma ought to be warned against aspartame use.

826

The superimposed effects of aspartame on other chemical and physical influences to which large segments of the population are constantly exposed deserve study. This realm remains highly charged. For example, long-term studies demonstrating that the electromagnetic fields from electric power lines can influence memory, behavior and even tumor formation in children generate considerable controversy.

XIII. <u>Genetic Engineering</u>

Advanced biotechnologies should be cause for concern when dealing with the incorporation of amino acids into genetic material (as recombinant DNA), and the synthesis of proteins by means of a protein synthesizer. The genetically engineered bacteria used in producing phenylalanine illustrate this issue. *The Independent* noted on its front page (June 20, 1999) that the bacteria used to make aspartame in American plants have an amino acid difference from the traditionally modified strain. (By way of reference, single amino acid differences are reported in sickle cell disease and diabetes.)

There is a paucity of published studies concerning certain metabolites of bacteria-generated phenylalanine and their metabolic/immunologic effects.

- Foreign DNA enters the body via the gastrointestinal tract, and can cross the placenta.
- Gene transfer occurs between transgenic plants and bacteria.
- Genes, like viruses, can infect the body and results in unanticipated side effects.
- The potential for contaminants has been raised, as was the case with certain batches of tryptophan products under comparable circumstances.

K. THE ISSUES OF SACCHARIN AND CYCLAMATES

The safety of saccharin and cyclamates as chemical sweeteners is inevitably raised in aspartame discussions.

I. <u>Saccharin</u>

The public perceives saccharin as unsafe, with emphasis on cancer. This stems from the mandated labels of foods and drinks containing it (Chapter XXVX). Such prejudice is indicated by the attitudes of women who were rated as being "very concerned" about saccharin (40 percent), and "slightly concerned" (35 percent) (Ebert 1987).

Saccharin ranked fifth in the list of negative attitudes to ingredients. (Cholesterol was first; salt third; and caffeine tenth.) In fact, the inference that products containing saccharin might cause tumors favored preference for aspartame on the grounds that it had been "proved safe."

The alleged carcinogenicity of saccharin stems from finding tumors of the urinary bladder in a few rats to which large doses had been given. This is consistent with the urogenous-contact hypothesis involving other carcinogenic substances (Michaud 1999).

Historically, saccharin was discovered in 1879, and found to be 300 times sweeter than sugar. President Theodore Roosevelt liked to sweeten his chewing tobacco with it. In apparent anticipation, he observed, "Anyone who says saccharin is injurious to health is an idiot."

The corporate advantages of this situation are obvious. The low price of saccharin contrasts sharply with the costs for aspartame, acesulfame-K and sugar. Some have suggested that this was the <u>primary</u> reason for continuing the "bogus cancer warning" on saccharin products.

Others share the author's skepticism relative to the validity of ensuing legislation.

- A position statement by the American Diabetes Association (1987) asserted

  > "Epidemiological studies show *no* evidence of a carcinogenic effect (of saccharin) in humans. The small risk, if any, from ingestion at moderate levels is considered to be *extremely small*. Because saccharin can cross the placenta, heavy use during pregnancy should be avoided." (Italics supplied)

- Researchers at the National Cancer Institute could NOT find evidence of bladder cancer in 20 monkeys given 25 mg per kg body weight five days a week for as long as 24 years (*Reuters*, January 6, 1998).
- Decades ago, *The Lancet* (1977) editorialized that banning saccharin for an as-yet-unrevealed compelling reason could lead to "mourning... the reputation of those responsible for its banishment."

- *The Wall Street Journal* (August 4,1 977, p. A-18) editorialized

  > "Saccharin may give rise to tumors in lab animals, but rodents are not real men. Diabetics have been relying on if for years – in high doses – with no ill effects. The proposed ban and Congress-enforced warning labels on saccharin was absurd in 1977, and is embarrassing now. The truth is that politicians have been afraid to eliminate the Delaney clause for fear of being labeled pro-cancer."

- Senator Samuel Nunn indicated in the *Congressional Record-Senate* of May 7, 1985: "It is my understanding that the many studies on human groups consuming large quantities of saccharin, such as diabetics, have never shown a correlation between human cancer and saccharin consumption."

- In the absence of new evidence for the carcinogenicity of saccharin, the Canadian government reconsidered its 1977 decision to ban saccharin as an additive in foods and soft drinks.

- Representative James G. Martin of North Carolina publicly accused the FDA for having acted "at the drop of a rat" in banning saccharin (*Science News* 112:12, 1977).

The FDA recognizes the daily saccharin intake of 1000 mg by adults and about 500 mg by children to be Generally Recognized As Safe (GRAS). This is the equivalent of 50-70 packets for adults, and 25-35 packets for children. (One teaspoon or packet of the powder contains 14-20 mg saccharin.)

The government **formally delisted** saccharin from its list of human carcinogens on May 15, 2000 in the biennial *Report on Carcinogens...* more than 20 years after the scare from limited tests in rats that cast doubt about its safety.

Criticisms Of the Rat Model

The initial studies indicating a statistically significant increase of bladder tumors in <u>male</u> rats were reported by the Wisconsin Alumni Research Foundation (1973).

The choice of rats for the pellet-implantation technique, however, has been criticized, especially by physicians treating diabetic and obese patients. Lindner (1979) titled an editorial on the subject, "The Laboratory Rat: Public Enemy Number One!"

- Dr. Freddy Homburger (1977), an authority on the experimental use of Sprague-Dawley rats, asserted, "Rats are not appropriate animals for the study of bladder cancer." He emphasized that extensive papillomatosis of the urinary bladder is caused by the parasite *Trichosomoides crassicauda*. Furthermore, naturally occurring carcinogens in food, microcrystals in the bladder, and hormonal imbalances may cause bladder cancer in these and other rodents.

- In their view of artificial sweeteners causing urinary bladder cancer, Bryan and Yoshida (1971) stated, "It appears that the pellet, as a foreign body, plays a role in the augmented sensitivity of the pellet method. The pellet does stimulate mitotic activity among the mucosal cells of the bladder." In two control groups, 13 percent and 12 percent of the mice developed bladder cancer from the implantation of cholesterol alone (*The Wall Street Journal* March 18, 1970).

- *The Lancet* (1977) observed, "Clearly, tumors may arise non-specifically as a consequence of the prolonged presence of solid bodies in the bladder." It further noted the absence of evidence for increased risk of tumors at <u>any</u> other site in the many animal studies reported.

Criticisms Based On The Consumption of Saccharin by Humans

Patients wishing to use saccharin in place of sugar have protested this artificial "mouse-to-man" dilemma. They emphasized the lack of evidence for saccharin-related tumors in humans, especially among diabetics who have taken saccharin since 1910.

A link between saccharin and urinary bladder cancer has <u>not</u> been convincingly shown in several large human epidemiologic studies.

- The president of the American Cancer Society stated, "There is no evidence that saccharin causes cancer in humans" (*Science* 196:276, 1977).

- Morgan and Jain (1974) examined the relationship of cancer of the urinary bladder to artificial sweeteners in a matched patient-control study. They were unable to identify an increased risk.

- Morrison and Burning (1980) sought a correlation between cancer of the lower urinary tract and the use of artificial sweeteners in a case-controlled study of 592 patients with lower-urinary-tract cancer (94 percent of whom had bladder tumors) and 536 controls (chosen from the general population of the study area). They concluded that users of artificial sweeteners, as a group, have "little or no excess rise of cancer of the lower urinary tract."

- Hoover and Strasser (1980) could find "no elevation in risk" among 3,010 patients with cancer of the urinary bladder and 5,783 controls from the general population of ten geographic areas in the United States relative to prior use of artificial sweeteners or artificially sweetened foods and beverages. (Aspartame was not commercially available then.) These investigators asserted that their data failed to support earlier reports of a relative risk as high as 1.6 for men using tabletop artificial sweeteners. They raised the possibility of increased risk among smokers from potentiation of the carcinogenic effect of smoking by sweeteners.

- *The Lancet* (1980; 1:855-856) editorialized on the foregoing study, as well as the subject in general. It concluded that "a moderate or strong carcinogenic effect of saccharin has been satisfactorily excluded."

- Winder and Stellman (1980) analyzed a case-control study of bladder cancer patients (302 males and 65 females) and an equal number of patients matched by age, sex, hospital and hospital-room status. They could find no association between bladder cancer and the use of artificial sweeteners or diet beverages. Moreover, t hey were unable to support the cited conjecture that artificial sweeteners promote a tumorigenic effect of tobacco.

Another criticism of the rat studies pertains to the enormous amounts of saccharin administered. Three of 20 rats evidencing bladder tumors had been fed a diet containing 5 percent saccharin over a two-year period (*The Wall Street Journal* January 31, 1972). The FDA noted that this was the equivalent of humans consuming 875 bottles of a typical diet soft drink daily. By contrast, persons who use saccharin-containing foods and sodas, and add saccharin to coffee, consume this chemical as an estimated 0.1 percent of their daily diet (*Science* 177:971, 1972).

Saccharin may be a carcinogen only for rodents because it combines with an alpha-2-u-globulin, which irritates the bladder lining. Humans do NOT have this particular globulin (Cohen 1992).

II. Cyclamates

Controversial research led to the withdrawal of cyclamates from United States markets in 1970. This artificial sweetener, discovered in 1937, is approximately 30 times sweeter than table sugar (sucrose). It has the added advantages of being heat-stable and devoid of saccharin's bitter aftertaste.

A 1969 study in rats given a saccharin/cyclamate mixture suggested that is might cause cancer in this rodent (Price 1970). The following subsequent conclusions, however, argue against human carcinogenesis by cyclamates taken in modest amounts.

- An expert panel on food safety an nutrition for the Institute of Food Technology submitted a summary statement on sweeteners in August 1986. It indicated that research had failed to prove the tumor-producing properties of cyclamate conclusively.
- The FDA's rejection in 1980 of a petition for cyclamate approval was based on the general safety clause of the Food, Drug and Cosmetic Act, not the Delaney Clause. Further petitions were introduced in the absence of these data and a convincing mutagenic effect.
- The Cancer Assessment Committee of the Center for Food Safety and Applied Nutrition of the FDA asserted in April 1984 that no further research into the question of cyclamate carcinogenicity was necessary.

SECTION 7

OBSTACLES TO INFORMATION, EDUCATION AND REGULATION

"The truth requires constant repetition because error is being preached about us all the time."
　　　Goethe

"Publicity and openness, honest and complete – that is the prime condition for the health of every society, and ours, too."
　　　Aleksandr I. Solzhenitsyn (1969)

"Falsehood flies and the truth comes limping after; so that when men come to be undeceived it is too late: the jest is over and the tale has had its effect."
　　　Jonathan Swift

Patients, physicians, consumers and consumer advocates have encountered disinterest or evasiveness when seeking information about aspartame reactions from professional, corporate and "official" sources. Another applicable term is "sponsored deception." This has been coupled with resistance by governmental bodies and Congress to suggestions that the safety of aspartame products be reevaluated.

- Barbara Mullarkey (*Wednesday Journal of Oak Park & River Forest* March 26, 1986) summarized her probes of aspartame reactions with this statement, "The FDA appears to align with industry, not the consumer."
- Senator Howard Metzenbaum was unable to get legislation passed that would require labeling the content of aspartame present in soft drinks accurately (Chapter XXVII-B). Without this information, for example, consumers could not determine that one brand of a popular diet cola contained only one-fourth the aspartame found in two other brands.

Other general attitudes and impediments proved vexing.

- The director of professional services for a major pharmaceutical company pointed out that "people do not read labels" (*The Wall Street Journal* April 22, 1987, p. 35).
- Dr. John Yudkin (1987), a British nutritionist, expressed concern that the public will continue to receive confusing dietary advice as long as "apparently authoritative bodies" issue selective or misrepresented reports.
- Slovic (1987) emphasized the necessity for communicating risk information to decision-makers and technical experts. Without understanding how the public thinks about and responds to risk, however, even well-intentioned policies are likely to prove ineffective.
- Pointing out that consumers do not need non-nutritive sweeteners, Lave (1987) elaborated upon "risk-risk" situations wherein a choice is required among alternatives. For example, the FDA considers the risk of a food additive increasing the chance of cancer by less than one case per million lifetimes as of little concern.

The primary intent of the Informed Consent Doctrine in "to protect the patient's right of self-determination, and to promote rational decision making" (Annis 1977). The latter is directly applicable to the proper labeling of ingredients in food products. It is a partial attempt to compensate for failure-to-disclose information about aspartame products in ads, everything-you-need-to-know features, and even scientific articles.

A. HISTORICAL MISGIVINGS ABOUT ASPARTAME

The extraordinary circumstances under which aspartame was approved by the FDA over objections by its senior scientists, especially in the case of beverages, have been documented in the public record (*Congressional Record-Senate* 1985a, b). Such approval also reflects the emphasis upon "deregulation" during the Reagan Administration.

A Bittersweet History

Senator Metzenbaum submitted the following "time-line" highlights of pertinent events and excerpts to Senator Orrin Hatch, Chairman of the Senate Labor and Human Resources Committee, on February 3, 1986. He unsuccessfully sought full subpoena power to investigate allegations about the concealment of "material facts" and the making of "false statements."

DOCUMENT LIST

<u>1965</u>: NUTRASWEET (ASPARTAME) DISCOVERED.

<u>MARCH 5, 1973</u>: SEARLE FILES PETITION FOR APPROVAL OF (NUTRASWEET) AS FOOD ADDITIVE.

<u>JULY 16, 1974</u>: FDA APPROVES NUTRASWEET AS FOOD ADDITIVE

<u>JULY 23, 1975</u>: FDA ESTABLISHES SEARLE INVESTIGATION TASK FORCE TO EXAMINE CERTAIN ANIMAL STUDIES CONDUCTED BY SEARLE, INCLUDING TESTS ON NUTRASWEET.

<u>DECEMBER 5, 1975</u>: BEFORE NUTRASWEET COMES ON THE MARKET, FDA STAYS ITS APPROVAL "BASED ON THE COMMISSIONER'S CONCLUSION IN JULY, 1975 THAT THE INTEGRITY OF CERTAIN ANIMAL STUDIES CONDUCTED BY SEARLE WAS QUESTIONABLE." (DOC #1, pg. 18)

<u>MARCH 24, 1976</u>: FDA'S SEARLE TASK FORCE OFFICIALLY REPORTS. CONCLUSIONS INCLUDE:

"AT THE HEART OF FDA'S REGULATORY PROCESS IS ITS ABILITY TO RELY UPON THE INTEGRITY OF THE BASIC SAFETY DATA SUBMITTED BY SPONSORS OF REGULATED

PRODUCTS. OUR INVESTIGATION CLEARLY DEMONSTRATES THAT, IN THE G. D. SEARLE COMPANY, WE HAVE NO BASIS FOR SUCH RELIANCE NOW." (DOC #2, pg. 1)

"WE HAVE NOTED THAT SEARLE HAS NOT SUBMITTED ALL THE FACTS OF EXPERIMENTS TO FDA, RETAINING UNTO ITSELF THE UNPERMITTED OPTION OF FILTERING, INTERPRETING, AND NOT SUBMITTING INFORMATION WHICH WE WOULD CONSIDER MATERIAL TO THE SAFETY EVALUATION OF THE PRODUCT. SOME OF OUR FINDINGS SUGGEST AN ATTITUDE OF DISREGARD FOR FDA'S MISSION OF PROTECTION OF THE PUBLIC HEALTH BY SELECTIVELY REPORTING THE RESULTS OF STUDIES IN A MANNER WHICH ALLAYS THE CONCERNS OF QUESTIONS OF AN FDA REVIEWER." (DOC #2, pg. 1)

THE TASK FORCE AUDITED 25 SEARLE STUDIES, 11 OF WHICH WERE ON NUTRASWEET.

REPORT INCLUDED A RECOMMENDATION THAT THE FDA ASK THE U.S. ATTORNEY IN THE NORTHERN DISTRICT OF ILLINOIS TO INSTITUTE GRAND JURY PROCEEDINGS "UTILIZING COMPULSORY PROCESS IN ORDER TO IDENTIFY MORE PARTICULARLY THE NATURE OF VIOLATION AND TO IDENTIFY ALL THOSE RESPONSIBLE FOR SUCH VIOLATIONS." (DOC #2, pg. 10)

APRIL 7, 1976: FDA WRITES TO U.S. ATTORNEY SKINNER CITING ITS TASK INVESTIGATION OF TESTS ON A NUMBER OF SEARLE FOOD ADDITIVES AND DRUGS. SKINNER IS INFORMED THAT FDA WANTS A GRAND JURY EMPANELED "TO INQUIRE INTO THE CAUSES AND SIGNIFICANCE OF THE DISCREPANCIES IN ANIMAL TEST DATA SUBMITTED IN SUPPORT OF SEARLE PRODUCTS." FORMAL REQUESTS FOR GRAND JURY TO FOLLOW. (DOC #3)

APRIL, 1976: SKINNER ASSIGNS BILL CONLON AND FRED BRANDING TO SEARLE INVESTIGATION. BILL CONLON WAS SKINNER'S DEPUTY CHIEF IN THE CIVIL DIVISION.

BRANDING, AN ASSISTANT U.S. ATTORNEY, WAS CONLON'S SUBORDINATE.

APRIL 15, 1976: BRANDING TO SKINNER. SEARLE HAS PROPOSED A MEETING WITH JUSTICE IN WASHINGTON "REGARDING THE FDA REFERRAL FOR CRIMINAL INVESTIGATION OF THE G. D. SEARLE COMPANY." BRANDING REQUESTS AUTHORIZATION TO ATTEND. (DOC #4)

OCTOBER 20, 1976: FDA HOLDS ADMINISTRATIVE HEARING ON G. D. SEARLE INVESTIGATION WHERE SEARLE PRESENTS ARGUMENTS AGAINST FURTHER PROCEEDINGS. FDA DECIDES TO PROCEED WITH RECOMMENDATION FOR CRIMINAL INVESTIGATION.

JANUARY 10, 1977: FDA WRITES A 33-PAGE LETTER TO SKINNER RECOMMENDING GRAND JURY INVESTIGATION OF G. D. SEARLE "FOR CONCEALING MATERIAL FACTS AND MAKING FALSE STATEMENTS IN REPORTS OF ANIMAL STUDIES CONDUCTED TO ESTABLISH THE SAFETY OF THE DRUG ALDACTONE AND THE FOOD ADDITIVE ASPARTAME (NUTRASWEET)". (DOC #1, pg. 1)

LETTER CITES 1970 SEARLE STRATEGY MEMO IN WHICH SEARLE COMMITS ITSELF TO OBTAINING FAVORABLE REVIEW OF NUTRASWEET BY FDA PERSONNEL BY SEEKING TO DEVELOP IN THEM A "SUBCONSCIOUS SPIRIT OF PARTICIPATION IN THE SEARLE STUDIES," MEMO SAYS.

SEARLE WANTS TO GET THE FDA IN THE HABIT OF SAYING "YES." FDA SAYS THEY WANT "THE TRUTH, NOT PSYCHOLOGICAL WARFARE." (DOC #1, pg. 26)

LETTER ALSO STRESSES IMPORTANCE OF SAFETY DATA ON NUTRASWEET SINCE "IF ULTIMATELY APPROVED FOR MARKETING, THIS SWEETENING AGENT CAN REASONABLY BE EXPECTED TO BE PART OF THE DAILY DIET OF EVERY AMERICAN"; "THE POTENTIAL COMMERCIAL VALUE OF ASPARTAME (NUTRASWEET) IS ENORMOUS." (DOC #1, pg. 18, pg.26)

FDA CITES TWO NUTRASWEET STUDIES FOR SPECIAL ATTENTION. A PRIMATE STUDY WHERE MONKEYS WHICH HAD SEIZURES WERE NEVER GIVEN AUTOPSIES AND A TOXICITY STUDY ON HAMSTERS. (DOC #1, pgs. 18-26)

SEARLE SUBMITTED THESE STUDIES TO THE FDA ON OCTOBER 10 AND DECEMBER 8, 1972. <u>SO, THE STATUTE OF LIMITATIONS ON ANY PROSECUTION (5 YEARS) WOULD EXPIRE ON OCTOBER 10 AND DECEMBER 8, 1977</u>.

FINALLY, THE FDA MADE IT CLEAR THAT THE GRAND JURY INVESTIGATION COULD COVER OTHER SEARLE TESTS WHOSE CREDIBILITY WAS BROUGHT INTO QUESTION BY THE 1976 TASK FORCE REPORT. "OUR SELECTION OF APPARENT VIOLATIONS, DOES NOT, OF COURSE, LIMIT THE INQUIRY BY YOUR OFFICE OR BY THE GRAND JURY." (DOC #1, pg. 30)

<u>JANUARY 24, 1977</u>: SKINNER CALLS MEETING IN U.S. ATTORNEY'S OFFICE TO DISCUSS "OUR NEXT STEP." (DOC #5)

<u>JANUARY 26, 1977</u>: SEARLE'S LAW FIRM, SIDLEY AND AUSTIN, WRITES TO SKINNER REQUESTING MEETING "PRIOR TO THE SUBMISSION TO A GRAND JURY OF ANY MATTERS RELATING TO THIS COMPANY" (SEARLE). (DOC #6)

<u>FEBRUARY 2, 1977</u>: LAWYERS FROM SIDLEY AND AUSTIN MEET WITH SKINNER. BRANDING TOOK NOTES. (DOC #7) NEWTON MINOW, A PARTNER AT SIDLEY AND AUSTIN, ATTENDS THE MEETING EVEN THOUGH HE IS NOT LISTED BY JUSTICE AS HANDLING THE SEARLE CASE. IT IS MINOW WHO OFFERS SKINNER A JOB AT SIDLEY AND AUSTIN. (DOC #8)

<u>FEBRUARY 7, 1977</u>: SIDLEY AND AUSTIN WRITE TO BRANDING TO CONFIRM THAT A MEETING WILL BE HELD IN THEIR OFFICES TO CONDUCT "A CALM AND ORDERLY BUT DETAILED FACTUAL REVIEW." REFERENCE IS MADE TO THE FACT THAT SKINNER WANTED SIDLEY AND AUSTIN TO ADDRESS INITIALLY MATTERS RELATING TO ALDACTONE. (DOC #9)

<u>MARCH 8, 1977</u>: SKINNER WRITES CONFIDENTIAL MEMO IN SEARLE CASE. (DOC #10) CITES HIS "PRELIMINARY EMPLOYMENT DISCUSSIONS WITH SIDLEY AND AUSTIN,", THE LAW FIRM DEFENDING SEARLE IN THE INVESTIGATION, AND THE FACT THAT IT IS

838

"INAPPROPRIATE FOR ME TO MAKE ANY DECISIONS IN THAT MATTER (SEARLE INVESTIGATION) WHILE I REMAIN IN OFFICE."

SKINNER STATES IT IS HIS UNDERSTANDING THAT CONLON AND BRANDING WILL DO ANY PRELIMINARY WORK THAT IS NECESSARY – BUT THAT A DECISION AS TO WHETHER OR NOT A GRAND JURY INVESTIGATION SHOULD BE CONDUCTED WILL AWAIT THE APPOINTMENT OF THE NEW U.S. ATTORNEY.

THE MEMO ALSO STATES:

"I HAVE ADVISED THE COUNSEL FOR G. D. SEARLE COMPANY (SIDNEY AND AUSTIN) OF MY DECISION TO RECUSE MYSELF IN THIS MATTER, BUT I WOULD APPRECIATE IT IF YOU WOULD KEEP THE FACT OF MY PRELIMINARY DISCUSSIONS CONFIDENTIAL TO AVOID ANY UNDUE EMBARRASSMENT UPON THE FIRM OF SIDLEY AND AUSTIN." (EMPHASIS SUPPLIED BY SENATOR METZENBAUM).

APRIL 13, 1977: OFFICIAL MEMO FROM KOCORAS TO SKINNER (DOC #11) CITES CONVERSATION WITH BRANDING AND CONLON. STATES "IT IS MY OPINION THAT A GRAND JURY INVESTIGATION BE UNDERTAKEN AT THE EARLIEST PRACTICABLE TIME." KOCORAS SAYS THE INVESTIGATION SHOULD NOT AWAIT THE APPOINTMENT OF A NEW U.S. ATTORNEY FOR TWO REASONS.

1. THE APPOINTMENT DATE IS UNCERTAIN. MAY NOT TAKE PLACE WITHIN NEXT TWO MONTHS.
2. "IT WOULD BE INAPPROPRIATE TO REFRAIN FROM CONDUCTING NECESSARY INVESTIGATION BY THE GRAND JURY DURING THE SUBSTANTIAL PERIOD OF TIME BETWEEN NOW AND MR. SULLIVAN'S APPOINTMENT."

KOCORAS TELLS SKINNER "IN LIGHT OF YOUR REFUSAL, THIS MEMORANDUM IS SOLELY TO ADVISE YOU OF MY DECISION TO PROCEED."

TWO POINTS SHOULD BE NOTED HERE. FIRST, THE GRAND JURY INVESTIGATION DOES NOT PROCEED AT THIS TIME. SECOND, THE STATUTE OF LIMITATIONS ON THE TWO NUTRASWEET TESTS CITED BY THE FDA EXPIRES IN OCTOBER-DECEMBER OF 1977. SO, THERE WAS A REAL URGENCY ASSOCIATED WITH THE INVESTIGATION.

APRIL 25, 1977: FDA LETTER TO BRANDING INFORMING HIM OF FDA FURTHER INSPECTION OF NUTRASWEET TESTS TO BE CONDUCTED AT SEARLE. ADVISING BRANDING THAT INSPECTION MAY GENERATE INQUIRES ABOUT "PENDING RECOMMENDATION" (GRAND JURY). ALSO TELLS BRANDING HE CAN CONTACT THE HEAD OF THE FDA INVESTIGATION TEAM, DR. BRESSLER, TO KEEP IN TOUCH WITH DEVELOPMENTS. (DOC #12)

MAY 4, 1977: FDA LETTER TO BRANDING RESPONDING TO SEARLE CHRONOLOGY OF EVENTS ON ALDACTONE WHICH THE U.S. ATTORNEY'S OFFICE HAD FORWARDED TO FDA. FDA SAYS "VERY LITTLE IS NEW AND NONE OF IT JUSTIFIES WITHHOLDING THIS MATTER FROM GRAND JURY AS RECOMMENDED IN OUR ORIGINAL TRANSMITTAL LETTER. (DOC #13)

MAY 25, 1977: BRANDING TO FDA. NOTES ANOTHER MEETING WITH SIDLEY AND AUSTIN. "THE SUBSTANCE OF THE MEETING WAS ESSENTIALLY THE SAME AS THE EARLIER MEETING (FEBRUARY 16, 1977) WITH MR. SKINNER PRIOR TO HIS REMOVING HIMSELF FROM ACTIVE PARTICIPATION IN THIS MATTER."

"AS BILL CONLON MAY HAVE ADVISED YOU VIA TELEPHONE, THREE ISSUES WERE RAISED IN 'DEFENSE' OF SEARLE'S POSITION..." BRANDING THEN ITEMIZES THE ISSUES AND REQUESTS WRITTEN RESPONSES FROM FDA. (DOC #14)

JUNE 2, 1977: FDA WRITES LETTER TO JUSTICE'S KOCORAS RESPONDING TO 3 SEARLE DEFENSES. AGAIN STATES THESE DEFENSES ARE "NOT NEW." FDA'S LEVINE SAYS HE HOPES THAT KOCORAS' RESERVATIONS "ARE ELIMINATED." IF ANY RESERVATIONS STILL EXIST, LEVINE OFFERS TO FLY TO CHICAGO "WHERE WE WOULD

HAVE THE BENEFIT OF THE KIND OF EXCHANGE AND PROBING FOLLOW-UP THAT CANNOT BE ACHIEVED IN WRITTEN COMMUNICATION." (DOC #15)

JULY 1, 1977: SAMUEL SKINNER LEAVES U. S. ATTORNEY'S OFFICE, JOINS SEARLE'S LAW FIRM, SIDLEY AND AUSTIN.

JULY 19, 1977: SULLIVAN BECOMES NEW U. S. ATTORNEY.

JULY 20, 1977: FDA CHIEF COUNSEL, MERRILL, WRITES TO SULLIVAN (DOC #16). STATES THAT HE HAS NOT HEARD FROM JUSTICE IN CHICAGO ABOUT GRAND JURY INVESTIGATION. CITES ALL THE RESPONSES FDA HAS GIVEN TO SEARLE'S DEFENSE AS RELAYED BY JUSTICE. NOTES SKINNER'S DEPARTURE TO SIDLEY AND AUSTIN, "WHICH HAS REPRESENTED SEARLE ON THE MATTERS INVOLVED IN THE CASE." ASKS SULLIVAN TO "PROCEED EXPEDITIOUSLY."

ALSO TELLS SULLIVAN THAT ANOTHER SEARLE TEST ON NUTRASWEET WHICH WAS REVIEWED BY FDA INSPECTORS RAISES ISSUES WHICH "COULD REQUIRE SUBMISSION TO THE GRAND JURY."

AUGUST 10, 1977: CHARLES MCCONACHIE, CONSUMER AFFAIRS ANTITRUST JUSTICE DEPARTMENT IN WASHINGTON, WRITES TO SULLIVAN. (DOC #17) CITES JULY 20,1977 LETTER FROM CHIEF COUNSEL OF FDA ASKING FOR GRAND JURY INVESTIGATION OF THE "PRIOR PRACTICES OF THIS FIRM" (SEARLE). MCCONACHIE STATES HIS SUPPORT FOR THAT REQUEST. SAYS IT SHOULD BE UNDERTAKEN "AS SOON AS POSSIBLE." (ALSO) SAYS HIS DIVISION IS RESPONSIBLE FOR CONDUCT AND SUPERVISION OF LITIGATION ARISING OUT OF ACTIONS RELATED TO FDA. HIS JOB TO ENSURE THESE CASES ARE HANDLED ON "AN EXPEDITED BASIS." "I AM BECOMING

CONCERNED AT THE AMOUNT OF TIME WHICH HAS TRANSPIRED BETWEEN FDA'S JANUARY, 1977, REFERRAL LETTER AND THE PRESENT. I KNOW OF NO REASON WHY THE GRAND JURY SHOULD NOT AT LEAST INVESTIGATE."

AUGUST 18, 1977: MEMO TO FILE. (DOC #18) MEETING BETWEEN SULLIVAN, BRANDING AND OTHER DEPARTMENT OF JUSTICE PEOPLE WITH SIDLEY AND AUSTIN. SULLIVAN ADVISES HE WILL SUBMIT ALDACTONE TO GRAND JURY. SIDLEY AND AUSTIN ASK IF GRAND JURY WILL INVOLVE ALL ISSUES RAISED BY FDA INCLUDING NUTRASWEET. SULLIVAN SAID AT THIS TIME ONLY ALDACTONE.

(NOTE: THIS IS AS CLOSE AS WE CAN COME TO THE DATE NUTRASWEET WAS DROPPED FROM THE INVESTIGATION.)

SULLIVAN ALSO SPOKE OF "PROCEDURES DESIGNED TO PERMIT PROMPT RESOLUTION OF THIS MATTER WITHOUT INCONVENIENCE AND UNDUE HARM TO THE PARTIES (SEARLE). MIGHT BE APPROPRIATE FOR NON-GOVERNMENTAL COUNSEL TO PROPOSE PROCEDURES THEY FELT WOULD BE APPROPRIATE."

SULLIVAN SUGGESTS RECEIPT OF SUBPOENAS BY COUNSEL. ALSO SUGGESTED COUNSEL CONSIDER OTHER "POSSIBLE SAFEGUARD PROCEDURES" AND RETURN IN A WEEK TO PRESENT SUGGESTIONS.

SEPTEMBER 13, 1977: LAWYERS FOR SOME OF THE TARGETS OF THE INVESTIGATION WRITE TO BRANDING SETTING UP A MEETING AT WHICH "NO WASHINGTON PERSONNEL WILL BE PRESENT." (DOC #19)

OCTOBER 3, 1977: FILE MEMO FROM CONLON ON "OFF THE RECORD" MEETINGS WITH SIDLEY AND AUSTIN LAWYERS REGARDING THE GRAND JURY INVESTIGATION. (DOC #20)

OCTOBER 10, 1977: STATUTE OF LIMITATIONS EXPIRES ON 52-WEEK MONKEY STUDY WHERE MONKEYS THAT HAD SEIZURES WERE NEVER GIVEN AUTOPSIES. THIS IS ONE OF

THE TWO TESTS SPECIFICALLY CITED IN FDA LETTER RECOMMENDING GRAND JURY INVESTIGATION OF NUTRASWEET ON JANUARY 10, 1977.

OCTOBER 12, 1977: SULLIVAN TO CONLON, BRANDING, REIDY. SULLIVAN SAYS CONLON WILL "NECESSARILY HAVE TO REDUCE OR END HIS INVOLVEMENT" IN SEARLE INVESTIGATION DUE TO "PRESS OF ADMINISTRATION DUTIES." REIDY TO TAKE OVER. (DOC #21)

OCTOBER 26, 1977: MCCONACHIE TO SULLIVAN. WE HAVE NOT BEEN KEPT ADVISED OF ANY GRAND JURY INVESTIGATION. GET US INFORMATION. (DOC #22)

NOVEMBER 7, 1977: SULLIVAN TO BRANDING ON SULLIVAN'S (DOC #23) CONVERSATION WITH MCCONACHIE. "I TOLD MCCONACHIE AT GREAT LENGTH HOW WE HAVE REPEATEDLY ASSURED THE

LAWYERS FOR SEARLE THAT WE DO EVERYTHING IN OUR POWER TO KEEP THE GRAND JURY INVESTIGATION SECRET."

IT SHOULD BE NOTED HERE THAT JUSTICE WILL NOT GIVE ANY DETAILS ABOUT THE GRAND JURY INVESTIGATION, WHEN IT WAS COMMENCED, HOW MANY WITNESSES WERE PRESENTED, ETC. ALL WE KNOW FOR SURE IS THAT THE GRAND JURY INVESTIGATION, SUCH AS IT WAS, INVOLVED ONLY ALDACTONE, NOT NUTRASWEET.

DECEMBER 8, 1977: STATUTE OF LIMITATIONS EXPIRES ON HAMSTER TOXICITY TEST, THE SECOND TEST CITED BY FDA IN ITS JANUARY 10, 1977 LETTER SEEKING A GRAND JURY INVESTIGATION OF NUTRASWEET.

DECEMBER 1977 - DECEMBER 1978: PERIOD IN WHICH GRAND JURY ACTION IS TAKEN ON ALDACTONE. NO DOCUMENTS ON GRAND JURY AVAILABLE.

DECEMBER 1978: SULLIVAN DECIDES NOT TO PROSECUTE SEARLE. INVESTIGATION DROPPED.

JANUARY 5, 1979: BILL CONLON LEAVES U.S. ATTORNEY'S OFFICE TO JOIN SIDLEY AND AUSTIN.

JANUARY 29, 1979: SULLIVAN WRITES TO FDA FORMALLY STATING HIS REASONS FOR NOT PROSECUTING SEARLE ON ALDACTONE. (DOC #24)

POSTSCRIPT

JUNE 1979: FDA ESTABLISHES PUBLIC BOARD OF INQUIRY TO RULE ON SAFETY ISSUES SURROUNDING NUTRASWEET.

OCTOBER 1980: PUBLIC BOARD OF INQUIRY REPORTS NUTRASWEET SHOULD NOT BE APPROVED PENDING FURTHER BRAIN TUMOR TESTS.

"THE BOARD HAS NOT BEEN PRESENTED WITH PROOF OF A REASONABLE CERTAINTY THAT ASPARTAME (NUTRASWEET) IS SAFE FOR USE AS A FOOD ADDITIVE UNDER ITS INTENDED CONDITIONS OF USE." (DOC #25)

MAY 1981: THREE OF THE SIX IN-HOUSE FDA SCIENTISTS ADVISING FDA COMMISSIONER HAYES ON WHETHER NUTRASWEET SHOULD BE APPROVED (THE SO-CALLED COMMISSIONER'S TEAM) ADVISE AGAINST APPROVAL. THEY STATE THAT THREE SEARLE TUMOR TESTS ARE UNRELIABLE (ONE INVOLVING DKP, A NUTRASWEET BREAKDOWN PRODUCT). QUESTIONS WERE ORIGINALLY RAISED ABOUT THESE TESTS BY THE FDA SEARLE INVESTIGATIVE TASK FORCE REPORT IN 1976, THE REPORT WHICH WAS TO FORM THE BASIS FOR A GRAND JURY INVESTIGATION OF NUTRASWEET. (DOC #26)

JULY, 1981: COMMISSIONER HAYES OVERRULES PUBLIC BOARD OF INQUIRY, AND APPROVES NUTRASWEET FOR DRY PRODUCTS.

JULY 8, 1983: NUTRASWEET APPROVED FOR USE IN CARBONATED BEVERAGES. (OVER 20 BILLION DIET SOFT DRINKS CONSUMED LAST YEAR).

B. BUREAUCRATIC-POLITICAL-CORPORATE COMPLEXES

"The slow reaction by the government agency responsible for protecting the food supply had major political ramifications. This experience reinforces lessons learned by some public health agencies in the USA. The folly of attempting to

withhold information or acting as departments of
public reassurance can result in a serious erosion of
public trust."
Richard Clapp and David Ozonoff (2000)

There have been repeated inferences about the ability of large companies to influence legislative and administrative decision-making, as can be inferred from the foregoing details. The gun lobby, the chemical-drug lobbies, and various coalitions are often cited in this regard. Furthermore, global corporate entities – with the sole goal of profit – can bypass governmental regulators. The Washington "revolving door" (Chapter XXX) also deserves mention. In *America, Inc.: Who Owns and Operates the Unites States*, Mintz and Cohen (1971) noted that many individuals who assume regulatory responsibilities intend to leave government, and subsequently work for corporations they had previously regulated. (See Document List under A)

Regulatory bodies tend to be partial to large corporations. This is illustrated by the EPA's action in halting distribution of its popular environmental guide, *The Environmental Consumer's Handbook*, (released in 1990). It came in the wake of corporate objections to "safer substitutes for household hazards" (steel wool; baking soda) to clean ovens, the use of natural soap flakes and vinegar to wash clothes, shunning insecticides in favor of natural repellents (e.g., Rosemary; eucalyptus) to treat pets for flea or tick problems, and polishing furniture with a mixture of lemon and mineral oil.

As a case in point, the National Yogurt Association proposed changes in yogurt standards during November 2000 that would rescind the warning label and other disclosure of aspartame and sweeteners. Such action is considered objectionable because of the frequency with which yogurt containing aspartame caused severe reactions.

The following commentaries are pertinent.

- Mintz and Cohen (1971) elaborated upon the ability of giant corporations to affect both the environment and the quality of life as much as elected officials. They noted that even "a discreet phone call" between a corporate officer and a bureaucratic official could "abort a necessary regulatory action" (p. 12).
- Beatrice Trum Hunter (1971) detailed the "unholy alliance" between science and the food industry in *Consumer Beware, Your Food and What's Been Done to*

It (Simon and Schuster). Over the ensuing decades, this problem assumed proportions that challenge professional ethics.

The American public has been almost desensitized to corporate exploitation or "misbehavior" as the cost of doing business in the wake of scandalous revelations involving lysine, pesticides, tobacco and other products by whistle-blowers. It may be less willing to do so in the case of aspartame disease.

"Scientific Proof"; Food Disparagement Bills

A coalition of the food industry and the National Feed Industry Association aims at intimidating those who assert that some "new and improved" food or agricultural product is unsafe through legislation requiring that "scientific proof" be provided. Many states adopted such food disparagement bills – over the violent objections of opponents who argue they are unconstitutional.

Professors of law became outraged over The Agriculture Deformation Act (S.B. 234). The sweeping implications of comparable bills not only were regarded as deeply flawed, but also a threat to the right of free speech for citizens in affected states. (This issue recalls an observation by Disraeli that it is easier to be critical than correct.)

The issue of "scientific proof" is addressed later in this section. George Orwell aptly warned that "scientific" can mean different things under different circumstances. The terms "scientific study" and "scientific validity" relating to clinical matters, such as aspartame disease, ought to be weighed carefully when the results fail to jibe with experience.

C. A RELUCTANT MEDICAL/SCIENTIFIC PRESS

"Any medical journal that would turn down an article on aspartame disease that had been fully researched and was needed for diagnostic reasons by physicians to help their patients does a great disservice to doctors and the medical community."

Betty Martini (Internet, August 8, 2000)

The prompt relay to journals of scientific information and medical insights, and their publication, ought to be an article of professional faith, especially in matters involving patient care and the public health. By contrast, the public-affairs staffs for industry can maintain "plausible deniability," or they may tell reporters, "That's none of your business" (Olsky 1986).

It remains an ethical obligation of physicians and scientists to make public observations they believe to have merit, preferably through publication. This does not make them Luddites. (reference to a band of workers who smashed machines two centuries ago in an attempt to halt the march of progress driven by technology and science.)

Editorial Policies and Decisions

The independence of medical journals and of Internet web sites having connections with profit-making organizations has been severely challenged by altruistic doctors and scientists. Their efforts to communicate could prove difficult or impossible in controversial subjects, such as aspartame disease.

Physicians encounter severe resistance from journals that preferentially publish "peer-reviewed" studies and editorials favorable to corporate-sponsored researchers and other groups. In turn, this could favor the prescription of new drugs and chemicals when reports of serious adverse effects do not appear, and overstating the benefits of popular drugs. One professor of medicine viewed the matter as tantamount to "a race to the ethical bottom."

As a frequent contributor to medical journals, and an occasional peer reviewer, the author values editorial trust. But the rejection of dozens of original articles and letters-to-the-editor dealing with aspartame disease, including detailed analyses of the flawed protocols of published "negative" studies, has heightened my concern.

> The departure of editors-in-chief of the *Journal of the American Medical Association* and the *New England Journal of Medicine* within a period of several months during 1999 suggested violation of their editorial independence. Dr. Jerome P. Kassirer (1999), resigned editor of the *New England Journal of Medicine*, underscored the matter of readers' trust when the views of a medical journal represent those of the owner or sponsoring medical society, including refusal to publish controversial subjects. He editorialized: "Medical journal editors walk a fine line. They must aspire to impartiality, open-mindedness, and intellectual honesty. They must try to select material for its merit, interest to readers, and originality alone." The subsequent naming of a pulmonologist with strong ties to the drug industry as editor of the *New England Journal of Medicine* added concern about the potential for subsequent corporate influence.

The gravity of this issue extends far beyond any personal sour-grapes attitude. When accused of being a "media terrorist" by a medical director of the NutraSweet Company, the author recalled a statement by Gandhi: "Remember, when you are pointing the finger at someone, three fingers are pointing back at you."

The "code of confidentiality" by reporters is understandable. Yet, some members of the general media who refused to disclose their private "scoops" pertaining to aspartame expected the author to divulge his researches in their entirety. Others expressed disinterest concerning the investigation and regulation of aspartame. One syndicated columnist wrote the concerned father of a young aspartame reactor, "I suggest that ill-health and even tragedy may be the result of too much government rather than too little."

The reluctance of the medical and scientific press to pursue aspartame reactions will be discussed in Chapter XXVIII. Another anecdote is germane.

> The author was scheduled to present a scientific exhibit, "Aspartame-Associated Confusion and Memory Loss: A Possible Human Model for Early Alzheimer's Disease," at the Annual Meeting of the American Association for the Advancement of Science held in Boston on February 13, 1988. I honored the request for an extended early-morning interview by the reporter of a scientific periodical. He later accosted me with this reservation from his editor, "I have to know where you have published the research before." It seemed extraordinary because this meeting had been purposefully chosen for the first presentation to scientists.

D. RELATED CONSIDERATIONS

"Unchecked giantism — be it political, religious or economic — has never been compatible with individualism."
Senator Philip Hart (1968)

A section of my book on traffic accidents (Roberts 1971b) was titled, "Obstacles and Resistance To Traffic Safety and Accident Prevention". If the reader were to substitute "aspartame disease" for "traffic safety," the following remarks under "Bureaucratic Resistance and Policies" would seem equally appropriate.

> "Regretfully, many of the critical comments in this section relate to policies pursued by local or federal government. Unless a compelling sense of urgency and innovation is infused into those civil servants charged with traffic safety, however, I fear that solutions for the transportation crisis will become increasingly elusive. Too much precious time and opportunities have been wasted by persons on every level of government who lack initiative, and who feel obliged only to maintain the status quo."

Physician Whistle-Blowers

Physicians who report serious adverse effects from products produced by billion-dollar companies can expect repercussions. This is particularly true when the science-for-sale issue is raised relative to publication of corporate-sponsored researches that regulatory agencies then use to approve safety.

Physicians and scientists have suffered striking professional and legal consequences after "blowing the whistle" on potentially harmful medical research. Some who had signed lengthy confidential clauses to receive funds for funding of drug studies anguished considerably when prevented from reporting their findings.

Under these circumstances, concerned doctors who serve as voluntary consumer advocates are likely to witness a collision between scientific opinion and corporate maneuvering involving different interpretations of "the facts" and "the truth." Considerable disinformation also may be coupled with denigrating personal attacks. Examples include assertions that fluoride is an essential mineral, and that there is more free methyl alcohol (methanol) in fruit juices than in aspartame products.

Corporate Sponsorship of Physician Lectures

The corporate financial arrangements of physicians who lecture to professional groups under the auspices of "speaker bureaus" can be impressive. The pro-aspartame attitude of most sponsored diabetes researchers is noteworthy. These affiliations become exposed when the listing of grant/research support becomes mandatory for compliance with state and federal regulations.

> The author attended a three-day seminar on neurology during February 2000 in which 13 of the lecturers listed *at least* three companies for which they served as consultants or researchers.

All emphasized the use of drugs One had 38(!) such associations. It is noteworthy that not a single person mentioned the possible contributory role of aspartame reactions for any of the neuropsychiatric problems discussed in Chapters VI and VII.

The current deficiencies relative to conflict-of-interest policies are so serious that some have suggested university-based investigators and research staffs be prohibited from holding stock and corporate decision-making in order to maintain scientific integrity (Lo 2000).

Self-serving conflicts of interest among physicians/researchers in this realm also exist abroad. Wilmhurst (2000) noted that several eminent British cardiologists profit handsomely from promoting the drugs of a pharmaceutical company in lectures to UK doctors. Speaker fees for members of this so-called Road Show exceed their annual hospital or university salaries, especially when engaged by multiple companies. Indeed, they may be so high that an agent negotiates such engagements! There are profound ethical implications, however. Some admitted that they remained silent about the adverse side effects of these drugs to avoid losing lucrative research contracts.

Resistance By Chemical and Drug Companies

The "party line" of the chemical industry, with reference to risk/benefit analysis, can be predicted. Blair and Hoerger (1979), representing Dow Chemical Company, offered the following corporate perspectives:

"All activity involves risk."
"Uncertainties exist in our total knowledge of benefits and risks."
"We tend to worry more and more about less and less."
"The more time and money we invest in toxicological testing of a compound, the more likely we are to generate overly restrictive regulations."
"Perspective on chemical risk is lacking, creating difficulty for the public in relating chemical risks to other societal risks."
"The 'zero-risk' concept of the Delaney Amendment, if applied universally, would markedly reduce industrial activity."

850

Consumer and employee advocates have countered the fallacies of such corporate analysis. Sheldon W. Samuels (1979) (Health, Safety and Environment Industrial Union Department, AFL-CIO) commented on "acceptable risk," "Determining an acceptable risk is like playing Monopoly with the Mafia: they always start the game owning the Boardwalk." He added

> "Thus, a citizen's <u>right to know</u> that his government attempts to ban the unnecessary proliferation of carcinogens in food (for example) derives from his <u>need</u> for this protection. This and all rights arise from the <u>need</u> to preserve life. This is the historic basis of the Delaney principle, not risk/benefit analysis in the parlor game of 'acceptable risk.' The fact that we often do not choose life is not an argument for the acceptance of risk. 'Threshold' implies that there is a dose below which there is no effect. None has ever been found for chemical or radiation carcinogenesis." (Reproduced with permission)

Self-Help vs. the Wellness Industry

The public should not expect the "health food" industry and "the wellness press" to dampen their evangelistic promotion of profitable products. The author previously made this assertion in discussing the potential toxicity of excess vitamin E (Roberts 1979a, 1981a, 1994c), dolomite/bonemeal (Roberts 1981b, 1983a), anti-static clothes softeners (Roberts 1986a), and fluoridation (Roberts 1992f).

The extensive over-the-counter promotion of phenylalanine and other single amino acids for their alleged benefit in relieving arthritis, migraine, depression, dyslexia and back pain falls in this category. Their potential side effects, and the need for restrictive legislation, were discussed in Chapter XXII and Section 6.

Increased Medical Costs; Indifferent Insurance Companies

The extraordinary costs associated with the incorrect diagnosis and treatment of aspartame disease – a decade ago averaging $1,719 personally, and $4,647 for insurance carriers – were noted in Chapter XIX. They have contributed to the rising cost of health care, and also undermine the emphasis on cost-effective preventive health care programs (*The Wall Street Journal* September 18, 1986, p. 1).

Even a random review of the medical histories in any chapter verifies this enormous financial burden, a theme also expressed by aspartame victims.

A professional man with aspartame-related seizures, severe mood swings, memory loss, and muscle symptoms stated, "Aspartame is wrecking havoc on HMOs and the medical insurance system, pushing up everyone's premiums. The winners seem to be the medical community and the manufacturers. The losers are the American people... Whether you are using the substance or not, you are affected."

Paradoxically, the insurance industry expressed minimal interest in studies on aspartame disease. Four major companies were indifferent to the unnecessary testing and treatment (including surgery) of aspartame reactors. An executive of one large insurance company "regrettably" explained that its guidelines for grants focused on "problems of urban public education, improving minority youth employment opportunities, urban neighborhood revitalization, public management and reform of the civil justice system."

Short-Sighted "Sugar Diplomacy"

The impact of escalating aspartame consumption on the sugarcane and sugarbeet industries of the United States was mentioned earlier. The incorporation of aspartame in soft drinks captured a large share of the market from milk, tea and other beverages (*The Palm Beach Post* August 1, 1987, p.B-1).

The United States price support program also encouraged the use of artificial sweeteners and high fructose corn syrup (HFCS) as sugar substitutes. For example, the domestic consumption of HFCS rose from 4.2 percent of the market in 1975 to 35.3 percent in 1986.

Grain farmers in the Dakotas added to the glut of sugar when they began growing sugar beets because of depressed grain prices. Additionally, the demand for sugar is "inelastic" as viewed by economists because users do not buy more when the price drops.

As the demand for sugar declined, U.S. sugar processors turned over 300,000 tons to the government during 1985 as their collateral under the sugar loan program (*Sun Sentinel* of Fort Lauderdale, August 31, 1986, p. F-1). Much of the 1985 surplus was then dumped onto an already-bulging world sugar market... at a loss of $77 million.

The United States was subsequently confronted with bumber domestic sugar crops, increased imports due to obligations under international trade agreements, and the widening use of non-sugar sweeteners. Taxpayers faced the prospect of paying for 250,000 tons to bolster the price and protect domestic growers (*The Palm Beach Post* March 28, 2000, p. B-6).

- With a decline in price by 23 percent, growers threatened to forfeit as much as $550 million in sugar pledged to the government as collateral on federal marketing loans.
- The U.S. Department of Agriculture then considered giving some of the huge surplus of sugar to farmers if they pledged to destroy part of their crop (*The Palm Beach Post* July 27, 2000. p. D-1).
- The government was paying $1.27 million a month to sugar growers for storing the sugar surplus.
- Two of Florida's major sugar growers forfeited $17 million in September 2000 to repay government loans, followed one week later by the loss of 300 jobs (including vice presidents) at U.S. Sugar Corporation (*The Palm Beach Post* September 9, 2000, p. A-1).

Contribution to illegal drugs. This revenue squeeze generated unforeseen consequences relative to the drug abuse epidemic. Sugar had held a central place in the economy of many Caribbean and Latin American countries. Accordingly, the combination of limited access to United States markets and removal of favorable quotas placed them in serious financial jeopardy. Facing concomitant restrictions on sugar imports by the United States, its allies had to close many sugar mills in Central America. A former President of the Dominican Republic, in which sugar production represented a major part of the economy, anticipated the loss of more than 60,000 jobs in his country (*The Evening Times* of West Palm Beach, March 10, 1987, p. A-15).

In order to survive, unemployed workers in these areas began or enlarged marijuana production (*The Wall Street Journal* September 26, 1986, p. 1). A vicious political cycle then undermined the ability of governments to dissuade farmers from growing marijuana on dry plots in mangrove swamps. In the wake of these events, the United States became inundated with marijuana.

XXVIII

CONFUSED HEALTH CARE PROFESSIONALS; FLAWED RESEARCH AND REPORTING

"The thing that bugs me is that the people think the FDA is protecting them — it isn't. What the FDA is doing and what the public thinks it's doing are as different as night and day."
> Dr. Herbert L. Ley (1969)
> (former FDA Commissioner)

"It will thus be seen that medical journalism is in a state of chaos... The greed for advertising patronage leads the editor only too often to prostitute his pen or his pages to the advertiser, so long as he can secure the coveted revenue."
> Dr. P. Maxwell Foshay (1900)
> (Editor, *Cleveland Journal of Medicine*)

The author included this chapter after considerable reflection. The decision largely stemmed from deliberate confusion of doctors concerning aspartame disease and related matters – most notably, flawed research and disinformation.

The title of a play by George Bernard Shaw, *The Doctor's Dilemma*, could apply to the confusion of physicians concerning the reality of aspartame disease. They and other health care professionals now wonder whom to believe concerning its frequency and severity. Most lack the background, time or motivation to analyze the voluminous and pertinent clinical scientific reports. Moreover, they have been conditioned to accept approval by the FDA and other authorities as proof of safety, especially when based on "negative" double-blind studies.

854

Practicing physicians, researchers and journal editors are at high risk for being duped by covert industry efforts aimed at subverting logical decisions they must make about profitable products that can pose public health hazards. Such was the case with lung cancer related to passive smoking. *The Lancet* (2000; 355:1197) editorialized: "All policymakers must be vigilant to the possibility of research data being manipulated by corporate bodies, and of scientific colleagues being seduced by the material charms of industry. Trust is no defense against an aggressively deceptive corporate sector."

The following items provide relevant examples of this form of "stonewall syndrome."

- A position paper of the American Dietetic Association (officially adopted on October 18, 1992) stated, "Long-term consumption of aspartame is safe and is not associated with any adverse effects." There was no reference in the bibliography, however, to any of the publications by the author and others concerning its clinical complications.
- In his review of a book dealing with food constituents and behavior, Dr. Malcolm A. Holliday (1986) reassured readers of the *New England Journal of Medicine* that aspartame intake by non-compulsive users has "no sinister effects." He did concede, however, that phenylalanine metabolism may be compromised among "compulsive users" of aspartame soft drinks. (See aspartame addiction in Chapter VII-G.)
- Fernstrom (1987) urged that more effort not be wasted on "being obsessive about something (aspartame disease) that isn't really there."
- Dr. F. Xavier Pi-Sunyer (1988), representing the American Diabetes Association (ADA) Board of Directors, told a Senate hearing on aspartame that he objected to this session because it might make the public needlessly apprehensive.

"We have no indication from these professionals (physicians treating diabetic patients) that there are significant problems with the use of aspartame, or, for that matter, that there is any pattern of complaints regarding this product... In conclusion, ADA supports the continued availability of aspartame. Our organization believes the product has been shown to be safe."

- The neurologist attending Case III-19B refused to entertain the possibility that her grand mal seizures on three occasions could have resulted from chewing ONE stick of aspartame gum. The details, along with his arrogant response to a doctor who concurred with such an association, appear in Chapter III.

- A study by Spiers et al (1998) (Massachusetts Institute of Technology and Harvard Medical School), "reaffirming the safety of aspartame," concluded: "Large daily doses of aspartame had no effect on neuropsychologic, neurophysiologic, or behavioral functioning in healthy young adults." The subjects were undergraduate graduate students to whom aspartame was administered chiefly in capsules. (The study was supported by a grant from the NutraSweet Company.) The "chronic" study consisted of a 20-day intake. This report was preambled by reference to "hundreds of unsolicited letters from concerned individuals after the publication of his (Dr. R. J. Wurtman) letter concerning aspartame and seizure susceptibility." Moreover, the bibliography of 42 references did not include any of the many papers and several books the author had written on aspartame disease.

Professional and Consumer Anguish

Health care professionals have anguished over the ongoing failure by their organizations to recognize aspartame disease.

- A 25-year-old dietitian who had experienced numerous reactions to aspartame products hoped that the American Dietetic Association would "some day accept the fact that aspartame is harmful" and issue professional warnings.
- A full-page advertisement for an aspartame tabletop "sugar substitute" appeared on the back cover of the February 1998 *Journal of the American College of Nutrition*.
- I have repeatedly encountered professors of rheumatology who were totally unaware of the severe bone and joint symptoms in aspartame disease.

Consumers have voiced comparable anguish. Ken and Jan Nolley (1987) stressed the limitations of physicians relative to chemical sensitivity, especially among children. "It is worth observing that most doctors are not research scientists, either. As clinicians, they are more predominantly technicians in their practice, applying 'medical knowledge,' only part of which has a solid experimental base." (Reproduced with permission)

856

A. SEEKING "THE TRUTH"

"Scientific truth, which I formerly thought of as fixed, as though
it could be weighed and measured, is changeable. Add a fact,
change the outlook, and you have a new truth. Truth is a
constant variable. We seek it, we find it, our viewpoint changes,
and the truth changes to meet it."
Dr. William J. Mayo (1861-1939)

Resistance to unpopular findings is not new. Jean-Martin Charcot, a famous neurologist, made this observation in 1888 about the delayed acceptance of new observations: "Such was the case for so many other ideas which are today universally accepted because they are based on demonstrable evidence, but which met for so long only skepticism and often sarcasm – it is only a matter of time."

In the case of aspartame disease, there **is** a pressing consideration: the ongoing harm from excessive delay by regulatory agencies in dealing with this perceived imminent public health hazard.

Another thorny issue confronts doctors, dietitians and consumers: "Who does one believe about the contested safety of popular products approved by the FDA?" At the November 3, 1987 Senate hearing on aspartame, FDA Commissioner Young defensively warned, "You will be dazzled, and at times confused, by a wide variety of scientific presentations."

The Cult of Information

A significant factor contributing to professional confusion concerning aspartame disease is conveyed by terms such as "the cult of information" (Horton 1999) and "misinformation in health care" (Jefferson 1999). Dr. Richard Horton (1999), editor of *The Lancet*, editorialized that physicians cannot escape the matter. It carries a real risk to patients when decisions are based largely on the selective citation of evidence in reviews and editorials. This commentary is germane to aspartame disease.

"In sum, judgment counts, even though the wish is that it did
not, even though there is frustration that it cannot be measured,
and even if, sometimes, it turns out to be wrong. Narrative
reviews develop connections between lines of evidence that

cannot be easily combined either systemically or quantitatively – e.g., between the biosciences and social sciences, between molecular medicine and epidemiology."

Commentary on The Truth

The search for truth always has proved an ongoing challenge. Confucius aptly stated, "Those who know the truth are not equal to those who love it." Roger Bacon (1220-1292) observed, "There are in fact four very significant stumbling blocks in the way of grasping the truth which hinder every man however learned, and scarcely allow anyone to win a clear title to wisdom, namely, the example of weak and unworthy authority, longstanding custom, the feeling of the ignorant crowd, and the hiding of our own ignorance while making a display of our apparent knowledge."

Embarrassing examples of the elusive nature of truth are readily recalled in virtually every realm – societal; political; legal; economic; scientific; religious. They caution against the legal dictum, "Truth is the ultimate defense."

Flaws in presumably inviolate "laws of nature," such as Einstein's theory of relativity, continue to be uncovered. Realizing that they risk being regarded as disrespectful or heretical, some dissenters admit that they would prefer to have believed "the party line," were it not for their conscience.

The author never set out to be a "majority of one." His stance in several perplexing areas evolved only after prolonged observation, inquiry and self-challenge. Encounters in this realm underscored the quip, "Truth is stranger than fiction, but not so popular." Several are cited.

- There are potential long-term medical consequences of vasectomy (Roberts 1994). The need for family planning and birth control under many circumstances is appreciated. On the other hand, the election of vasectomy by healthy young men who are not informed about the extraordinary immunologic responses from this "simple" operation remains of profound concern. The subsequent publication of "scientific" rebuttals has not diminished such anguish because analysis of their protocols usually disclosed major loopholes.
- There is potential harm from various "supplements" aggressively marketed to professionals and consumers. This applies, for example, to the recommendation of megadoses of vitamins C and E as therapeutic antioxidants," when in fact each might actually promote oxidation in high doses (Roberts 1981a, 1994c).

B. THE REJECTION OF ANECDOTAL EVIDENCE

Disparaging comments about "anecdotal evidence" by editors of medical journals and reviewers in academia have contributed significantly to the ongoing lack of awareness of aspartame disease. The great tradition of the clinical anecdote, dating back to Hippocrates, has been forsaken. Borgstein (1999) observed: "Have you noticed that the clinical anecdote has almost disappeared?... We have statistics now, and no case is worthwhile unless we can collect a series and apply some complex statistical formula to it to make it significant somehow."

Defining anecdotal evidence as "what really happens to real people and they tell you about it," the editors of *Diabetic Reader* (Fall/Winter 1996) stated, "We find anecdotal evidence, especially in diabetes, is often ahead of the scientific pack and is often right!"

Pro-industry physicians and investigators have consistently attempted to put a favorable spin on aspartame safety by denigrating published clinical observations as "merely anecdotes." Corporate-sponsored critics reflexively scorn "anecdotal evidence" as invalid and unreliable.

Physician Criticism of the Internet

Numerous aspartame reactors first became aware of the nature of their problem by searching the Internet, and connecting with an informative link. Yet, this remarkable achievement by afflicted "lay persons" has been challenged by physicians. They express dismay over "pseudoscience," selective reporting, oversimplification of complex issues, the attractiveness of web site names (for example, *aspartamekills.com*), and "anecdotal" information from "anonymous" sources.

- A Massachusetts Institute of Technology graduate student became interested in aspartame toxicity. He was mortified that his institution "had been ensnared into a web of deadly deception... Were it not for the Net, and the heroic efforts of a few volunteers, the plight of untold thousands would be virtually hopeless." He urged a professor at his Alma Mater, previously involved in aspartame research, to oppose the propaganda "portraying the aspartame opposition as cranks, and denying them funding and publication"

- A letter by Zehetner and McLean, published in the July 3, 1999 issue of *The Lancet* (page 78), relates to the matter. My commentary of July 14 about an inaccurate pro-aspartame communication was not published in *The Lancet* itself, but subsequently did appear on its August 10, 1999 Interactive Discussion Group pages.

Representative Case Report

Case XXVIII-1

A male aspartame reactor was taken to an emergency room after experiencing seizures, severe vertigo and other symptoms. In a desperate search for the cause, he found references to aspartame disease. There was marked improvement following aspartame abstinence. In a letter to the manufacturer, he wrote

> "The real kicker came when I stopped using any type of aspartame. It was about the closest thing to a miracle I will ever experience in my lifetime. Within weeks I was more than 50% recovered. I am very angry at the way your product has affected my overall quality of life. I have read your comments about all the bunk information on sites like www.dorway.com. If it was not for these people and my Internet search, I would probably be dead today."

C. MISLEADING STATISTICS, META-ANALYSES AND EVIDENCE-BASED REPORTS

"A half truth is a whole lie."
Author unknown

Statistical Projections

Physicians and other health care professionals must be wary of "safety" projections based on clinical studies that involve relatively small numbers of subjects. Statisticians recognize "beta error" wherein the probability of an adverse effect might not have been identified because of small sample size.

> It has been estimated that 229 subjects are required for a 90 percent chance of finding a one percent incidence – or "90

percent confidence" – of harm. For a 95 percent chance of finding a one percent incidence, 298 subjects are needed, while 458 subjects are required for a 99 percent chance.

The public health implications of this matter are enormous. A one percent incidence of harm among 100 million users of aspartame products (an underestimate) translates into **one million** cases! The gravity becomes compounded when the test subjects had been healthy young adults (as college students) to whom aspartame or other substances were given for only several days or weeks. The potential disaster inherent in such false claims of certitude <u>must</u> be argued for <u>every</u> product before and after approval.

A prime example of flawed design in this context is the contention by some investigators that aspartame products do not cause headaches, based on administering encapsulated aspartame only <u>one day</u>. This contrasts with the occurrence of severe headache in 43 percent of 1200 aspartame reactors (Chapter V).

<u>Evidenced-Based Reports</u>

Concerned physicians have expressed indignation concerning the current emphasis on "evidence-based medicine." Sweeney, MacAulay and Gray (1998) stated

"Evidence-based medicine is the new deity of clinical medicine: physicians worship it, managers demand it, and policy makers aspire towards it... Patients are not passive recipients waiting for doctors to make decisions about their health; the evidence suggests that the more actively patients participate in consultation, the better controlled are their chronic diseases... What we need to concentrate on now is clarifying these issues at the level of the recipient of clinical messages – the patient."

The evidence-based demand invites reflexive denial of manuscripts submitted by practicing physicians on the part of editors and reviewers. Sackett et al (1996) editorialized that its intent is to assist doctors in making decisions about the care of patients. However, they warned: "Without clinical expertise, practice risks becoming tyrannised by evidence."

Dr. Michael O'Donnell (2000) addressed this issue in *The Lancet* with a feature titled, "Evidence-Based Illiteracy: Time to Rescue 'the Literature.' " He wrote, "Our modern 'literature' needs more writing by people who want to share the lessons they have learned... in the hope of provoking readers to think afresh about their work and its implications, and more writing that sharpens our professional scepticism."

Meta-Analyses

Physicians and other professionals place considerable emphasis on meta-analyses to provide evidence supporting clinical strategies. It applies to aspartame use as well as the evaluation of drugs and various measures alleged to be of therapeutic value.

This "scientific approach" has been severely challenged, with special criticism directed to the influence of industry sponsors.

- La Lorier et al (1997) demonstrated marked discrepancies between beta-analyses and subsequent large randomised controlled trials. An example involves the use of tacrine for treating Alzheimer's disease.
- Koepp and Miles (1999) underscored the failure of some investigators to consider the potential influence of such sponsorship, stressing that studies without corporate support almost unanimously were unable to detect a clinical effect. They concluded, "There is no compelling need for industry-supported meta-analyses in the peer-reviewed literature."

D. DISINFORMATION FROM A POWERFUL INDUSTRY

The healing professions are deluged with reports and symposia featuring famous physicians and scientists who were funded, directly or indirectly, by the drug industry. Moreover, these "players" serve on committees that help set public health policy.

A realm coming under increased criticism involves new vaccines manufactured by multiple pharmaceutical firms in the face of "anecdotal" links between various immunizations and a host of chronic illnesses. The latter include multiple sclerosis, asthma, inflammatory bowel disease, diabetes, and even intussusception (especially with rotavirus vaccine). The incorporation of formaldehyde (Chapter XXI) and mercury as preservatives in vaccines also concerns some critics.

Industry's "information tyranny" was mentioned in the introduction to this section. Physicians are among its prominent victims owing to the readiness with which large pharmaceutical and chemical companies currently monopolize both research and advertising. A contributory element has been the corrupted passion for seeking "the truth" by corporate-subsidized spin doctors. For example, a major food producer concluded its pamphlet on what health professionals should know about aspartame: "The ingredients of aspartame (aspartic acid and phenylalanine methyl ester) occur naturally in the normal diet and, hence, our metabolism is well adjusted to their utilization... Aspartame, even at abuse doses, is safe for adults and children."

Pro-aspartame apologists have become proficient in deflecting the warnings from health professionals and anti-aspartame activists. Their rhetoric employs terms and phrases such as "pseudoscience," "bogus scare tactics," "self-proclaimed prophets of this hoax who twist the facts," and "a conspiracy babble by flat-earthers."An anti-aspartame activist regarded the apparent addiction to diet sodas of highly critical persons in the media and government as "drinking on the job."

Various industries have used propagandists posing as consumer advocates in attempts to undermine grassroot organizations of concerned consumers by disseminating disinformation. In the aspartame controversy, they include watchdog organizations touted to be "food police." Similarly, professors of nutrition have asserted the safety of large amounts of aspartame as sodas and tabletop sweeteners taken for a "lifetime." In *The Ordeal of Change* (Harper & Row 1963), Eric Hoffer emphasized that propaganda and advertising reflect a "general relentless drive to manipulate men."

The control of medical information by the pharmaceutical industry should be cause for great concern. This has been achieved through the financing of medical research, placing expensive ads in medical journals that otherwise could not stay in business, compiling package inserts for the *Physician's Desk Reference*, the training of many "detail" men and women, expensive freebies for prescribing physicians, and the selection of physicians with significant prior ties to this industry as editors-in-chief of major journals. The problem becomes compounded by an incestuous relationship between drug firms and the FDA. Ambitious professionals use this agency as a stepping stone to six-figure salaries within the pharmaceutical industry. While on their "tour of duty" at the FDA, they are likely to focus more on relatively minor issues (e.g., denigrating alternative-care practitioners) than disinformation concerning new drugs and supplements.

E. CONTRIBUTORY FACTORS

There are major reasons for the confusion of health care professionals concerning aspartame disease.

I. Limited Clinical Publications

E. O. Wilson (1998) correctly observed, "One of the strictures of the scientific ethos is that a discovery does not exist until it is safely reviewed and in print."

The paucity of published information about reactions to aspartame products from practicing doctors largely reflects editorial attitudes and the influence of vested interests. The vacuum so created lends credence to the assertion that aspartame intolerance exists in only a small segment of the population, akin to infrequent sensitivity to shell fish and strawberries. For example, the disbelief of a professor of pediatrics that aspartame in breast milk might injure infants appears in Chapter XI. This was in response to <u>his</u> challenge at a seminar to name <u>any</u> substance consumed by breast-feeding infants that could harm them.

The "sins of omission" in scientific investigations may be as important as "sins of commission." Dr. Iain Chalmers (1990) (National Perinatal Epidemiology Unit, Oxford, England) amplified this theme in his address to the First International Congress on Peer Review in Biomedical Publication. It was titled, "Underreporting Research Is Scientific Misconduct."

The retraction of a corporate-sponsored study planned for publication in the *Journal of the American Medical Association* illustrates the issue. It pertained to the bioavailability of inexpensive generic forms of synthetic thyroxine, compared to a well-known brand. When the results proved comparable, the investigators were forced to retract their report because a clause in the 21-page research contract stated that the data were not to be published, or otherwise released, without written consent by the company and sponsoring university. Editorializing on this "morality play of our times," *Science* (July 26, 1996, p.411) stated, "It highlights the potential pitfalls of corporate-funded university research when the results are antithetical to the interests of the funder."

The author agrees with Dr. Chalmers' misgivings on the basis of his researches involving several types of widely used products on which experimental studies and clinical trials were minimal or absent. A case in point involves antistatic clothes softeners. Another was my inability to uncover publications of subsequent attempts aimed at proving or disproving the high incidence of brain tumors in rats fed aspartame (Chapter XXVII-F) in the <u>three years</u> between expiration of the statute of limitations for two studies, and approval of this chemical for human consumption by the FDA. Chalmers observed

> "Substantial numbers of clinical trials are never reported in print, and among those that are, many are not reported in sufficient detail to enable judgments to be made about the validity of their results. Failure to publish an adequate account of a well-designed clinical trial is a form of scientific misconduct that can lead those caring for patients to make inappropriate treatment decisions. Investigators, research ethics committees, funding bodies, and scientific editors all have responsibilities to reduce underreporting of clinical trials."*

Other battles over the publication of negative or ineffective results have made headlines, especially biotechnology products and vaccines. Commenting on the frantic efforts of companies to get out positive results, *The Wall Street Journal* noted the great difficulty in having neutral or negative results published (November 1, 2000, p. B-1).

Another threat to the spread of new ideas involves conglomeratized publishing companies having links with drug manufacturers.

II. Anticipated Litigation

The prospect of litigation has deterred publication on this subject, particularly abroad where there is no First Amendment protection. Researchers, practicing physicians, and publishers are restrained from criticizing drugs, foods and food additives for fear of being sued, especially by companies having enormous budgets for legal representation. *U.S. News & World Report* (December 8, 1986, p. 68) categorized this threat as "defamation or anticompetitive activities."

- Dr. James Todd of the American Medical Association asserted, "Physicians aren't going to put themselves out on a limb."
- An aspartame reactor with multiple neurologic and ocular symptoms was told by an ophthalmologist at a university center: "They could possibly have been caused by aspartame... but I couldn't put it in writing for fear of a lawsuit."

---

* © 1990 *American Medical Association*. Reproduced with permission

- Even gross errors found in published research may be understated by reviewing scientists who fear libel suits (*Science* 1987; 235: 422-423).

Such inhibited communication can paradoxically contribute to subsequent risk of suit. For example, neurologists and other physicians who incorrectly diagnose multiple sclerosis because they lack important related information about aspartame disease could face legal difficulties. For example, the Supreme Court of Israel affirmed a prior conviction of malpractice resulting from ignorance of the current medical literature that offered alternative diagnoses, opinions and recommended treatments (Fishman 1998). This judicial opinion emphasized that doctors have "personal responsibility" in their "professional duties to remain updated with the medical literature."

In this regard, many outraged patients with unrecognized aspartame disease misdiagnosed as multiple sclerosis have expressed the desire to sue. Such outrage will intensify if powerful new drugs having potentially severe side effects are administered to patients with incorrectly-presumed "early" multiple sclerosis, as is being currently recommended.

III.   Professional Ethics

Professional concern involving public policy ought to mount when corporate public-relations activities stress the improved "quality of life" afforded diabetics by aspartame products, without any mention of their adverse effects on this disease (Chapter XIII).

- Dr. Thomas A. Preston (1986), Professor of Medicine at the University of Washington in Seattle, editorialized on this general subject.

    "But news releases also may give one-sided, distorted, or even inaccurate information because private interests tend to underinvest in research and development, and to funnel resources to areas of greater profitability... The ethical need for full and unweighted information should make us wary of this growing influence on public opinion." *

* © 1986 *Medical World News*. Reproduced with permission

- Dr. Arthur D. Silk (1971) asserted

> "Organized medicine as represented by the AMA will either have to publicly disavow its role as the ultimate medical authority or adopt an ethical code insuring a pre-publication preview of what is to be released to the public – before the fact. Inaction or laissez-faire will serve only to increase the medical credibility gap".**

Another ethical commitment involves the discovery by expert witnesses that previous research, especially when corporate-funded, was never published or presented at appropriate scientific assemblies. They should inform retaining counsel, and suggest interrogatories for full clarification of the matter. This ought to include the submission of unpublished data and manuscripts considered as "disappointing," "uninteresting," or potentially damaging to corporate interests.

IV. Failure to Obtain Grants

Physicians on the faculty of medical schools who expressed interest in various facets of aspartame disease became discouraged because of their inability to obtain research grants. For example, a professor of otolaryngology wrote: "Since I have not received funding to continue my investigations into the link between aspartame and dizziness, I have not pursued this problem."

V. FDA Input

Health care professionals regarded the extended use of aspartame as an all-purpose general sweetener as FDA affirmation of its safety (*The Wall Street Journal* November 26, 1986, p. 9). The dubious role of the FDA therein was amplified in Section 6.

An FDA representative sent a long letter of reassurance to the author's congressman, dated September 8, 1986, in reply to a request for copies of correspondence from aspartame complainants. He asserted

> "In conclusion, the physiological and neurological effects of aspartame have been comprehensively studied, and most of the issues raised (by Dr. Roberts) were substantially identical to issues that FDA has already examined and resolved in its prior determination of aspartame's safety."

Therein lies an enigma: aspartame reactors had <u>volunteered</u> their case histories to the FDA and Centers for Disease Control in the hope that information would prove helpful to interested researchers.

> Yolles, Connors and Grufferman (1986) editorialized on the difficulties encountered by researchers in obtaining access to data about government-sponsored medical research, even through the Freedom of Information Act. Initially, they could not gain information concerning the alleged association between aspirin and Reye's syndrome because it was held by a private contractor... and therefore not subject to disclosure! Other excuses included possible violation of patients' privacy and the potential for lawsuits.

F. Edward Scarborough, Ph.D. (1989), Acting Director of the FDA, commented

> "Although protection and promotion are both part of the same coin, there is a creative, dynamic tension between the two that is now, as never before, being brought to the forefront of public health policy... However, it has become increasingly apparent that certain aspects of the s a f e t y   o f   f o o d additives cannot be addressed adequately by non-human investigations or from existing population exposure data... (The Red Book) does not contain guidelines for human clinical studies involving food additives... *Predicting the intake of a truly novel ingredient prior to its introduction into the food supply is virtually impossible."* (Italics provided)

F. SOURCES OF POTENTIALLY MISLEADING INFORMATION

In seeking reliable data, interested physicians have encountered questionable statements and misleading information that contributed to their confusion.

A U.S. federal judge ruled that regulations limiting what drug companies can disseminate to health care providers about unapproved uses of medicines unconstitutionally restricts freedom of speech, as guaranteed by the First Amendment. This further impacts the medical profession. *The Lancet* (1999; Volume 354, page 446) editorialized: "The judgment shifts the job of protecting patients from adverse drug reactions from the government to the prescriber, and means that medical schools, professional bodies and journals must intensify their efforts to ensure that doctors are able to interpret correctly the material, commonly biased, that they receive from drug companies."

I. Corporate "Front" Groups

Front groups often serve the interests of major corporations under the guise of offering impartial educational material. Moreover, the description of such organizations as "neutral" and "independent" can be misleading. Dr. Thomas E. Lindow (1988) averred that most of the health care "information" given by industry to the public is advertisement aimed at enticing rather than informing.

A high-level FDA physician told the author that the Epilepsy Foundation of America had studied allegations about aspartame causing or aggravating seizures, and implied the findings were "negative." The Director of Research and Professional Education of this Foundation subsequently wrote me on July 28, 1986:

> "In checking with our information and referral service, I have learned that, since January, we have received an estimated 15 to 20 inquiries on the subject. Our information is not kept in such a way that I am able to tell the substance of the inquiry. However, our director of information and referral informs me that these calls were generally for information only and did not involve reports of seizures. I hope this information is helpful."

I subsequently received a printout of data on 149 persons who had reported aspartame-induced convulsions to the FDA (Chapter III).

II. Professorial Denials

Industry-sponsored doctors at respected institutions have appeared on national television shows and elsewhere to counter or deny consumer complaints related to aspartame products. Their views were incompatible with the data presented in Sections 2 and 3.

III. Corporate Representatives

A glaring example of biased information about aspartame reactions was the answer printed in the *Journal of the American Medical Association* (1994; 272:1543) to a

869

physician's inquiry: "Is there any evidence that aspartame causes memory loss?" Dr. Robert Moser, a consultant to The NutraSweet Company, answered, "Aspartame does not cause memory loss." The author questioned the physician who submitted this question. She stated that she had done so for personal reasons, and because of a related severe problem involving an anesthesiology colleague.

The scores of patients in my medical and consultation practice, and the many correspondents who experienced marked confusion and memory loss that were unequivocally related to use of aspartame products, appear in Chapters VI-D and XV. Relatively young adults in this category repeatedly expressed concern about the possibility of early Alzheimer's disease. Indeed, the contention that aspartame may accelerate Alzheimer's disease has been elaborated in a book (Roberts 1995b).

G. PUBLISHED "NEGATIVE" REPORTS

"Negative" evaluations of reports about reactions to additives generally ought to be interpreted with caution. This caveat does not detract from some important investigations undertaken or sponsored by manufacturers.

The professional pressures and financial inducements confronting investigators in "controlled clinical trials" have been described (Sparro 1986; Lipper 1986). Their undesirable aftermaths include distorted physician-patient relationships, and an undermining of true informed consent.

In the present context, "negative" studies that discount the behavioral and cognitive effects of aspartame products must be scrutinized. This reservation is underscored when the nature of the placebo is not known to investigators in placebo-controlled tests (see below). Furthermore, independent confirmation of all aspects (including the amount of aspartame in the test substance) is desirable when studies are financed by contract rather than grant.

A decade ago, the author concluded that the majority of studies asserting the safety of aspartame were funded by this industry or organizations subsidized by it. Dr. Ralph G. Walton (1999), Professor of Psychiatry at Northeastern Ohio University College of Medicine, independently also expressed the same conviction after analyzing 166 relevant studies. One hundred percent (!) of 74 industry-funded reports attested to the safety of aspartame; by contrast, 91 percent of 92 independently-funded researches identified significant problems.

More on Conflicts of Interest

The Lancet (1997; volume 349: page 1112) editorialized on conflicts of interest in clinical research. It emphasized that (a) financial relationships and their effects are not easily detectible, and (b) the credibility of manuscripts decreases when projects are funded by companies having an interest in their outcome.

- The editors of the *New England Journal of Medicine* apologized to its readers for having violated the financial conflict-of-interest policy of this prestigious journal <u>19 times</u> during a three-year period relative to the selection of doctors who wrote its Drug Therapy articles (Angell 2000). They had received grants or served as consultants to drug companies in realms pertinent to this book – including multiple sclerosis, insulin, asthma, attention-deficit/hyperactivity, lipid disorders and diabetic retinopathy.
- The financial arrangements and corporate affiliations of physician-lecturers who emphasize the use of drugs, without making any reference to diet and other contributory factors, have been impressive. One professor of psychiatry who addressed a recent seminar listed 38 such associations!
- The current deficiencies relative to conflict-of-interest policies are so serious that university-based investigators and research staffs should be prohibited from holding stock and corporate decision-making in order to maintain scientific integrity (Lo 2000).

The author has been criticized for suggesting confirmatory corporate-neutral research when implications about the devastating consequences of certain foods, drugs or supplements arise. The notion of a widespread "new McCarthyism in science" (Rothman 1993) involving granted researchers also has been raised. Rothman defined "conflict of interest" as "any situation in which an individual with (professional) responsibility to others might be influenced, consciously or unconsciously, by financial or personal factors that involve self-interest." He argued against this being the equivalent to an accusation of wrongdoing because "no one works in a vacuum."

H. FLAWED "PLACEBO-CONTROLLED" STUDIES

Physicians and scientists are conditioned to seek the results of placebo ("dummy" administration) studies when evaluating drugs and additives. Double-blind studies in humans – that is, wherein neither the investigator nor subjects know the nature of the substance given – assume great significance in the present context. Anti-aspartame activists have ridiculed the alleged "inert" nature of aspartame, especially when in placebos, by asserting that it is as inert as Mount Vesuvius when erupting.

There are serious reservations about some placebo-controlled studies aimed at evaluating reactions to aspartame.

- An increase of gastrointestinal side effects was noted among a group of young overweight persons given a placebo of lactose (milk sugar) for 13 weeks, compared to others receiving aspartame (Visek 1984). The high incidence of lactase deficiency in the general population might explain the occurrence of gastrointestinal symptoms in the control group.
- More frequent adverse reactions were reported among diabetics receiving a placebo of corn starch (nine capsules swallowed daily) than aspartame (Nehrling 1985). One patient had to stop the aspartame, however, because of severe diarrhea; it recurred on rechallenge with aspartame (see Chapter IX).
- In a randomized double-blind crossover trial by Suarez et al (1995), aimed at evaluating lactose intolerance, the subjects received 240 ml milk daily with breakfast for two one-week periods – either as a two per cent fat-and-lactose-hydrolyzed milk or two per cent fat milk plus Equal®. Inasmuch as there were no statistically significant differences in the severity of gastrointestinal symptoms, the investigators concluded that persons who identified themselves as being lactose-intolerant had mistakenly attributed their problem to lactose intolerance. The possible role of aspartame in the control group apparently was not considered.

Studies in which aspartame was administered as a freshly-prepared cool solution (see Chapter XXVI) also introduce confusion.

Elsas (1988) challenged the accuracy of administering aspartame as capsules in commenting on a report that concluded it did not cause headache more often than a placebo. He indicated that absorption is less than 50 percent when aspartame is encapsulated. Moreover, administration as an "acute" load of 30 mg/kg in capsules during four hours could not be equated with the long-term ingestion of aspartame drinks and other products. (At least seven days are required for blood concentrations of phenylalanine to reach a new equilibrium.) Another problem with the gelatin capsules used in placebo studies concerns their ability to induce headache by themselves (Strong 2000). The gelatin is partially hydrolyzed animal protein, which is known to precipitate migraine in susceptible individuals.

<u>Selection of the lunchtime feeding paradigm to assess the effect of aspartame on food intake has several inherent shortcomings.</u> For example, more insulin tends to be secreted – with concomitant stimulation of appetite – as the day advances (Roberts 1964d, 1968).

<u>The testing protocols and control subjects have been challenged in some instances.</u>

- Walton et al were unable to obtain aspartame from a manufacturer for a proposed double-blind study on depressed patients (Chapter VII-B). They then had to procure it from a chemical company.
- Dr. Anthony Kulczycki, Jr. had studied aspartame-induced urticaria, but declined to take part in a proposed corporate-sponsored study of aspartame-induced hives because of several flaws in the protocol (Kulczycki 1995). They included the methods of recruiting subjects, the tendency to discourage participation of subjects likely to be allergic to aspartame, and the inclusion or exclusion criteria and challenged design (such as failure to exclude other recognized causes of chronic urticaria).

Input From Researched Patients

Enlightening correspondence was received from perceptive patients who had participated in double-blind studies involving aspartame administration. An instance is cited.

Case XXVIII-2

A female aspartame reactor worked for a major investment firm. She experienced "undiagnosed" grand mal seizures for two and a half years. This patient received considerable medication to control the attacks. She stated

> "I was one of the lucky souls chosen by NutraSweet and the FDA in 1989 to participate in a study performed at the V.A. Hospital in the Bronx to determine if there was any relation between aspartame use and neurological disorders. It was a double-blindfold study that required my being studied at a hospital for seven days under close monitoring of substance intake with a battery of tests. The reason for risking my health for the sake of this study was simple: my medication was killing me, and my doctor agreed that if I had a reaction, I could be phased off of it. Well guess what? My left arm went numb on the second substance day. Needless to say, it was later

confirmed that I received aspartame that day, not a placebo. My doctor phased off my meds shortly thereafter. I have not had a problem since."

There was a pertinent added comment. "I then tried – unsuccessfully – to file a product liability suit against the manufacturer through three different attorneys."

I. MORE ON SCIENCEGATE

Misleading research reports dealing with the safety of aspartame, a chemical initially designed as a drug for treating peptic ulcer, were cited earlier. This aura of sciencegate is likely to expand as aspartame analogs and other powerful faux sugars are introduced for consumer use. There is an underlying theme: doctors and scientists cannot simultaneously serve industry and the public interest.

An overview by others of the sciencegate issue underscores some general problems encountered by aspartame reactors and their advocates. These introductory commentaries are germane.

- Dorothy Nelken (1998), New York University, observed that the shift in power within science, with "the promise of profits," now motivates many scientists.
- Gail Heriot (1997) pondered, "When doctors are torturing data to make a political point, whom can you trust?"
- A feature appearing in *USA Today* (September 25, 2000) indicated that 54 percent of scientific advisors for the FDA concerning the issues of safety and effectiveness had financial ties to the drug industry.

Selected Commentaries

FDA Commissioner David Kessler (1991) stressed that physicians employed by drug companies should "do their best to avoid becoming unwitting participants in promotional activities." He urged physicians who give presentations to reveal the source of corporate sponsorship "as well as the extent to which a sponsor has exercised control over the material."

Stephen Fried (1998) analyzed "the hazardous world of legal drugs." He noted (a) the potential fallacy of using relatively healthy individuals or patients in most trial designs, (b) the delay of information about serious side effects in a diverse population until the postmarketing period, (c) the conduct of considerable research on drugs by doctors and scientists who are on the payroll of drug companies, and (d) the frequency with which members on key advisory committees receive grants from the pharmaceutical industry.

Reviewing his book for *The Lancet*, Barbehenn (1998) asked the question relative to preventing history from repeating itself, "The question, as always, is: will anyone listen?"

Miller, Rosenstein and De Renzo (1998) analyzed the relationship between investigators and patient-volunteers. A major issue is the moral conflict posed by clinical research that requires considerable professional integrity. They concluded, "The roles of clinician and scientist must be integrated to manage consciously the ethical complexity and ambiguity tensions between the potentially competing loyalties of science and care of volunteer patients."

Campbell et al (1998) analyzed the effects of research-related gifts on academic scientists. Many recipients feel obligated to keep the results of their research confidential or to provide donors with prepublication manuscripts... thereby significantly delaying publication. In effect, this constitutes *an academic-industrial complex*.

"Research For Hire"

Eichenwald and Kolata (1999) detailed the enormous conflicts involving doctors engaged in "clinical trials" to make money – perhaps $500,000 to $1 million annually. They focused on physicians in practice who had been recruited, or whose services had a premium because of private patients. Industry treated the research agreements as corporate secrets, the doctors being forbidden to disclose them.

- Emphasis was placed on the rapid recruitment of patients to expedite studies for drugs being sought for licensure.
- There were glaring revelations about the inadequate and inappropriate background of some clinical investigators – e.g., psychiatrists performing pap smears.
- Patients were enticed by their physicians into taking unapproved drugs having potentially serious but undisclosed side effects. The ethical issue escalated when they had medical disorders contraindicating such use.
- Participants are invited to attend seminars without cost, and have their names put on manuscripts written by drug companies.
- Walton (1999) emphasized the clear relationship between corporate funding of aspartame studies and favorable reports by investigators.

- Stelfox et al (1998) demonstrated a strong association between the favorable published positions concerning the safety of calcium-channel antagonists and the authors' financial relationships with drug manufacturers.

<u>When biomedical research is negotiable, it risks being undermined by corporate funding</u>. Such "research for hire" has proved an embarrassment for physicians owing to the inherent conflicts of interest and potential fraud. The extent of this matter can be inferred from expensive ads for clinical studies appearing daily in newspapers. A wide range of specialists participate. They include rheumatologists, neurologists, dermatologists, gastroenterologists, cardiologists, allergists and psychiatrists. If their integrity is challenged, the researchers involved react like outraged virgins being propositioned.

J. BIASED REVIEWS

"As good as almost killing a man is killing a good book. Who kills a man kills a reasonable creature, God's image; but he who destroys a good book kills reason itself."

Milton *(Areopheitica)*

Biased reviews of books warning about reactions to aspartame, monosodium glutamate and other suspected neurotoxins are not uncommon. A case in point is the hostile review of *Aspartame (NutraSweet): Is It Safe?* (Roberts 1988) appearing in the *New England Journal of Medicine* (1990; 232:1495-1496). Dr. Arturo R. Rolla concluded

"This type of book raises many questions for the medical community. Is it right for a physician with a hypothesis to write a book of this nature without first seeking scientific proof and presenting the data to a medical journal or society? I appreciate the concern and effort of the author, but my reaction to his book is as negative as it is strong. There is no place for a publication such as this one. It only adds to public misinformation, confusion, and mistrust. There are many other medical and scientific avenues available. I hope the author will continue his effort using more rigid scientific methods, in order to be able to present it to his peers. He has a right to write, but he also has a responsibility as a physician. Freedom of the press relies as much on the honesty and responsibility of the writer as on the government that supports it." (Reproduced with permission).

The reply I submitted, containing these following criticisms of this review, was **not** published.

- "The statement, 'There is no place for a publication such as this one,' would deny my responsibility as a practicing physician and clinical researcher." For perspective, I indicated that (a) I was a Board-certified internist, a member of the Endocrine Society, and author of five medical texts, (b) the research had been done at my own expense, and (c) this information <u>was</u> presented to peer groups, and <u>had been</u> published in a peer-reviewed journal – contrary to the "without previous scrutiny by his peers" allegation.
- A search of the reviewer's publications failed to uncover a single article or abstract indicating personal research of this subject.

Two independent commentaries on this review argue against solely a sour grapes attitude on the part of the author.

- Beatrice Trum Hunter, food editor of *Consumer's Research*, wrote a letter criticizing this review. She took exception to dismissing the evidence so summarily, and listed several persons who seemed to have far more expertise. I received a copy of her letter that the journal also failed to publish. It contained this commentary (reproduced with permission).

> "Is every clinician who reports on adverse health effects from substances expected to take time from a busy practice to seek funding, conduct costly and time-consuming double-blind studies, and then seek journals willing to publish the results? If so, this would have a chilling effect on medical reporting of adverse effects suffered from a variety of consumer substances. Rather, the Food and Drug

Administration, which approved aspartame and has allowed it to proliferate wildly in the market place, should have mandated the manufacturer to conduct double-blind human studies before approval... Let's not kill the messenger, but instead address ourselves to the cautionary message."

- Frank Murray, Editor of *Better Nutrition for Today's Living*, received a letter from the senior medical consultant of The NutraSweet Company on June 21, 1994 in response to an editorial about sugar and aspartame. He took exception to the results of a recently published study pertaining to the effects of sugar and aspartame on hyperactivity in children. (My letter to the *New England Journal of Medicine* offering similar criticism was not published.) The corporate spokesman added that all of my information was "based on anecdote, hearsay and personal opinion... the worst kind of non-science." Mr. Murray replied on July 8, 1994.

"I find Dr. Roberts' book extremely well researched. If the book is as odious as you indicated, I am curious why the *New England Journal of Medicine* devoted space to it. Surely there were more important books to be reviewed. Was the book reviewed objectively, or was it merely a 'hatchet job' by someone who wanted to make brownie points with NutraSweet?... Obviously, aspartame is not one hundred percent safe for all people. Our concern is that, now that NutraSweet does not hold the exclusive patent for aspartame, it is turning up everywhere... Regardless of whether or not double-blind studies with aspartame have been done extensively, one would have to be extremely naive, in our opinion, to believe that all of these sweeteners are not causing health problems."

K. PROBLEMS CONCERNING PUBLICATION

878

> "Loyalty to petrified opinion never yet broke a
> chain or freed a human soul."
> Mark Twain

Health care professionals who encountered aspartame reactions were beset by hurdles in getting their observations published. Such difficulty was not limited to physicians and neurophysiologists. Dr. Kenneth Bada, a respected peptide chemist, informed the author of the considerable resistance he encountered getting basic studies published in scientific journals (personal communication March 2, 1988).

Most articles that cast suspicion on the safety of aspartame trigger unyielding objections by consultants from prestigious institutions available to this industry. One aspect of these "scientific" rebuttals is further regulatory delay. In turn, this enables greater corporate profits for a perceived "imminent public health hazard.

Encounters By the Author

The author submitted many of short manuscripts on specific aspartame-associated problems – e.g., joint pains; "dry eyes"; pseudotumor cerebri, aspartame addiction – to appropriate peer-reviewed specialty of journals. They were coupled with the request that reviewers selected not be employees or consultants for the aspartame industry.

Even though strict clinical criteria for such associations had been set forth, these submissions were rejected. The reasons included "absence of controls," "failure to study subjects in a prospective, double-blind fashion," "lack of objective or quantifiable observations" (as the absence of joint scans in patients with rheumatologic symptoms), and "lack of credentials as an investigative or clinical rheumatologist."

- In the case of joint pains (Chapter IX-G), one reviewer stated that the induction of these symptoms by food products "is no longer novel, and is familiar to rheumatologists."
- Another aspect that disturbed reviewers of earlier manuscripts was the paucity of references, notwithstanding absence of a related literature.
- A detailed manuscript on 157 patients titled, "Aspartame-Associated Confusion and Memory Loss: A Possible Human Model for Early Alzheimer's Disease," was submitted to *Neurology*. It was promptly returned with this one-sentence letter from the editor: "The conclusions in your paper were not derived by a replicable objective controlled study, and therefore we cannot consider your paper for publication." Considering the increasing magnitude of Alzheimer's disease, the extraordinary relevance of my observations to newer biochemical

findings therein (Chapter XV), and my membership in the American Academy of Neurology, the readers of this publication were denied access to perspectives considered original and constructive.

Getting acceptance of original manuscripts on aspartame disease by conventional medical journals proved a daunting task. This is illustrated by editor/reviewer reactions to my original report on aspartame addiction (Chapter VII-G). It centered on 33 persons who characterized themselves in this manner, and repeatedly experienced severe withdrawal reactions after attempts to stop aspartame products. Pro-aspartame reviewers for the *Southern Medical Journal*, for example, expressed the following criticisms of "this most curious manuscript."

- "It is unusual to read a medical manuscript predicated on anecdote in the modern era of evidence-based medicine... The kindest interpretation is that it represents an anachronism."
- My objectivity was questioned because some experiences noted in the completed questionnaire (Section 4) had been used, even though the term "addiction" did <u>not</u> appear therein. Such use inferred that "investigator bias" equated with "When will you stop beating your wife?"
- Even though the manuscript had been limited to 22 typed pages to conform with journal policies, a reviewer criticized it for failing to have included the <u>entire</u> nine-page survey form.
- "Methanol toxicity cannot occur with aspartame ingestion" (see Chapter XXI). The only two references offered by this critic had been published in 1984 and 1987, contrasting to more recent ones cited in the bibliography.
- The FDA found "no cases of blindness even alleged to be caused by aspartame" (see Chapter IV).
- "Publishing this piece in any form would be an embarrassment to the *Southern Medical Journal*."

The excited response of physicians and addictionologists throughout the world to this article, when finally published (Roberts 2000), contrasted with that of the reviewers. Complimentary calls from the United Kingdom and Australia also requested permission to copy it for colleagues.

The foregoing and other critical commentaries on my aspartame manuscripts **always** were studied carefully by the author in the hope of finding valid constructive information and overlooked references. This was rarely the case.

880

I. The Obstacle of Peer Review

The peer review process of major journals, noted above, posed a formidable obstacle in reporting aspartame disease. Even many short letters-to-the-editor were refused. Others concur with this issue.

- In a "J'accuse" letter, Dr. Frederick Hecht (1987) criticized the *New England Journal of Medicine* for "not providing an equal forum for the debate of issues. Fair journalism calls for equal coverage." He emphasized the potential jeopardy to health care and research in the United States stemming from such policies.
- Southgate (1985) editorialized in the *Journal of the American Medical Association* on potential for conflict of interest involving the peer review process. Since this system is based on "a network of trust among colleagues," she averred that it must be "purer than Caesar's wife."

Dr. Lawrence K. Altman (1987), health editor of *The New York Times*, offered a critical analysis of the peer review process by many scientific journals. He concluded with the caveat that the present system risks giving physicians a false sense of security when they use such information as a basis for patient care.

- Some prestigious medical and scientific journals that boast the quality of their peer review do publish material and advertisements that have not been subjected to peer review.
- Forbidding authors to disclose their data before publication has become a form of self-serving "scoop journalism," largely because this policy increases circulation, advertising and profits – directly or indirectly.
- In the real world, "medical politics" tends to influence the peer review of referees, particularly when chosen **because of** certain biases. As a result, those having vested interests as researchers or consultants are likely to reject disconcerting manuscripts.

Dr. Altman (1988) later expressed concern over the extraordinary power exerted by one American journal relative to the flow of information (or lack thereof) on medical research, government policy, financial markets, and the treatment of patients. He cited the criticism of a respected Princeton health economist, who opined that such manipulation of data and information "is all in the name of peer review. But it really is in the name of profit." Comparable anxiety was expressed concerning the "degree of suppression of information there."

The foregoing extreme resistance by editors of peer-reviewed journals to publish articles on aspartame reactions invites additional reflection. This applies in particular to magazines and book publishers supported or owned by corporations having vested interests in foods, drugs and chemicals. The Supreme Court ruled in *Red Line Broadcasting Co. Inc. v. Federal Communications Commission* (89 S. CT 1794) (1969): "It is the purpose of the First Amendment to preserve an uninhibited marketplace of ideas in which the truth will ultimately prevail, rather than to countenance monopolization of that market, whether it be by the Government itself or a private licensee."

The plight of medical and scientific editors in selecting controversial manuscripts was summed in a *Journal of the American Medical Association* commentary by Dr. James L. Mills (1987) titled, "Can We Publish 'Hot' Papers Without Getting Burned?" He noted that authors of such material have the options of discarding their findings, "burying" them in a small-circulation journal, reporting the findings as a letter to the editor, or seeking publication by a major journal. *One of the problems with "burial" is its effectiveness in concealing important data*, as was the case with the fetal alcohol syndrome.

Concerning editorial boards, the use of volunteer reviewers does not ensure high-quality reviews. Easterbrook et al (1991) emphasized the potential "publication bias in chemical research." They suggested the cautious interpretation of conclusions based only on a review of published data.

Editors have been confronted with the embarrassment of having rejected classic papers. This is illustrated by the address of Dr. Rosalyn Yalow to the Endocrine Society after winning the Nobel Prize. She noted that the key manuscript leading to this achievement had been rejected by a well-known journal!

II. Corporate Challenges

Challenge to publications on aspartame disease by producers, with emphasis upon the absence of double-blind studies, has become routine. These and other strategies are understandable in light of the enormous economic stakes involved. As a point of reference, saccharin cost less than $4 a pound when aspartame was selling for $70 or more a pound.

> The response to a letter by Dr. Donald Johns (1986), published in the *New England Journal of Medicine*, illustrates this issue. He described a 31-year-old woman who predictably developed migrainous headaches within one to two hours after ingesting several cans of a diet cola, or when challenged with 500 mg pure aspartame in solution. They did not occur when she

swallowed comparable amounts of saccharin and sucrose in solution. Dr. Gerald E. Gaull (1986), representing the NutraSweet Company, suggested the study be repeated by administering these sweeteners in capsules inasmuch as solutions of these products "are easily distinguished by taste. Thus, the study of this patient was not truly blinded." (The problem with capsules was emphasized in Chapter XX).

This industry and several institutions to which it gave much support leveled attacks on persons concerned about the safety of aspartame (Chapter III and Section 7).

- Shortly after my initial press interview, a letter was received from Dr. Robert H. Moser, Vice-President for Medical Affairs of the NutraSweet Company. He asserted that anything short of "double blind provocative testing of these subjects" was not in "...the nature of the scientific method. To do less – especially to go directly to the press with alarming allegations – is not in consonance with the scientific foundation where both of us cut our intellectual teeth."

  This correspondence seemed a strange twist of fate! Dr. Moser and I had been fellow residents in Washington D.C. At the time, I also held an appointment as instructor and research fellow in medicine at Georgetown University Medical School.

- A corporate press release on October 16, 1986 accused an attorney associated with the Community Nutrition Institute of "creating media events" and engaging in "media terrorism."

III. Conflicts Involving Advertising

Warner et al (1992) concluded that magazines which advertise potentially hazardous products tend to reduce their editorial coverage of such hazards. This is not limited to cigarettes. There has been similar corporate economic influence against publishers in the case of aspartame-containing products, and antistatic clothes softeners (Roberts 1986, 1990). Such exposés were decried as "ambush journalism."

Some citizens in Palm Beach County reached the point of utter dismay over "practiced deception" and the "erosion of ethics" by the media. They set forth these grievances in a statement to the *News/Sun-Sentinel* (December 15, 1987, p. E-10) about the "increasing number of advertisements that digress from the facts and indulge in misleading innuendo."

Large sums are received for advertising in medical journals. The account of a personal experience is germane.

> The *Journal of the American Medical Association* published approval of aspartame by its Council on Scientific Affairs in 1985 (1985; 254:400-402). The author submitted his initial report on aspartame reactions to this periodical the following year. It reviewed 157 patients, and presented a succinct clinical review. The companion letter stated, "I am <u>preferentially</u> submitting this manuscript to the *Journal of the American Medical Association* because the A.M.A. Council on Scientific Affairs published its approval of aspartame therein. The present investigation therefore seems to warrant the same forum."
>
> The article was rejected within two weeks, coupled with this editorial comment: "Obviously this is a subject of great interest and importance at this time. I am sorry that the paper does not seem to contain original observations or substance that would withstand critical scrutiny." The author then counted **17** observations in the manuscript that had never been published previously to his knowledge.
>
> A full-page color ad for an aspartame tabletop sweetener appeared in **that** week's edition (September 26, 1986). This one and others for aspartame products appeared in subsequent weekly editions of the *Journal of the American Medical Association*. The statement therein that aspartame is "better than sugar for your diabetic patients" was <u>diametrically opposite</u> to my experience (see below and Chapter XIII).

<u>The enormous revenues reaped by medical journals and lay periodicals from the advertising of aspartame products likely influenced the choice of manuscript publication</u>. Another encounter is relevant.

The publisher of a household-name magazine made an **urgent** call to my home one evening, requesting an article on aspartame that "positively" would be printed. I was asked to send the manuscript "collect" by Federal Express. There was another reason: <u>two</u> children of this publisher had suffered severe reactions to aspartame products. I received a call one week later. After several minutes of beating around the bush, this publisher confided, "When I showed it to my advertising people, they hit the ceiling because much income could be jeopardized if companies making or using aspartame pulled their ads!"

L. EXCLUSION FROM SCIENTIFIC PROGRAMS

Denying participation as a presenter for the scientific session of a medical association is properly the decision of program committees. On the other hand, refusal to publish a relevant <u>abstract</u> in its proceedings submitted by an active member requires sober explanation.

- I submitted an abstract intended for presentation at the June 1987 annual scientific program of the American Diabetes Association. It was titled, "Complications Associated With Aspartame In Diabetics." This abstract summarized observations in 58 diabetic aspartame reactors. The cover letter stated, "This represents a nationwide research of aspartame reactors. I believe the study is of practical and immediate interest to every physician caring for diabetics."

  The Committee on Medical and Scientific Programs refused to print the abstract in the section for abstracts submitted but not presented. The Chairman replied that his committee "...does not find it suitable for publication in the program supplement... It is our policy to publish only those which are judged to be of clear scientific merit." The case for "scientific merit" in this instance appears in Chapter XIII.

- An abstract on aspartame-associated epilepsy was submitted for the 1988 Annual Scientific Program of the American Academy of Neurology. It dealt with 250 cases — 101 from my data, and 149 cases reported to the FDA (Chapter III). Presentation was denied.

M. REFLECTIONS ON IBSEN:
EMOTIONAL BACKLASH BY THE PUBLIC

The emotional backlash of the public against physicians who suggest that popular products may be harmful can be intense. Henrik Ibsen captured this intimidating phenomenon in his play, *An Enemy of the People*. This literary work ought to be required reading for doctors who challenge the safety of products manufactured and distributed by billion-dollar corporations.

Ibsen focused on Dr. Thomas Stockmann, the medical officer of the municipal Baths in a small community. It anticipated an economic revival because of their increasing popularity. But Stockmann became alarmed over the poisons contained therein, describing the Bath establishment as "a whited, poison sepulchre... the gravest possible danger to the public health!" On the basis of personal observations in patients, coupled with confirmation by independent scientific analysis, he concluded "all that stinking filth" coming from tanneries had been affecting water in the conduit pipes leading to the reservoir.

Dr. Stockmann felt compelled to exercise "the duty of a citizen to let the public share in any new ideas." Instead of appreciation for having brought to light "such an important truth" in the *People's Messenger* (the community newspaper), however, he was humiliated and stigmatized – especially by those in power having self-serving interests. Within days of expressing his view, Stockmann was declared "an enemy of the people." He and members of his family were ostracized. The doctor was even denounced by his brother... mayor of the town, and chairman of the Bath's Committee.

In an attempt to understand the scope of this matter, the physician made his "great discovery" – namely, "all the sources of our *moral* life are poisoned, and the whole fabric of our civic community is founded on the pestiferous soil of falsehood."

N. SUPPORT FROM MEDICAL COLLEAGUES

The author acknowledges the appreciation expressed by health care professionals for his lectures and publications on aspartame disease. A number of such references appear in previous chapters, especially from physicians so afflicted or members of their family.

This personal communication, dated August 13, 1991, was received from Dr. Derrick Lonsdale (Editor, *Journal of Advancement in Medicine*).

"I, for one, am grateful for your drawing attention to this matter which has been perpetrated on the innocent public. I believe

886

that it is our job as physicians to try to educate our patients to these dangers, served up, as it were, like 'the wolf in sheep's clothing'... We are dedicated to the truth as much as we can decipher it in this crazy world of so-called science."

XXIX

THE PLIGHT OF CONFUSED CONSUMERS

"Whom can I blame, how can I function, When I am the source
of my own destruction?"
                    Avraham ben Shmuel
                    (13th Century Spain)

"If we do not pay proper attention to the nutritional problems
associated with food technology, we run the risk of eventually
producing an abundance of palatable, convenient staple foods
that are not capable of meeting man's nutrient needs. We run
the risk of undermining the nutritional well-being of our
nation."
                    O. Stewart (1964)

Most health professionals remain confused about aspartame disease (Chapter XXVIII). It is therefore little wonder that health-conscious consumers fare no better. FDA's approval of the extended use of aspartame as an all-purpose sweetener compounded the problem. (Food producers now can get these new improved items on the shelves within weeks.) An aspartame reactor who suffered severe symptoms perceptively reflected, "It would be a miracle if I survive to 65!"

Downey and Macnaughton (2000) have emphasized the value of anecdotal evidence for doctors and their patients. Unfortunately, the scorn of anecdotal evidence by researchers, coupled with the impact of consumerism, has blocked physicians from having adequate access to information about aspartame disease. An anti-aspartame activist also noted the apparent addiction to diet sodas of media and government workers, which she regarded as "drinking on the job."

Informed consumers in the post-thalidomide era realize another danger: acceptance by bureaucracies of the proposition that the marketplace serves as an ultimate correcting

887

888

force. The reason: it may be too late. As a result, they try to minimize dietary risk. A feature on personal fitness appearing in *The Philadelphia Inquirer* (March 15, 1987) carried the apt title, "Think before you sweeten."

Consumer v. Citizen

Darden Asbury Pyron (1987), Professor of History at Florida International University, noted that the meaning of "to consume" could be "to destroy; to spend wastefully; to squander; to engross." On the occasion of the Constitution's 200th anniversary, a humorous cartoon of Mt. Rushmore depicted Thomas Jefferson with a diet cola, and George Washington with a regular cola beverage. Pyron indignantly perceived this erosion of our noble heritage in these terms:

> "The title of consumer has almost completely supplanted that of citizen in contemporary American society... However one cuts it or describes it, citizenship is the antithesis of consumption... From its inception in the polis and political order of classical Greece, citizenship has always entailed the subordination of our appetites and individual whims to the law, the larger good, the commonwealth... citizenship is not a salable commodity. The Constitution is not a joke. And Mr. Jefferson is not a diet cola.*

The author concurs with the need for a nonpolitical and corporate-neutral board charged with clearing ads for sweeteners and other food additives. The Canadian Pharmaceutical Advertising Advisory Board serves such a function in the case of drugs.

The Yo-Yo Consumer

Consumers have been subjected to frustration over the past four decades when some favorite food or additive was maligned or removed because laboratory animals evidenced clinical or laboratory changes after being given huge doses. It becomes more intensive when the original studies could not be reproduced in more suitable animal models. The unproved bias against saccharin as a possible cause of urinary bladder cancer in humans (Chapter XXVII) is a case in point.

---

* Reproduced with permission of Professor Darden Asbury Pyron and *The Palm Beach Post*.

On the other hand, some persons cherish their sweet tooth, and will continue using aspartame products until shown <u>absolute</u> proof that it poses a health threat. In fact, a few aspartame reactors in this series used aspartame products, albeit in smaller amounts (Chapter XIX), on this premise.

The Plight of Merchants

The managers of reputable stores are confronted with difficult decisions concerning the alleged hazards of aspartame products they carry. A British retailer commented on this matter to the author.

> "As a retailer, we have to appeal to a wide customer base, some of whom are diabetic, and some who are slimming and wish to consume low-sugar products. We consider ourselves responsible retailers, and would not sell any products likely to be of detriment to a consumer. We are aware of the concerns surrounding aspartame, but as yet feel the evidence is weighted against it. If the situation should change, we would have no hesitation in reviewing our position relative to aspartame."

CONSUMER DISTRUST

The aspartame fiasco has generated extreme distrust by consumers against a number of professional, organizational, business and regulatory groups. Further details appear later in this chapter.

I. The Medical Profession

Every chapter describes the desperate search for causation by severe aspartame reactors after repeatedly encountering "clueless" physicians. A computer professional described himself as "an avid diet cola drinker." He had been "diagnosed with just about every mental disorder you can imagine, including anxiety, panic attacks, depression, bipolar disorder, ADHD, etc." He listed <u>ten</u> psychotropic drugs that proved ineffective. Other problems included chest pains, dizziness, numbness, tremors, cramps and infertility. Seeking an alternative health practitioner, he explained his case to a friend who was the medicine man for a native American tribe. After carefully listening to the history, the healer stated, "Stop drinking the diet pop! It's doing great harm to you physically and spiritually." Dramatic improvement occurred after going "cold turkey," including the conception of his first child.

Mention was made in the Preface of an ongoing revolution in doctor-patient relationships created by the Internet. Many persons now check out their symptoms, diagnoses, prescribed drugs and related information derived from various web sites and chat groups, seeking to present the fruits of such research to their doctors. A number of aspartame reactors changed physicians when told by uninformed or disinterested ones that these printouts were "ridiculous" or too time-consuming to review.

II. Corporate Platitudes

Some consumers who complained about reactions to aspartame products received platitudes about having a rare idiosyncrasy and the meaningless nature of "anecdotal" reports. One company spokesman denigrated such persons (*The Miami Herald* February 16, 1986, p. A-18).

- A woman with fructose intolerance was advised, "You shouldn't have a problem with aspartame." She proceeded to take it... and had a severe reaction.
- Relatives concerned about the considerable consumption of aspartame products by children have been repeatedly told that (a) it is one of the most tested products in history, and (b) the FDA's limit for a person weighing 30 pounds is the equivalent of six quarts of soft drinks containing aspartame, or 130 packets of an aspartame tabletop sweetener.

The National Yogurt Association proposed changes in yogurt standards during November 2000 that would rescind the warning label and other disclosure of aspartame and sweeteners. I consider such action highly objectionable because of the frequency with which yogurt containing aspartame has caused severe reactions. For example, one aspartame reactor found by rechallenge that the near-fatal "choking sensation" she experienced when traveling was specifically due to the sugar-free yogurt she ate at airports.

Consumers having aspartame disease have been subjected to added frustration when reassured by corporate representatives that their problem had "nothing to do" with using aspartame products, coupled with receiving coupons to purchase more of the goods in question! One was advised in July 1990 by the consumers affairs manager of a major food producer: "There are no documented reports in the medical literature of seizures or any of the symptoms you describe after consumption of aspartame."

Representative Case Report

Case XXIX-1

An aspartame reactor concluded. "I know beyond a shadow of a doubt that aspartame has bothered me." She repeatedly experienced "terrible headaches" for which she was "living off aspirin." She discontinued the use of aspartame, based on her own deductions, and sought further information. Her encounter was described in this letter.

"I had not read or heard anything adverse about aspartame – this is not why I stopped using it. I just tried to think back when my headaches started, and what I was doing differently. The weather had gotten warmer, and I started to drink pop. I immediately stopped using any form of aspartame to see if this was the cause.

"It has been over a month now, and I have had no headaches at all.

"I called the company that makes aspartame, and was referred to another company to get information about aspartame. I did get a large stack of data, but nothing to really answer my inquiry.

"I called a large cola producer to inquire as to whether they might bring back saccharin in their drinks – but they wouldn't answer."

III. FDA Correspondence (see below and Chapter XXXI)

The author has many letters from patients with aspartame disease who had written the FDA about their reactions to aspartame products. In turn, they received intimidating correspondence and "scientific evidence" aimed at proving them wrong.

IV. Inadvertent Consumption

Inadvertent exposure to aspartame products (Chapter I) poses a sufficient danger for some severe reactors that they refuse to dine out, even in health-oriented restaurants. The tendency for some chefs to replace corn syrup with aspartame enhanced their anxiety.

Aspartame is also administered to sick infants and children with fever. Many parents are not aware of its presence in "delicious" chewable acetaminophen and flavored antibiotics, or fail to understand the significance of labels stating that the product contains phenylalanine or warning "phenylketonurics."

A woman in Austria with severe gastrointestinal and other reactions to aspartame wrote of another problem she was encountering: "All the syrups for fountain machines contain aspartame and acesulfame-K even if they are not 'light' or for diabetics!"

FDA RESISTANCE AND DISINFORMATION
(also see Chapter XXXI)

An aspartame reactor expressed the sentiments of many victims in these terms: "The FDA is as interested in protecting the public against aspartame as Ahab was in saving whales."

Donald Kennedy (1987), President of Stanford University and a former FDA Commissioner, expressed his increasing concern about public confusion over claims and counterclaims regarding scientific issues... coupled with the extent of scientific illiteracy. In the case of aspartame disease, such "illiteracy" can be attributed in part to FDA reluctance to provide **any** statement about aspartame disease. Indeed, ninety-five (23.9 percent) of 397 aspartame reactors who initially completed the survey questionnaire (Chapter XIX) had written or called the FDA... generally to no avail. Those who requested information about the safety and prudent limits of aspartame intake received incomplete or misleading replies.

- A member of Senator Howard Metzenbaum's staff received assurance that children could safely consume large amounts of aspartame (*Congressional Record-Senate* 1985a, p.S 5491).
- Peter Dews, a Harvard psychologist and consultant for the International Life Sciences Institute, told a Senate hearing on aspartame (November 3, 1987) that the public may be confused if provided with too much information. (This Institute is funded by the food industry, including a manufacturer of aspartame.)
- As of December 1987, there was no "aspartame hotline" for consumers. The Senate hearing on November 3, 1987 revealed that persons calling about aspartame-related complaints were informed by the FDA, or by the AIDS hotline, that there was "no problem" with aspartame.

The challenged record of the FDA within these realms was summarized in this report by the Committee on Government Operations of the 101st Congress (November 14, 1990) titled, *FDA's Continuing Failure to Prevent Deceptive Health Claims for Food.*

"Whereas drugs are subjected to a rigorous expensive, and sometimes lengthy premarket approval process, foods may be marketed with no such prior review. Thus, food companies who are allowed to make explicit disease-prevention claims have a distinct advantage over drug companies who must obtain FDA permission for any labeling claims." (p. 3)

"This remarkable concession from an official agency charged with policing the food label is both alarming and pathetic. It makes no sense for FDA to allow companies to make health claims on food labels if the agency admits it lacks the resources to enforce its regulations in a way that will deter manufacturers from making deceptive claims." (p. 13)

"During his appearance before the subcommittee, Commissioner Young displayed a very cavalier attitude about his violations of FDA's recording requirements. When confronted with his repeated violations of the regulation, Commissioner Young suggested that this was not a "substantive" issue and refused to give the subcommittee any assurance that these violations would cease." (p. 22)

"The Food and Drug Administration is perhaps the most important regulatory agency in the Federal Government charged by Congress with the responsibility to protect the public's health. Over the last ten years, political interference has stripped FDA of its ability to function as a credible and independent entity." (p. 22)

"This abdication of responsibility was coupled with a complete failure to employ even a token amount of enforcement resources to combat the proliferation of deceptive health claims. FDA's top food labeling compliance official admitted the agency had not allocated adequate resources to police the food label. He was reduced to pleading, if not begging, with industry representatives to voluntarily cease deceptive labeling practices."

Premature Reassurance

Inquiring consumers generally receive reassuring statements about the safety of aspartame from the FDA, the manufacturer, and their physicians. An FDA consumer safety officer asserted, "We conclude that there was no cause-and-effect relationship between the complaints and aspartame... There are always individual people who have idiosyncratic reactions to different substances" (*The Miami Herald* July 31, 1986, p. PB-4).

By contrast, Senator Howard Metzenbaum wrote this opinion to Senator Strom Thurmond (Chairman, the Senate Judiciary Committee) in a letter dated February 3, 1986)

"The average consumer assumes that all safety questions surrounding this sweetener have been resolved long before it found its way onto every grocery shelf in America. A recent investigation undertaken by my office raises serious questions as to whether this is, in fact, the case."

These reservations also apply to media comments by FDA officials. For example, *The Palm Beach Post* (December 10, 1991) carried a reassuring statement under "Health Notes" about concern over "the amount of aspartame that could be consumed by 2-to 5-year-old children." Its source: Dr. Linda Tollefson, a veterinarian and chief of clinical nutrition assessment at the FDA, who stated, "We have never found a problem." But this author found enough problems to devote an entire chapter to reactions among infants and children in his first book on aspartame reactions (Roberts 1988). They included convulsions, headaches, rashes, asthma, anorexia and gastrointestinal problems.

Consumer Attitudes

Many aspartame reactors, or their families, encountered "passing the buck" while attempting to obtain pertinent information.

- The father of a severe aspartame reactor requested information from the Bureau of Alcohol, Tobacco and Firearms concerning the methanol content of two popular colas. The chief of its Industry Compliance Division wrote him, "We understand your interest in this matter; however, the Bureau's jurisdiction extends only to the importation, production, labeling and advertising of alcohol beverages. The production of soda products is regulated by the U.S. Food and Drug Administration (FDA)."
- Parents and grandparents of children with congenital deformities and other disorders born to mothers who consumed aspartame during pregnancy expressed related encounters. The grandfather of a 5-year-old boy with spina bifida asked, "Who do we believe?"

The following illustrate consumer/patient attitudes to the FDA on this matter.

- A 28-year-old aspartame reactor expressed concern that "there is too much money to be made on the disabled. How can I maintain good health if we are continually deceived into bad health?"

- "After ten years of being addicted to diet cola, and suffering progressively worse migraine headaches daily, someone suggested that I stop drinking it. Guess what! No more daily headaches. I'm so mad at the government for allowing this poison to be considered safe!"

- Paul R. Ruggles, the father of a daughter whose severe aspartame disease had been diagnosed as multiple sclerosis, replied to a disbelieving journalist on August 14, 1987.

> "What I believe happened in the saga of aspartame certification by the FDA was actually a result of the spirit of deregulation, and the FDA implementing less-than-adequate scientific judgement. Unfortunately, the damage has been done, and now 100 million consumers are unfolding." (Reproduced with permission)

- Julie Kelly wrote this letter to Dr. David Kessler, FDA Commissioner, in July 1996.

> "How could you approve the poison aspartame in everything in the supermarket when you receive more complaints on this chemical than all other food additives? The masquerade is over.

> "I am a diabetic, and tried aspartame when it was approved. I had severe headaches, nausea, vomiting, blurred vision, was incoherent, couldn't remember, lost my equilibrium, and my blood sugar climbed. I then got off aspartame.

> "My sister, also a diabetic, continued to get worse on aspartame. Her blood sugar was out of control. She had such severe numbness in her feet and legs that she had to keep them wrapped. As soon as she stopped the aspartame, her blood sugar came under control, and she improved.

> "I am a hair dresser and see many people. It gives me an opportunity to see how many persons are stricken because of this poison, but don't associate the problems. For example, Mae F. often brings in her five-year-old child. He is a hyperactive. As soon as she gives him a diet cola,

he goes wild. When I asked Mae why she gives it to him,
she said, "He loves it! He's addicted to it."

Blistering attacks have been directed to the FDA about perceived hidden political agendas affecting important decisions involving drugs and additives. A feature titled, "Politics Trumps Science at the FDA," was published by *The Wall Street Journal* (July 21, 1997, p. A-22).

Betty Martini, founder of Mission Possible (Chapter XXX), repeatedly criticized the FDA for tenaciously advocating the safety of aspartame products. She wrote, "They knew the gun was loaded! Is aspartame sweet? Yes, it is a sweet poison. Roaches won't eat it; cats and dogs won't eat it; ants won't eat it; and flies won't eat it. But the FDA serves it to you with its approval."

PROFESSIONAL RESISTANCE AND DISINFORMATION

Consumers have received considerable disinformation concerning the safety of aspartame products from health professionals. This section focuses on several groups contributing to their confusion.

I. Physicians

Consumer-patients who raise pertinent questions about the safety of aspartame products can expect difficulty when following this advice of the FDA or manufacturers, "Ask your doctor." Disappointment is the rule if they presume their physicians are interested and knowledgeable about aspartame disease.

Aspartame reactors have leveled severe criticism against doctors who ignored or ridiculed their observations concerning a perceived relation between the use of these products and their symptoms. Case III-I, a nurse who was hospitalized with aspartame-induced convulsions, found comparable reports when researching this subject in the hospital's library, but was told by her neurologist, "Stop reading!

Similarly, patients misdiagnosed as having multiple sclerosis had to endure remarks by their physicians about being "in denial" after exhibiting dramatic improvement with aspartame abstinence.

Ken and Jan Nolley (1987) commented on the plight of patients with chemical sensitivities, especially the parents of such children. They asserted: "These dismissals often reveal a disdain for patients' abilities to assess their own symptoms rationally, as well as subtle, unexamined cultural biases." They were critical of physicians whose "own interest makes it easiest to deny patient-reported symptoms, and their training reinforces the perceived superiority of their own judgements over patient perceptions."

The **Internet** has been a diagnostic blessing for numerous patients whose doctors were unaware of aspartame disease. For example, a 55-year old woman experienced severely slurred speech. She typed "slurred speech" in a search engine on the Internet and out of desperation, and found an appropriate reference. Her symptoms promptly improved after avoiding aspartame products.

A number of aspartame reactors, however, found that obtaining vital information on the Internet backfired on them when they relayed it to physicians and other health care professionals. Their greatest anguish entailed being bluntly told they were "the worried well" for whom the Internet reinforced hypochondriasis – or terms to that effect. To the contrary, physicians should react positively and gratefully when patients bring them valid Internet information that enhances their knowledge.

This theme is also conveyed in various health/wellness letters published by prestigious organizations that soundly "debunk" rumors about aspartame disease spread by e-mail campaigns.

Aspartame reactors expressed outrage when aspartame foods and liquids were recommended – and even sold – by "diet doctors." The latter include authors of popular books on weight reduction. Some aspartame reactors were introduced to aspartame products by complimentary coupons sent to their doctors for purchasing them, especially diet drinks.

Numerous case histories in this book reflect such professional indifference and hostility. The following letters are representative.

- An engineer with aspartame disease wrote, "I have wasted hundreds of hours and thousands of dollars trying to get well from totally clueless doctors! My legacy for not having been informed is maddening tinnitus, massive memory loss (things I did for 42 years in electronics I couldn't even recall the names of)... It makes me wonder how many others just don't care."
- Case IV-13 C suffered severe visual damage attributed to the use of aspartame sodas. Several consulting ophthalmologists denied any causative or aggravating role of aspartame. "One looked at me as if I was a little nuts when I told him I was sure that it was the sweetener."

898

A remission followed aspartame abstinence. She wrote three years later, "These doctors don't want to hear or admit to anyone that there is a problem."

- A 49-year-old woman experienced severe joint pains after consuming aspartame products for ten years. She had been treated with prednisolone and methotrexate while consuming aspartame, but without benefit. The patient experienced dramatic relief of these and other systemic symptoms after avoiding aspartame. When she related this experience to her rheumatologist, he not only denied any association, but increased the dosage of methotrexate!

- Some patients who discovered that aspartame products were the basis for their misery (after considerable personal research and experimentation) refused to revisit prior consultants. One executive with recurrent aspartame-induced hives stated, "I figure that I am wasting my time educating a medical specialist who will likely not take the time to read up on this poison."

- A secretary developed a recurrent rash and "a deep red color on my face" for which she consulted several physicians, including an allergist. She had been drinking "tons" of a diet soda to lose weight. Out of desperation, she resorted to drinking only bottled water for fluid. Her condition improved until "just sipping a diet soda" while doing errands. A rash on the arms and "a deep flushing red" of the face developed. She immediately drove to her doctor's office. "He just looked at me, patted me on the knee, and said I was making too much of everything. In other words, it was all in my head. I came home humiliated, frustrated and angry."

- A diabetic woman with severe aspartame reactions stated that a physician had dismissed her as a patient after she expressed concern about his lack of knowledge on aspartame disease – particularly when handing him considerable information obtained from the Internet. She wrote, "Can you believe that he would not admit he might be wrong in his stance on this subject? And he is supposed to be a diabetes specialist!"

Representative Case Report

Case XXIX-2

This aspartame reactor was the wife of a food scientist engaged in research and development for a major snack food company. She experienced tremors, a faint feeling, and weakness in the lower limbs of sufficient severity to force her to lie down – even in the aisle of a grocery store! As a result, she refused to drive or go anywhere by herself. During this time, she also suffered intense headaches, extreme intolerance to noise, depression, and uncharacteristic behavior. All tests proved inconclusive.

Her husband stocked their pantry with aspartame products because she had been diagnosed as having reactive hypoglycemia. Moreover, their three-year-old daughter would become hyperactive after consuming sugar.

Once aware of aspartame's potential side effects, the couple removed all such products from their home. The patient resumed sugar in small amounts. Her symptoms totally subsided within ten days. Her physician then scolded her for having discontinued his medication when she became symptom-free!

III. Dietitians and Nutritionists

Numerous patients with diabetes or reactive hypoglycemia (low blood sugar attacks) have expressed exasperation over the advice of dietitians – both while hospitalized under my care, and as patients of other physicians – relative to their approval of aspartame products. The author has had to check their dietary intake **personally** when patients' blood sugar values became erratic under these circumstances. A case in point was the serving of "dietetic" yogurt containing aspartame, notwithstanding **specific** written instructions that no patient of mine was to receive aspartame products!

This issue is illustrated by the statement of Dr. Jean Mayer, a prominent nutritionist. He and Jeanne Goldberg (1988), writing as members of the Washington Post Writers Group, summarized "the safety of aspartame" in these terms: "So far it has come up with a clean bill of health... there seems to be no evidence that aspartame used in moderation poses any threat to health."

The consequences of nutritional deception to our society are profound. Professor Alfred E. Harper (1988) emphasized the "extensive self-deception" created by "authorities" who generate nutritional strategies aimed at preventing or minimizing chronic degenerative diseases that variously focus on calories, carbohydrates, fats, proteins, minerals and vitamins. They undermine confidence in the American diet, causing widespread fear of food ("trophophobia"), and spawning a nation of "healthy hypochondriacs." An extreme of such perversion is manifest by undernourished small children of affluent parents who regard certain foods rich in nutrients (as dairy products and meats) as potentially hazardous.

900

Representative Case Report

Case XXIX-3

A female athlete developed intense thirst, fatigue, and drowsiness that caused her to sleep at the wheel. She wrote, "I used to run three to four miles a day. I drank six or more diet drinks a day, up to five cups of coffee with a tabletop sweetener, and everything diet that I could buy. I never thought I had to read the labels because of the belief the FDA was protecting me."

She developed marked blurring of vision, itching of the skin, numbness of the fingers and toes, and became unsteady. As a result, she repeatedly injured herself from falls.

A diagnosis of type II diabetes mellitus was made. She began surfing the Internet to learn more about diabetes and an appropriate diet, especially after the nurses who taught diabetics had been laid off by her managed care company. She became increasingly convinced that aspartame products precipitated her clinical diabetes, and aggravated the complications.

This patient contacted her local American Diabetes Association chapter. The nurse instructor encouraged her to take diet drinks and food. In fact, diet products were available as refreshments for everyone. This frustrating experience motivated her to write a booklet about diabetes for other patients seeking advice on the Internet.

Health-Related Organizations

The pro-aspartame attitudes of various organizations that focus on specific diseases – for example, epilepsy and diabetes – appear in previous sections. Many receive funds and support from the aspartame industry, both directly and indirectly. An instance is cited.

The American Diabetes Association offered these "Facts About Aspartame."

> "People of all ages, including pregnant or breast feeding women, teens, and children over two years old, can enjoy products sweetened with aspartame while maintaining a healthful diet... and, aspartame has special benefits for people with diabetes, either insulin-dependent or non-insulin-dependent, because it lets them satisfy their taste for sweets without affecting blood sugar... Consuming products sweetened with aspartame is no different than consuming other foods."

Another shortcoming involves the failure of organizations to impart information requested by consumers. For example, the father of a three-year-old child with severe dermatitis repeatedly induced by aspartame products wrote to London's National Eczema Society. He was informed that this society could find "no published research reporting a link between aspartame and eczema." (See Chapter VIII)

CORPORATE INFLUENCES

I. Aggressive Promotion

Consumers are bombarded with slick "advertorials" and other public relations campaigns for selling aspartame products. These packaging efforts are tantamount to manufactured consent of the mass media. The public's increasing concern about aspartame sodas, however, has influenced promotional efforts, such as replacing the word "diet" with "one calorie."

> The father of a 3-year-old girl who had developed a severe rash from using aspartame products became infuriated after receiving a sample of "sugar free gum." He termed this "a totally inappropriate and irresponsible marketing ploy."

The touting of aspartame as "the most tested additive in history" and "virtually totally safe" is mentioned in other chapters. Victims of aspartame disease resent these nothing-but-good promos on television as "ads that try men's souls". They become highly incensed by those aimed at pregnant women (Chapter X) and children (Chapter XI).

Such unrestrained advertising may backfire. For example, a reactor included in her decade-long list of medical consultants a neurologist (migraine), a cardiologist (heart palpitations), a psychiatrist (depression), her general practitioner (fatigue), and "etc." She was "tipped off" to aspartame disease because of the intensity with which pro-aspartame sites on the Web denied ANY side effects.

II. Inadequate or Misleading Labels

"Deception by omission" is not infrequently encountered. The incomplete labeling of aspartame-containing products was reviewed in Chapters XIX, XXVII and XXX. In point of fact, one ought to be able to judge a food by its cover.

Many aspartame products no longer are identified by the familiar corporate "swirl." Consumers can request a Material Safety Data Sheet from the manufacturers of products they suspected contain aspartame. They are entitled to receive this information under the Community Right to Know Law and worker exposure laws.

Patients seeking to avoid sugar have been confused by other forms of labeling. For example, many use a popular tabletop aspartame sweetener on the assumption it contains no sugar – a reference to sucrose. The label, however, lists "dextrose with dried corn syrup" as the first ingredient.

Of the 397 aspartame reactors who initially completed the survey questionnaire (Chapter XIX), 375 (94.4 percent) felt the actual content by weight of aspartame should be required on food and beverage labels. Furthermore, 340 (85.6 percent) indicated they would study such labels.

Exasperated aspartame reactors who were unable to find this chemical listed among product ingredients have repeatedly vented their frustration.

- One product listed only aspirin, sodium bicarbonate and citric acid as active ingredients, citing aspartame as an "inactive ingredient." This infuriated a patient who had been diagnosed as having Crohn's disease. She experienced a prolonged remission after abstaining from aspartame products.
- The presence of aspartame may appear in the insert, but not on the box of some products.
- Some "diet" bakery products indicate "contains artificial sweeteners" without identifying their nature.

III. Failure to Impart Negative Information

The aspartame industry has received considerable correspondence from consumers about perceived aspartame reactions, coupled with requests for pertinent information. Without legal pressure, however, corporate unwillingness to provide this information is likely to be encountered.

The following letter embodies the frustration of numerous persons with aspartame disease under these circumstances.

"I'm a 33-year-old diabetic with kidney disease. Two years ago, I had numerous tests at Duke University to find out why I had so many headaches. I was told I had an allergic reaction to the aspartame that is found in most diet products. Several of my letters to the Company have gone unanswered. God help all that are using these products to try and make themselves thin and beautiful! I learned the hard way that they're putting themselves in the grave."

IV. Saccharin: A Scapegoat

Consumers who decide to shift back to saccharin-containing beverages must come to grips with this caveat on labels: "Use of this product may be hazardous to your health. This product contains saccharin which has been determined to cause cancer in laboratory animals."

The serious limitations of this unproved warning were discussed in Chapter XXVII-K. Others concur.

- Scientists have been unable to demonstrate "a significant human health risk" warranting removal of saccharin from the market after the Saccharin Studies and Labeling Act of 1978 (*Congressional Record-Senate* 1985a).
- Dr. Frank Young, the FDA Commissioner in April 1985, stated that any link between saccharin consumption and the development of cancer in humans had **not** been proved after years of intensive research (*Congressional Record-Senate*, 1985a, p. S 5512).
- Dr. Neil Solomon (1986), a syndicated health columnist, regarded the risk of cancer from saccharin use as "extremely small or nonexistent."

When saccharin was temporarily withdrawn from the market, persons seeking a sugar substitute regarded the introduction of aspartame as a godsend. The manufacturer vigorously pushed aspartame products to market as soon as possible – in part to diminish incentives by others working on new sweeteners. When saccharin consumption was subsequently allowed, its use became subject to renewed approval by Congress every two years.

Another paradox may be emerging: the possible carcinogenicity of aspartame (Chapter XXVII-E and F).

904

V. Intimidation By a Perceived Economic Goliath

Most patients, health professionals, bureaucrats and elected officials are unwilling to tackle the issue of aspartame toxicity because they fear challenge by a multibillion-dollar industry.

Case III-6 experienced severe memory loss and a grand mal convulsion after drinking considerable aspartame sodas. Believing that aspartame products should be "removed from the market," his mother added, "Given the kind of earnings it generates, however, it is going to be a tough battle."

This perception has undermined the public's attitude about expecting protection from the medical profession (see above). There are precedents. Sinclair Lewis criticized physicians and health care in his famous 1925 novel *Arrowsmith*. It depicted the greed, commercialism and bureaucratic obstacles encountered by Dr. Martin Arrowsmith throughout his career in medical practice, bacteriologic research and epidemiology.

The food and "supplement" industries have intensified suppression of free speech in this sphere through libel laws in more than a dozen states that could criminalize citizens and journalists who express concern about food safety. This is illustrated by the suit against Oprah Winfrey for her remarks concerning "mad cow disease in a 1996 show .

VI. Personal Vilification

The inflammatory rhetoric used by pro-aspartame apologists was discussed in Chapter XXVIII-D. Outrageous disinformation contributing to consumer and professional confusion has involved vilification.

With reference to the author, one critic wrote, "Palm Beach County, Florida, is the largest sugar-producing county in the United States. So how is Dr. Roberts 'corporate neutral?' And how come the references to his own books? Is that neutral too?" (*Author's response: I have not received a cent from the sugar industry for my researches.*)

THE MEDIA

The confusion of health care providers resulting from disinformation by their "professional" media was considered in Chapter XXVIII. The same applies to information read or viewed by consumers.

I. Inadequate Research

The general press has inaccurately reported on many aspartame research studies. This reflected a lack of awareness of basic methodologic and scientific considerations by some investigative reporters. As a result, they failed to probe for them and ask fundamental questions.

II. Cancellation of Projected Exposés

There has been intimidation of the media (newsprint; radio; television) relative to newsworthy features on the aspartame issue that their staff wished to pursue. This constitutes a gross disservice to audiences. The matter became uniquely hypocritical when investigative reporters were eager to obtain corporate-neutral views after soliciting and actually programming the author and others for interviews. It could be logically inferred that the ensuing cancellations after such considerable effort reflected coercion by top-level management. One example suffices.

> KPFK is the major public radio station (110,000 watts) in the Los Angeles area. Its popular co-hosts requested a 30-minute interview of the author for February 3, 1999. This required shifting two important appointments by visitors from Paris and Amsterdam.
>
> The station also requested that multiple copies of my books, position papers and biographical material be sent <u>overnight</u> by Federal Express. I complied... at considerable personal expense. Furthermore, it wished to receive 50(!) <u>gratis</u> copies as gifts to callers during its fundraising week. Having been the first Vice-President of Palm Beach County's Friends for Public Broadcasting two decades earlier, I was sympathetic to this request.
>
> The producer left a message on my answering machine the evening of February 2, stating that he had decided to cancel the interview! No apology or explanation was offered.

III. Fear of Litigation

Fear of litigation (see above) also has intimidated the media here and abroad, especially in the United Kingdom where dissenters are not protected by a First Amendment. As a result, few newspapers are willing to risk expensive suits by covering "the aspartame story."

In the same vein, researchers involved within this realm are disinclined to become involved.

Consumers have been denied safety information about products containing other sugar substitutes when ads by consumer groups were rejected. For example, one deploring the promotion of sugar-coated cereals for children had been prepared on behalf of Public Advocates, a public interest law firm. It was turned down by *The Wall Street Journal* which insisted upon certain changes and a letter of indemnification protecting the periodical against "any liabilities" (Moskowitz 1984). Advocates for the public regarded this "double standard" as hypocritical because the paper had been running ads for cigarettes.

An apparent breakthrough occurred when the *Sunday Express* carried a front-page feature titled, "Prove That Diet Drinks Are Safe," in its January 9, 2000 edition. It included my separate interviews with investigative journalists Lucy Johnston and Hazel Courtney. Norman Baker, a Liberal Democrat Member of Parliament, was reported to have called for the immediate withdrawal of aspartame products pending a full investigation.

IV. Intended Ridicule

Features have been published in both local newspapers and syndicated columns that view concern about aspartame use as false "urban legends." They reinforce comparable corporate denigration of serious studies describing aspartame disease (Chapter XXXI).

A staff writer of *The Palm Beach Post* (June 19, 2000, page E-1) singled out such concern as a primary "health myth." She equated the suspect contributory role of aspartame in brain tumors (Chapter XXVII-F), multiple sclerosis (Chapter VI-D) and lupus (Chapter VIII-E) with "alligators in the sewers, bananas carrying flesh-eating bacteria, or asbestos in tampons."

XXX

ANTI-ASPARTAME CONSUMER ADVOCATES

"Ye shall know the truth, and the truth shall make you mad."
Aldous Huxley

"It's the sugar-substitute, stupid!"
(Revision of the campaign slogan
"It's the economy, stupid!")
Carolyn Baldas Gray

"Never doubt that a small group of thoughtful, committed
citizens can change the world. Indeed, it is the only thing that
ever has."

Margaret Mead

Two basic consumer-oriented issues deserve emphasis. First, *aspartame disease primarily represents a medical and public health problem, not a legal one.* Second, *even if only one-tenth of one percent of persons consuming this chemical in the United States currently suffer reactions, at least 140,000 are being victimized!*

The FDA had already received nearly 4,000 <u>volunteered</u> consumer complaints about aspartame products as of December 1987. Its ho-hum attitude on the matter infuriated aspartame victims and their relatives. This contrasted with only several dozen complaints about the formaldehyde present in home insulation that effectively banned such use. Similarly, fewer than a score of adverse reactions resulted in removing prior liquid protein formulas promoted for weight loss from the market.

Indignant aspartame reactors reacted both individually and as members of newly-created consumer groups. They began exploiting the Internet to compare notes and to take action against manufacturers and the FDA. Activists who became enraged at the "piggies" who let this poison go to market sought their exposure and prosecution. An aspartame reactor who had not had a seizure for 12 years until consuming aspartame asserted in a letter to the manufacturer, "But, is it not better to be honest about the possible bad effects of aspartame, or must you change only after the company is slapped with a huge lawsuit?"

These groups also attempted informing the general public about aspartame disease, and obtaining injunctions barring the distribution of aspartame products predicated on imminent-public-health hazard and food additive legislation (Section 6). Anti-aspartame activists seeking to remove "Frankenstein foods" have had several significant achievements abroad. Iceland, a major UK grocery chain, announced that it would ban aspartame from its own-label products, largely out of concern for the apparent link to brain tumors (*The Sunday Times* October 25, 1999.)

The unfettered access of patients to pertinent medical information obtained from the Internet dismayed many uninformed physicians who were caught off-guard when presented with reams of information about aspartame disease (Chapter XXIX). These diligent sleuths became outraged when the initial "professional" reaction was to "debunk this myth."

The multiplicity of corporate and bureaucratic obstacles confronting these individuals and groups will be described in Chapter XXXI. Morton Mintz and Jerry S. Cohen discussed the general subject in *America, Inc.: Who Owns and Operates the United States*? (Dell Publishing Company, New York, 1971). In his introduction to their book, Ralph Nader emphasized that corporate institutions and their friends in governmental regulatory bodies tend to be relentless in combating adversaries through various strategies. He noted "harmful food additives" amount the products of such concern.

Despite daunting challenges, these anti-aspartame advocates persisted and became remarkable "epicenters of activism." With few resources other than committed persons and the Internet, they continued challenging disinformation in the media ("deceitful journalism") and the marketplace. Several favored the quote of Mohammed Ali, "They can run, but they can't hide." Others cited the U.S. Code (Title 18, Part I, Chapter 47, Section 1001) concerning purposeful misinformation. One activist suggested the acronym JAAA for a press conference: "Just Avoid All Aspartame!"

INPUT FROM INDIVIDUAL ASPARTAME VICTIMS

I. The Driving Force of Consumer Anger

Many expressions of anger by aspartame reactors against companies and the FDA appear throughout this book. Several other examples are offered.

- David Rietz expressed the sentiments of many afflicted with aspartame disease in this reply to a corporate apologist on the internet.

> "I am all too familiar with the deceit, subterfuge, bogus tests, fraud... not to mention the players switching sides to work for the manufacturer and its representatives. Those bogus test results do not negate the truth. To your dogma-bound dismay, you will, sooner than later, have this national disgrace shown in the total light of day – despised in the same manner as those who were prosecuted for war crimes after World War II. Mass international poisoning makes those crimes against humanity pale in comparison!"

- A 32-year-old woman with aspartame-induced convulsions stated

> "My children are not allowed to drink diet soda soft drinks or have anything that contains the chemical. I feel that aspartame is a dangerous food additive and should be taken off the market. I have had no problems at all with saccharin. I am angry because I was not given a choice."

- An aspartame reactor expressed his anger in these terms: "Make them pay for what they are doing to so many unsuspecting victims!"
- A 48-year-old professor had severe reactions to aspartame products that resulted in permanent disability. She wrote, "Stop its use! We, the American people, should not be guinea pigs, or duped for corporate capitalist profits."
- "I am 29 and the father of one. I went through hell the last four years of my life with chest pains, anxiety, and thousands of dollars worth of treatment, only to find that stopping diet cola seemed to cure all of my ailments. I'm 1000% better now."

II. The Need To Expiate Guilt

Awareness of aspartame disease caused considerable guilt among relatives and friends who had encouraged young persons to use aspartame products. The mother of a 16-year-old daughter wrote

"She was a member of the swim team, the snow ski team, the basketball, volleyball and softball teams, and on the cheerleading squad. She had even been offered a deal with the _____ Modeling Agency. She was always a good student. In 1995, we started to drink a soda sweetened with aspartame. In the mornings, I would make a gallon of it. My daughter started to have leg cramps, headaches, muscle aches, and was always very tired. She dropped out of sports, one by one, and started to miss a lot of school. At one point, the truant officer even came by to my home with a deputy to try and force me to send my daughter to school. You will never know the guilt a mother feels after finding out she has been poisoning her child for five years!!"

III. Pleas for Regulation

The clamor for regulation of aspartame products by persons with aspartame disease is detailed in Chapters XIX and XXX. Additional examples are cited.

- A 42-year-old registered nurse with severe aspartame-associated depression and irritability, urged Aspartame Victims and Their Friends to "do something." She wrote, "My worry is that they'll possibly just put a warning label on the product, and not take it off the market completely."
- A 27-year-old data processing coordinator had experienced recurrent abdominal pain after drinking a diet cola. He asserted that Congress or the FDA "should take it off the market until it has been further tested."

IV. Criticism of Disinterested or Uninformed Physicians

Aspartame reactors often vented hostility toward physicians who had ignored or ridiculed detailed assertions they provided (see above) that aspartame products might be causing their problems. The theme, "doctors have been brainwashed about aspartame," was repeatedly encountered. Several concurred with the assertion in *Medical Nemesis* by Ivan Illich (1975) that the medical establishment itself has become "the major threat to health."

- There was sarcastic reference to "M.D." as "medical deity."

- A 29-year-old businessman with aspartame-induced seizures was seen in consultation after having <u>five</u> CT scans and <u>three</u> MRI studies of the brain, and <u>five</u> electroencephalograms! The author suggested to his neurologist that both follow the patient, and try to reduce the medications if he remained seizure-free. The neurologist promptly called the patient and told him that I was "on the wrong track" Furthermore, he insisted that his two potent antiepileptic drugs be continued in full doses <u>indefinitely</u>.

- A Boston physician had written the FDA about several patient experiences involving aspartame-associated hyperactive behavior in children, and severe indigestion mimicking an acute heart attack. The father of one severe aspartame reactor asked him for further information. He received this startling lecture-reply from the doctor: "I do not fully endorse the hazards of aspartame. I think you have to be careful how you interpret various reports. It's important not to over-interpret anecdotal reports without having further information."

- The mother of a 13-year-old boy who had suffered severe abdominal and chest pains for nine months (Case XI-5) described this "nightmare experience." He had been subjected to multiple gastrointestinal x-rays, gastroscopy, gallbladder ultrasound, electrocardiograms, and numerous other studies. All proved normal. The physicians concluded the problem was psychological, and insisted that he needed counseling for "puberty" and "stress." The mother suspected a relationship between these complaints and aspartame intake. <u>All</u> symptoms disappeared after avoiding aspartame. She wrote, "The doctors would not believe me. Their response was, 'I've never heard of that!' "

The ongoing failure of the medical profession to delve deeply into aspartame disease seems inexcusable to many affected consumers. Their resentment increased on learning that the National Soft Drink Association had been prepared to oppose the incorporation of aspartame into soft drinks. (It did not, however, when producer/members found it more profitable to do so.)

V. Criticism of Disinterested or Uninformed Dietitians

Dietitians who enthusiastically recommended aspartame products to clients were severely criticized.

A prominent businesswoman developed aspartame-associated headaches, depression, bloat and difficulty in voiding. Her symptoms disappeared after avoiding aspartame products. She had expressed concern previously about the possible role of aspartame to a dietitian, but was assured, "Aspartame is perfectly safe."

VI. Criticism of the PR Barrage

Concerned parents and young adults often found themselves in a hopeless situation when deluged by a sophisticated media blitz for aspartame products. They felt outraged by its potential psychologic and physical impact on a highly impressionable younger generation. The caption of a humorist's column in *The Palm Beach Post* (August 26, 1986, p. F-2), "TV commercials disguised as the real America," could apply.

Oft-repeated television commercials for diet beverages intensified consumer frustration. Aspartame reactors objected to less-than-candid advertising, such as picture-of-health actors rejoicing over this preference.

- A registered nurse with violent aspartame reactions wrote

  "In a state of innocence, we are poisoning our bodies with supposedly safe substances that are advertised as natural. However, in truth, it is produced in a factory and is not extracted from natural substances such as 'milk and bananas' as advertised."

- A 43-year-old aspartame reactor resented several particular pitches.

  "I hate the ad, 'Mother will never know it's (aspartame) rather than sugar, Dear,' on the radio. And the TV ad with the cow that implies aspartame is natural. PHOOEY!"

VII. Criticisms of Irresponsible Journalism

Victims of aspartame disease were revolted by "irresponsible journalism scraping the bottom of the barrel" when newspapers featured pro-industry denials of any association between aspartame products and major contemporary problems.

A woman had to quit medical school in her third year because of presumed multiple sclerosis. She wrote to one major paper: "How dare you intentionally misinform readers that the aspartame/MS association is a hoax! Aspartame disease shattered by life. Had I not been referred to Dr. Roberts' paper, 'Aspartame Mimics MS' by my former biochemistry professor, I would probably be dead. Today I am 90 percent improved, and am ovulating at 45 years."

VIII. Personal Demonstrations

There were remarkable altruistic efforts by outraged aspartame victims who took it upon themselves to "spread the word," at times in an evangelical manner. Their theme is embodied in the expression, "The right to know includes the right to say no."

Victims of aspartame disease forged their own campaigns for warning relatives and friends. An example: "If it says 'sugar free' on the label, don't even think about it!!!" Others are listed.

- An anti-aspartame advocate suggested writing "Aspartame Is Poison" on one-dollar bills "to get the message out."
- Aspartame victims resorted to printing the dangers of aspartame on business cards, which they would hand to persons drinking diet sodas, especially pregnant women. One suggested use of the acronym CAPS for "chronic aspartame poisoning syndrome."
- After dramatic improvement following aspartame avoidance, one grateful reactor conveyed her experience to others by ending her letters as "Things are looking up" rather than "As always."
- A 49-year-old woman with severe aspartame disease developed a brain tumor (glioblastoma) after using large amounts to lose weight. She wrote the author about her attempts to warn others: "If I can't get this crap off the market through legal means, I will do it all by myself by scaring the hell out of anyone who uses it. I can't even tell you how many people have sworn off it because of my persistence. I cringe when I see parents getting their children sugar-free anything. So I have to open my big mouth."
- Elaine F. read a newspaper advertisement that offered coupons for an aspartame recipe booklet. She responded by submitting considerable literature on the potential hazards of aspartame products. Her note stated, "I hope you realize you are sending out recipes for devastation."

- A Florida businesswoman sent hundreds of envelopes stuffed with information about aspartame disease, as well as sugar-free and aspartame-free recipes. One of her customers was astonished when a friend requested diet soda at a retreat. She replied, "You don't want to drink <u>that</u>!" When the fellow asked the reason, she gave him a dissertation on aspartame's side effects. Others at this session promptly imparted their personal adverse experiences.

- The well-meaning efforts of persons who had suffered severe aspartame reactions occasionally led to embarrassing confrontations in markets. Several <u>literally</u> took aspartame soft drinks out of the hands of pregnant women and exclaimed, "If you want to have a healthy baby, you shouldn't be drinking this stuff!"

- A neonatal nurse suffered multiple severe aspartame reactions. She reported that "someone" had been placing red hazardous-substance stickers on all the diet cola buttons in the vending machines on her hospital floor. The diabetes educator-nurse removed these stickers, which magically reappeared in the same spots about two minutes later.

Many of these anti-aspartame activists remained frustrated by the inability to convince high-risk consumers about their message – as pregnant women who continued to use aspartame products. Physicians are familiar with this phenomenon of self-destructiveness in dealing with alcoholic patients and habitual smokers.

Representative Case Report

Case XXX-1

A 42-year-old educator suffered severe dizziness, confusion, slurred speech, rashes, lightheadedness and exhaustion while consuming aspartame. Her symptoms disappeared within eight days after stopping such products. They recurred within three days on the one occasion she retested herself. She related her "righteous indignation" in these terms.

> "I no longer eat foods with aspartame in them. I read labels and ask questions. This includes foods, sodas (I now drink water), gum, candy, etc. Within eight days of being off aspartame on two separate occasions, all symptoms disappeared. Playing golf became a pleasure. Within weeks, I was back to riding my bike at least 12 miles a day.

"Two years ago, I attended an ice-skating championship sponsored by an aspartame product. I wore a T shirt that said in bold letters, 'Aspartame Is Dangerous to Your Health,' and passed out flyers. The company wasn't too happy nor was the Capital Center."

IX. Expressions of Support From Irate Consumers

The author has received many hard-hitting letters from frustrated consumers who implored me to continue my studies (Chapter XIX). One aspartame reactor stated, "Aspartame contains nothing but trouble." A reader of the *New Orleans Times-Picayune* wrote

"I want to thank you for speaking out about aspartame causing medical problems... When a mere patient tries to speak out to defend his health against chemical additives, he meets deaf ears and closed doors. But when a doctor such as yourself is brave enough to speak out for us, we are encouraged that there may yet be a chance to get some of the chemicals out of our food.

"Thanks again. Please don't let 'them' silence you."

ANTI-ASPARTAME GROUPS

Consumer advocates are keenly aware of the obstacles they face in this "Disinformation Age." Our nation should be grateful for the efforts of various consumer groups that gathered facts about perceived environmental hazards, and analyze them carefully before launching into action.

Most are not "frightmongers" bent on recklessly attacking industries. A few examples of this genre involving issues other than aspartame are cited.

A feature in *Medical World News* (March 9, 1987, pp. 44-45) carried the title, "Is Government Suppressing Health Data?" It noted the dramatic undermining of concerted attempts to reduce lead poisoning in the United States. The Reagan Administration "essentially demolished" the Federal Lead Poisoning Prevention Program during October 1981 by making the reporting of lead poisoning voluntary rather than mandatory. The number of reported cases of lead poisoning predictably and precipitously declined. Similar trends involved information on the nutritional status of children and the over-65 population, and infant mortality rates, when this Administration severely reduced the funding required by appropriate agencies.

- The urethane present in a number of alcoholic beverages, particularly fruit-flavored brandies, causes cancer in experimental animals. Accordingly, Canada limits this chemical in liquor and wine. The Center for Science in the Public Interest decried alleged footdragging by the FDA, claiming it had "kept the danger secret" (*Newsweek* December 22, 1986, p. 60-61).
- Other consumer watchdog groups do not pull punches about corporate disinformation. One referred to "corporate lying" (*The Wall Street Journal* May 11, 1999, p. A-10).

Background Perspectives

Aspartame victims became highly incensed over (a) the seeming minimal interest and disinclination to act on the matter by most members of Congress and the FDA, (b) the laissez faire attitude toward related regulation, and (c) tolerance for bureaucratic stalling. Moreover, motivated anti-aspartame individuals had to endure a barrage of personal attacks by self-serving corporate and bureaucratic interests. They included being labeled as "media terrorists" and "cyber-terrorists." One wrote, "Are we really toxic cyber-terrorists frightening people? I don't think so unless it takes a great surge of fear to wake people up."

Frustration from negative encounters with physicians (see above) increased the determination of these persons to persevere and combine their efforts.

> An anti-aspartame activist was appalled by an experience while attending a Passover Seder in 2000. A leading neurologist at the National Institute of Health involved in researching degenerative brain diseases was drinking diet cola. When this aspartame reactor mentioned the neurotoxicity of aspartame, the physician adamantly refused to believe it in an insulting manner.

The Evolution of Groups

The formation of informal anti-aspartame groups became inevitable under these circumstances, and as aspartame disease took an increasing toll on the population. When confronted with insistence that aspartame products are "completely safe" for most consumers, these consumer advocates acknowledge the advice of Goethe: "The truth requires constant repetition because error is being preached about us all the time."

The Aspartame Consumer Safety Network was begun by Mary Stoddard in August 1987, and Mission Possible several years later by Betty Martini. Both had previously read the author's publications, and discussed them at length with him.

Persons with aspartame disease were pleased to learn that such groups existed. This was especially welcome by those who had been repeatedly told their reactions were a figment of the imagination or some rare idiosyncracy. Having the opportunity now to compare notes, they felt relieved that their own assessments were correct.

> Mary Stoddard (see below) was seen in consultation by an internist, neurologist, ear specialist, gynecologist and audiologist – "but nothing concrete was found." She described her reaction after discovering herself to be an aspartame reactor by using the central character in the movie, *Close Encounters of the Third Kind*, as an analogy. He felt extreme relief in finding that others had shared his vision of Devil's Monument, and now "the entire world knew that we were not crazy."

Scores of aspartame reactors expressed gratitude for these groups. One Internet correspondent stated

> "A friend of mine gave me a paper from Mission Possible with the title, 'Warning! Aspartame is a Neurotoxin.' It changed my life!!! I was drinking a 12-pack of diet cola daily for 2 years. Thanks to that letter, I quit!"

The Question of Proper Representation

The question has been raised, "Who should represent the consuming public if aspartame disease constitutes an imminent public health hazard?"

In the author's opinion, they ought to encompass aspartame victims, concerned health care professionals, properly motivated attorneys, and not-for-profit consumer organizations capable of coping with legalistic maneuvering. The latter involves such basic issues as alleged violations of product liability statutes. (Courts and legislators are mindful of the legal dictum: "When the facts are bad, argue the law. When the law is bad, argue the facts.")

I. Mission Possible

Mission Possible became a highly effective international group of volunteers committed to providing information about the hazards of aspartame products. It addressed the public, the media, health professionals, elected officials, pilots, air traffic controllers, and chat groups on the Internet. Its motto: "We are dedicated to the proposition that we will not be satisfied until death and disability are no longer considered an acceptable cost of business."

This corporate-neutral organization was founded by Betty Martini of Atlanta. Her amazing efforts stimulated the author to write the "profile of a super volunteer activist" (Roberts 1996c). In reply to an interested German television production company, she explained its genesis.

> "Mission Possible rose out of a desperate need to warn the world. It is estimated that three out of five people using aspartame already have the symptoms or some disease. Why don't physicians and people know? Because the manufacturers fund trade organizations like the American Diabetic Association, the American Dietetic Association, the American Medical Association, and persons in Congress. The trade organizations tell the physicians this is a safe sweetener. Mission Possible sends packets of information to physicians containing the independent studies not funded by manufacturers and other information so they can associate the symptoms seen in practice with aspartame use."

Betty initially confined her activities to assembling "kits" of literature detailing the hazards of aspartame products. These contained more than a dozen articles and letters published in various journals and periodicals, and "position" statements by the author dealing with the potential complications of aspartame products in pregnant women, young children, persons with diabetes and hypoglycemia, ear problems, and presumed "early" multiple sclerosis (see Appendix Section).

She then produced flyers on this subject which were personally distributed to thousands of interested persons. Concomitantly, she had April declared "Anti-Aspartame Month" in Georgia.

Betty's engaging next-door-neighbor behavior, coupled with a delightful Southern accent, captivated many. A religious person teaching Bible classes twice weekly, she seemed to embody "the great need for a love standard rather than a gold standard."

Betty's previous contacts with health care professionals were formidable. When she expressed the wish to attend the annual meeting of the American College of Physicians held at the Georgia World Congress Center in 1995, the author balked. But there was no question about her intent to learn. She listened attentively at EVERY lecture, making extensive and highly perceptive notes.

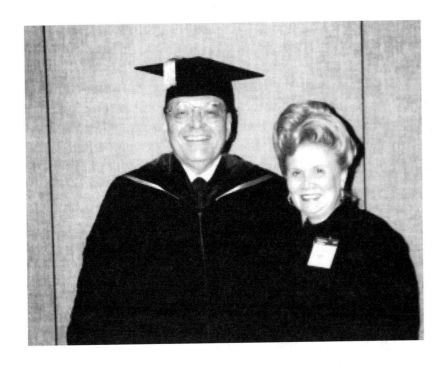

Betty Martini and H.J. Roberts, M.D. at the March 16, 1995 convocation of the American College of Physicians.

Without fear or embarrassment, Betty cornered many physicians in attendance – including professorial lecturers – about various topics, and usually ended up explaining aspartame disease. Most expressed gratitude for orienting them to this disorder about which they had been unaware.

Betty's first-hand encounter with "the arrogance of ignorance" at this meeting proved a sobering eye-opener to the author, a Fellow of the American College of Physicians. It was embodied in the reflexive behavior of doctors who regarded her comments as "nonsense," and the biases of "authorities" on topics such as reactive hypoglycemia, the chronic fatigue syndrome, and lupus erythematosus.

Betty willingly paid a high price for her ambitious activities as an unsalaried activist. They often consumed 18 hours a day. With reserved approval of Don, her talented husband, she transformed several areas of their home into "war rooms" for copying, storing and distributing anti-aspartame literature on a vast scale. Betty's "kits" had now evolved into "packages."

Betty and several affected friends finally formed Mission Possible (M.P.) They reached the four corners of the earth through their own networks, the distributing of flyers to flight attendants and pilots on planes, and mastery of the Internet. Hundreds of e-mail messages were then received every day!

Every Doubting Thomas on the Internet became a personal challenge for this feisty advocate, especially when his or her sarcasm was signed by some provocative pen name (e.g., "Uncle Wolf"). But there were limits to Betty's patience. She responded to one person: "So I say, go ahead and drink all the diet cola you want, and don't worry about silly things like your health. Some things are worse, like an arrogant attitude."

When an impasse had been reached, Betty resorted to her ultimate weapon: poetry.

- One ditty read

    Aspartame. It's the Devil's treat,
    It's poured on everything you eat.
    Don't mind if you go blind
    Or leave your brains behind.

- "Rockhead" received this opus (slightly modified) titled, *Educated Fool.*

    I love my chemo poison
    I'm a modern guy, you know,
    Every day consuming "foods"
    Like the ads all tell me to.

I argue, fight and persevere
Defending toxins others fear...
No matter that you've spent 2 years
Researching, hearing others' tears.

I know so much with my degree
No evidence will alter me!
I did my thinking back in school,
But since haven't used a mental tool.

Your new ideas just hurt my pride
And so your evidence I deride.
I've got to struggle hard, you see
To keep someone from teaching me!

The audacity of Mission Possible's activities commanded respect.

- A market manager objected to the passing out of anti-aspartame flyers by a member of M.P. He shouted, "THIS IS BUSINESS!" The consumer advocate replied with their motto, "I'm sorry, but death is not an acceptable cost of doing business!"
- Members of M.P. staged their version of the Boston Tea Party before the media by dumping diet colas and other aspartame sodas in front of a large health food store. (On learning of this escapade in Atlanta, headquarters of the Coca-Cola Company, the author recalled the line by John Milton in *Lycidas:* "Look homeward Angel now.")
- The Olympic games were held in Atlanta during 1996. This venue provided M.P. with a perceived opportunity to inform the world. Its members distributed tens of thousands of flyers warning athletes, visitors and the media about aspartame disease.
- Betty Martini offered this concise response to a large producer of aspartame in China who wished to be contacted: "Please close down your factory." (Internet, April 8, 2001).

M.P. members also inundated their congressmen and other elected officials with information about aspartame disease, clamoring for another congressional hearing. Rachel H. Blehr of Marietta, Georgia, wrote Newt Gingrich (her representative and Speaker of the House of Representatives) a forceful letter on July 18, 1995. It contained this excerpt (reproduced with permission).

"If you read the politics, the sell-outs and the power behind aspartame approval, you will realize this is the greatest atrocity ever committed by the FDA affecting millions of people, as confirmed by Dr. Roberts in his June letter to you. This courageous physician has stood before the world and warned of the impending doom caused by this toxin. Welcome to OUTBREAK ASPARTAME!

"This is not simply a national scandal – it's genocidal! There are so many layers of coverup that federal indictments should be entered against the perpetrators of this pestilence who ruthlessly reduce intelligence of children and destroy the unborn. This is a criminal conspiracy between a conscienceless chemical conglomerate and the FDA, dietitians, and other pushers for hire...

"This is the most important matter that may ever come before you. It involves the poisoning of millions of people!"

II. The Aspartame Consumer Safety Network

Mary Stoddard, a marketing consultant in Dallas, organized the Aspartame Consumer Safety Network in the wake of her own severe reactions to aspartame products (see above). She distributed a booklet of published articles about aspartame disease, and established a "hot line" for pilots who believed they had suffered reactions.

III. The Community Nutrition Institute

The Community Nutrition Institute, a consumer organization in Washington, D.C., attempted to curb aspartame use as early as 1983. (Its efforts were unknown to the author during the early phases of his research.) The following statement by Rodney E. Leonard, issued on July 17, 1986, indicates the frustrations that beset this and other groups.

"The continued use of aspartame... as a food additive endangers the health of too many Americans and should be stopped immediately. The Community Nutrition Institute is petitioning the Commissioner of the Food Drug Administration (FDA) to declare that aspartame is an imminent hazard, and to ban the chemical sweetener from use as a food additive.

"The danger is real: aspartame causes harm to some people. It is not a harmless substance.

"We have held this belief for some time. We did not believe in 1981 that FDA had sufficient or credible scientific data to make a finding that aspartame would cause no harm. We said in 1983 that the introduction of aspartame in soft drinks would greatly increase the health risk for an apparent health benefit. By late 1983 and early 1984, individual users began to contact us with complaints of adverse reactions. FDA and Searle, which markets aspartame... dismissed those complaints as simply the normal "placebo" effect that follows the introduction of any new additive. We did not accept that argument.

"Those complaints continued, however, and grew steadily – severe, unrelenting headaches; seizures; blurred vision, and partial blindness; skin lesions; hyper behavior; menstrual disorders. FDA now has almost 3,000 complaints, and new injuries are reported almost every day.

"By 1985, clinical studies had begun to link aspartame with specific injuries. Dr. Richard Wurtman, for example, has now begun a clinical investigation of some 80 persons who experience grand mal seizures after consuming aspartame. A more detailed description of this study is attached as part of a report he presented earlier this year to FDA.

"Following revelation by Dr. Wurtman of these tragic and needless injuries, FDA has requested proposals for a research project to develop criteria, guidelines and standards to use in evaluating the safety of substances that consist of amino acids, particularly aspartame.

"FDA said in its request: 'Resolving the persistent questions about the potential effects of aspartame and other dietary components on the central nervous system is one aspect of food safety which the FDA must address... The relatively inconclusive state of knowledge in this field of science explains in part the difficulties of formulating a regulatory strategy. The question is... can dietarysubstances produce abnormal physiological and/or neurobehavorial changes.'

"We are angry. We are disheartened. FDA now has the clinical evidence that people are harmed. It is evidence acquired in the most brutal and heartless way: an experiment has been conducted using the American people as guinea pigs, as test animals...

"FDA acknowledged in its request for studies of aspartame that it has yet to acquire adequate data on which to determine whether aspartame should be used as a food additive.

"We believe that if the Commissioner of FDA were truly concerned with health and safety, the facts support a finding of imminent hazard. He has demonstrated a willingness to interpret the law in novel ways. For example, he has introduced the 'de minimis' concept as an interpretation of the Delaney clause in the food safety law. This interpretation allows the use of any carcinogen as a food additive if FDA determines it is present in amounts so small as to be inconsequential. The Delaney clause specifies that any substance causing cancer in test animals or humans is prohibited from use as a food additive.

"The Commissioner could act to protect public health as easily as he has chosen to introduce carcinogens, and we urge him to use his power in the service of public health."*

James S. Turner, an attorney representing the Community Nutrition Institute, filed the following petition to the Food and Drug Administration on July 17, 1986 with the assistance of Diane T. Dean. It requested "Reconsideration and/or Repeal" in reference to aspartame as an imminent hazard.

Turner's interest initially had been generated by a casual remark of the then-director of the Division of Food and Color Additives. As they walked in an FDA warehouse, he said, "By the way, you might want to take a look at this aspartame stuff. There are some problems with it" (*The Sunday Journal* of Kankakee, Illinois, May 4, 1986, p. 5).

* * * * * * * * * * *

---

*Reproduced with permission of Mr. Rodney E. Leonard

CITIZENS PETITION: Request, in accordance with Food, Drug and Cosmetic Act Section 409(b), (c), (e), (f), (g), and (h) and 21 CFR 10.25 and 10.33, that the Commissioner (1) reconsider 21 CFR 172.804 Aspartame (c) (17) and (d) and, based on new evidence, repeal them, as creating an imminent hazard, or for failure to meet the legal safety standard, and (2) convene a public hearing to consider the evidence supporting each request.

Action Requested

The undersigned, James S. Turner and Diane T. Dean, on behalf of the Community Nutrition Institute, submit this petition to request the Commissioner of the Food and Drug Administration to reconsider and repeal 21 CFR 172.804 (c), and (d) by deleting the following:

Aspartame: 21 CFR 172.804

(c) The additive may be used as a sweetener in the following foods:
(1) Dry, free-flowing sugar substitutes for table use (not to include use in cooking) in package units not to exceed the sweetening equivalent of 2 teaspoonfuls of sugar.
(2) Sugar substitute tablets for sweetening hot beverages, including coffee and tea. L-leucine may be used as a lubricant in the manufacture of such tablets at a level not to exceed 3.5 percent of the weight of the tablet.
(3) Cold breakfast cereals.
(4) Chewing gum.
(5) Dry bases for:
(i) Beverages.
(ii) Instant coffee and tea.
(iii) Gelatins, pudding and fillings.
(iv) Dairy products analog toppings.
(6) Carbonated beverages and carbonated beverage syrup bases.
(7) Chewable multivitamin food supplements.
(d) The additive may be used as a flavor enhancer in chewing gum.

Statement of Factual Grounds

926

I. Repeal as an Imminent Hazard

On April 21, 1986 Dr. Richard Wurtman and his associates, Dr. Donald Schomer and Ms. Leuann Hazarjian, presented FDA scientists with information connecting NutraSweet (aspartame) with seizures in more than 80 patients. (See attached "Introductory Comments" by Dr. Wurtman and supporting case summaries).

The previously healthy young adult subjects of Wurtman's report had a variety of symptoms including headache, personality changes, and déjà vu experiences for days or weeks followed by the onset of seizures. Some consumed "surprisingly small" amounts while most consumed in excess of three grams a day.

Dr. Wurtman asserts that the average consumption level of aspartame is far in excess of the average daily intake (ADI) established by FDA. He believes that the symptoms preceding seizures may make it possible to identify potential seizure victims in advance; he therefore recommends that FDA issue a warning to physicians that patients who report headaches or seizures after using aspartame should be told to discontinue use to prevent development of or additional seizures.

Dr. Wurtman further recommends that quantity labeling be provided for aspartame containing products, particularly to limit consumption by pregnant women. He reports one to two new subjects are referred to him weekly as potential study candidates for aspartame reactions.

The existence of these 80 cases meets the FDA definition of an imminent hazard to the public health requiring the FDA Commissioner to expeditiously remove a product from the market without an administrative hearing. (See attached memorandum of law in support of this citizens petition.)

II. Repeal for Failure to Meet Legal Safety Standard

In addition to receiving more than 80 NutraSweet-related seizure cases from Dr. Richard Wurtman, the FDA has issued a request to physicians for reports linking disabilities in patients to the ingestion of aspartame, and has issued a request for proposals (RFP) on the establishment of an animal model to test the impact on the brain of substances such as aspartame and other dipeptide amino acids. (See Attached RFP Section "C" Scientific Justification.)

The RFP demonstrates that FDA cannot say that aspartame has been shown to be safe. It calls for the development of animal testing procedures to identify the appropriate questions that must be answered to evaluate the safety of food chemicals which, like aspartame, may affect neurological and neurobehavioral functions. It characterized existing knowledge relating diet, neurotransmitters and brain function as "insufficient": "Although statistically significant changes in brain regions of rats and mice have been observed following very high doses of aspartame, it is not yet possible to know whether these changes are behaviorally or otherwise biologically significant, or typical... The fact that so little is known at this time about the inter-relationships between diet, neurochemistry, and brain function underscore the need for the type of information sought in this contract."

The Commissioner acknowledges that previous studies in this area have been deficient, that there is little consensus among researchers, and that persistent questions remain about the potential effects of aspartame on the central nervous system. A substance about which these questions are only now being proposed to be addressed cannot be said to have been shown to be safe.

III. Hearing

Whether aspartame is removed from the market by repeal of CFR 172.804 (c) and (d) because it fails to meet the basic safety standard under the Food, Drug and Cosmetic Act and is an imminent hazard or solely because it fails to meet the safety standard, a public hearing should be held so FDA can systematically receive the evidence that aspartame is implicated as a possible – indeed probable – cause of neurological damage in a significant portion of its users establishing that the additive has not been shown to be safe as the food additive laws require and therefore establishing that properly it should be banned from the market.

IV. Conclusion

Petitioners request the Commissioner to immediately repeal 21 CFR 172.804 (c) and (d) as an imminent hazard or repeal them for failure to meet the basic standard of safety of the Food Additive Amendments to the Food, Drug and Cosmetic act and that the Commissioner convene a public hearing to receive and evaluate evidence that aspartame is causing neurological damage in a significant portion of its users.*

GROUP ACTIVITIES

The following summary of volunteered activities by the foregoing and other anti-aspartame groups indicates the scope of their commitment. They repeatedly considered

---

*Reproduced with permission of James S. Turner, Esquire.

symbolic acts and "processions" that would arouse the country – akin to Gandhi's march to the sea, and the Boston Tea Party.

I. Distributing Information

The "unfriendly takeover" of the food industry by large timber companies and giant food cartels incensed anti-aspartame activists. Through education, letter-writing campaigns, and calls to elected public officials, they urged consumers, "organic" food stores and fine clubs to champion the safety of food and water.

II. Product Boycotts

Aspartame reactors who manifested severe allergies, or the parents of allergic children, wrote to companies in the United States and England when they learned that aspartame was present in popular chewable antihistamines and related medicinal products. Their anger heightened on discovering the many skin, respiratory and other allergies to aspartame products – including my report titled, "Aspartame As Cause of Allergic Reactions, Including Anaphylaxis" (Roberts 1996a). Failing to receive replies, they attempted to boycott these aspartame products using the Internet.

III. Product Returns

Anti-aspartame activists urged aspartame reactors to return aspartame products to the original point of sale for a refund or exchange, thereby raising the issue of their toxicity. They also suggested that such persons send detailed complaints to the FDA.

IV. FDA Correspondence

Aspartame victims did not mince words with the FDA over its failure to address aspartame disease. One irate aspartame reactor wrote its acting director, "What is going on is criminal. If you don't do something, I hope they dissolve the FDA. I suggest you get your act together, and get this garbage off the market!"

V. Countering Apathy by Diabetes Organizations

Convinced that aspartame products can aggravate diabetes and its complications (Chapter XIII), individuals and groups faulted diabetes organizations for not having taken a stand on this matter. They did so at diabetes walk-a-thons, and by sending "open letters" on the Internet.

929

VI. Multinational Correspondence with Producers

Consumers abroad, most notably in Europe, expressed outrage to the manufacturers of aspartame products and other "multinationals of foul food." This reflected concern about safety as much as cultural/culinary preferences. The Additives Survivors' Network, formed in the United Kingdom during March 2000, publishes facts sheets about aspartame problems, and "learning to live additive-free."

Anti-aspartame activists throughout the world have requested that many companies avoid adding aspartame to their products. A notable example involved chewing gum – in part because of repeated reference by the author to severe neuropsychiatric complications associated with the prolonged chewing of aspartame gum (Chapter II-E).

This issue was reinforced by Directive 96/83/EC, wherein the European Union banned aspartame in any food used by infants and small children.

VII. Use of the Internet

Anti-aspartame vigilantes utilized the Internet to inform about aspartame disease, to express their indignation, and to effect political regulatory changes. For aspartame victims unable to elicit information from physicians and manufacturers, access to cyberspace soulmates – especially bettym19@mindspring.com and dorietz@awod.com – proved a blessing. Dr. M. Faith McLellan (1997) aptly observed

> "Whether they recount their tales in journals, to friends in letters or e-mail, in a printed book, or in an electronic form, the authors of illness narratives have common goals: They are all trying to make sense of what is happening to them, to set some boundaries that will confine the experience of illness in their lives, to fend off chaos and the darkness that sometimes threatens to overwhelm... For physicians, care givers, and ethicists, they are a window on the ways illness can permeate lives and relationship, and on the ways the experience affects thinking and decision making."

The Internet proved the diagnostic salvation of many aspartame victims. For example, Case IX-D-15 had gone through needless surgery (removal of the gallbladder), and continued to suffer nausea, abdominal pain and other symptoms of aspartame disease. In desperation, this 38-year-old woman recounted her ordeal to a friend. The latter listed her complaints on an Internet chat group, and promptly came up with the correct diagnosis.

A "Roberts' Angel" (see below) chose the Internet designation of "Paula Revere" in attempting to "fire shots heard around the world" about aspartame disease.

Anti-aspartame activists held their ground, and refused to let insults on the Internet go unanswered. Betty Martini did so in this retort to the suggestion that the author was not corporate-neutral because he lives in a sugar-producing county.

> "You must stay up nights thinking of dumb things to say. If Dr. Roberts lived in Alaska, does that assure him of being in oil? Perhaps if he lived in Hawaii, he would have an interest in orchids or palm trees. Why would a world-famous physician and diabetic specialist have a side interest in sugar? You are talking about a man who has practiced medicine many years taking care of the sick and healing, while you whine because you are loyal to the manufacturer who makes the poison... Just remember, those who cook up stories usually find themselves in hot water!"

Problems were encountered. First, anti-aspartame advocates using the Internet found they must maintain vigilance after receiving "viruses" capable of erasing all documents in their hard drive. Second, persons interested in sending or receiving information about aspartame disease encountered obstacles apparently created by corporate interests. They variously entailed blocked access to relevant sites, or the absence of reference material on major search engines (e.g., "no abstract"). An additional cause for outrage was the automatic appearance of banners advertising aspartame products when the subject of aspartame reactions was being sought.

VIII. Challenging the Press

Anti-aspartame activists attempted to rebut pro-industry features published in newspapers and magazines, but generally to no avail – even with the threat of membership in their "Media Hall of Shame."

They focused on reporters, and attempted to lay down some ground rules before being interviewed. Betty Martini encapsulated these assertions: "You believe that the public has a right to the truth, and you believe you have an obligation to report hte truth as you find or discern it." She made the following suggestion to a reporter on the Internet (July 18, 2000).

"If you think aspartame is safe, why not conduct a personal study? Start ingesting lots of it yourself. It's in quite an array of foods, so you wouldn't be doing anything more than many people today. Drink a 6-pack or more of your favorite aspartame-laden diet soda. Buy a box of tabletop sweetener in the blue packet, and sprinkle liberally on your cereal, in your coffee, on your yogurt, and in your iced tea. Keep a diary for two months of your intake <u>and</u> how you feel... If your symptoms get really bad, stop the study early. (We don't want to kill you.) ... Then, 'cure' yourself. Sixty days from the beginning of the study, remove all traces of aspartame from your diet. Record what you eat, as well as how you feel for the next 60 days."

IX. Other Activities

A tactic used to increase public awareness of aspartame disease was <u>Aspartame Awareness Day</u>, first held in several cities on August 28, 1999.

Anti-aspartame activists in the United Kingdom held an <u>Additives Awareness Weekend</u> that emphasized additive-free picnics.

Various <u>"Boston Tea Parties"</u> were sponsored. One featured a large brass band. Its organizer jokingly expressed concern over exposing fish to dumped aspartame... likening the activity to polluting water with run-off motor oil.

In a somber vein, the bioconcentration of aspartame and its metabolites in the aquatic food chain – as occurs with dioxins (Roberts 1990b; Clapp 2000) – requires clarification. Even in parts per <u>trillion</u>, delayed developmental consequences have been reported with dioxin, especially exposure before and during puberty (Mocarelli 2000).

The term "aspartame warriors" is used for persons <u>fighting "the cola wars"</u> on behalf of children, especially through seeking accountability of school boards that condone the marketing of sodas on school property through vending machines. One approach has been the study of their Comprehensive Annual Financial Reports (CAFRs) rather than estimated budgets, which may fail to indicate fiscal/business partiality.

Blistering humor provided an outlet for many aspartame victims and their groups. Repetitious denial of aspartame disease by the manufacturers and distributors of these products so infuriated persons who had suffered severe reactions that they felt the need for such retort. One journalist sarcastically commented: "Denial is not a river in Egypt." Others referred to the ostrich syndrome – a reference to "don't bother me with the facts."

Outraged by corporate hype, aspartame reactors resorted to a broad spectrum of humor in attempts to discourage the use of these products.

- The prefix "Nutra" was termed an oxymoron. Many persons with aspartame disease substituted "nutrapoison" for what they considered a "witches' brew of poison."
- An aspartame reactor stated, "Aspartame contains nothing but trouble."
- Some of the rebuttals to believers in aspartame's safety were blunt. For example, "Aspartame is as natural as polyethylene or nerve gas." Similarly, when the amino acids in aspartame were referred to as being "natural," some countered that arsenic, lead and other toxic metals are also "natural."
- Dr. William Campbell Douglass jested to readers of *Second Opinion* (April 1999) with foods in their pantry containing aspartame: "Donate them to your local IRS Office. Most of them could use a little sweetening."
- One victim suggested that the manufacturers of aspartame products be indicted for "crimes against humanity."
- Activists concerned over the perceived enormity of aspartame disease dubbed its victims as members of the "International Society of Guinea Pigs and Lab Rats."
- Activists utilized the female preponderance in aspartame disease (Chapter II-H) for "dumb blonde" jokes. Example: "How many dumb blondes are needed to change a bulb?" "Two – one for calling the landlord, and the other to get a diet soda."
- A physician afflicted with aspartame disease warned that the continued use of aspartame in the face of awareness of its many adverse effects because of assertions by "pseudo-scientists" could be likened to talking with Mr. Ed. (a horse comedian that appeared to talk like a man), and thinking one is having a real conversation.
- Anti-aspartame activists have ridiculed the presumed "inert" nature of aspartame by asserting, "It is as inert as Mount Vesuvius when erupting."

- Activists criticized aspartame reactors who avoided such products themselves, but who kept diet sodas in their refrigerators "for visiting guests," as hypocritical.

X. Litigation As an Ultimate Expression of Frustration

Persons afflicted with severe aspartame disease were delighted when they experienced considerable improvement after stopping aspartame products... but also shocked by this revelation. While some were willing to join class action suits, they could not do so because of inability to find law firms willing to undertake the litigation. Several wealthy individuals, however, persisted.

> Case VI-D-2, a 40-year-old woman, had been diagnosed for eleven years as having multiple sclerosis. Her weakened foot and ankle culminated in injury for which fusion surgery was performed in October 1997. An amazing turn of events then occurred in December 1998 when she learned about aspartame disease, and became asymptomatic after _two_ days of abstinence from aspartame products! The author later called to check the details, which she reaffirmed. She added: "I can't walk now because of my fusion. I am so mad! What I want to do is sue the company for $11 million... one million for each year I lost of my career, home life and mental state. I realize it is a big company I am dealing with, but I _can_ afford to do this and will try!"

"ROBERTS' ANGELS"

"Do you not think an Angel rides in the whirlwind
and directs this storm?"
                John Page (Letter to Thomas Jefferson, July 1776)

It came as a dramatic surprise to the author that a number of anti-aspartame activists had been calling themselves "Roberts' Angels." This term – a takeoff on the television series _Charlie's Angels_ – had been concocted by two "Angels" in Dallas and Chicago.

The "angel theme" has become popular in both business and entertainment. There is a vast difference in motivation, however, between altruistic Roberts' Angels and "the angle market." The latter term refers to high-net-worth investors sought by companies needing start-up or expansion capital.

Other Expressions of Gratitude

The author has received hundreds of appreciative letters and e-mail messages from persons afflicted with aspartame disease.

- David Rietz, a "Roberts' Angel," wrote on November 13, 1996

  "I can truly give special thanks to the concerned folks who helped me find the truth of my 'afflictions'... not arthritis, not fibromyalgia, not in my head, not incurable – just by stopping to poison myself with aspartame!"

- The daughter of an aspartame victim stated

  "I am convinced that you had a hand in saving my mom's life. After discontinuing all aspartame products, the pain in her legs went away, her vision improved, and her blood sugar levels returned to normal. Our family thanks you for your role in helping her get back her health!"

- The wife/receptionist of a physician wrote: "Nutra-Poison (aspartame) is the most horrible item since arsenic. The stuff nearly killed me the first time I used it. I placed your article on our office front desk."

- An aspartame reactor in Hawaii sent this message.

  "I appreciate all the information you sent. My life is wonderful now! I am spreading the word! I provided info for the health editor of a local university paper. She is writing an article to be published in the next issue!"

An Ultimate Expression of Gratitude

An ultimate form of personal satisfaction involved grateful aspartame sufferees who had experienced infertility or multiple problems during pregnancy. After abstaining from aspartame and having a normal pregnancy thereafter, they named their babies *Robert* and *Roberta*.

XXXI

MORE LEGAL, CORPORATE AND
BUREAUCRATIC OBSTACLES

"Let us not, I beseech you, sir, deceive ourselves longer."
Patrick Henry

"Government is a trust, and the offices of the government
are trustees; and both the trust and the trustees are created
for the benefit of the people."
Henry Clay (1777-1852)

Health care professionals, consumers and consumer groups mentioned in the preceding chapters became increasingly appalled by the severity and magnitude of aspartame disease. They tried addressing the problem in different ways, only to meet seemingly insurmountable legal, corporate and bureaucratic resistance. Disregard of the legal petition by the Community Nutrition Institute, requesting the reevaluation of aspartame as an "imminent hazard" (Chapter XXX), illustrates the matter.

These obstacles have a common denominator detrimental to the public health: delay that enables greater corporate profits. The thalidomide tragedy and a complication of aspirin were previous examples of comparable delay.

The Centers for Disease Control provided conclusive evidence for a link between aspirin and Reye's syndrome in its 1980 report. In 1984, the federal government urged manufacturers to adopt warning labels cautioning about the administration of aspirin to children and teenagers with influenza-like illnesses and chickenpox. Such labeling, however, was not mandated until 1986. Editorializing in the *Journal of the American Medical Association*, Dr. Edward Mortimer, Jr. (1987) asked, "Why did it take so long?" He decried additional "irresponsible" actions – as the ability of manufacturers to delay public warnings or package labeling, the sending of misleading reassurances to doctors, and the threat of a lawsuit against the American Academy of Pediatrics if it published a warning about this association.

936

This chapter addresses some of the issues. The considerable research involving such complex realms serves as an orientation not only to aspartame disease, but also related public health matters. The formidable obstacles by the FDA are discussed in Chapter XXXII.

PERTINENT LEGAL ISSUES

This section is preambled with the fact that the author heretofore has **not** testified as an expert witness, through deposition or at court, in any litigation involving alleged reactions to aspartame products.

Causation

Proof of causation is required for recovery under any legal theory of liability in litigation involving the liability of manufacturers. Causation may be demonstrated by epidemiologic studies, and the documentation of a so-called "signature effect" (or syndrome) by an expert witness. Considerable time is often required. For example, it took more than five years to prove that thalidomide really caused severe birth defects.

The nature of a "defective" product, whether a chemical or machine, has been addressed by many courts relative to imposing strict liability. There are three functionally distinct types of defect: those involving defective design; defects in construction; and inadequate warnings. In *Phillip v. Kimwood Machine co.* (1974), the Supreme Court of Oregon noted

> "[A] dangerously defective article would be one which a reasonable person would not put into the stream of commerce if he had knowledge of its harmful character. The test, therefore, is whether the seller would be negligent if he sold the article knowing of the risk involved. Strict liability imposes what amounts to constructive knowledge of the condition of the product."

The opinion by an individual medical or scientific expert concerning causation can be crucial in a strict tort liability action against the manufacturer of a product. The following commentary by the Court of Appeals of Idaho in *Earl v. Cryovac, A Division of W. R. Grace Company* (1989) is germane.

> "Accordingly, when the courts apply medical and scientific evidence to a question of causation, they must interpret the evidence carefully in light of the applicable standard. They may not assume that a causal relationship is probable merely because a physician deems it significant in his diagnosis and treatment of a patient's condition. Neither may they assume that a causal

relationship is improbable merely because it has not been documented in a body of research literature where a high degree of certainty is demanded. These distinctions are particularly important in a toxic tort case where, as here, the issue of causation is framed by the expert opinions of scientists and treating physicians." (p.727,728)

Duty to Warn

Courts have emphasized the nature of duty to warn with a degree of intensity for reasonable persons. Since this issue is germane to aspartame-product reactions, several related rulings are cited.

- In *Spruill v. Boyle-Midway, Inc.* (1962), the Court stated

  "To be of such character the warning must embody two characteristics: first, it must be in such form that it could reasonably be expected to catch the attention of the reasonably prudent man in the circumstances of its use; secondly, the content of the warning must be of such a nature as to be comprehensible to the average user and to convey a fair indication of the nature and extent of the danger to the mind of a reasonably prudent person."

- In *Barson v. E. R. Squibb & Sons, Inc.* (1984), the Supreme Court of Utah asserted

  "... the drug manufacturer is held to be an expert in its particular field and is under a 'continuous duty ... to keep abreast of scientific developments touching upon the manufacturer's product and to notify the medical profession of any additional side effects discovered from its use.' The drug manufacturer is responsible therefore for not only 'actual knowledge gained from research and adverse reactions reports,' but also for 'constructive knowledge as measured by scientific literature and other available means of communication.' "

Related Legal Issues

It has been asserted that sale of the decomposed or otherwise adulterated breakdown products of aspartame is unlawful, according to Section 402 (a) (3) of the FDA Act 21, U.S.C. 342 that deals with unfit food.

Consumer groups also have contended that the FDA and producers of aspartame products are in violation of U.S. Code Title 18, Section 1001. This pertains to any matter involving the falsification or concealment of material facts, making any materially false, fictitious or fraudulent statement or representation, or any false writing or document known to contain any materially false, fictitious, or fraudulent statement or entry.

Statistical Significance

Failure to demonstrate a "statistically significant" association cannot be interpreted as meaning there is no biological association. In *Allen v. United States* (1984, 1988), the court ruled: "The cold statement that a given relationship is not 'statistically significant' cannot be read to mean 'there is no probability of a relation.' "

The "Implied Warranty" Issue

Several aspartame reactors focused on the "implied warranty" relative to the safety of aspartame-containing products (*The Grand Rapids Press* March 6, 1986, p. C-6). Under Florida law, it is necessary to prove that a defect was present in the product causing injury at the time the supplier parted possession with it when arguing an alleged breach of implied warranty. This also directs responsibility to the federal agencies that licensed aspartame.

The inference of warranty by advertisements is governed by Article 2 of the Uniform Commercial Code. In general, it provides that affirmations of fact and promises could create a warranty when the seller makes statements about goods to potential buyers. Such a warranty about safety applies to a wide variety of products that humans ingest or contact.

LEGAL CHALLENGES CONFRONTING CONSUMER ADVOCATES

The "legal shield" afforded manufacturers and distributors against consumer advocates must be convincingly addressed to protect society against the ever-increasing number of profitable chemicals, drugs and additives having potential neurotoxic, fetotoxic and carcinogenic hazards.

Major legal challenges can be anticipated when chemical manufacturers and distributors are sued on the basis of selling environmental hazards. They include formidable corporate defense, the intimidation of treating physicians and potential medical experts, the unethical behavior of some corporate experts, legal doctrines concerning causation (see above), judicial decrees, and courtroom secrecy. The value of a corporate-neutral expert medical witness can become paramount. Moreover, he or she may be the first, or one of the first, to testify in the matter of product liability as problems with newer technologies surface. A "majority of one" opinion could become an essential part of landmark decisions by the trial court and an appeals court when comparable disorders are encountered by practicing physicians.

The Supreme Court has emphasized the need to keep "junk science" out of the courtroom by targeting the reliability of testimony by "experts." To this end, some jurists have exercised the option of enlisting independent experts under the Federal Rules of Evidence, as in the silicone breast implant litigation (Roberts 1999).

Public interest groups have referred to defective products as "societal malpractice" (Claybrook 1989). Most resent corporate power that allows courts to issue protective orders, and governmental agencies to ignore petitions for informing the public about defective products or insisting upon their recall.

Similarly, corporate expert witnesses have undertaken regional or nationwide studies on defective products and toxic chemicals. This state of affairs stems from the need for trial lawyers to persuade juries and appellate courts with admissible facts, some not known to the appropriate regulatory agency. As a result, the paradox arises that trial lawyers tend to accrue more and better information about product defects than governmental agencies.

Formidable Corporate Legal Defense

It is axiomatic that wealthy corporations will try to obtain the best defense attorneys in suits involving profitable popular products, such as those containing aspartame. This theme extends centuries back.

The many precedents include the thalidomide disaster, revelations in 1978 about the Love Canal tragedy, and vehicle defects (Roberts 1971b).

Notable instances of public health problems, such as leukemia and congenital defects, have been argued by altruistic attorneys representing victims on a contingency basis. But they proved no match for the power of corporate defenders.

Anti-aspartame groups face another impediment. The denigration or criticism of food products and additives can constitute a civil crime in a dozen states having "food slander"

941

("food disparagement") laws promoted by pro-industry lobbyists. Although considered unconstitutional by some, their primary aim is to intimidate activists and concerned consumers.

THE INTIMIDATION OF TREATING PHYSICIANS; THE BEHAVIOR OF RETAINED MEDICAL EXPERTS

> "The most sensible man, therefore, as soon as he
> sees the dole being brought in, runs from the
> theatre; for he knows that one pays a high price for
> small favors."
>
> Seneca (*Epistles*)

Most physicians who treated patients alleging injury from aspartame products are easily intimidated against testifying about a causal relationship for several reasons. The same applies to expert witnesses for plaintiffs.

A 44-year-old woman developed blindness in the left eye, and decreased vision in the right eye while consuming aspartame. Her ophthalmologist felt it represented "methyl alcohol poisoning." Two days before being scheduled to testify, however, the plaintiff's expert witness could not be located because he was "away for three weeks." Thereafter, he refused to give testimony in the case!

Comparable suits never went to trial because of difficulty in finding a qualified expert witness, or eleventh-hour settlements. Others have commented on these phenomena.

- On the basis of their experiences in raising two chemically sensitive children, Ken and Jan Nolley (1987) observed that "the current unrelenting threat of malpractice litigation produces pressure to avoid diagnoses not clearly and unambiguously validated by the tests the physicians have at their disposal."
- Mills (1987) noted the increasing difficulty facing both authors and editors relative to publication of "provocative results" and "hot papers" in "our current litigious and socially volatile climate."

Strong statements that favor decisions by both regulatory agencies and industry relative to the safety of foods, drugs and other substances also may intimidate witnesses.

This is likely when made by persons on the highest rungs of academia. For example, an overview of food additives and contaminants from the Massachusetts Institute of Technology and Boston University School of Medicine stated, "Evidence to date indicates that those responsible for food safety are doing an admirable job, and as a society, our food supply has never been better or safer, and, as a population, we have never been healthier" (Newberne 1986).

Another obstacle confronting plaintiff expert witnesses in a product liability action is the introduction of published editorials by "authorities" who had been solicited to write them. Dr. Herbert L. Fred (1990) expressed indignation about such "credence by fiat," especially when an unbalanced opinion was based on the reviewers' own contributions and opinions. This matter assumes great significance when the subject is a drug or other product alleged to be harmful.

OTHER JUDICIAL OBSTACLES

"Truth is a passion. One cannot learn it; one must possess it."
Ernst Toller (1893-1939)

The Supreme Court clearly stated in *William Daubert v Merrell Dow Pharmaceuticals* that judges are responsible for both the accuracy and the reliability of scientific evidence presented at court. Specifically, "any and all scientific testimony or evidence admitted is not only relevant, but reliable." Accordingly, the advisability of case histories and related correspondence sent to the FDA, the CDC and producers is essential for medical and public health professionals investigating aspartame disease, and the courts.

In turn, courts should not hamper the disclosure of such valuable information, as unfortunately has happened. In the case of toxic shock syndrome associated with use of tampons, the manufacturer and its consultant not only initially refused to release the data, but persuaded a presiding judge to prohibit the attorneys of one victim from disseminating pertinent information (Sun 1984).

In the present context, consumer advocates were placed at a disadvantage by the Supreme Court's refusal to investigate the manner in which the government approved aspartame for public use (*The New York Times* April 22, 1986). Specifically, it would not hear claims from the Community Nutrition Institute (Chapter XXX) and other consumer groups during the spring of 1986 when they again challenged the safety of aspartame in soft drinks, and an adverse ruling by the U.S. Circuit Court of Appeals for the District of Columbia the previous September.

Plaintiffs who had experienced severe reactions to aspartame products generally hit a blank wall in their product liability actions.

Ballinger v. Atkins (947 F.Supp 1925, December 16, 1996) involved a plaintiff who claimed that the use of aspartame, in conjunction with a ketogenic diet, caused neurologic injuries. His complaints included tachycardia, dizziness, anxiety, panic attacks, blurred vision, inability to concentrate, memory loss, and shooting pains in the left arm. Most subsided after avoiding aspartame products, but his poor concentration persisted. The United States District Court excluded the expert testimony presented because "(1) biochemist was not qualified to give expert testimony, and (2) internists lack sufficient basis to provide expert testimony that plaintiff suffered neurological injury or that those injuries were caused by consuming artificial sweetener in conjunction with diet." This court did not accept the "working hypothesis" on causation because it was "not well accepted in any scientific or medical field."

Courtroom Secrecy

Consumer advocates and appellate judges must contend with the ability of corporate defendants to avoid the production or disclosure of "smoking gun" documents. Joan Claybrook (1989) classified the techniques in these categories:

- Secrecy and settlement. This dual obstacle refers to prohibiting discussion of a case or outcome, the destruction or return of documents, and restrictions on the trial attorney from taking similar cases.
- Protective orders. Such orders are issued on a wholesale basis, and may not be removed with the ending of the case. Many believe that this process does not serve the public interest.
- Federal preemption. This tactic is employed by defense attorneys to prevent the litigation of worthy cases. In essence, federal regulatory statutes allegedly prevent state courts from making decisions.
- The destruction of documents. This can be done systematically by large companies, such as disposing of key design documents and the labeling of safety-standard compliance tests as "research."

These tactics handicap subsequent plaintiffs and their attorneys, as well as the courts.

POLITICAL AND BUREAUCRATIC OBSTACLES

A pun avers that "money talked, government listened, and business reaped the rewards." This theme could be invoked in the present context. Several events are noteworthy.

- The National Soft Drink Association initially lobbied **against** the incorporation of aspartame in soft drinks. Its document (dated August 8, 1983) for the U.S. Senate (*Congressional Record* S5507-S5511) detailed the basis for such objections, including startling deficiencies in the stability studies using aqueous media.
- Senator William Proxmire severely criticized the attempt to rapidly license aspartame, especially allowing only 30 days for scientific and public comment on the enormous amount of information requiring analysis (*Federal Register* July 26, 1974).
- The political aspects of aspartame approval, especially through Republican Party connections, have been reviewed elsewhere (Roberts 1989). G.D. Searle & Company reapplied for the approval of aspartame on January 21, 1981 – the day after Ronald Reagan took office as President.
- Democratic Senator Howard Metzenbaum introduced the Aspartame Safety Act of 1985 (S. 1557). Its purpose was "To provide the public with information concerning the use of products containing aspartame, to provide for the conduct of studies to determine the health effects of using products containing aspartame, and for other purposes." The Senate defeated his proposal by a 68-27 vote.
- Senator Metzenbaum later pleaded with Republican Senator Orrin Hatch (Chairman, Senate Labor and Human Resources Committee) to hold follow-up hearings concerning the safety of aspartame. Hatch rejected this request because "it would serve no useful purpose" (*The Tampa Tribune* February 11, 1986, p. A-4.)
- There have been other inferences concerning political influence relativeto the licensing of aspartame. Gregory Gordon, an investigative reporter for United Press International, listed the significant campaign contributions received by several senators **after** passage of legislation favorable to aspartame, or following their opposition to the aspartame labeling bill.

The exercise of comparable political clout in other realms repeatedly surfaces. Several instances are cited.

- Noting the increased politicization of science and medical journals, Fumento (1999) commented: "But the role these journals play is so incredibly important, and the cost of malfeasance so terribly high, that politics must not be allowed to worm into the science."

- The Senate Comprehensive Regulatory Reform Act of July 19, 1995 in effect overturned the Delaney clause (Chapter XXVII-E). It asserted that a substance or product shall not be prohibited or refused approval when it "presents a negligible or insignificant foreseeable risk to human health"... but without defining "negligible" or "insignificant."

- Dr. Woodrow Monte sought to have the State of Arizona ban aspartame after researching its adverse effects, especially those attributed to methanol (Chapter XXI). Using a rare maneuver to change State Law without public notice, the Legislature barred the state regulation of FDA-approved food additives.

The Washington "Revolving Door"

The cynicism of anti-aspartame consumer groups was fanned when several government lawyers who had made the decision not to prosecute the manufacturer of aspartame for alleged falsification of test results joined a law firm representing **that** company (*The Wall Street Journal* February 7, 1986, p.4). Furthermore, the statute of limitations for related prosecution was allowed to expire **during** the interval wherein one of the attorneys left the government, and **before** his replacement could become fully operational on the matter.

Senator Howard Metzenbaum pointed out during the November 3, 1987 Senate hearing that **ten** ranking FDA and other federal officials involved with the regulation of aspartame had subsequently taken jobs in the private sector linked to that industry. They included former chiefs and acting chiefs of the Bureau of Foods, and the commissioner who first approved aspartame for use in dry foods and as a tabletop sweetener! Official records indicate that he left the FDA to become a senior medical consultant for the public relations agency representing the manufacturer (*Congressional Record - Senate* 1985a, p.5494).

CORPORATE OBSTACLES

The current and future culinary landscapes will feature many staples presweetened with faux sugars. Despite United States laws against monopolies, a few companies have gained considerable control over the food supply. The soft drink industry, a $58 billion enterprise, is also dominated by several giant corporations. Dr. David Kessler (2001), former FDA Commissioner, asserted, "I had underestimated the enormous power of industry. I don't think people know the extent to which their tentacles really reached."

The following perspectives are pertinent.

- The sales of aspartame products used for "controlling" weight are so huge that this industry will battle attempts to have them regulated or removed.

- The use of soda vending machines that can change prices according to the weather, as during summer championship games, evidences corporate opportunism.

- The marketing of diet sodas to young individuals has become fierce. For example, the director of marketing for a major producer of diet sodas offered (March 23, 2000) four cases of its diet cola free to every person contacted by Internet viewers "as a promotion to get our name to young people around the world." But manufacturers of low-calorie soft drinks recognize the increasing concern about such beverages, especially among "transitioners" – that is, persons from 18 to 30 who turn to them for the first time. Accordingly, they attempt to avoid the word "diet" when naming new products containing aspartame, its analogs, and sweeteners such as acesulfame potassium.

- Pharmaceutical and chemical companies increasingly avoid the term "drug" relative to sweeteners because of the enormous expense involved. It costs up to $350 million at present to bring a new drug to market (Gale 2000). This may have been a factor in removing the drug application for aspartame as possible therapy for peptic ulcer.

- Industry has been given even more clout through the Multilateral Agreement on Investment (MAI) by which empowered foreign corporations and investors could sue governments directly for policies or actions that undermine profits.

Disinformation

The widespread nature of disinformation about aspartame products was reviewed in Chapter XXIX. The media have been supplied with a multitude of reports for debunking "health rumors" and "urban legends" about reactions to these products.

Altruistic persons associated with the aspartame industry have confided the reluctance of manufacturers to impart information about the adverse effects of aspartame and its breakdown products.

The mother of a diabetic patient had worked as an executive for a major soft drink producer when aspartame was being introduced. The patient wrote, "Based on upper-level management memos that she read discussing the possibility of brain tumors and neurological disorders with the use of aspartame in dry and wet forms, my mother decided to tell the family, even though each one had to be signed and returned in compliance with non-disclosure. She had no reason to lie to me."

There are many examples of comparable corporate resistance to having the side effects of drugs, ingredients, and contaminants revealed.

Instances of companies attempting to repress or change the results of studies they had sponsored, but did not welcome, have been reported in the general press.

Damage Control About Aspartame Reactions

Lawyers representing persons with aspartame disease have been subjected to considerable personal criticism when they expressed "righteous indignation" over reactions to aspartame products. A manufacturer issued this statement to the press on October 16, 1986 denouncing the efforts of James Turner, Esquire, and the Community Nutrition Institute (Chapter XXX) for

"... their repeated efforts to gain publicity: for their thoroughly discredited views on aspartame. Over the past decade, Turner and CNI have made numerous defamatory allegations about aspartame before regulatory agencies and the courts... The only thing notable about today's actions is Turner's and CNI's ingenuity in creating media events on anecdotal reports and unsupported allegations... It is simply a form of media terrorism."

The projected introduction of aspartame analogs is bound to invite extreme criticism by concerned physicians and others who use the "lessons" of aspartame disease as arguments against approval. There have been comparable instances involving drugs and supplements. One is the extreme corporate resistance to research indicating the bioequivalence of generic and brand-name levothyroxine products for treating hypothyroidism (Dong 1997).

948

Ethical Considerations

Not-for-profit organizations and "health charities" ought to avoid the pressures of marketplace competition. They include groups that focus on diabetes, arthritis, heart disease and cancer. Unfortunately, many undermined their reputation by providing "seals of approval" for aspartame and other products in accepting corporate money.

The reverberations of aspartame disease have engendered negative behavior. Upton Sinclair made the pertinent observation: "It is difficult to get a man to understand something when his salary depends on his not understanding it."

An aspartame reactor attended a diabetes conference in San Diego. After asking two representatives of a major insulin manufacturer about their advice to diabetic patients concerning aspartame, he stated, "I've never seen educated people profess such ignorance of a term in my life." He projected the probable decrease of diabetes drugs and testing units "if diabetics were to swear off diet drinks and aspartame-laden foods." As an example, he had calculated the cost of $550 million just for diabetes strips – based on only one test per day – with 10 million diabetics doing the testing, and 50 test strips costing $55 per month.

The ethical facets of "sciencegate" were considered in Chapter XXVIII. The matter extends to the regulatory realm as well. As an example, a former acting FDA commissioner had been bombarded with numerous complaints from consumers concerning their reactions to aspartame products, but largely remained silent on the matter. In June 1999, he announced that he would be joining a drug firm linked to aspartame as its senior vice-president for clinical affairs.

Physicians Employed or Sponsored by the Aspartame Industry

FDA Commissioner David Kessler (1991) stressed that physicians employed by drug companies should "do their best to avoid becoming unwitting participants in promotional activities." He also urged physicians who give presentations to reveal the source of any corporate sponsorship "as well as the extent to which a sponsor has exercised control over the material."

The author analyzed the data and statements submitted by some aspartame reactors on the "NutraSweet Consumer Medical Complaint Report" wherein multiple complaints ttributed to ingesting aspartame products were documented in detail. The "reply" by an associate medical director to one such sufferer stated: "Thank you for the information you provided regarding your complaint. I appreciate the time you took to supply me with more details of your medical history and symptoms. I am presently evaluating these data and will incorporate this information into our records."

Some researchers who conducted studies, or gave reports on testimony favorable to aspartame, received the largesse of this industry in various forms. They include fees as well-paid consultants, large research grants, funds for laboratory equipment, and honoraria for media interviews and appearances at public forums. Paradoxically, Dr. Richard Wurtman (1987c) told a Senate hearing on November 3, 1987 that a number of prestigious investigators paid by industry as private consultants chose not to attend the pertinent international conference he had chaired six months earlier.

XXXII

THE FOOD AND DRUG ADMINISTRATION (FDA)

"If the FDA violates its own laws, who is left to
protect the people?"
                    Dr. M. Adrian Gross

"I am not going to tell you that the FDA has
devised the perfect system for keeping hazardous
chemicals out of our foods... You'll simply have to
live with it."
                    Herbert L. Ley, Jr.
                    (Former FDA Commissioner)

Sections 6 and 7 contain references to many pro-industry decisions by the FDA. The request by its chief legal officer for an investigation concerning aspartame by a grand jury was the first, and apparently only, such action to date in this agency's history.

Concern over the failure to hold persons in authority at this and other regulatory agencies responsible for gross blunders had led to the characterization of an "era of no-fault government."

- Betty Martini, founder of Mission Possible, expressed her exasperation over the FDA in an open letter. She asserted, "The aspartame fiasco, in my opinion, is the greatest scandal in U.S. history – the mass poisoning of the American public."
- One anti-aspartame activist wore a button about the FDA stating, "THEY LIE AND DENY!"
- F. Edward Scarborough, Ph.D.(1989), then Acting Director of the FDA, emphasized that "predicting the intake of a truly novel ingredient prior to its introduction into the food supply is virtually impossible."

- On the occasion of Passover 2000, an anti-aspartame activist wrote, "The Food and Drug Administration is Pharaoh, and the American people are slaves to a system of exploitation. We have had many plagues. The worst of all will be FDA's legacy: biotechnology's angel of death."

Physicians ought to scrutinize the ambivalent position of the FDA when they encounter aspartame disease in their practices. At the very least, Congress should insist upon an "early warning system" relative to medical side effects or complications attributed to aspartame products... with manufacturers being required to inform the FDA promptly of such occurrences.

GENERAL CONSIDERATIONS

I. The Quantitative and Qualitative Limitations of the FDA

The Wall Street Journal noted that the FDA is "an agency under stress" whose limited funds cast doubt on its "ability to perform its many tasks satisfactorily" (September 28, 1990, p. B-4).

- Joseph Levitt (2000), Director of the FDA Center for Food Safety and Applied Nutrition, stated that the dietary supplement program "represents our biggest mismatch between the resources we have available and the job we have to accomplish."
- The FDA, which employs 8900 persons, faces a constant exodus of experienced staffers, including statisticians. This is due in part to psychological and verbal abuse by members of Congress or their representatives. The issues involve deadlines for drug reviews, limited resources, and a barrage of constituent complaints (as in the case of aspartame reactors).
- The FDA allegedly hesitates to prosecute for erroneous advertising because of the considerable expense entailed. Its Deputy Commissioner previously stated that each criminal prosecution costs the agency from $200,000 to $300,000 (*U.S. News & World Report* December 8, 1986, p. 69).

Historically, an FDA Commissioner asserted the following in June 1983 – one month before the FDA approved adding aspartame to soft drinks – in a reply to questions about the safety of aspartame breakdown products.

"The agency also concludes that the allegation that all possible reaction products have not been tested for safety is not a tenable issue in terms of regulatory food additive safety evaluations. Such a requirement for the demonstration of safety would necessitate an unlimited amount of experimental data (48 RF 142 P 31383)."

II. The Agency's Partiality to Aspartame

This revealing exchange occurred in the United States Senate on November 3, 1987 during a hearing by the Committee on Labor and Human Resources.

- Senator Orrin Hatch: "Do you persist in your opinion that the 3,000 adverse reaction reports you have received are of no clinical significance?"
- Frank Young, M.D., FDA Commissioner: "Yes, I do, and this is a relatively low incidence of adverse reactions compared to the large number of individuals who are using the product."
- Senator Hatch: "Has the Center noticed an increase in adverse reaction reports associated with the publicity on aspartame?"
- Commissioner Young: "Yes, we have. We usually see a peak of adverse reactions with publicity."

III. Deficiencies in Documenting and Tracking Aspartame Reactors

Thomas Wilcox, FDA epidemiology branch chief, informed the Community Nutrition Institute in its May 26 edition of *Nutrition Week* that *aspartame complaints constituted 75 percent of all reports of adverse reactions to substances in the food supply received by the FDA since 1981*! Yet, the FDA severely curtailed its tracking of complaints attributable to aspartame products by the end of 1995. Furthermore, *Food & Chemical News* (June 12, 1995) stated that the FDA had no further plans to continue collecting adverse-reaction reports on aspartame and for periodical monitoring.

Betty Martini of Mission Possible (Chapter XXX) enlightened the acting director of the FDA after he told *The Wall Street Journal* that his agency had received only 11 adverse complaints in 1995. She stated that her group had already received that many in **one day**!

The predictable sequence of complaints experienced by aspartame reactors described in this book contradicts these statements by FDA Commissioner Dr. Frank E. Young:

- "As of October 23, 1987, the ARMS has evaluated 3,511 of the 3,679 aspartame consumer complaints received by the FDA. There still is no consistent pattern of symptoms reported that can be attributed to the use of aspartame."

- "Moreover, because the reports are most frequently anecdotal in nature, it is not possible, without other data such as medical records, to eliminate factors other than aspartame consumption as possible causes of the reported effects." (The author had personally given an FDA investigator the medical records of a nurse [Case III-1] who experienced her first seizure one week after she began drinking aspartame.)

IV. Lowered Approval Standards for Supplements

The passage of several laws – the Prescription Drug User Fee Act of 1992 and 1997, and the Food and Drug Administration Modernization Act of 1997 – served to lower drug and supplement approval standards. In fact, the PDUFA allows the FDA to collect fees from manufacturers for reviewing new drug applications, thereby transforming this presumably regulated industry into an FDA client! The expanded use of "accelerated approval" reviews is a case in point.

V. Perceived Corporate Relationships

There has been a perceived symbiotic relationship between major corporations and the FDA. It is illustrated by the ability of a large firm to have a job created for one of its researchers wherein the person essentially reviewed her own studies!

The acceptance of millions of dollars annually by the FDA since 1993 from the drug industry to expedite drug and supplement approval (*The Wall Street Journal* April 20, 1999, p. A-24) concerns scientists at this agency because such a policy could compromise safety.

Unfortunately, regulatory bodies frequently become easy targets for "industry capture" – that is, the interests of citizens become subverted to those of big business. One prominent anti-aspartame advocate stated that the health of populations has become hostage to this "devious sellout of public interests."

VI. Congressional Criticism of the FDA

The Committee on Government Operations of the 101st Congress (2d Session) published a report on November 14, 1990 titled, *FDA's Continuing Failure to Prevent Deceptive Health Claims For Food.* It contained these statements:

- "Whereas drugs are subjected to a rigorous, expensive, and sometimes lengthy premarket approval process, foods may be marketed with no such prior review."
- "FDA had improperly permitted companies to make health claims based on the vague guidelines in the proposed rule, even before FDA received public comment on the proposal."
- *"FDA has admitted it lacks the resources to initiate enforcement action... It makes no sense for FDA to allow companies to make health claims on food labels if the agency admits it lacks the resources to enforce its regulations in a way that will deter manufacturers from making deceptive claims."* (italics supplied)
- "During his appearance before the subcommittee, Commissioner Young displayed a very cavalier attitude about his violations of FDA's recording requirements. When confronted with his repeated violations of the regulation, Commissioner Young suggested that this was not a 'substantive' issue and refused to give the subcommittee any assurance that these violations would cease."

VII. Consumer Criticism of the FDA

Numerous communications critical of FDA policies appear in Chapter XXX and other sections. Consumer advocates have bitterly attacked an attempt by the FDA to stop "unauthorized" use of information about supplements and other products through its "gag rule."

The challenge to the FDA for an honest reevaluation of aspartame products was boldly penned in this letter by an irate consumer.

"As might be expected, only a small fraction of people who experience problems with aspartame bother to contact the FDA, their congressmen, friends, or anyone else. So don't tell me that you have had only so many complaints. This is only the number of people that have bothered to write."

"I would estimate that about 90 percent of my female friends have had problems with aspartame and have quit using diet drinks and other products."

"This may not represent a health problem to the FDA or any other organization, but it certainly has to these people who have been to doctor after doctor, given up their activities and their jobs, plus the mental and monetary problems. What does the FDA consider a health problem anyway?"

"You haven't received millions of complaints because people don't know that aspartame is causing their health problems. Erroneously, they think that the food and drinks they consume are safe."

VIII. Criticism of FDA by the Scientific Community

Regulators have adopted a permissive "prove harm" philosophy whereby virtually all chemicals are considered innocent until proven harmful. This is a potentially dangerous attitude relative to the public health because it assumes that every ecosystem and species has some "assimilative capacity" whereby the induced harm can be absorbed without irreversible damage.

A different philosophy – variously termed "clean technology" and "clean industrial ecology" – ought to be emphasized. "The principle of reverse onus" argues that chemicals should be considered guilty until proven innocent... **not** the other way around. The International Joint Commission (1250 23rd Street N.W., Suite 100, Washington, D.C. 20440) in its Sixth and Seventh reports on Great Lakes water quality recommended the principle of precautionary action relative to toxic chemicals that bioaccumulate or have a half life greater than eight weeks in any medium (water, air, soil, or living things). It defined toxic substances as those that can "cause death, disease, behavioral abnormalities, cancer, genetic mutations, physiological or reproductive malfunctions, or physical deformities in any organism – or its offspring – or which can become poisonous after concentrating in the food chain or in combination with other substances."

Dr. M. Adrian Gross, a Senior Science Advisor at the Office of Pesticide Program, castigated the FDA in his concluding summary relative to aspartame that was submitted and sworn on November 3, 1987.

> "Although in their report the GAO express the view that the FDA 'followed its required process in approving aspartame (for marketing),' I would sharply disagree with such evaluation. Although the FDA may have gone through the motions or it may have given the appearance of such a process being in place here, the people of this country expect and require a great deal more from the agency charged with protecting their public health. In addition to mere facade or window-dressing on the part of the FDA, they require a <u>thorough</u> and <u>scientifically based</u> evaluation by the Agency on the safety of the products it regulates. Unfortunately, this has clearly not been the case here. And without this kind of assurance, any such 'process' or dance represents no more than a farce and a mockery of what is truly required."

IX. Approval of Low-Calorie Products

The FDA regulates the labeling of most foods. In the author's opinion, its actions tend to support both the safety and implied health claims for "low-calorie" and "reduced-calorie" products containing aspartame, notwithstanding denials to the contrary.

- The inference that nonnutritive sweeteners will have an impact on the incidence and severity of obesity could be misleading. In fact, persons consuming these products often **gain** weight because they consume increased calories (Stark 1987) and for other reasons (Chapter IX).
- The *FDA Drug Bulletin* of November 1986 requested "information from the medical community about clinically significant toxicity suspected to be associated with the consumption of excessive amounts of nutrients or food components in dietary supplements, including vitamins and minerals." It failed, however, to identify aspartame specifically.

X. Deficiencies of Pre-Marketing Tests

The shortcomings of aspartame testing in animals and humans prior to approval were reviewed in Section 5. They include the potential for brain tumors and birth defects, and the unknown long-term biologic effects of aspartame's breakdown products.

The issues were published in the *Congressional Record – Senate* (1985a,b). For example, it noted deficiencies of stability tests relative to the degradation of aspartame in soft drinks after exposure to temperatures higher than those used in company-sponsored studies.

Dr. Frank Young, FDA Commissioner, complained at a Senate hearing held on November 3, 1987 about (a) the grossly excessive monies spent for aspartame research, and (b) the FDA's "poor facilities" for such evaluation. The ominous nature of these comments is evidenced by the fact that more than half the population now consumes aspartame products.

OTHER FDA ACTIONS AND POLICIES

"Public and Congressional confidence in the ability of the Food and Drug Administration to carry out its statutory responsibilities has unquestionably been undermined."
Peter Barton Hutt (1973)
(Former Assistant General Counsel, FDA)

Instead of imposing a moratorium on additional uses of aspartame – whether in foods, beverages or drugs – until the availability of a corportate-neutral reevaluation of aspartame toxicity, the FDA approved its expanded uses in November 1986 (Overview), and later as a general all-purpose sweetener.

The FDA denied requests for a further hearing on the incorporation of aspartame in carbonated beverages and carbonated beverage syrup bases (*Federal Register* July 8, 1983, p. 31382) in its final approval of such use (*Federal Register* February 22, 1984, pp. 6672-6682).

The FDA denied requests for a public hearing on the approved uses of aspartame in a variety of products that the Aspartame Consumer Safety Network sought on January 30, 1992. The Agency demanded a "threshold burden of tendering evidence suggesting the need for a hearing." It further indicated that a hearing would be justified only if the objections were made in good faith and "draw in question in a material way the underpinnings of the regulation at issue." The ACSN objected to the reliability of prior double-blind tests, and pointed to "hundreds of pilots who have reported adverse reactions, including grand mal seizures."

- The Agency also objected to "anecdotal case reports."
- The Agency denied that aspartame should have been tested as a drug inasmuch as it felt the substance had met the definition of a food additive.
- The Agency refused to entertain the objection that aspartame products should have a warning label for pregnant women.

The FDA was reluctant to supply pertinent information. Truth in Labeling Campaign (TLC) President Jack L. Samuels, an opponent of MSG marketing, commented that "Freedom of Information gives one freedom to request information from the FDA; unfortunately, the FDA has freedom either to ignore such requests or turn them down."

The ambivalent attitude of the FDA on the issue of aspartame-induced tumors was considered in Chapter XXVII-E and F. It contrasts with mounting suspicion by the EPA concerning a number of chemicals and pesticides linked to cancer in laboratory animals to which food and water are exposed (*The Wall Street Journal* November 20, 1986, p. 37).

The FDA's opposition to Stevia as an alternative sweetener is discussed in Chapter XXXIV. This agency forced Stevita, a small company in Arlington, Texas to stop selling books mentioning it. Moreover, it ordered the destruction of 2,500 books about Stevia on May 20, 1998!

The FDA reversed the 1994 Dietary Supplement Health and Education Act, effective February 2000. This allowed manufacturers to sell products without approval of the agency as long as they did not make claims related to disease. The issue of herb-aspartame interactions (Chapter IX-I) assumes further significance in this context.

RELATED ISSUES

The Methyl Alcohol Issue

The author asked a senior FDA physician to furnish recent data supporting his contention that there is more free methanol in fruits and fruit juices than in aspartame, as the agency repeatedly alleged (Chapter XXI). The references supplied pertained to studies published decades earlier (chiefly in the European literature) with older assay methods.

Requested Complaints

The author requested copies of complaints the FDA had received from aspartame reactors, including the 2,800 consumers who submitted them _after_ the CDC analysis. It was necessary to invoke the Freedom of Information Act.

After repeated requests, I received a computer printout of 149(!) aspartame consumers who had suffered grand mal convulsions. (It was made available by Dr. David G. Hattan, Chief of the Regulatory Affairs Staff.)

Dual Sensitivities to Aspartame and MSG

The author's testimony to an FDA committee about dual sensitivity to aspartame and MSG (Chapter VIII-E) (Roberts 1993a) was of no avail. Dr. Adrienne Samuels (1991) concluded that no study nor a preponderance of the literature "proved" that ingested free glutamate is safe in _any_ form. She took the FDA to task over the matter of "judges" it appointed to review data concerning the safety of MSG.

Comments by Aspartame Reactors

Ninety-nine (23.9 percent) of 397 aspartame reactors who initially completed the survey questionnaire (Section 4) had either written or called their complaints to the FDA. The failure of its professionals to respond approximately, or at all, frustrated many – especially those consumers who had figured out the role of aspartame _by themselves_ (Chapter I). Their poignant criticisms appear in Chapter XIX. Several asked the same question, "Is the FDA supposed to represent the public or the manufacturer?"

- A 48-year-old woman developed two grand mal convulsions after drinking up to eight cans of aspartame-containing soft drinks daily. She was forbidden to drive by her physician, even after remaining seizure-free when she stopped aspartame. (This insight resulted from reading a newspaper article.) Her emotional wounds were exacerbated when she sought to submit her medical records to the FDA, but encountered total disinterest.
- A 27-year-old retail manager suffered violent aspartame-associated headaches for one year. She expressed outrage over a recent commercial inferring that aspartame was natural and healthy. She

added, "My experience taught me a lot. Too bad it is not enough for the FDA to see its potential harm."

- A correspondent with aspartame disease had two close relatives who also suffered severe aspartame reactions. She wrote the FDA as early as 1982, "This problem is too serious to let go on any longer. The FDA doesn't need to waste any more time on research that has been made to show the side that someone wants it to show."

- A 37-year-old diabetic with severe aspartame reactions expressed her outrage to several FDA staff members. "When will you pull this product from the shelf? How many innocent people must die? Will it take one of your close family members or a close friend having reactions to aspartame to take this problem seriously? WHEN WILL THIS INSANITY BE STOPPED?"

Brave Souls in the Federal Bureaucracy

An occasional frank response concerning aspartame reactions surfaced from members of the FDA staff.

A 64-year-old secretary attributed her previous severe headaches, dizziness, insomnia, depression, hair changes, visual problems, and ear symptoms to the consumption of one liter of aspartame-containing soft drinks daily. She wrote

"It was by the grace of God that I found out what was causing my trouble... aspartame.

"I contacted the FDA and told them what happened to me. I told them I was in pretty good health before I took aspartame, and if this happened to me it must be happening to others who do not realize what is causing their problem.

"I also asked how they could let this product on the market. His answer to me was, 'This is off the record, but we do not think the public should consume as much as they do.' "

SECTION 8

POINTERS FOR PHYSICIANS AND CONSUMERS

"There's No Free Lunch: The Benefits and Risks of Technologies."
>   Dr. William R. Hendee (1991)
>   Editorial, *Journal of the American Medical Association*

"This is what we must learn in relation to helping others. Because we care, we would like to spare them our misfortune by warning them to beware. However, owing to human nature, rarely is this possible. Usually our advice is scorned even to the point of ruining our friendship if we should persist."
>   T. S. Eliot

"I will be harsh as truth and as uncompromising as justice.
I am in earnest.
I will not equivocate.
I will not excuse.
I will not retreat not a single inch, and I will be heard."
>   William Lloyd Garrison

XXXIII

POINTERS FOR PHYSICIANS

"All professions are conspiracies against the laity."
George Bernard Shaw

"Risk assessment does not address ethical issues
of safety – people do. People make political and
moral decisions about how much risk is
acceptable."
Gail Charnley

The proverbial smoking gun demanded by health care professionals who doubt the existence of aspartame disease can be readily found among myriads of patients with this disorder who flock to their offices and hospitals IF they are willing to seek it.

Physicians must question **every** patient presenting with challenging disorders, especially those listed in Sections 2 and 3, about aspartame use. When encountered, it is prudent to recommend a brief trial of abstinence **before** ordering expensive tests and consultations, and embarking upon risky interventions.

Specific Caveats

- *Every evaluation of difficult allergic, dermatologic, gastrointestinal and metabolic problems should incorporate queries about aspartame consumption.*
- *Recent visual, neurologic or bowel problems in diabetics should not be attributed to a complicating retinopathy or neuropathy until there has been time to observe the response to abstinence from aspartame products.*
- Diabetics who experience unaccountable loss of "control" must be asked about concurrent aspartame use. *Changes in vision ought not be attributed solely to cataracts, multiple sclerosis, or toxic amblyopia from smoking or alcohol without aspartame disease also being considered.*

962

- *Cataract surgery should be deferred in heavy aspartame consumers until it is determined whether spontaneous improvement of vision occurs after avoiding such products.*
- *Patients with "refractory" neurological and psychiatric problems must be asked about aspartame use before ordering invasive studies and potent medications. They include unexplained seizures, headache, facial or eye pain, depression and dizziness. Aspartame reactors in these categories have suffered extreme anguish over initial misdiagnoses such as brain tumor, cerebral aneurysm and multiple sclerosis.*
- *Individuals who express concern about "early Alzheimer's disease" because of unexplained confusion and memory impairment should be observed at least several months after abstaining from aspartame before this ominous diagnosis is rendered.*
- *Cystoscopy, prostate surgery, uterine curettage, and hysterectomy should be deferred in aspartame consumers having unexplained urinary-tract complaints and altered menses pending observation for remission after stopping aspartame products.*

The Issue of Persistent Symptoms

The persistence or recurrence of symptoms in patients having aspartame disease poses a formidable diagnostic challenge. Under these circumstances, physicians should consider **all** the following possible explanations:

- Is the patient really aspartame-free because of failure to identify its presence in a number of products? They include drugs, yogurt, gum, mouthwashes, mints, antacids and various "supplements"... particularly when labels are vague or deceitful about their aspartame content.
- Is the patient being exposed to other definable neurotoxins (e.g,. MSG) and adverse environmental chemicals or influences?
- Have other major diagnose, such as hypothyroidism and reactive hypoglycemia, been overlooked or inadequately treated?Has enough time lapsed for affected organs to vidence optimum improvement – especially the brain, eyes and joints?
- Has some new disorder unrelated to aspartame disease been evolving?

The persistence of psychiatric and neurologic symptoms requires a careful search for **other** neurotoxins to which aspartame reactors may be exposed. This can be a major undertaking that involves a host of dietary offenders and toxic substances rarely suspected by physicians. The more common ones have been amplified in *Defense Against Alzheimer's Disease* (Roberts 1995b). For example, excessive fluoride intake is unlikely to be considered in this context.

- Flavor enhancers added to diet products, especially in liquid form, should be regarded with much suspicion relative to their excitotoxin content.
- The L-cysteine added to some breads (as a dough conditioner) is converted to yet another powerful excitotoxin.

The multiple <u>chemical sensitivity syndrome</u> was considered in Chapter VIII-G, including the neurotoxic effects of monosodium glutamate (MSG). The latter could be inadvertently consumed, as in barleygreen and powdered stevia products containing maltodextrin.

Lengthy lists of <u>products containing MSG</u>, and its synonyms, have been published (Samuels 1991, 1994; Roberts 1995b). Many "hidden sources," however, escape detection because they do not appear on labels. Jack Samuels, a pioneer in this realm, cited these instances:

- Binders, fillers and carriers used in "enriched" products, and flowing agents
- Poultry and meat "basted" with substances containing MSG
- "Broth" used as an ingredient for products other than broth
- Soaps, shampoos, hair conditioners, and cosmetics containing "hydrolyzed" ingredients and amino acids
- Drinks, candy and chewing gum
- Medications, especially for children

"Negative" Reports

Health care professionals should avoid being misled by published reports denying aspartame disease that were based on corporate-sponsored studies, especially if the approving "peer" reviewers or editors have had connections with this industry. Clues to such "fine print" appear in Section 7.

Vivid Dreams: A Warning by the Brain

Physicians ought to regard recurrent waking with intense dreams in aspartame reactors (Chapter VII-F) as a warning. On the basis of the author's prolonged clinical observations and researches, several protective responses are warranted. They include (a) taking full breaths after wakening to counter reduced oxygen intake resulting from diminished respirations during deep sleep, (b) eating a small snack to minimize glucose deprivation in the near-fasting state, and (c) total abstinence from aspartame products.

Conversely, the reflexive prescription of hypnotic drugs under these circumstances can set a vicious new neurodegenerative cycle in motion, particularly among diabetics and persons prone to nocturnal hypoglycemia (Chapter XIV). It involves oxygen deprivation from sedative-induced hypoventilation, and decreased brain glucose. Aspartame and other neurotoxins compound the damage.

Treatment of Methanol Poisoning

The manifestations of methanol toxicity were detailed in Chapter XXI. They are largely attributable to the effects of formic acid. Prior therapies of severe poisoning entailed hemodialysis for the removal of methanol, and intravenous ethanol as a competitive substrate to inhibit methanol metabolism.

Fomepizole (4-methylpyrazole) given intravenously as an inhibitor of alcohol dehydrogenase appears to be a safe and effective treatment for methanol poisoning (Brent 2001). It may be considered for patients presenting with severe metabolic acidosis, cardiovascular instability or acute blindness following the ingestion of considerable aspartame. The decline of formic acid concentrations, resolution of metabolic abnormalities, and improved vision in methanol poisoning caused by other agents have been dramatic.

XXXIV

CONSUMER PRECAUTIONS AND OPTIONS

"The rights of physicians and patients are
recklessly violated by frauds in foods and drugs...
The subject of food ethics is one of the most
important of all that come before this Section in
my opinion."
                              Dr. Ephraim Cutter (1893)

"But the interesting thing – or better, the tragedy
– is that the most dangerous items provoke no
fear at all. We decide <u>caveat emptor</u> when, but
only when, it is convenient to do so."
                              John B. Thomison, M.D. (1983)

*The most important precautionary measure aimed at preventing aspartame
disease is knowledge that it exists. A corollary is the careful study of labels on foods,
drinks, medications and other products for the presence of aspartame.* Their avoidance
is especially important for persons in high-risk groups (Section III). Unfortunately,
consumers are challenged because of inadequate or misleading labels (Chapter XXVII-
B).

Consumers concerned about aspartame can exercise various options to satisfy their
"sweet tooth." This poses a special challenge for patients with diabetes mellitus (Chapter
XIII) and severe hypoglycemia (Chapter XIV) who ought to avoid sugar. Furthermore,
hypoglycemia is frequent among persons who use considerable aspartame. The problem
of caffeinism (introduction to Section 2) poses an added consideration.

The following perceptive advice concerning the fallacies and shortcomings of ads promoting over-the-counter drugs, offered by Federal Judge William C. Conner (1987), is also valid for additives.

- "Don't be fooled by headlines and pictures."
- "Beware of every small word, even the smallest ones."
- "Numbers don't mean much, even the big ones."
- "Know the ingredients behind the brands."
- "Repeating a slogan doesn't make it true."

The names given new products can be a challenge. Recognizing the increased concern over aspartame beverages, especially among "transitioners" – that is, persons from 18 to 30 who turn to them for the first time – manufacturers of low-calorie soft drinks now tend to avoid the word "diet."

Concerned consumers should pay special attention to the <u>labels and inserts</u> of these items that **frequently** contain aspartame:

All "diet" drinks
All "reduced calorie" drinks
All protein drinks
All "diet" sauces and other preparations
All pre-packaged foods
All "sugar-free" gum and candy
All "patient-friendly" medicines for infants and children

A man with swelling of the gums caused by aspartame-containing toothpaste noted a paradox. It concerned the previous incorporation of sugar in toothpaste which had been "the laugh of the dental profession."

Unfortunately, FDA policies and standards may change under corporate pressure. The National Yogurt Association proposed changes in yogurt standards during November 2000 that would rescind the warning label and other disclosure of aspartame and sweeteners. I consider such action highly objectionable because of the frequency with which yogurt containing aspartame caused severe reactions. For example, one aspartame reactor found by rechallenge that the near-fatal "choking sensation" she experienced when traveling was <u>specifically</u> due to the sugar-free yogurt she ate at airports.

Individual aspartame reactors have evolved their own empiric dietary regimes based on considerable study and personal experiences. They may include vegetables, breast of fowl, salmon, blueberries, red grapes, garlic, red onions, colored bell pepper, decaf green tea, and "nothing white."

Reactors generally are wary of alternative "aspartame free" products until they have studied their labels. Even so, they could encounter a problem in which aspartame-free cans arrive at producers sooner than the aspartame-free drink – and filling the former with the old aspartame product.

The combination of phenylpropanolamine and aspartame in a number of "appetite suppressant" products – including "maximum strength" appetite control formulas and diet gums – may induce or aggravate hypertension (Chapter IX-C) and its complications... even among children.

Aspartame addicts

Aspartame addicts (Chapter VII-G) face an additional problem. One stated, "I'm convinced I have an aspartame problem, but just don't know for sure how to get it out of my life." Some adopted the Alcoholics Anonymous principle of "one day at a time" to get through aspartame withdrawal.

Some of the successful non-drug methods used by persons to free themselves from aspartame addiction are listed.

- Drinking considerable water (at least 2-3 liters daily), even carrying it at all times if necessary.
- Tapering the amount of aspartame products consumed daily – for example, from seven drinks to six drinks, to five drinks, etc.
- Avoiding the location of vending machines, and of areas where considerable diet sodas are usually being imbibed.
- Avoid carrying much loose change needed for vending machines.
- Utilizing a support system – whether family, a chat group on the internet, or an interested health care professional.
- Reinforcement from the gradual loss of symptoms and regained energy.

Products for Children

When treating infants and children for colds and other disorders, it is preferable to split and grind the "adult" form of a drug that does not contain aspartame, and administer it in apple sauce, ice cream or another acceptable vehicle. The author's researches in the toxicity of pentachlorophenol and other pesticides (Roberts 1990b) reinforce his dictum about aspartame-containing solutions: "dilution is not the solution." (Pesticides have evidenced adverse effects among animals in concentrations as little as several parts per <u>trillion</u>.)

Consumers have literally "hunted" for products that do not contain aspartame... especially concerned parents. It is a daunting task because they are likely to encounter "label games" (Chapter XXVII), but persistence can pay off. In response to numerous requests, there are current efforts to list the more than 9000 products containing aspartame for on-line posting.

Here are examples of products found to be aspartame-free prior to the publication of this book.

- Walgreen-brand <u>acetaminophen</u> drops do not contain aspartame. On the other hand, it is present in virtually all chewable acetaminophen products. Another approach for managing fever or pain in children with acetaminophen is crushing Junior Tylenol Caplets in a teaspoon to which baby pears or applesauce is added, or placed in diluted juice for infants. (This approach also obviates ingesting colorings and sodium/potassium benzoate.)
- A few brands of <u>children's vitamins</u> "contain no artificial sweetener;" the matter must be double-checked, however. Several children's liquid vitamin preparations are sweetened only with stevia.

Issuing Advance Warnings

Individuals who suffered severe aspartame reactions had to adopt preventive tactics similar to those used by MSG reactors when dining out. They would inform managers of restaurants about their problem, and warn – in the presence of witnesses – that the serving of food or beverages misrepresented as being aspartame-free would result in legal action if emergency hospitalization became necessary.

CONSUMER OPTIONS

The following precautionary choices are based on many observations and patient experiences. They should not replace the sound recommendations of informed physicians.

Aspartame reactors ought to view their options as "the lesser of several evils." For example, a 41-year-old dental receptionist with severe reactions to aspartame products wrote, "Many times I long for a soft drink, especially on a hot day or when we go out for pizza. Many companies now use aspartame, and I can't have any. I drink only water."

I. Water

Water – whether from the tap, filtered, or as "pure" bottled water – can be taken alone or with lemon or lime juice and other flavorings. Care should be take to avoid aspartame-laden water currently being promoted. Glass bottles are preferrable to plastic containers because a suspect carcinogen in the latter may leech into the water.

Individual bottles of seltzer water have become popular, but should be used with caution by persons having esophageal reflux.

Adding Stevia (see below) is another variation. Some are partial to the Sunrider brand with its squeeze bottle.

Fluoridated water ought to be minimized or avoided. I have detailed the neurotoxic and other adverse effects of fluoride (Roberts 1992f, 1995b, 1998h). Fluoridation has also contributed to excess arsenic in water.

II. Unsweetened Beverages

Modest amounts of tea, coffee (regular or decaffeinated), and other beverages (such as unsweetened tea mixes) generally are satisfactory. Lemon, lime, various flavorings or saccharin may be added.

III. Saccharin

The prudent use of saccharin seems safe (Chapters XXVII and XXIX). The calcium form (if available) is preferred by some because it has no bitter aftertaste.

Women have less concern. The debatable matter of experimental urinary bladder tumors ascribed to saccharin involved only male rats.

Saccharin-presweetened soft drinks are still available. *Aspartame reactors must constantly remain on alert, however, because producers have substituted or added aspartame.*

IV. Fruits and Juices

Juices provide another option, albeit with some reservations.

- "Unsweetened" prune juice and grape juice contain excessive "natural" sugar for diabetics and persons subject to severe hypoglycemia.
- Orange juice can release more insulin than eating an orange, and may provoke a "hypoglycemic attack," especially when taken at breakfast.
- There are reservations about carbohydrate-derived sweeteners, such as honey, sucanat (whole cane sugar with water removed), products sweetened with fruit juice, and fructooligosaccharides.

Fruits less likely to precipitate hypoglycemia can serve as satisfactory snacks. Examples include pears, peaches, strawberries and grapefruit. On the other hand, certain fruits that contain considerable carbohydrate (mangos; prunes; raisins) should be avoided, or taken with adequate fat and protein.

Robert Cohen, an anti-aspartame activist, recommends this variation of an acceptable substitute: "Put any fruit (cantaloupe, honeydew, peaches) in a blender, and then puree. Freeze the puree in ice cube trays. Keep orange or other juice in the refrigerator. Fill a glass with the frozen ice cubes, and add juice to fill the glass. The mixture can be placed in the blender for a 'smoothie.' The ice cubes also can be taken as snacks."

V. Laxatives

Several popular psyllium hydrophilic mucilloid preparations used for managing constipation contain dextrose or aspartame. A few have neither, such as Hydrocil Instant® (Rowell).

VI. "Dietetic Diabetic Products"

Some aspartame-free "diet" foods, candies, cookies and ice creams are sweetened with saccharin, sorbitol, mannitol and other non-sugar sweeteners. Their number and palatability have been less in the United States than Europe. These products are generally innocuous when used with discretion. Large amounts, however, may cause considerable "gas," indigestion and diarrhea due to their osmotic effects within the gastrointestinal tract. They also may trigger "reflex hypoglycemia."

A granular sweetener (Sweet Balance®) resembling ivory-colored sugar is made from organically grown kiwis.

VII. Other Sweetening Agents

Sweetener options, perhaps as much as 10,000 times sweeter than sucrose (table sugar), increasingly will become available as "blessed friends" of dieters. There are several caveats.

- Considerable insulin released because their sweet taste triggers the cephalic phase of insulin secretion (Chapter XIV).
- Persons sensitive to barley malt have reacted to hidden MSG.
- The excessive and prolonged use of licorice should be avoided because of water retention and hypertension.

VIII. Acesulfame Potassium (K)

Acesulfame K stimulates insulin secretion directly from the pancreatic islets, and potentiates glucose-induced insulin release (Liang 1987). Its carcinogenicity has not been resolved. Moreover, there is evidence that acesulfame-K induces significant dose-dependent chromosomal aberrations in mice with doses in the "no-toxic-effect" range (Mukherjee 1997).

IX. Sucralose

Sucralose (Splenda®), a trichloro derivative of sucrose produced from selective chlorination of the hydroxyl groups, is being used as an artificial sweetener. Sucralose has been approved for use in 15 food and beverage categories. There is 2 percent sucralose in the major product for use in home recipes, the rest being dextrose and maltodextrin.

Despite claims to the contrary, as much as 40 percent of sucralose IS absorbed in humans. From 20-30 percent of the absorbed compound is metabolized, and then excreted in the urine.

Animal research indicates that sucralose causes shrinking of the thymus gland, enlargement of the liver and kidneys, renal mineralization, diarrhea, reduced growth rate, decreased red blood cell count, aborted pregnancy, and decreased placental weight. It was also found to be weakly mutagenic in a mouse lymphoma mutation assay.

Impurities found in sucralose include lead, arsenic, chlorinated disaccharides, chlorinated monosaccharide, and triphenilphosphine oxide methanol. The human consequences of 1, 6-dichlorofructose require clarification. Having researched chlorinated pesticides (especially pentachlorophenol) more than three decades (Roberts 199b, 1997d), the author awaits the results of long-term clinical studies.

Another disconcerting finding is the significant increase in glycosylated hemoglobin (an important indicator of lessened long-term control) among diabetic patients using sucralose.

X. Cyclamates

The use of cyclamates was banned in the United States for several controversial reasons. One involved a study released by Abbott Laboratories showing that eight of 240 rats fed a mixture of saccharin and cyclamates (in large doses) developed bladder tumors. Another pertained to malformed chicks injected with cyclamate.

The National Academy of Sciences concluded from an analysis of all the available evidence that cyclamate and its metabolite are **not** carcinogenic for humans (Chapter XXVII-K).

XI. Stevia

Stevia rebeaudiana Bertoni is a perennial shrub native to a mountain region of Paraguay. The local population used it for hundreds of years to sweeten herbal tea. Moises Santiago Bertoni, an Italian botanist, "rediscovered" Stevia in 1899. Grower plantations throughout South America flourished thereafter.

Stevia has been referred to as "Paraguay's sweet herb." Its preserved leaves remain intensely sweet for more than six decades. A pure white crystalline extract, stevioside, isolated in 1931, was characterized by a U.S. government researcher as "the sweetest natural product yet found."

To the author's knowledge, there are no significant side effects. One aspartame reactor contrasted the comparison of Stevia to aspartame by comparing peaches to plutonium.

There have been regrettable related events in the United States. The recall of more than 6500 books on this subject in 1994 reminded some of tactics practiced by Nazi Germany. After years of bureaucratic resistance, the FDA finally approved its use as a supplement.

Stevia is preferably taken in a liquid form because the packets may contain maltodextrin and MSG.

Aspartame reactors can place a few drops of liquid Stevia in 8-12 ounces water and add lemon, thereby making a "lemonade" without aftertaste. Others have mixed club soda and cranberry or other unsweetened juices, and then added drops of Stevia and ice. The mixing of herbal teas or fruit juices with club soda, and sweetened with liquid Stevia, offers another variation.

Many recipes using Stevia powder or drops of the concentrate can be found in *The Stevia Story* (BED Publications Company, Atlanta, Georgia), and *Sugar-Free Cooking With Stevia* by James and Tanya Kirkland (Crystal Health Publications, Arlington, Texas).

XII. Sugar As An Option

Patients with diabetes and hypoglycemia generally should avoid or minimize the consumption of sugar (sucrose), especially in "foods of commerce." Other issues involve the critical role of sugar-stimulated insulin secretion in depositing body fat, and elevating triglyceride (fat) and cholesterol concentrations (Roberts 1967a, 1968b, 1969c). The blending of aspartame with sugar in an attempt to hide its taste constitutes yet another potential danger for consumers.

In the wake of severe reactions to aspartame products, some patients understandably ask: "Doctor, which is worse... sugar or aspartame?" After prolonged reflection, the author concluded that sugar in small amounts is preferable, provided the meals contain adequate protein, fat and fiber. Following prior abstention from sugar, the taste buds of diabetic and hypoglycemic patients are usually satisfied with minimal quantities.

"DETOXIFICATION"

Persons who have suffered chronic aspartame disease often ask about "detoxification." This issue is likely to be raised when neurologic, psychiatric and visual symptoms persist or recur after avoiding aspartame. Unfortunately, aspartame reactors must guard against exploitation in the guise of detoxification.

It is obvious that there must be TOTAL avoidance of aspartame products under these circumstances, with emphasis on products that may have been overlooked. Examples are gum, breath mints, toothpaste, laxatives, instant breakfasts, vitamins, and various medications.

Other diagnostic considerations facing physicians under these circumstances were discussed in Chapter XXVIII – with particular reference to incompletely treated disorders or the emergence of a new disease.

Drinking Water

One reasonable measure is the drinking of considerable non-fluoridated water unless there are contraindications to doing so. Indeed, the body may be attempting to rid itself of aspartame breakdown products through intense thirst and frequent urination (Chapter IX-F).

There is evidence that high fluid intake lessens toxic risk. The reduction of urinary bladder cancer in men presumably reflects greater dilution and excretion of carcinogens (Michaud 1999). Drinking considerable water (preferably distilled) as part of a detoxification program also tends to keep formaldehyde in solution within the blood stream, thereby minimizing addition to formaldehyde adducts (Chapter XXI).

Related Considerations

Some suggested forms of "detoxification" could pose risks. Concerning chronic methanol poisoning, the use of ethyl alcohol is not recommended (as is the case in acute methanol intoxication.)

Similarly, there are misgivings about taking considerable amounts of these and other amino acids. The issue of reactions to aspartate preparations was repeatedly raised by correspondents. Several aspartame reactors whose symptoms persisted after the avoidance of such products (notably ringing in the ears or tinnitus) after avoiding aspartame products found as a result of considerable personal research that various preparations chelated with aspartic acid caused or exacerbated their problems. Examples are vitamins, minerals (most notably magnesium, potassium and calcium), "enzyme therapies," and "fitness" powders/supplements.

Several aspartame reactors used Noni juice as part of their "detoxification" process. The fruit is derived from the *Morinda citrifolia* plant, known by various names in different countries (e.g., Indian mulberry; Nono), which traditional healers use for a variety of disorders. Proxeronine, its active component, stimulates the alkaloid xeronine. In turn, this activates various enzymes that presumably enhance the absorption and utilization of amino acids, vitamins and minerals.

Several researchers have emphasized the ability of Noni juice to bind with serotonin in a safe manner. Its benefit in various psychiatric disorders and in drug/alcohol addiction is attributed to this pharmacologic property. Unfortunately, labels must be studied because one noni fruit extract contains "natural flavors."

APPENDICES

APPENDIX A

STATEMENT BY H. J. ROBERTS, M.D.
FOR U.S. SENATE HEARING

S. HRG 100-567

'NUTRASWEET"—HEALTH AND SAFETY CONCERNS

HEARING
BEFORE THE

COMMITTEE ON
LABOR AND HUMAN RESOURCES
UNITED STATES SENATE
ONE HUNDREDTH CONGRESS
FIRST SESSION

ON

**EXAMINING THE HEALTH AND SAFETY CONCERNS OF NUTRASWEET
(ASPARTAME)**

NOVEMBER 3, 1987

466

PALM BEACH INSTITUTE FOR MEDICAL RESEARCH, INC.
300 27th Street
West Palm Beach, Florida 33407

H.J. Roberts, M.D.
Medical Director

THE ASPARTAME PROBLEM

STATEMENT FOR SENATE HEARING

NOVEMBER 3, 1987

I am concerned over the escalating number of aspartame-related complaints documented by or reported to interested investigators, the FDA, and consumer groups such as Aspartame Victims And Their Friends and the Community Nutrition Institute.

The most serious reactions I have encountered among 551 aspartame reactors in my nationwide computerized study include severe headaches (45.2%), dizziness (39.4%), decreased vision or blindness (27.9%), epileptic attacks (17.8%), profound confusion and memory loss (28.5%), extreme depression (25.2%), and marked personality changes (16%). Hives, other rashes, itching, mouth reactions, hyperactivity, extreme fatigue, insomnia, menstrual disorders, diarrhea, intense thirst, ringing in the ears, aggravated hypoglycemia, loss of diabetic control, severe weight loss (suggestive of anorexia nervosa), a paradoxic gain of weight, and joint pains also have been prominent. These observations, which have been reported in the references listed, are supported by FDA data.

An unexpected finding has been the occurrence of reactions to aspartame in the relatives (up to 7) of 22 percent of persons so affected.

The causative or contributory role of aspartame is supported by (1) the gratifying relief or disappearance of these complaints (except for blindness and severe neuropsychiatric features) after its cessation, and (2) their predictable recurrence on rechallenge.

Damage to the retina, optic nerves and brain can be caused by methyl alcohol in heavy consumers. (Aspartame promptly releases 10 percent methanol by weight when metabolized.) Other complications may reflect the combination of high levels of phenylalanine within the brain, altered neurotransmitter function, severe caloric reduction, and increased release of insulin and other hormones. Recent data also raise the possibility that selective amino acid imbalance of phenylalanine and aspartic acid may accelerate or aggravate Alzheimer's disease, Parkinsonism, behavioral abnormalities, and other neuropsychiatric afflictions.

The problems of aspartame reactions assume even greater importance for certain high-risk groups. They include infants, children, pregnant women, older persons, and patients with diabetes, migraine, hypoglycemia, epilepsy, allergies, and liver or kidney disease who consume large amounts of such products.

467

Severe deficiencies pertaining to the evaluation, licensing, promotion and surveillance of aspartame must be addressed in the face of this potential "recipe for disaster." They encompass (1) the need for accurate clinical data collected by the responsible governmental agencies, including an analysis of tumors (especially brain and urinary bladder) and blood disorders, (2) the arbitrarily high maximum allowable daily intake, (3) the prior resistance by Congress to enactment of legislation that would mandate the proper labeling of aspartame products, (4) the failure to challenge the alleged safety and effectiveness of aspartame in massive promotional campaigns, especially for long-term weight loss, and (5) unfounded bias against saccharin based on limited and controversial studies concerning urinary bladder tumors in male rats.

It is now the burden of regulatory agencies that have minimized or denied the accumulated clinical data to convincingly explain them in terms other than isolated idiosyncratic reactions.

The informational gap caused by the biases and other misgivings of reluctant editors, publishers, and chairmen of major medical conferences is a public health and scientific disservice.

Concerning my credentials, I have been certified and recertified by the American Board of Internal Medicine, and am a member of the Senior Active Staff of the Good Samaritan Hospital and St. Mary's Hospital in West Palm Beach. I have authored more than 200 original scientific publications and five texts, and am listed in The Best Doctors in the U.S. and Who's Who in the World.

REFERENCES

Roberts, H.J.: *Is Aspartame (NutraSweet®) Safe?* On Call (publication of the Palm Beach County Medical Society), January 1987, pp. 16-20.

Roberts, H.J.: *Neurologic, Psychiatric and Behavioral Reactions to Aspartame in 505 Aspartame Reactors.* In Wurtman R.J., Ritter-Walker E. (eds) Proceedings of the First International Conference on Dietary Phenylalanine and Brain Function. Washington, D.C., 1987, May 8-10, pp. 477-481.

H.J. Roberts, M.D.

APPENDIX B

PROFESSIONAL OPINION OF H. J. ROBERTS, M.D., F.A.C.P., F.C.C.P. CONCERNING THE USE OF PRODUCTS CONTAINING ASPARTAME BY PERSONS WITH DIABETES AND HYPOGLYCEMIA

I have treated many patients with diabetes mellitus and hypoglycemia (low blood sugar) in my capacity as a Board-certified internist and an endocrinologist (member of the Endocrine Society). Since both groups should abstain from sugar, I initially was pleased that these persons had an acceptable – and presumably safe – sugar substitute in aspartame.

Unfortunately, many patients in my practice, and others seen in consultation, developed serious metabolic, neurologic and other complications that could be <u>specifically</u> attributed to using aspartame products. This was evidenced by:

> *The <u>loss of diabetic control</u>, the <u>intensification of hypoglycemia</u>, the <u>occurrence of presumed "insulin reactions"</u> (including convulsions) that proved to be aspartame reactions, and <u>the precipitation, aggravation or simulation of diabetic complications</u> (especially impaired vision and neuropathy) while using these products.

> *<u>Dramatic improvement of such features after avoiding aspartame</u>, AND the <u>prompt predictable recurrence of these problems when patients resumed aspartame products</u>, knowingly or inadvertently.

I have cited many instances of severe complications in patients with diabetes and hypoglycemia caused by the use of aspartame products in my books and scientific articles. Here are few illustrations.

> <u>A 21 year-old insulin-dependent teacher</u> suffered more frequent insulin reactions, both at school and home, while drinking many aspartame colas daily. He reported, "When I cut down on aspartame, I stopped having so many reactions."

> <u>A diabetic man</u> suffered severe changes in vision when he was drinking liters of aspartame soft drinks daily. An ophthalmologist assured him that there was no detectable diabetic retinopathy. The patient then chanced to read an article about aspartame-related eye problems. He promptly improved after avoiding these beverages, an unlikely event if the problem was primarily a diabetic retinopathy.

> <u>A 46 year-old man with insulin-dependent diabetes</u> had been in good control for three decades until he began ingesting several aspartame sodas and many packets of tabletop sweetener daily. He summarized his experience in these terms: "My diabetes went haywire, and I had terrible insulin reactions." His diabetes was fully controlled within one week after abstaining from aspartame products.

> <u>A 12 year-old boy with known diabetes</u> required multiple hospitalizations for diabetic coma whileconsuming considerable aspartame. Physicians at a university hospital had difficulty in stabilizing his insulin requirements while he used these products.

In the light of this experience, <u>I advise ALL patients with diabetes and hypoglycemia to avoid aspartame products</u>. A number of acceptable alternatives are available.

I regret the failure or unwillingness of other physicians and the American Diabetes Association (ADA) to sound appropriate warnings based on these repeated findings which have been described in my corporate-neutral studies and publications. This is largely due to these factors:

(1) It has been virtually impossible to present these observations on the programs for national meetings of diabetologists and other professional groups. Indeed, the ADA (of which I had been a member for over three decades) even refused to print an <u>abstract</u> of the adverse reaction I encountered in 58 diabetic patients submitted for its 1987 annual meeting. (This abstract subsequently appeared in CLINICAL RESEARCH – Vol. 3:489A, 1988.)

(2) Journals devoted to diabetes and internal medicine refused to publish my manuscripts on this subject due to negative "peer review" comments. The likelihood existed that some of these reviewers had self-serving interests in denying publication.

(3) The AMA, the FDA, and the ADA dogmatically continue to express the <u>unequivocal</u> opinion that aspartame is "completely safe" for diabetics... and nearly everyone else.

(4) Manufacturers and producers accomplished the "marketing miracle of the 1980's" through highly effective PR campaigns, the underwriting of numerous research projects (a number involving flawed protocols) by investigators they granted, and enormous biopolitical clout in order to protect their billion-dollar market."

I detailed these matters in ASPARTAME DISEASE: AN IGNORED EPIDEMIC and SWEET'NER DEAREST: BITTERSWEET VIGNETTES ABOUT (NUTRASWEET®) (Sunshine Sentinel Press (P.O. Box 17799, West Palm Beach, Florida 33416; 1-800-814-9800), and ASPARTAME (NUTRASWEET®): IS IT SAFE? (The Charles Press). They are also summarized in my audio cassette set, IS ASPARTAME (NUTRASWEET®) SAFE? A MEDICAL, PUBLIC HEALTH AND LEGAL OVERVIEW (Sunshine Sentinel Press).

The possible mechanisms for aggravation of diabetes and hypoglycemia include the following:

*Excessive insulin secretion and depletion of the "insulin reserve"

*Possible alteration of cellular receptor sites for insulin, with ensuing "insulin resistance"

*Neurotransmitter alterations within the brain and peripheral nerves

*The toxicity of <u>each</u> of the three components of aspartame (phenylalanine; aspartic acid; the methyl ester, which promptly becomes <u>free</u> methyl alcohol or methanol), and their multiple breakdown products after exposure to heat or during prolonged storage.

I have asserted in my publications, and in testimony to Congress and an FDA advisory group, that the current wholesale ingestion of aspartame products by over half the adult population constitutes an "imminent public

982

health hazard." Yet, this warning continues to be ignored by the medical profession and the FDA. Informed and concerned consumers <u>are</u> justified in criticizing this bureaucratic-industrial-medical complex that refuses to acknowledge the existence of aspartame disease, and fails to warn high-risk groups about the potential dangers. In addition to patients with diabetes and hypoglycemia, they include pregnant women, children, patients with epilepsy, liver, kidney disease and eating disorders, older persons with memory impairment, and the relatives of aspartame reactors, diabetics and patients with phenylketonuria.

APPENDIX C

PROFESSIONAL OPINION OF H. J. ROBERTS, M.D., F.A.C.P., F.C.C.P. CONCERNING THE USE OF PRODUCTS CONTAINING ASPARTAME BY PREGNANT WOMEN, INFANTS AND CHILDREN

It is my firm opinion that pregnant women, infants and children should avoid ALL products containing aspartame – including diet foods/sodas, vitamins, drugs and "supplements."

This corporate-neutral summary statement has been prepared in response to numerous requests from concerned patients, parents and consumers. There is no bias or malice intended against any company, distributor, researcher or individual who may hold a contrary view.

The statement is based on considerable observation, research and correspondence published in more than a score of articles and these books:

- ASPARTAME DISEASE: AN IGNORED EPIDEMIC (Sunshine Sentinel Press, P.O. Box 17799; West Palm Beach; 1-800-814-9800)
- ASPARTAME (NUTRASWEET®): IS IT SAFE? (Charles Press)
- SWEET'NER DEAREST: BITTERSWEET VIGNETTES ABOUT ASPARTAME (NUTRASWEET®) (Sunshine Sentinel Press)

This subject is also reviewed in my audio cassette set, IS ASPARTAME (NUTRASWEET®) SAFE? A MEDICAL, PUBLIC HEALTH AND LEGAL OVERVIEW (Sunshine Sentinel Press).

AN OVERVIEW OF ASPARTAME

<u>Each of the three components of aspartame</u> – <u>phenylalanine; aspartic acid; the methyl ester, which promptly becomes free methyl alcohol or methanol</u> – <u>and their multiple breakdown products after exposure to heat or during prolonged storage is potentially toxic, especially to the developing brain.</u>

Such toxicity and other serious physiologic derangements are evidenced by the serious reactions that persons who used these products have suffered. The neurotoxic and metabolic complications are likely to affect the fetus and young children more severely.

In my publications, and testimony to Congress and an FDA advisory group, I expressed the belief that the current wholesale ingestion of aspartame products by over half the adult population constitutes an "imminent public health hazard." This concern is intensified by (1) evidence that these products may play a causative or aggravating role in many medical disorders (including headaches, dizziness, confusion, impaired vision, convulsions, and probably brain tumors), (2) the flawed nature of most "scientific" studies cited to "prove" the alleged safety of these products, and (3) reports of serious reactions volunteered to me and the FDA by thousands of irate consumers.

PREGNANT WOMEN AND NURSING MOTHERS

I urge ALL pregnant women and mothers who breast-feed to avoid aspartame products... without exception! This message also has been given to obstetricians.

The medical and scientific grounds for such advice include:

- Exposure of the fetus to considerable phenylalanine and methyl alcohol
- Maternal malnutrition associated with nausea, vomiting, diarrhea and reduced calories
- Transmission of aspartame and its byproducts via the mother's milk
- Increasing the "allergic load," thereby risking future hypersensitivity diseases

INFANTS AND CHILDREN

Many adverse effects of aspartame products have been experienced by young persons. They include severe headache, convulsions, rashes, asthma, gastrointestinal problems, and weight loss or gain. The neuropsychiatric features encompass irritability, hyperactivity, attention deficit, depression, antisocial behavior, deterioration of intelligence, poor school performance, and aspartame addiction.

These complications tend to be magnified in children with unrecognized hypothyroidism (underactive thyroid), hypoglycemia (low blood sugar reactions), diabetes, and phenylketonuria or PKU. Persons with PKU lack the enzyme needed for handling phenylalanine, which can cause severe neurological and other damage if dietary precautions aimed at preventing excessive levels are not instituted.

BIRTH DEFECTS

The issue of aspartame-related birth defects has not been resolved by reliable epidemiologic studies. I remain concerned about this possibility because of reports about severe problems in the fetus or infant of parents (including fathers) who consumed much aspartame at the time of conception and/or during pregnancy. Several animal studies support such concern.

APPENDIX D

PROFESSIONAL OPINION OF H. J. ROBERTS, M.D., F.A.C.P., F.C.C.P. CONCERNING THE USE OF PRODUCTS CONTAINING ASPARTAME BY PERSONS WITH EAR AND EQUILIBRIUM PROBLEMS

It is my opinion that individuals with the following symptoms who consume products containing aspartame – including diet sodas/foods, drugs and "supplements" – should avoid them when no specific cause can be found.

* "Ringing" or "buzzing" of the ears (tinnitus)... sometimes described
    as hissing, humming or whistling
* Marked intolerance to noise
* Impairment or loss of hearing
* Marked unsteadiness or dizziness

The same precaution is reasonable for persons in whom these complaints may be due to other disorders because the latter could be aggravated by aspartame, even in minimal amounts.

My corporate-neutral suggestions are based on considerable observations, research and correspondence published in more than a score of articles, and these titles:

* ASPARTAME DISEASE: AN IGNORED EPIDEMIC (Sunshine Sentinel Press,   P.O. Box 17799, West Palm Beach; FL 33416; 1-800-814-9800)
* ASPARTAME (NUTRASWEET®): IS IT SAFE? (Charles Press)
* SWEET'NER DEAREST: BITTERSWEET VIGNETTES ABOUT ASPARTAME (NUTRASWEET®) (Sunshine Sentinel Press)
* IS ASPARTAME (NUTRASWEET®) SAFE? A MEDICAL, PUBLIC HEALTH AND LEGAL OVERVIEW – audio cassette set (Sunshine Sentinel Press)

These represent hard-won insights in the trenches of medical practice. Patients and consumers should not be misled by the "negative" conclusions of flawed studies sponsored by vested interests.

There is no bias or malice intended against any company, distributor, researcher or professional who may hold contrary views.

THE ROLE OF ASPARTAME

Each of these components of aspartame – phenylalanine; aspartic acid; the methyl ester, which promptly becomes <u>free</u> methyl alcohol or methanol – and their multiple breakdown products after exposure to heat or during prolonged storage is potentially toxic to the brain and inner ear. These organs are highly vulnerable to metabolic disturbances and neurotoxins because of their unique metabolic requirements.

REPRESENTATIVE CASE REPORT

A 30-year-old woman drank five or more cups or glasses of aspartame beverages daily for 17 months. She experienced ringing and pain in both ears, dizziness, a severe headache, and considerable loss of hearing in the left ear by audiometric studies. When brain tumor was ruled out by CT scans, otology and neurology consultants made the diagnosis of Meniere's disease. The patient **herself** deduced that the aspartame sodas were responsible because she could <u>predictably</u> reproduce these symptoms on rechallenge with them.

AN OVERVIEW

In my publications, and in testimony to Congress and an FDA advisory group, I have expressed the belief that the current wholesale ingestion of aspartame products by over half the population constitutes an "imminent public health hazard." My concern is bolstered by (1) evidence that these products may play a causative or aggravating role in many other medical disorders (including headaches, dizziness, confusion, impaired vision, convulsions, and probably brain tumors), (2) the flawed nature of most "scientific" studies being cited to prove the alleged safety of these products, and (3) numerous reports of serious reactions volunteered to me and the FDA by thousands of irate consumers.

In the present context, these statistics are pertinent.

> *In my earlier report on 551 aspartame reactors (the data base is now doubled), dizziness was a major problem in 217 (39%), tinnitus in 73 (13%), severe intolerance for noise in 47, and marked impairment of hearing in 25.
> *The FDA (as of August 1995) had received complaints about dizziness and problems with balance from 737 consumers, and a change of hearing from 36.
> *The American Tinnitus Association was unable to find a cause for tinnitus in one-third of 18,000 sufferers.

These complications tend to be magnified in persons with unrecognized hypothyroidism (underactive thyroid), hypoglycemia (low blood sugar reactions), diabetes, hypertension, reactions to MSG, treatment with aspirin and other drugs that can irritate the auditory nerves, and problems associated with aging. They become compounded because of the threat of falls and driving accidents.

APPENDIX E

PROFESSIONAL OPINION OF H. J. ROBERTS, M.D., F.A.C.P., F.C.C.P. CONCERNING THE USE OF PRODUCTS CONTAINING ASPARTAME BY PERSONS WITH EYE PROBLEMS

It is my opinion that individuals who consume products containing aspartame – including diet sodas/foods, drugs and "supplements" – should avoid them when no specific cause can be found for these eye problems:

* Decreased vision or blindness in one or both eyes
* Blurring, "bright flashes"; tunnel vision; "black spots"
* Double vision
* Unexplained retinal detachment or bleeding
* Pain in one or both eyes
* Decreased tears
* Difficulty wearing contact lens

The same precaution is reasonable for persons in whom the above complaints may be due to other disorders because the latter could be aggravated by aspartame, even in minimal amounts.

* Surgery of immature cataracts should be deferred in patients who consume aspartame until after they have abstained from it for at least 2 months to determine if spontaneous improvement of vision occurs.
* Impaired vision of diabetic patients who consume these products should not be assumed to represent diabetic retinopathy without a "no aspartame test" trial.
* A similar trial is warranted in persons diagnosed as having "macular degeneration."
* The diagnosis of "early multiple sclerosis," based on concomitant eye and neurologic features, should be deferred pending a "no aspartame test."

These corporate-neutral suggestions are based on considerable observation, research and correspondence published in more than a score of articles, and these titles:

* ASPARTAME DISEASE: AN IGNORED EPIDEMIC (Sunshine Sentinel Press, P.O. Box 17799, West Palm Beach; FL 33416; 1-800-814-9800
* ASPARTAME (NUTRASWEET®): IS IT SAFE? (Charles Press)
* SWEET'NER DEAREST: BITTERSWEET VIGNETTES ABOUT ASPARTAME (NUTRASWEET®) (Sunshine Sentinel Press)
* IS ASPARTAME (NUTRASWEET®) SAFE? A MEDICAL, PUBLIC HEALTH AND LEGAL OVERVIEW – audio cassette set (Sunshine Sentinel Press)

These represent hard-won insights in the trenches of medical practice. Patients and consumers should not be misled by the "negative" conclusions of flawed studies sponsored by vested interests.

There is no bias or malice intended against any company, distributor, researcher or professional who may hold contrary views.

THE ROLE OF ASPARTAME

Each of the components of aspartame – phenylalanine (50%); aspartic acid (40%); the methyl ester, which promptly becomes <u>free</u> methyl alcohol or methanol (10%) – and their multiple breakdown products after exposure to heat or during prolonged storage are potentially toxic to the retina and optic nerves. These organs are highly vulnerable to metabolic disturbances and neurotoxins because of their unique metabolism. Methanol, a severe metabolic poison, causes swelling of the optic nerve and degeneration of ganglion cells in the retina.

Particular attention is directed in this regard to the formaldehyde and formate (formic acid) that result from the breakdown of methyl alcohol, and the D-aspartic acid stereoisomer.

AN OVERVIEW

In my publications, and in testimony to Congress and an FDA advisory group, I have expressed the belief that the current wholesale ingestion of aspartame products by over half the adult population constitutes a probable "imminent public health hazard." My concern is bolstered by (1) evidence that these products may play a causative or aggravating role in many other medical disorders (including headaches, dizziness, confusion, memory loss, impaired hearing, ringing in the ears, convulsions, and brain tumors), (2) the flawed nature of most "scientific" studies being cited as evidence for the alleged safety of these products, and (3) reports of serious reactions volunteered to me and the FDA by thousands of irate consumers.

In the present context, these statistics are pertinent.

* In my series of 1,200 aspartame reactors, decreased vision was a major problem in 302 (25%), severe pain in 87 (7%), and "dry eyes" or trouble wearing contact lens in 95 (8%). Furthermore, 27 lost vision in one or both eyes.

* The FDA (as of August 1995) had received complaints about change in vision from 384 consumers, and "eye irritation" from 30.

These complications tend to be magnified in persons with diabetes, hypertension, unrecognized hypothyroidism (underactive thyroid), hypoglycemia (low blood sugar), MSG reactions, treatment with drugs that can damage the optic and auditory nerves, individuals who smoke or drink alcohol, and problems associated with aging. They are compounded by the threat of falls and driving accidents.

© 2001 H. J. Roberts, M.D.

APPENDIX F

PROFESSIONAL OPINION OF H. J. ROBERTS, M.D., F.A.C.P., F.C.C.P.
CONCERNING ASPARTAME DISEASE
SIMULATING MULTIPLE SCLEROSIS

Aspartame disease refers to symptoms and signs attributable to the use of products containing aspartame, a chemical commonly known as NutraSweet® and Equal®. In my opinion, it afflicts many consumers of such products based on a database of over 1,200 aspartame reactors, extensive research, and the many thousands of complaints volunteered by consumers to the Food and Drug Administration (FDA). Over half of adults in the U.S. currently consume aspartame!

The areas most vulnerable to aspartame are the brain, eyes, inner ear and peripheral nerves. Frequent clinical features include headache, dizziness, poor equilibrium, confusion, impaired vision or double vision, convulsions, ringing in the ears, slurred speech, tremors, extreme fatigue, motor and sensory disturbances affecting the limbs, and other neuropsychiatric complaints.

I have encountered scores of patients with aspartame disease in whom combinations of these features were diagnosed as multiple sclerosis. This has been particularly impressive in the case of weight-conscious young women using considerable aspartame as soft drinks, tabletop sweeteners, and gum. The causative or contributing role of aspartame was indicated by (1) dramatic improvement within several days or weeks after avoiding aspartame products, and (2) the prompt and predictable recurrence of complaints after resuming aspartame (often inadvertently).

Each component of aspartame - phenylalanine (50%); aspartic acid (40%); the methyl ester, which promptly becomes free methyl alcohol or methanol (10%) - and their multiple breakdown products after exposure to heat or during prolonged storage are potentially toxic to the brain, retina and nerves.

The details appear in ASPARTAME DISEASE: AN IGNORED EPIDEMIC, my audio cassette set, IS ASPARTAME (NUTRASWEET®) SAFE? A MEDICAL, PUBLIC HEALTH AND LEGAL OVERVIEW, and SWEET'NER DEAREST: BITTERSWEET VIGNETTES ABOUT ASPARTAME (NUTRASWEET®) – all published by the Sunshine Sentinel Press (P.O. Box 17799, West Palm Beach, Florida 33416; 1-800-814-9800).

An erroneous diagnosis of multiple sclerosis can penalize persons in numerous ways. Accordingly, it is my opinion that the diagnosis of "early" multiple sclerosis should not be made in individuals consuming aspartame products until they have been observed for many months after total abstinence. Some minor finding by imaging (CT or MRI) scans of the brain does not justify this diagnosis in an aspartame reactor.

APPENDIX G

PROFESSIONAL OPINION OF H. J. ROBERTS, M.D.,   F.A.C.P., F.C.C.P.
CONCERNING CARDIAC AND CHEST COMPLAINTS
ATTRIBUTABLE TO ASPARTAME

Many patients and correspondents have inquired whether products containing aspartame can cause or aggravate symptoms relating to the heart, blood pressure and chest. Based on my experience, as detailed in multiple publications and books (see below), the answer is YES.

Hundreds of such instances have been documented in my database of over 1,200 aspartame reactors. There was dramatic improvement after avoiding aspartame, and a prompt and predictable recurrence of these problems when the patient resumed aspartame products... knowingly or inadvertently.

ABNORMAL HEART ACTION

190 (16%) reactors experienced detectable changes in their heart rate or rhythm after consuming aspartame – including gum – and products that did not contain caffeine. They consisted of "fluttering" (palpitations), skipped beats, and rapid heart action (tachycardia). A number underwent heart monitoring (Holter testing) and other studies, especially when there had been associated weakness and faint.

One patient developed a slow pulse and complete heart block within hours after consuming an aspartame drink for the **first** time. His attack spontaneously subsided within one day (without requiring a pacemaker). There has been no recurrence with aspartame avoidance.

This subject has relevance to reports of unexplained sudden death in persons who had been consuming considerable aspartame.

HYPERTENSION

64 aspartame reactors were found to have elevation of their blood pressure – systolic, diastolic, or both. Some were in their twenties. While aspartame products unequivocally cause headache, superimposed hypertension can be a contributing factor.

Other patients who had been treated for hypertension could not be adequately controlled on their maintenance medication as long as they used aspartame. This reflects its interaction with various drugs. (Aspartame was originally devised as a drug to treat peptic ulcer.)

The rapid heart action and the elevation of blood pressure presumably reflect the effects of phenylalanine (an aspartame component) and its metabolic products – dopamine, norepinephrine and epinephrine.

ATYPICAL CHEST PAIN

85 aspartame reactors (7%) experienced unexplained pain in the chest. (Many others have atypical pain

elsewhere in the body.) A number were subjected to stress tests and angiography for coronary heart disease, which proved normal in the majority.

SHORTNESS OF BREATH

110 aspartame reactors (9%) who complained of otherwise-unexplained "shortness of breath" promptly improved after avoiding these products. They predictably suffered a recurrence on rechallenge.

Clinical <u>sleep apnea</u> dramatically stopped in three patients after they avoided aspartame.

RELATED COMMENTS

I asserted in my publications, testimony to Congress, and letters to Congressmen and the FDA that the current wholesale ingestion of aspartame products by over half the adult population constitutes an"imminent public health hazard" because of the frequency and severity of reactions to them. This warning should be of particular concern for high-risk groups – most notably, patients with diabetes and hypoglycemia, pregnant women, children, patients with epilepsy, liver, heart, kidney disease and eating disorders, older persons with memory impairment, the relatives of aspartame reactors, and patients having phenylketonuria.

These issues are elaborated in ASPARTAME DISEASE: AN IGNORED EPIDEMIC, and SWEET'NER DEAREST: BITTERSWEET VIGNETTES ABOUT ASPARTAME (NUTRASWEET®) (Sunshine Sentinel Press, P.O. Box 17799, West Palm Beach, Florida 33416, 1-800-814-9800), and ASPARTAME (NUTRASWEET®): IS IT SAFE? (Charles Press). They are summarized in my audio cassette set, IS ASPARTAME (NUTRASWEET®) SAFE? A MEDICAL, PUBLIC HEALTH AND LEGAL OVERVIEW (Sunshine Sentinel Press).

APPENDIX H

PROFESSIONAL OPINION OF H. J. ROBERTS, M.D., F.A.C.P., F.C.C.P. CONCERNING ALLERGIC REACTIONS TO PRODUCTS CONTAINING ASPARTAME

Allergic reactions occurred in one-fifth of 1,200 aspartame reactors in my database. They include hives (urticaria), severe itching, lupus erythematosus-type rashes, other skin eruptions (including yeast infections in women), marked swelling of the lips, tongue and throat, the aggravation of upper and lower respiratory tract allergies, and severe swelling of the salivary glands.

These relationships were documented by improvement on ceasing such products, and their prompt recurrence on rechallenge – deliberate or inadvertent.

The FDA has reported comparable reactions among over 7300 aspartame reactions who volunteered their case histories to this agency (Department of Health and Human Services: Summary of Adverse Reactions Attributed to Aspartame, April 20, 1995).

These reactions may reflect sensitivity to the aspartame molecule, its three components, or the multiple breakdown metabolites (including stereoisomers and the diketopiperazine derivative) during heating and prolonged storage. The latter are likely to be absent when aspartame is administered as a capsule or freshly prepared cool solution in "scientific" studies being cited used to reassure concerned consumers.

I also have warned the FDA of dual sensitivities to both aspartame and monosodium glutamate (MSG), especially as convulsions (Testimony to Federation of American Societies for Experimental Biology: Analysis of Adverse Reactions to Monosodium Glutamate. Bethesda. April 8, 1993).

RELATED COMMENTS

These issues are elaborated in ASPARTAME DISEASE: AN IGNORED EPIDEMIC, and SWEET'NER DEAREST: BITTERSWEET VIGNETTES ABOUT ASPARTAME (NUTRASWEET®) (Sunshine Sentinel Press, P.O. Box 17799, West Palm Beach, Florida 33416, 1-800-814-9800), and ASPARTAME (NUTRASWEET®): IS IT SAFE? (Charles Press). They also are summarized in my audio cassette set, IS ASPARTAME (NUTRASWEET®) SAFE? A MEDICAL, PUBLIC HEALTH AND LEGAL OVERVIEW (Sunshine Sentinel Press).

APPENDIX I

PROFESSIONAL OPINIONS OF H. J. ROBERTS, M.D., F.A.C.P., F.C.C.P. CONCERNING SACCHARIN AND ASPARTAME LABELING

I. THE LISTING OF SACCHARIN AS A CANCER-CAUSING AGENT

A subcommittee of the National Toxicology Program's Board of Scientific Counselors voted on October 31, 1997 to keep saccharin on the federal government's list of cancer-causing substances. As a corporate-neutral physician and researcher, I question this decision.

The committee also demonstrated reluctance to remove an unwarranted cancer scare that exists on the labels of saccharin products. This attitude now seems inappropriate, especially when based largely on studies involving a few male rats that developed urinary bladder tumors after receiving large amounts of saccharin. They are unconvincing for the following reasons:

* Use of this rat model has been challenged.
* Humans lack a critical protein in the urine that causes saccharin to form jagged irritating crystals in the male-rat bladder.
* There has been no convincing increase in the frequency of urinary bladder cancer since the introduction of saccharin over a century ago.
* A 23-year monkey study failed to evidence a cancer-causing effect of saccharin in primates.

II. THE ISSUE OF ASPARTAME LABELING

I believe that the FDA ought to recommend the removal of products containing aspartame as an "imminent public health hazard." This is based on the chemical's adverse neurotoxic, metabolic, fetotoxic and probable carcinogenic effects.

Short of such action, aspartame products ought to carry labels indicating their potential adverse effects for high-risk individuals. They include pregnant women; infants; children; (older) persons with memory problems; patients with migraine, epilepsy, multiple sclerosis, diabetes, hypoglycemia, hypertension, hypothyroidism (underactive thyroid), and liver/kidney disease; and the relatives of persons with aspartame disease.

Labels also should mention brain tumors. The FDA's arbitrary approval of aspartame in 1981 had been delayed a number of years because of the **high** incidence of brain tumors among animals given aspartame.

The details for these observations and conclusions appear in my publications. They include ASPARTAME DISEASE: AN IGNORED EPIDEMIC, SWEET'NER DEAREST: BITTERSWEET VIGNETTES ABOUT ASPARTAME (NUTRASWEET®) (Sunshine Sentinel Press, P.O. Box 17799, West Palm Beach, Florida 33416, 1-800-814-9800), and ASPARTAME (NUTRASWEET®): IS IT SAFE? (Charles Press). They are summarized in an audio cassette set, IS ASPARTAME (NUTRASWEET®) SAFE? A MEDICAL, PUBLIC HEALTH AND LEGAL OVERVIEW (Sunshine Sentinel Press).

BIBLIOGRAPHY

Abelson, P. H.: Dietary carcinogens. *Science* 1983; 221:1249.

Abrams, F. R.: Patient advocate or secret agent? *Journal of the American Medical Association* 1986; 256:1784-1785.

Adamkiewicz, V. W.: Glycemia and immune responses. *Canadian Medical Association Journal* 1963; 88:806.

Adamsons, K.: Obesity and Fad Diets. Testimony for the U.S. Senate Select Committee on Nutrition and Human Needs, April 12, 1973, p. 34.

Agnati, L. F., et al.: Evidence for cholecystokinin-dopamine receptor interactions in the central nervous system of the adult and old rat. In *Neuronal Cholecystokinin*, edited by J. Vanderhaegagn and J. N. Crawley, *Annals of the New York Academy of Sciences* 1985; 448:315-333.

Alexander, E.: Cited by *Medical Tribune* November 1986, p.11.

Allen v. United States, 588 F.Supp. 246, 416-18 (D. Utah 1984, rev'd on other grounds, 816 F.2d 1417 (10th Cir. 1987), cert. denied, 484 U.S. 1004 (1988).

Altman, L.: Leaked story raises questions about medical journal's power. *The Palm Beach Post* January 29, 1988, p. E-5.

Altschule, M. D.: Hypothesis in medicine. *Medical Science* 1966; 17:94.

American Cancer Society. Cancer Prevention Study II: An epidemiological study of lifestyles and environment. *CPS II Newsletter*, Spring, 4/1:3, 1986.

American Diabetes Association: Position Statement: Use of Noncaloric Sweeteners. *Diabetes Care* 1987; 10:526.

Amiel, S. A., et al.: Effect of antecedent glucose control on cerebral function during hypoglycemia. *Diabetes Care* 1991; 14:109-118.

Anderson, A. E., Watson, T., Schlechte, J.: Osteoporosis and osteopenia in men with eating disorders. *Lancet* 2000; 355:1967-1968.

Anderson, J. W., Zettwoch, N., Feldman, T., et al.: Cholesterol-lowering effects of psyllium hydrophilic mucilloid for hypercholesterolemic men. *Archives of Internal Medicine* 1988; 148:292-296.

Anderson, K. K., Perez, G. L., Fisher, G. H., Man, E. H.: Effect of aluminum ingestion on aspartame racemization in the protein of rat brain. *Neuroscience Research Communications* 1990; 6:45-50.

Angell, M.: Do breast implants cause systemic disease? *New England Journal of Medicine* 1994; 330:1748-1749.

Angell, M.: Reply by Dr. Angell. *New England Journal of Medicine* 1996; 335:1154-1156.

Angell, M.: Is academic medicine for sale? *New England Journal of Medicine* 2000:342:1516-1518.

Angell, M., Utiger, R. D., Wood, A. J. J.: Disclosure of authors' conflicts of interest: A follow-up. *New England Journal of Medicine* 2000; 342:586-587.

Antener, L., Verwilghen, A. M., Vangeert, C., Mauron, J.: Biochemical study of malnutrition. 5. Metabolism of phenylalanine and tyrosine. *International Journal of Vitamin and Nutrition Research* 1981; 51:296-306.

Antonios, T. F. T., MacGregor, G. A.; Salt – more adverse effects. *Lancet* 1996; 348:250-251.

Associated Press: Feature. *The Palm Beach Post* 1995; June 17:A-2.

Atkinson, R. L.: Opioid regulation of food intake and body weight in humans. *Federation Proceedings* 1987; 46(1):178-182.

Atroshi, I., Gummesson, C., Johnsson, R., et al.: Prevalence of carpal tunnel syndrome in a general population. *Journal of the American Medical Association.* 1999; 282:153-158.

Avoli, M., Olivier, A.: Bursting in human epileptogenic neocortex is depressed by an N-methyl-D-aspartate antagonist. *Neurosciences Letter* 1987; 76:249-254.

Awata, T., Kuzuya, T., Matsuda, A., et al.: High frequency of aspartic acid at position 57 of HLA-DQ β-chain in Japanese IDDM patients and non-diabetic subjects. *Diabetes* 1990; 39:266-269.

Ballinger v. Atkins 947 F. Supp. 1925 (December 16, 1996).

Bandow, D.: Many torts later, the case against implants collapses. *The Wall Street Journal* November 30, 1998, A-23.

Barbehenn, E. K.: Book review. *Lancet* 1998; 352:1155.

Barker, R.: *And The Waters Turned to Blood: The Ultimate Biological Threat.* New York, Simon & Schuster, 1997.

Barnes, E. A.: Some causes of congenital deformities. *Journal of the American Medical Association* 1897; 29:1298-1301.

995

Barson v. E. R. Squibb & Sons, Inc., 682 P.2d 832 (Utah 1984).

Baumbach, F. L., Cancilla, P. A. Martin-Amat, G., Tephly, T. R., McMartin, K. E., Maker, A. B., Hayreh, M. S.: Methyl alcohol poisoning. IV. Alterations of the morphological findings of the retina and the optic nerve. *Archives of Ophthalmology* 1977, 95:1859-1865.

Beckman, H. B., Frankel, R. M.: The effect of physician behavior on the collection of data. *Annals of Internal Medicine* 1984; 101:692-696.

Bender, D. A.: *Amino Acid Metabolism.* Chichester/New York, Wiley, 2nd Edition, 1985.

Bender, R., Jockel, K., Trautner, C., Berger, M.: Effect of age on excess mortality in obesity. *Journal of the American Medical Association* 1999; 281:1498-1504.

Ben-Shlemo, D., et al.: Enhancement of glucose uptake in a muscle cell line: A mechanism for phenylpyruvic induced hypoglycemia and mental retardation in phenylketonuria. Presented at 81st Annual Meeting of the Endocrine Society, San Diego, June 12, 1999, P3-127.

Bennett, I. L., Jr., Nation, T. C., Olley, J. F.: Pancreatitis in methyl alcohol poisoning. *Journal of Laboratory and Clinical Medicine* 1952; 40:405-409.

Bennett, I. L., Jr., Carey, F. H., Mitchell, G. L., Jr., Cooper, M. N.: Acute methyl alcohol poisoning. A review based on experiences in an outbreak of 323 cases. *Medicine* 1952; 32:431.

Berger, M.: Safety of insulin glargine. *The Lancet* 2000;356:2013-2014.

Berkovitz v. United States, 100 L.Ed.2d 531 (1988).

Bernard, C.: *Introduction to the Study of Experimental Medicine.* MacMillan Publishing Company, New York, 1927, p. 82.

Bigby, M., Gick, S., Gick, H., Arndt, K.: Drug-induced outaneous reactions. *Journal of the American Medical Association* 1986; 256:3358-3360.

Blackburn, H.: Olestra and the FDA. *New England Journal of Medicine* 1996; 334:984-986.

Blair, E. H., Hoerger, F. D.: Risk/benefit analysis as viewed by the chemical industry. In *Public Control of Environmental Health Hazards,* edited by E. C. Hammond and I. J. Selikoff, *Annals of the New York Academy of Sciences* 1979; 329:253-262.

Blum v Merrell Dow Pharmaceuticals, Common Pleas, 1927 (Phil Ct 1996).

Blumenthal, F., Lundin, A. P.: The safety of di(2-ethylhexyl) phthalate in patients receiving hemodialysis treatment. *Journal of the American Medical Association* 1986; 256:2817-2818.

Blumenthal, H. J., Vance, D. A.: Chewing gum headaches. *Headache* 1997; 37:685-686.

Blundell, J. E., Hill, A. J.: Paradoxical effects of an intense sweetener (aspartame) on appetite. *Lancet* 1986; 1:1092-1093.

Blundell, J. E., Hill, A. J., Rogers, P. J.: Effects of aspartame on appetite and food intake. In *Proceedings of the First International Meeting on Dietary Phenylalanine and Brain Function,* edited by R. J. Wurtman and E. Ritter-Walker, Washington, D.C., May 8-10, 1987, pp. 299-309.

Boecker, H., Brooks, D. J.: Functional imaging of tremor. *Movement Disorders* 1998; 13 (Supplement 3):64-72.

Boehm, M. F., Bada, J.L.: Racemization of aspartic acid and phenylalanine in the sweetener aspartame at 100°C. *Proceedings of the National Academy of Sciences USA* 1984; 81:5263-5266.

Bombeck, E.: Give me some real motivation to be thin. *The Palm Beach Post* December 11, 1988, p. F-12.

Borgstein, J.: The end of the clinical anecdote. *Lancet* 1999; 354:2151-2152.

Bortz, W. P. M., Howat, P., Holmes, W. L.: The effect of feeding frequency on diurnal plasma free fatty acids and glucose levels. *Metabolism* 1969; 18:120.

Bowie, J. U., Reidhaar-Olson, J. F., Lim, W. A., Sauer, R. T.: Deciphering the message in protein sequences: Tolerance to amino acid substitutions. *Sciences* 1990; 247:1306-1310.

Brayne, C., Calloway, D.: Normal ageing, impaired cognitive function, and senile dementia of the Alzheimer's type: A continuum? *Lancet* 1988; 1:1265-1266.

Brent, J., McMartin, K., Phillips, S., et al: Fomepizole for the treatment of methanol poisoning. *New England Journal of Medicine* 2001;344:424-429.

Bressler, J., et al.: FDA Report on Searle. August 4, 1977.

Bridges, A. J., Conley, C., Wang, G., et al.: A clinical and immunologic evaluation of women with silicone breast implants and symptoms of rheumatic disease. *Annals of Internal Medicine* 1993; 118:929-936.

Broad, W. J.: Fraud and the structure of sciences. *Sciences* 1981; 212:137-141.

Brosens, J. J., Mak, I. Y., White, J. O.: Interaction between cyclic AMP and progesterone in the activation of the decidual prolactin promoter in human endometrial stromal cells. Presented at 81st Annual Meeting of the Endocrine Society, San Diego, June 12, 1999, OR26-4.

Brown, E. S., Waisman, H. A., Swanson, M.A., Colwell, R. E., Banks, M. E., Gerritson, T.: Effects of oral contraceptives and obesity on carrier tests for phenylketonuria. *Clinica Chimica Acta* 1973; 44:183-192.

Brown, W. D.: Present knowledge of protein nutrition, Part 3, *Postgraduate Medicine* 1967; April:119-126.

Brownstein, N. J., Rehfeld, J. F.: Molecular forms of cholecystokinin in the nervous system. In *Neuronal Cholecystokinin*, edited by J. Vanderheagagn and J. N. Crawley, *Annals of the New York Academy of Sciences* 1985; 448:9-10.

Brunner, R. L., Vorhees, C. V., Kinney, L., Butcher, R. E.: Aspartame: Assessment of developmental psychotoxicity of a new sweetener. *Neurobehavioral Toxicology* 1979; 1:79-86.

Bryan, G. T.: Artificial sweeteners and bladder cancer: Assessment of carcinogenicity of aspartame and its diketopiperazine derivative in mice. In *Aspartame: Physiology and Biochemistry*, edited by L. D. Steqink and L. J. Filer, Jr., Marcel Dekker, Inc., New York, 1984, pp. 321-348.

Burget, S. L., Andersen, D. W., Steqink, L. D., et al.: Aspartame and phenylalanine methyl ester metabolism by the porcine gut. (Abstract) *Clinical Research* 1984; 32:762.

Bryson, D. D.: Health hazards of formaldehyde. *Lancet* 1981; 1:1263.

Burton, T. M.: Implant makers get a boost from report. *The Wall Street Journal* December 2, 1998, B-1,4.

Butcher, S. P., Bulleck, R., Graham, D. R., McCulloch, J.: Correlation between amino acid release and neuropathologic outcome in rat brain following middle cerebral artery occlusion. *Stroke* 1990; 21:1727-1733.

Caballero, D., Wurtman, R. J.: Control of plasma phenylalanine levels. In *Proceedings of the First International Meeting on Dietary Phenylalanine and Brain Function*, edited by R. J. Wurtman, Washington, D.C. May 8-10, 1987, pp. 9-23.

Caballero, D., Gleason, R. E., Wurtman, R. J.: Plasma amino acid concentrations in healthy elderly men and women. *American Journal of Clinical Nutrition* 1991; 53:1249-1252.

Caldecott, R.: Cited by *Science Newsletter* November 18, 1961.

Callaway, C. W.: Nutrition. *Journal of the American Medical Association* 1986; 256:2097-2098.

Callander, T. J.: Multiple chemical sensitivity syndrome and neurological abnormalities. (Abstract) 26th Annual Meeting, American Academy of Environmental Medicine, Jacksonville, October 28, 1991, p. 19.

Camfield, P. R., Camfield, C. S., Dooley, J. M., et al.: Aspartame exacerbates EEG spike-wave discharge in children with generalized absence epilepsy: A double-blind controlled study. *Neurology* 1992; 42:1000-1003.

Campbell, E.G., Louis, K. S., Blumenthal, D.: Looking a gift horse in the mouth. *Journal of the American Medical Association* 1998; 279-995-999.

Carlson, H. E., Hyman, D. B., Blitzer, M. G.: Evidence for an intracerebral action of phenylalanine in stimulation of prolactin secretion: Interaction of large neutral amino acids. *Journal of Clinical Endocrinology and Metabolism* 1990; 70:814-816.

Ceci, F., et al.: Oral 5-hydroytryptophan promotes weight loss in bulimic obese subjects. *Clinical Research* 1986; 34:866A.

Centers for Disease Control: Evaluation of consumer complaints related to aspartame use. *Morbidity and Mortality Weekly Report* 1984;(Nov 2):605-7.

Centers for Disease Control: Prevalence of chronic migraine headaches – United States, 1988-1989. *Morbidity and Mortality Weekly Report* 1991; May 24, 331-338.

Chalmers, I.: Underreporting research in scientific misconduct. *Journal of the American Medical Association* 1990; 263:1405-1408.

Chapman, A. G., Engelsen, B., Meldrum, B. S.: 2-Amino-7-phosphonoheptanoic acid inhibits insulin-induced convulsions and striatal aspartate accumulation in rats with frontal cortical ablation. *Journal of Neurochemistry* 1987; 49:121-127.

Charnley, G.: Book review. *American Scientist* 2000; 88:366.

Choi, T. B., Yang, J., Pardridge, W. M.: Phenylalanine transport at the human-blood-brain barrier: Studies with isolated brain capillaries. *Diabetes* 1986; 35 (Suppl.1):196.

Christensen, H. N.: Dual role of transport competition in amino acid deprivation of the nervous system. In *Proceedings of the First International Meeting on Dietary Phenylalanine and Brain Function*, edited by R. J. Wurtman and E. Ritter-Walker, Washington, D.C., May 8-10, 1987, pp. 95-104.

Clapp, R., Ozonoff, D.: Where the boys aren't: Dioxin and the sex ratio. *Lancet* 2000; 35:1838-1839.

Clark, L. H., Jr.: How protectionism soured the sugar market. *The Wall Street Journal* November 4, 1987, p. 36.

Claybrook, J.: Going public about defective products. *Trial* November 1989, pp. 34-36.

Cloninger, M. R., Baldwin, R. E.: Aspartylphenylalanine methyl ester: A low calorie sweetener. *Science* 170:81, 1970.

Cohen, S.: Cited by *The Palm Beach Post* April 9, 1992, p. A-2.

Cole, G. C., Wilkins, P. R., West, R. R.: An epidemiological survey of primary tumors of the brain and spinal cord in South East Wales. *British Journal of Neurosurgery* 1989; 3:487-493.

Collings, M.: Testimony for the Committee on Labor and Human Resources, U.S. Senate, Hearing on *"NutraSweet"-Health and Safety Concerns*, November 3, 1987. 83-178, U.S. Government Printing Office, Washington, 1988, pp. 305-307.

Committee Nutrition Institute, et al. V. Dr. Mark Novitch, Acting Commissioner, Food and Drug Administration, United States court of Appeals for the District of Columbia Circuit (fill in)

a. Congressional Record-Senate: *Saccharin Study and Labeling Act Amendments of 1985*. 1985; 131(May 7):S 5489-5519.

b. Congressional Record-Senate: *Aspartame Safety Act*. 1985; 131(August 1):S 10820-10847.

Cook, R. R., Delongchamp, R. R., Woodbury, M. A., et al.: The prevalence of woman with breast implants in the United States – 1989. *Journal of Clinical Epidemiology* 1995; 48:519-525.

Coon, J. J.: Food toxicology: Safety of food additives. *Modern Medicine* 1970; November 30:105.

Cornell, R. G., Wolfe, R. A., Sanders, P. G.: Aspartame and brain tumors: Statistical issues. In *Aspartame: Physiology and Biochemistry*, edited by L. D. Stegink and L. J. Filer, Jr., Marcel Dekker, Inc., New York, 1984, pp. 459-479.

Council of Scientific Affairs: Aspartame: Review of safety issues. *Journal of the American Medical Association* 1985; 254:400-402.

Coyle, J.: More dimensions for glutamate toxicity. Cited by *Science* 1988; 242:1509-1510.

Craft, I. L., Peters, T. J.: Quantitative changes on plasma amino acids induced by oral contraceptives. *Clinical Science* 1971; 41:301-307.

Crawley, J. N.: Comparative distribution of cholecystokinin and other neuropeptides. In *Neuronal Cholecystokinin*, edited by J. Vanderhaegagn and J. N. Crawley, *Annals of the New York Academy of Sciences* 1985; 448:1-8.

Cross, A. J., Slater, D., Simpson, M., et al.: Sodium dependent D- (3H) aspartame binding in cerebral cortex in patients with Alzheimer's and Parkinson's disease. *Neurosciences Letter* 1987; 79:213-217.

Csernansky, J. G., Bardgett, M. E., Sheline, Y. I., Miorris, J. C., Olney, J. W.: CSF excitatory amino acids and severity of illness in Alzheimer's disease. *Neurology* 1996; 46:1715-1720.

Curran, D. A., Lance, J. W.: Clinical trial of methysergide and other preparations in management of migraine. *Journal of Neurology, Neurosurgery & Psychiatry* 1964; 27:463.

Cutter, E.: Address on dietetics – medical food ethics now and to come. *Journal of the American Medical Association* 1893; 20:239-244.

D'Adamo, A. F., Jr., Yatsu, F. M.: Acetate metabolism in the nervous system. $\underline{N}$-acetyl-L-aspartic acid and the biosynthesis of brain lipids. *Journal of Neurochemistry* 1966; 13:961-965.

D'Arienzo v. Clairol, Inc., 310 A2d 106 (1973).

a. Davoli, E., et al.: Serum methanol concentrations in rats and in men after a single dose of aspartame. *Food and Chemical Toxicology* 1986; 24:187-189.

b. Davoli, E., et al.: Trace analysis of methanol in rat serum by headspace high resolution gas chromatography/selected ion monitoring. *Journal of Chomatographic Science* 1986; 24:113-116.

Department of Health and Human Services. Summary of Adverse Reactions Attributed to Aspartame. April 20, 1995.

Deschodt-Lanckman, M.: Enzymatic degradation of cholecystokinin in the central nervous system. In *Neuronal Cholecystokinin*, edited by J. Vanderhaegagn and J. N. Crawley, *Annals of the New York Academy of Sciences* 1985; 448:87-98.

Devesa, S. S., Blot, W. J., Stone, B. J., et al.: Recent cancer trends in the United States. *Journal of the National Center Institute* 1995; 87:172-182.

998

Devinsky, O.: Patients with refractory seizures. *New England Journal of Medicine* 1999; 340:1565-1570.

De Vivo, D. C., et al.: Defective glucose transport across the blood-brain barrier as a cause of persistent hypoglycorrhachia, seizures, and developmental delay. *New England Journal of Medicine* 1991; 325: 703-709.

Dews, P.: Testimony for the Committee on Labor and Human Resources, U.S. Senate, Hearing on *"NutraSweet"-Health and Safety Concerns* November 3, 1987. 83-178, U.S. Government Printing Office, Washington, 1988, pp. 374-376.

Diaz-Sanchez, D., Morimoto, S., Peza, N. M., et al.: Testosterone effect on insulin biosynthesis, mRNA levels, promoter activity and secretion. Presented at 81st Annual Meeting of the Endocrine Society, San Diego, June 12, 1999, P1-268.

Dhont, J. L., Kapatos, G., Parniak, M., Wilgus, H., Kaufman, S.: Biopterin metabolism and phenylalanine hydroxylase activity during early liver regeneration. *Biochemical and Biophysical Research Communications* 1982; 106:786-793.

Diamanti-Kandarakis, E., Kouli, C., Vergiele, A., et al.: Hyperinsulinemia and breast cancer: Evidence of postreceptor defect in insulin action. Presented at 81st Annual Meeting of the Endocrine Society, San Diego, June 12, 1999, P3-199.

Dingell, J. D.: Shattuck lecture – misconduct in medical research. *New England Journal of Medicine* 1993; 328:1610-1615.

Dolan, G., Godin, C.: Phenylalanine toxicity in rats. *Canadian Journal of Biochemistry* 1966; 44:143-145.

Dong, B. J., Hauck, W. W., Gambertoglio, J. G., et al.: Bioequivalence of generic and brand-name levothyroine products in the treatment of hypothyroidism. *Journal of the American Medical Association* 1997; 277:1205-1213.

Downham, T. F. II: Possible hypersensitivity reactions to aspartame. *Clinical Cases in Dermatology* 1992;4 (Number 4):12-15.

Downie, R.S., McNaughton, J.: *Clinical Judgement: Evidence in Practice.* New York, Oxford University Press, 2000.

Dozio, N., Sarugeri, E, Scavini, M., et al.: Insulin receptor antibodies inhibit insulin uptake by the liver. *Journal of Investigative Medicine* 2001; 49(#1): 85-92.

Drake, M. E.: Panic attacks and excessive aspartame ingestion. *Lancet* 1986; 2:631.

Duffy, J.: Eosinophilia-myalgia syndrome. *Mayo Clinic Proceedings* 1992; 67:1201-1202.

Dunbar, P. V.: Statement to the U.S. House of Representatives Select Committee to Investigate the Use of Chemicals in Food Products, 81st Congress, 2nd Session, 1950.

During, N. J., Acworth, I. N., Wurtman, R. J.: An in vivo study of dopamine release in iron striatum: The effects of phenylalanine. In *Proceedings of the First International Meeting on Dietary Phenylalanine and Brain Function*, edited by R. J. Wurtman and E. Ritter-Walker, Washington, D.C., May 8-10, 1987, pp. 395-403.

Eby, N. L, Grufferman, S., Flannelly, C. M., et al.: Increasing incidence of primary brain lymphoma in the U.S. *Cancer* 1988; 62:22461-22465.

Ebner, S. A., Badonnel, M., Altman, L. K., Braverman, L. E.: Conjugal Graves disease. *Annals of Internal Medicine* 1992; 116:479-481.

Edmundson, A. B., Manion, C. B.: Treatment of osteoarthritis with aspartame. *Clinical Pharmacology & Therapeutics* 1998; 63:580-593.

Eelos, J. T., et al.: Formate-induced alterations in retinal function in methanol-intoxicated rats. *Toxicology and Applied Pharmacology* 1996; 140:58-69.

Ehrlich, J. P.: Cholesterol awareness. (Editorial) *Medical Tribune* November 11, 1987, p. 32.

Eichenwald, K., Kolata, G.: Drug trials hide conflicts for doctors. *The New York Times* May 16, 1999, pp. 1, 28.

Elble, R. J.: Origins of tremor. *Lancet* 2000; 355:1113-1114.

Elliott, K. A. C., Page, I. H., Quastel, J. H.: *Neurochemistry.* Charles C Thomas, Springfield, 1962.

Elsas, L. J., II, and Trotter, J. F.: Changes in physiological concentrations of blood phenylalanine-produced changes in sensitive parameters of human brain function. In *Proceedings of the First International Meeting on Dietary Phenylalanine Brain Function*, edited by R. J. Wurtman and E. Ritter-Walker, Washington, D.C., May 8-10, 1987, pp. 263-273.

Elsas, L. J., II: Aspartame and headache. (Letter) *New England Journal of Medicine* 1988; 318:1201.

El-Serag, H. B., Mason, A. C.: Rising incidence of hepatocellular carcinoma in the United States. *New England Journal of Medicine* 1999; 340:745-750.

Engler, R. L., Covell, J. W., Friedman, P. J., et al.: Misrepresentation and responsibility in medical research. *New England Journal of Medicine* 1987; 317:1383-1388.

Epstein, S. S.: Letter. *The Wall Street Journal* March 15, 1999, p. A-19.

Erlanson, P., et al.: Severe methanol intoxication. *Acta Medica Scandinavica* 1965; 177:393.

Farkas, C. S., Forbes, C. E.: Do non-caloric sweeteners aid patients with diabetes to adhere to their diets? *Journal of the American Dietetic Association.* 1965; 46:482-484.

Feingold, B. F.: Adverse Reactions to Food Additives. Address to Section on Allergy, American Medical Association, New York City, June 19, 1973, p. 5.

Felback, H., Wiley, S.: Free D-amino acids in the tissues of marine bivalves. Cited by Man and Bada (1987).

Felig, P., Marliss, E., Cahill, G. F.: Plasma amino acid levels and insulin secretion in obesity. *New England Journal of Medicine* 281:811-816, 1969.

Ferbee v. Chevron Chemical Company, 736 F2d 1529 (D.C. Cir.), Cert. denied, 469 U.S. 1062 (1984).

Ferguson, J. N.: Interaction of aspartame and carbohydrates in an eating-disordered patient. *American Journal of Psychiatry* 1985; 142:271.

Fernstrom, J. D., Wurtman, R. J., Hammarstrom-Wirklund, D., et al.: Diurnal variations in plasma neutral amino acid concentrations among patients with cirrhosis: Effect of dietary protein intake. *American Journal of Clinical Nutrition* 1979; 32:1923-1933.

Fernstrom, J. D.: Letter. *American Journal of Nutrition* 1987; 45:801-803.

Ferrannini, E.: Insulin resistance, iron, and the liver. *Lancet* 2000; 355:2181-2182.

Filer, L. J., Jr., Stegink, L. D.: Effect of aspartame on plasma phenylalanine concentration in humans. In *Proceedings of the First International Meeting on Dietary Phenylalanine and Brain Function*, edited by R. J. Wurtman and E. Ritter-Walker, Washington, D.C., May 8-10, 1987, pp. 25-26.

Filer, L. J., Jr., Stegink, L. T.: Aspartame metabolism in normal adults, phenylketonuric heterozygotes, and diabetic subjects. *Diabetes Care* 1989; 12 (Suppl. 1):67-74.

Finkelstein, M. W., Daabees, T. T., Stegink, L. D., Applebaum, A. E.: Correlation of aspartame dose, plasma dicarboxylic amino acid concentration, and neuronal necrosis in infant mice. *Toxicology* 1983; 29, 109-119.

Finley, J. W., Schwass, D. E.: *Xenobiotics in Food and Feeds. American Chemical Society Symposium Series*, No. 234, Washington, D.C., 1983.

Fishman, R. A.: The glucose-transporter protein and glucopenic brain injury. *New England Journal of Medicine* 1991; 325:731-732.

Fishman, R. H. B.: Israel's doctors obliged to read journals. *Lancet* 1998; 252:1765.

Floyd, J. C., Jr., Fajans, S., Conn, J. W., Kropf, R. F., Rull, J.: Stimulation of insulin secretion by amino acids. *Journal of Clinical Investigation* 1966; 45:1487-1502.

Floyd, J. C., Fajans, S. S., Pek, S., et al: Synergistic effect of certain amino acid pairs upon insulin secretion in man. *Diabetes* 1970; 19:102-108.

Food and Drug Administration: *Aspartame: Summary of Commissioner's Decision.* Docket No. 75F-0355. 1981; July 15.

Food and Drug Administration: *Food Additives Permitted for Direct Addition to Food for Human Consumption; Aspartame. Federal Register* 21 CFR Part 172. 1983; July 8.

Forbes, A. L.: Dimensions of the issue of explicit health claims on food labels. *American Journal of Clinical Nutrition* 1986; 43:629-635.

Forney, R. B., Hughes, F. W.: *Combined Effects of Alcohol and Other Drugs.* Charles C Thomas, Springfield, 1968, pp. 92-95.

Foshay, P. M.: Medical ethics and medical journals. *Journal of the American Medical Association* 1900; 34:1041-1043.

Francot, P., Geoffroy, P.: Le methanol dans les jus de fruits, les boissons, fermentees, les alcools et spiritueux. *Rev. Ferment, Inc. Ailment.* 1956; 11:279-287.

Frank, R. E., Serdula, M. K., Adame, D.: Weight loss and bulimic eating behavior: Changing patterns within a population of young adult women. *Southern Medical Journal* 1991; 84:457-460.

1000

Franzblau, A., Werner, R. A.: What is carpal tunnel syndrome? *Journal of the American Medical Association.* 1999; 282:186-187.

Fred, H. L.: Solicited editorials: Credence by fiat. *Southern Medical Journal* 1990; 83:734.

Freedman, D. X., Grouse, L. D.: Physicians and the mental illnesses: The nudge from ADAMHA. *Journal of the American Medical Association* 1986; 255:2485-2486.

Fried, S.: *Bitter Pills: Inside The Hazardous World Of Legal Drugs* New York, Bantam Books, 1998.

Froehling, D. A., et al.: Benign positional vertigo: Incidence and prognosis in a population-based study in Olmsted County, Minesota. *Mayo Clinic Proceedings* 1991; 66:596-601.

Fudenberg, H. H., Singh, V. K.: Chemical stress, thyroid dysfunction, and aberrant-cell mediated immunity. Presented at the annual meeting of the American Association for the Advancement of Science, Boston, February 12, 1988.

Fugh-Berman, A.: Herb-drug interactions. *Lancet* 2000; 355:134-138.

Fumento, M.: Medical journals give new meaning to "political science". *The Wall Street Journal* January 21, 1999, p. A-18.

Fürst, P., Alvesstrand, A., Bergatröm, J.: Effects of nutrition and catabolic stress on intracellular amino acid pools in uremia. *American Journal of Clinical Nutrition* 1980; 33:1387-1395.

Gabriel, S. E., O'Fallon, W. M., Kurland, L. T., et al.: Risk of connective-tissue diseases and other disorders after breast implantation. *New England Journal of Medicine* 1994; 330:1677-1702.

Gaby, A. R.: Literature Review & Commentary. *Townsend Letter for Doctors* 1992; December:1048.

Gale, E. A. M., Clark, A.: A drug on the market? *Lancet* 2000; 355:61-63.

Garibotto, G., Deferrari, G., Robaudo, C., et al.: Effect of amino acid ingestion on blood amino acid profile in patients with chronic renal failure. *American Journal of Clinical Nutrition* 1987; 46:949-954.

Gauguier, D., Bihoreau, M., Ktorza, A., Berthault, M., Picon, L.: Inheritance of diabetes mellitus as consequence of gestational hyperglycemia in rats. *Diabetes* 1990; 39:734-739.

Germain, B. F.: Silicone breast implants and rheumatic disease. *Bulletin of Rheumatic Diseases* 1991; 41:1-5.

Genazzani, A. R., Facchinette, F., et al.: Hyperendorphinemia in obese children and adolescents. *Journal of Clinical Endocrinology & Metabolism* 1986; 62:36-40.

Gilger, A. P., Farkas, I. S., Potts, A. M.: Studies on the visual toxicity of methanol X. Further observations on the ethanol therapy of acute ethanol poisonings in monkeys. *American Journal of Ophthalmology* 1959; 48:153-161.

Giugliano, D., Salvatore, T., Cozzolino, D., et al: Hyperglycemia and obesity as determinants of glucose, insulin, and glucagon responses to β-endorphin in human diabetes mellitus. *Journal of Clinical Endocrinology and Metabolism* 1987; 1122-1128.

Go, V. L. W., Hofmann, A. F., Summerskill, W. H. J.: Pancreozymin bioassay in man based on pancreatic enzyme secretin: Potency of specific amino acids and other digestive products. *Journal of Clinical Investigation* 1970; 49:1558-1564.

Goldfinger, S. E., et al: Physician paper: Physicians and pharmaceutical industry. *Annals of Internal Medicine* 1990; 112:624-626.

Goldstein, D. S., Udelsman, R., Eisenhofer, G., et al: Neuronal source of plasma dihydroxyphenylalanine. *Journal of Clinical Endocrinology and Metabolism* 1987; 64:856-861.

Goltermann, N. R.: The biosynthesis of cholecystokinin in neural tissue. In *Neuronal Cholecystokinin*, edited by J. Vanderhaegagn and J. N. Crawley, *Annals of the New York Academy of Sciences* 1985; 448:76-86.

Gomez, C. M., Gammack, J. T.: A leucine-to-phenylalanine substitution in the acetylcholine receptor ion channel in a family with the slow-channel syndrome. *Neurology* 1995; 45:982-985.

Goodman, E.: Fat may be just a state of mind. *The Palm Beach Post* May 3, 1984, p. A-18.

Goodman, L. S., Gilman, A.: *The Pharmacological Basis of Therapeutics* 6th Ed. MacMillan Publishing Company, New York, 1980, pp. 386-387.

Gordon, G.: UPI investigative report: NutraSweet: Questions swirl. Committee on Labor and Human Resources, U.S. Senate, Hearing on *"NutraSweet"-Health and Safety Concerns* 83-178, U.S. Government Printing Office, Washington, 1988, pp. 483-510.

Gordon, G. S., Elliott, H. W.: Action of diethylstilbestrol and some steroids on respiration of rat brain homogenates. *Endocrinology* 1947; 41:517.

Gould, G. M.: Epilepsy and other diseases due to albumin-starvation and sugar poisoning. *Medical Review of Reviews* 1919; July:1-4.

Gourch, A., Orosco, M., Rodrigues, M., et al.: A cholecystokinin agonist/antagonist according to dose and time of action: Effect on food intake. *Neuropeptides* 1990; 17:187-191.

Graves, F.: How safe is your diet soft drink? *Common Cause* Magazine. 1984; July/August 24-43.

Grater, W. C.: Cited by *Medical Tribune* August 18, 1969, p. 10.

Greenberg, D. S.: All expenses paid, Doctor. *Lancet* 1990; 336:1568-1569.

Greening, J., Smart, S., Leary, R., et al.: Reduced movement of median nerve in carpal tunnel during wrist flexion in patients with non-specific arm pain. *Lancet* 1999; 354:217-218.

Gulya, A. J., Sessions, R., B., Troost, T. R.: Aspartame and dizziness: Preliminary results of a prospective, nonblinded, prevalence and attempted cross-over study. *American Journal of Otology* 1992; 13:438-442.

Gurney, J. G., Davis, S., Severson, R. K., et al: Trends in cancer incidence among children in the U.S. *Cancer* 1995; 78:532-541.

Gusella, J. F.: Molecular genetic studies on familial and sporadic Alzheimer's disease. Presented at annual meeting of the American Association for the Advancement of Science, Boston, February 12, 1988.

Hadjidassiliou, M., Grünewald, R. A., Chattopadhyay, A. K., et al.: Clinical radiological, neuropsychological, and neuropathological characteristics of gluten ataxia. *Lancet* 1998; 352:1582-1585.

Hagenfeldt, L., Bollgren, I., Venizelos, N.: N-acetylaspartic aciduria due to aspartoacylase dificiency – a new aetiology of childhood leukodystrophy. *Journal of Inherited and Metabolic Diseases* 1987; 10:135-141.

Haier, R. J.: Cerebral glucose correlates of personality & intelligence. Presented to the Annual Meeting of the American Association for the Advancement of Science, Boston, February 14, 1988.

Haley, R. W.: Chronic multisystem illness among Gulf War veterans. *Journal of the American Medical Association* 1999; 282:327.

Hardcastle, J. E., Bruch, R. J.: Effect of L-aspartyl-L-phenylalanine methyl ester on leukotriene biosynthesis in macrophage cells. *Prostaglandins, Leukotrienes and Essential Fatty Acids* 1997; 57:331-333.

Hardell, L.: Case-control study on radiology work, medical X-ray investigations, and of cellular telephones as risks factors for brain tumors. *Medscape* (www.medscape.com) May 4, 2000.

Harper, A. E., Benevenga, N. J., Wohlhueter, R. M.: Effects of ingestion of disproportionate amounts of amino acids. *Physiological Reviews* 1970; 50:439-448.

Harper, A. E.: Killer french fries: The misguided drive to improve the American diet. *The Sciences* 1988; January/February:21-28.

Harris, C.: Chelation: Anecdote vs science. *Medical Tribune* September 16, 1987, p. 14.

Hart, P.: Remarks to National Council of Salesmen's Organization, Inc., New York City, December 2, 1968.

Hayreh, M. S., Hayreh, S. S., Baumbach, G. L., Cancilla, P., Martin-Amat, G., Tephly, T. R., McMartin, K.E., Makar, A. B.: Methyl alcohol poisoning III. Ocular toxicity. *Archives of Ophthalmology* 1977; 95:1851-1858.

Hattan, D. G.: Regulations of food additives with neurotoxic potential. In *Proceedings of the First International Meeting on Dietary Phenylalanine and Brain Function*, edited by R. J. Wurtman and E. Ritter-Walker, Washington, D.C., May 8-10, 1987, pp. 337-346.

Health and Public Policy Committee: Eating disorders: Anorexia nervosa and bulimia. *Annals of Internal Medicine* 1986; 105:790-794.

Heberer, M., Talke, H., Maier, K. P., Gerok, W.: Metabolism of phenylalanine in liver diseases. *Klinische Wochenschrift* 1980; 58:1189-1196.

Hendee, W. R.: There's no free lunch: The benefits and risks of technologies. *Journal of the American Medical Association* 1991; 265:1437-1438.

Heriot, G.: Doctored affirmative-action data. *The Wall Street Journal* October 15, 1997, p. A-22.

Herishanu, Y., Rosenberg, P.: β-blockers and myasthenia gravis. *Annals of Internal Medicine* 1975; 83:834-835.

Hernandez-Diaz, S., Werler, M.M., Walker, A.M., Mitchell, A.A.: Folic acid antagonists during pregnancy and the risk of birth defects. *New England Journal of Medicine* 2000; 343:1608-1614.

Hertzler, A. E.: *Ventures in Science of a County Surgeon.* 1994, private printing.

Heybach, J. P., Allen, S. S.: Resources for inferential estimates of aspartame intake in the United States. In *Proceedings of the First International Meeting on Dietary Phenylalanine and Brain Function*, edited by R. J. Wurtman and E. Ritter-Walker, Washington, D.C., May 8-10, 1987, pp. 421-435.

1002

Hillman, A. L., Eisenberg, J. M., Pauly, M. V., et al.: Avoiding bias in the conduct and reporting of cost-effectiveness research sponsored by pharmaceutical companies. *New England Journal of Medicine* 1991; 324:1362-1365.

Hines, L.M., Stampfer, M.J., Ma, J., et al: Genetic variation in alcohol dehyrogenase and the beneficial effect of moderate alcohol consumption on myocardial infarction. *New England Journal of Medicine* 2001; 334:549-555.

Hodge, H. C.: Research needs in the toxicology of food additives. *Food and Cosmetics Toxicology* 1963; September 31.

Hoffer, E.: *First Things, Last Things.* New York, Perennial Library, 1971.

Hoi Sang U., Kelly, P. Y., Hatton, J. D., Shew, J. Y.: Proto-oncogene abnormalities and their relationship to tumorigenicity in some human glioblastomas. *Journal of Neurosurgery* 1989; 71:83-90.

Holden, C.: Depression research advances, treatment lags. *Science* 1986; 233:723-726.

Holliday, M. A.: Book review. *New England Journal of Medicine* 1986; 315:654.

Homburger, F.: Saccharin and cancer. *New England Journal of Medicine* 1977; 297:560-561.

Hommes, F. A., Matsuo, K.: Effect of phenylalanine on brain maturation: Implications for the treatment of patients with PKU. In *Proceedings of the First International Meeting on Dietary Phenylalanine and Brain Function,* edited by R. J. Wurtman and E. Ritter-Walker, Washington, D.C., May 8-10, 1987, pp. 229-236.

Honorof, I.: St. Louis Medical Prof Critical of FDA Ruling on Synthetic Sweetener. *National Health Federation Bulletin.* 1975; March:25-29.

Horton, R.: The information wars. *Lancet* 1999; 353:164-165.

Horwitz, D. L., Bauer-Nehrling, Cohen, J. K.: Can aspartame meet our expectations? *Journal of the American Dietetic Association* 1983; 83:142146.

Hotchkiss, W. S.: Doctor as patient advocate. *Journal of the American Medical Association* 1987; 258:947-948.

Hussein, N. M., D'Amelia, R. P., Manz, A. L., Jacin, H., Chen, W. T. C.: Determination of reactivity of aspartame with flavor aldehydes by gas chromatography, HPLC and GPC. *Journal of Food Science* 1984; 49:520-524.

Huff, J., Haseman, J., Rall, D.: Scientific concepts, value, and significance of chemical carcinogenesis studies. *Annual Review of Pharmacology and Toxicology* 1991:31:621-652.

Hutt, P. B.: Safety Regulation in the Real World. Address to the First Academy Forum on the Design of Policy on Drugs and Food Additives, National Academy of Sciences, Washington, D.C., May 15, 1973.

Huttenlocher, P. R.: Morphometric study of human cerebral cortex development. *Neuropsychologia* 1990; 28:517-527.

Hyland, K., Fryburg, J. S., Wilson, W. G., et al: Oral phenylalanine loading in dopa-responsive dystonia. *Neurology* 1997; 48:1290-1297.

Ishii, H.: Incidence of brain tumors in rats fed aspartame. *Toxicology Letters* 1981; 7:433-437.

Ismail, K., Everitt, B., Blatchley, N., et al.: Is there a Gulf War syndrome? *Lancet* 1999; 353:179-182.

Ivanitskiy, A. M.: Evaluation of the content of methanol formed in certain beverages by fermentation hydrolysis of pectin. (Translated from the Russian) Nutrition Institute, USSR Academy of Medical Sciences, Moscow, March 3, 1973.

Jacobson, M.F., Brown, M.A., Whorton, E.B.., Jr.: Gastrointestinal symptoms following Olestra consumption. *Journal of the American Medical Association* 1998; 280:385-326.

Jaffe, G. J., Burton, T. C.: Progression of nonproliferative diabetic retinopathy following cataract extractions. *Archives of Ophthalmology.* 1988; 106:745-749.

Jagenburg, R., Olsson, R., Regardh, C. G., Rödjer, S.: Kinetics of intravenously administered L-phenylalanine with cirrhosis of the liver. *Clinica Chimica Acta* 1977; 78:453-463.

James, O., Day, C.: Non-alcoholic steatohepatitis: Another disease of affluence. *Lancet* 1999; 353:1634-1636.

Jansco, G.: Selective degeneration of chemosensitive primary sensory neurons induced by capsaicin: Glial changes. *Cell Tissue Research* 1978; 195:145-152.

Javier, Z., Gershberg, H., Hulse, M.: Ovulatory suppressants, estrogens, and carbohydrate metabolism. *Metabolism* 1968; 17:443.

Jefferson, T.: What are the benefits of editorials and non-systematic reviews? *British Medical Journal* 1999; 318:135.

Jenkins, R., Hunt, S. P.: Long-term increase in levels of c-jun mRNA and jun protein-like immunoreactivity in motor and sensory neurons following axon damage. *Neuroscience Letters* 1991; 129:107-110.

Joachim, J., Kalantzis, G., Delonca, H., et al.: The influence of particle size on the strain applied on the punches during compression concerning effervescent tablets of aspartame. (Translation of the French title) *Journal de Pharmacie de Belgique* 1987; 42:17-28.

Jobe, P. C., and Dailey, J. W.: Role of monoamines in seizure predisposition in the genetically epilepsy-prone rats. In *Proceedings of the First International Meeting on Dietary Phenylalanine and Brain Function*, edited by R. J. Wurtman and E. Ritter-Walker, Washington, D.C., May 8-10. 1987, pp. 143-160.

John, P. J.: Can plagues be predicted, prevented? *Lancet* 2000; 354:54.

Johns, D. R.: Migraine provoked by aspartame. *New England Journal of Medicine* 1986; 315:456.

Johns, D. R.: Aspartame and headache. In *Proceedings of the First International Meeting on Dietary Phenylalanine and Brain Function*, edited by R. J. Wurtman and E. Ritter-Walker, Washington, D.C., May 8-10, 1987, pp. 311-325.

Johnson, P. E.: Cited by *Chemical and Engineering News* March 9, 1970.

Johnson, R.: Nutritionists detect a dark side in new world of food substitutes. *The Wall Street Journal* February 3, 1988, p. 25.

Kahn, E.: Ephraim Kahn replies. *The Journal of Pesticide Reform* 1987; 7:37.

Kako, K.: Relationship between endogenous fuel and performance of isolated hearts of fed, starved and alloxan diabetic rats. (Abstract) *Circulation* 1965; 31 (II):121.

Kalaria, R. N., Harik, S. I.: Reduced glucose transporter at the blood-brain barrier and in cerebral cortex in Alzheimer's disease. *Journal of Neurochemistry* 1989; 53:1083-1088.

Kamm, T.: Soft drinks get the hard sell in Europe. *The Wall Street Journal* November 21, 1988, p. B-7.

Kang, S., Brange, J., Burch, A., et al.: Absorption kinetics and action profiles of subcutaneously administered insulin analogues (Asp ^{B9}Glu^{B}27, Asp ^{B10}, Asp ^{B28}) in healthy subjects. *Diabetes Care* 1991; 14:1057-1065.

Kasamaki, A., Uraswa, S.: The effect of food chemicals on cell aging of human diploid cells in an in vitro culture. *Journal of Toxicologic Sciences* 1993; 18:143-153.

Kassirer, J. P., Angell, M.: Losing weight – an ill-fated New Year's resolution. *New England Journal of Medicine* 1998; 338:52-4.

Kassirer, J. P.: Editorial independence. *New England Journal of Medicine* 1999; 340:1671-1672.

Kemp, S. F., Lockey, R. F., Wolf, B. L., Lieberman, P.: Anaphylaxis: A review of 266 cases. *Archives of Internal Medicine* 1995; 155:1749-1754.

Kennedy, D.: The anti-scientific method. *The Wall Street Journal* October 29, 1987, p. 32.

Kenney, R. A., Tidball, C. S.: Human susceptibility to oral monosodium L-glutamate. *American Journal of Clinical Nutrition* 1972; 25:140-146.

Kessler, D. A.Drug promotion and scientific exchange. *New England Journal of Medicine* 1991; 325:201-203.

Kessler, D. A.: Cancer and herbs. *New England Journal of Medicine* 2000; 342:1742-1743.

Kessler, D.: Cited in *The Palm Beach Post* 2001; January 7:A-13.

Kim, K. C., Tasch, M. D., Kim, S. H.: The effect of aspartame on 50% convulsion doses of lidocaine. In *Proceedings of the First International Meeting on Dietary Phenylalanine and Brain Function*, edited by R. J. Wurtman and E. Ritter-Walker, Washington, D.C., May 8-10, 1987, pp. 431-435.

Klahr, S., Purkerson, M. L.: Effects of dietary protein on renal function and on the progression of renal disease. *American Journal of Clinical Nutrition* 1988; 47:146-152.

Klavins, J. V.: Pathology of amino acid excess: VII. Phenylalanine and tyrosine. *Archives of Pathology* 1967; 84:238-250.

Koch, R., Blaskovics, M.: Four cases of hyperphenylalaninemia: Studies during pregnancy and of the offspring produced. *Journal of Inherited and Metabolic Diseases* 1982; 5:11-15.

Koehler, S. M., Glaros, A., Fennell, E. B., et al.: The effects of aspartame consumption on migraine headache. In *Proceedings of the International Meeting on Dietary Phenylalanine and Brain Function*, edited by R. J. Wurtman and E. Ritter-Walker, Washington, D.C., May 8-10, 1987, pp. 441-447.

Koepp, R., Miles, S. H.: Meta-analyses of tacrine for Alzheimer disease: The influence of industry sponsors. *Journal of the American Medical Association* 1999; 281:2287.

Koivusalo, M.: Effect of disulfiram (tetraethylthiuram disulphide) on the elimination rate of methanol. (Abstract) *Quarterly Journal of Studies on Alcoholism* 1958; 19:363.

1004

Konno, R., Isobe, K., Niwa, A., et al.: Excessive urinary excretion of methionine in mutant mice lacking D-amino acid oxidase activity. *Metabolism* 1988; 37:1139-1142.

Koob, G.: Cited by *Lancet* 1998; 352:1290.

Korte, D.: Is the FDA only guessing? *The Wall Street Journal* January 26, 1989, p. A-15.

Kraemer, H. C.: "Lies, damn lies, and statistics" in clinical research. *The Pharos* 1992; Fall:7-12.

Krause, W. L., Halminski, M., Naglak, M., et al.: Effects of high phenylalanine in older early-treated PKU patients: Performance, neurotransmitter synthesis, and EEG power frequency. In *Proceedings of the First International Meeting on Dietary Phenylalanine and Brain Function*, edited by R. J. Wurtman and E. Ritter-Walker, Washington, D.C., May 8-10, 1987, pp. 237-246.

Krebs, H. H.: Metabolism of amino acids. III. Deamination of amino acids. *Biochemical Journal* 1935; 29:1620-1644.

Krebs, H. H.: The D- and L-amino acid oxidases. *Biochemical Society Symposium* 1948; 1:2-19.

Krempf, M., Hoerr, R. A., Pelletier, V. A., et al.: An isotopic study of the effect of dietary carbohydrate on the metabolic fate of dietary leucine and phenylalanine. *American Journal of Clinical Nutrition* 1993; 57:161-169.

Kreusi, M. J. P., Rapoport, J. L., Cummings, E. M., et al.: Sugar or aspartame: Effects on aggression and activity. Presented at 139th Annual Meeting of the American Psychiatric Association, Washington, D.C., May 12, 1986.

Krinke, G., Naylor, D. C., Schnid, S., Frönlich, E., Schnider, K.: The incidence of naturally-occurring primary brain tumors in the laboratory rat. *Journal of Comparative Pathology* 1985; 95:175-192.

Kulczycki, A., Jr.: Aspartame-induced urticaria. *Annals of Internal Medicine* 1986; 104:207-208.

Kulczycki, A., Jr.: Aspartame allergy. *Allergy Observer* 1987; June:6.

Kulczycki, A., Jr.: Aspartame induced hives. (Letter) *Journal of Allergy & Clinical Immunology* 1995; 95:639-640.

Lajtha, A.: The "brain barrier system." In *Neurochemistry*, edited by K. A. C. Elliott, I. H. Page, J. H. Quastel, Charles C Thomas, Springfield, 1962, p. 410.

La Lorier, J., Gregoire, G., Benhaddad, A., et al.: Discrepancies between meta-analyses and subsequent large randomized, controlled trials. *New England Journal of Medicine* 1997; 337:536-542.

Landau, R. L., Lugibihl, K.: The effect of progesterone on the concentration of plasma amino acids in man. *Metabolism* 1967; 16:1114-1122.

Lawrence, J. F., Inyengar, J. R.: Liquid chromatographic determination of beta-aspartame in diet soft drinks, beverage powders and pudding mixes. *Journal of Chromatography* 1987:404, 261-266.

Ledley, F D., Woo, S. L. C.: Reconsidering the genetics of phenylketonuria: Evidence from molecular genetics. In *Proceedings of the First International Meeting on Dietary Phenylalanine and Brain Function*, edited by R. J. Wurtman and E. Ritter-Walker, Washington, D.C., May 8-10, 1987, pp. 217-227.

Lehmann, W. D., Heinrich, H. C.: Impaired phenylalanine-tyrosine conversion in patients with iron-deficiency anemia studied by a L- ($^2H_5$) phenylalanine-loading test. *American Journal of Clinical Nutrition* 1986; 44:468-474.

Leibel, R. L., Hirsch, J.: Site- and sex-related differences in adrenoreceptor status of human adipose tissue. *Journal of Clinical Endocrinology & Metabolism* 1987; 64:1205-1210.

Le Moan, M. G.: Methanol in fruit juices: Methanol analysis in official fruit juices and in various preparations based on vegetable juice. (Translation) *Annales Pharmaceutiques Francaises* 1956; 14:470-475.

Levine, J., Baukol, P., Pavlidis, I.: The energy expended in chewing gum. *New England Journal of Medicine* 1999; 341, 2100.

Levitt, J.: Cited by *The Wall Street Journal*, February 22, 2000, p. B-1.

Levy, H. L., Waisbren, S. E.: Effects of untreated maternal phenylketonuria and hyperphenylalananemia on the fetus. *New England Journal of Medicine* 1983; 309:1269-1274.

Levy, H. L., Waisbren, S. E.: The safety of aspartame. *Journal of the American Medical Association* 1987; 258:205.

Lewis, S. A., Lyon, I. C., Elliott, R. B.: Outcome of pregnancy in the rat with mild hyperphenylalinaemia and hypertyrosinaemia: Implications for the management of "human maternal PKU." *Journal of Inherited and Metabolic Diseases* 1985; 8:113-117.

Ley, H. L.: Address to the 12th Annual Food and Drug Law Institute, FDA Educational Conference, December 3, 1968, p. 4.

Ley, H. L.: Cited by *The New York Times* December 30, 1969.

Liang, Y., Maier, V., Steinbach, G., et al.: The effect of artificial sweetener on insulin secretion. II. Stimulation of insulin release from isolated rat islets by Acesulfame K. *Hormone and Metabolism Research* 1987; 19:285-289.

Lieblich, I., Cohen, E., et al: Morphine tolerance in genetically selected rats induced by chronically elevated saccharin intake. *Science* 1983; 221:871-873.

Lindow, T. E.: What is quality care? *New England Journal of Medicine* 1988; 318:859.

Lipton, R. B., Newman, L. C., Solomon, S.: Aspartame and headache. (Letter) *New England Journal of Medicine* 1988; 318:1200.

Lipton, S. A., Rosenberg, P. A.: Excitatory amino acids as a final common pathway for neurologic disorders. *New England Journal of Medicine* 1994; 330:613-622.

Lissner, L., et al.: Variability of body weight and health outcomes in the Framingham population. *New England Journal of Medicine* 1991; 334:1839-1844.

Little, R. E., Anderson, K. W., Ervin, C. H., et al.: Maternal alcohol use during breast-feeding and infant mental and motor development at one year. *New England Journal of Medicine* 1989; 321:425-430.

Lo, B., Wolf, L.E., Berkeley, A.: Conflict-of-interest policies for investigators in clinical trials. *New England Journal of Medicine* 2000; 343:1616-1620.

Lockey, S. D.: Cited by *Medical Tribune*, June 6, 1973.

Longcope, C., Gorbach, S., Goldin, B., et al.: The effect of a low-fat diet on estrogen metabolism. *Journal of Clinical Endocrinology and Metabolism* 1987; 64:1246-1250.

Lou, H. C.: Increased vigilance and dopamine synthesis by large doses of tyrosine or phenylalanine restriction in phenylketonuria. In *Proceedings of the First International Meeting on Dietary Phenylalanine and Brain Function*, edited by R. J. Wurtman and E. Ritter-Walker, Washington, D.C., May 8-10, 1987, pp. 275-282.

Lu, L. B., Shoaib, B. O., Patten, B. M.: Atypical chest pain syndrome in patients with breast implants. *Southern Medical Journal* 1994; 87:978-984.

Lubec, G.: D-amino acids and microwaves. (Letter) *Lancet* 1990; 335:792.

Luby, E. D., Frohman, C. E., Grisell, J. L., Lenzo, J. E., Gottlieb, J. S.: Sleep deprivation: Effects on behavior, thinking, motor performance, and biological energy transfer systems. *Psychosomatic Medicine* 1960; 22:182.

Luby, E. D., Grisell, J. L., Frohman, C. E., Lees, H., Cohen, B. D., Gottlieb, J. S.: Biochemical, physiological, and behavioral responses to sleep deprivation. *Annals of the New York Academy of Sciences* 1962; 96:71.

Lund, E. D., Kirkland, C. L., Shaw, P. E.: Methanol, ethanol, and acetaldhyde contents of citrus products. *Journal of Agriculture, Food and Chemistry*, 1981; 29; 361-366.

Maher, T. J., Kiritsy, P. J.: Aspartame administration decreases the entry of a-methyldopa into the brain of rats. In *Proceedings of the First International Meeting on Dietary Phenylalanine and Brain Function*, edited by R. J. Wurtman and E. Ritter-Walker, Washington, D.C., May 8-10, 1987, pp. 467-472.

Maher, T. J., Pinto, J. M. B.: Aspartame, phenylalanine, and seizures in experimental animals. In *Proceedings of the First International Meeting on Dietary Phenylalanine and Brain Function*, edited by R. J. Wurtman and E. Ritter-Walker, Washington, D.C., May 8-10, 1987, pp. 161-172.

Maller, O., Kare, M.R., Welt, M., Bohrman, H.: Movement of glucose and sodium chloride from the oropharyngeal cavity to the brain. *Nature* 1967; 213:713.

Man, E. H., Sandhouse, M. E., Burg, J., Fisher, G. H.: Accumulation of D-aspartic-acid with age in the human brain. *Science* 1983; 220:1407-1408.

Man, E. H., Bada, J. L.: Dietary D-amino acids. *Annual Review of Nutrition* 1987; 7:209-225.

Mapelli, C., Stammer, C. H., Lok, S., et al.: Synthesis, taste properties, and conformational analysis are four stereoisomeric cyclopropane analogs of aspartame. *International Journal of Peptide Protein Research* 1988; 3:484-495.

Marshall, J.: Internet message, July 20, 1999.

Martensson, E., Olofsson, U., Heath, A.: Clinical and metabolic features of ethanol-methanol poisoning in chronic alcoholics. *Lancet* 1988; 1:327-328.

Matalon, R., Michals, K., Sullivan, D., Levy, P.: Aspartame consumption in normal individuals and carriers for phenylketonuria (PKU). In *Proceedings of the First Meeting on Dietary Phenylalanine and Brain Function*, edited by R. J. Wurtman and E. Ritter-Walker, Washington, D.C., May 8-10, 1987, pp. 81-93.

1006

Matsuzawa, Y., O'Hara, Y.: Tissue distribution of orally administered isotopically labeled aspartame in the rat. In *Aspartame: Physiology and Biochemistry*, edited by L. D. Stegink and L. J. Filer, Jr., Marcel Dekker, Inc., New York, 1984, pp. 161-199.

Maugh, T. H.: Shortage of chemical causes aggression, studies confirm. *Los Angeles Times* November 13, 1995.

Maus, M. B., Rially, S. C., Clevenger, C. B.: Prolactin as a chemoattractant for human breast carcinoma. Presented at 81ˢᵗ Annual Meeting of the Endocrine Society, San Diego, June 12, 1999, OR18-1.

McGinley, L.: Of mice and men. *The Wall Street Journal* September 26, 1997, p. A-8.

McLain, D.: Cited by *The Miami Herald* October 23, 1986, p. A-15.

McLean, D. R., Jacobs, H., Mielke, B. W.: Methanol poisoning: A clinical and pathological study. *Annals of Neurology* 1980; 8:161.

McLellan, M. F.: Literature and medicine: Narratives of physical illness. *Lancet* 1997; 349:1618-1620.

Megalli, M., Friedman, A.: *Masks of Deception: Corporate Front Groups in America*. Essential Information, Washington, D.C., 1991.

Mehigan, D.: A controlled trial of controlled trials. *New England Journal of Medicine* 1981; 305:347.

Melchior, J. C., Ragaud, D., Colas-Linhart, N., et at.: Immunoreactive beta-endorphin increases after an aspartame chocolate drink in healthy human subjects. *Physiology and Behavior* 1991; 50:941-944.

Mellanby, E.: The chemical manipulation of foods. *British Medical Journal* 1951; October 13; 864.

Menne, F. R.: Acute methyl alcohol poisoning: A report of 22 incidences with post-mortem examination. *Archives of Pathology* 1938; 26:77.

Merkel, A. D., Wayner, M. J., Jolicoeur, F. B., Mintz, R. B.: Effects of glucose and saccharin solutions on subsequent food consumption. *Physiological Behavior* 1979; 23:791-793.

Metzenbaum, H. M.: Discussion of S.1557 (Aspartame Safety Act). *Congressional Record-Senate* 1985; August 1, p.S 10820.

Metzenbaum, H. M.: Statement for Committee on Labor and Human Resources, *NutraSweet: Health and Safety Concerns* United States Senate, November 3, 1987. 83-178, U.S. Government Printing Office, Washington, 1988, pp. 1-3.

Michals, K., Matalon, R.: Phenylalanine metabolities, attention span and hyperactivity. *American Journal of Clinical Nutrition* 1985; 42:361-365.

Michaud, D. S., Spiegelman, D., Clinton, S. K., et al.: Fluid intake and the risk of bladder cancer in men. *New England Journal of Medicine* 1999; 340:1390-1397.

Miller, A. B., Howe, G. R.: Artificial sweeteners and bladder cancer. *Lancet* 1977; 2:1221.

Miller, F. G., Rosenstein, D. L., De Renzo, E. G.: Professional integrity in clinical research. *Journal of the American Medical Association* 1998; 280:1449-1454.

Mills, J. L.: Reporting provocative results: Can we publish "hot" papers without getting burned? *Journal of the American Medical Association* 1987; 258:3428-3429.

Mintz, D. H., Finster, J. L., Taylor, A. L., Fefer, A.: Hormonal genesis of glucose intolerance following hypoglycemia. *American Journal of Medicine* 1968; 45:187.

Mintz, M., Cohen, J. S.: *America, Inc.: Who Owns and Operates the United States*. Dell Publishing Company, New York, 1971.

Mocarelli, P., Gerthoux, P. M., Ferrari, E., et al.: Paternal concentrations of dioxin and sex ratio of offspring. *Lancet* 2000; 355:1858-1863.

Mokdad, A. H., Serdula, M. K., Dietz, W. H., et al.: The spread of the obesity epidemic in the United States, 1991-1998. *Journal of the American Medical Association* 1999; 282:1519-1522.

Monte, W. C.: Aspartame: Methyl alcohol and the public health. *Journal of Applied Nutrition* 1984; 36:42-54.

Morton, J. H.: Premenstrual tension. *American Journal of Obstetrics and Gynecology* 1950; 60:343.

Morton, J. H., Addison, H., Addison, R. G., Hunt, L., Sullivan, J. J.: A clinical study of premenstrual tension. *American Journal of Obstetrics and Gynecology* 1953; 65:1182.

Moser, R. H.: *Diseases of Medical Progress: A Study of Iatrogenic Disease*. 3ʳᵈ edition. Charles C Thomas, Springfield, 1969.

Moskowitz, M.: Ad deploring sugared cereal given tough time in journal. *The Evening Times* (West Palm Beach), August 6, 1984, p. B-6.

Mukherjee, A., Chakrabarti, J.: In vivo cytogenic studies on mice exposed to acesulfame-K, a non-nutritive sweetener. *Food and Chemical Toxicology* 1997:35:1177-1179.

Murphy, C.: Effects of age and biochemical status on preference for amino acids. In *Olfaction and Taste IX*, edited by Stephen D. Roper and Jelle Atema, *Annals of the New York Academy of Sciences* 1987; 510:515-518.

Murrell, J., Farlow, M., Gagtti, D., Benson, M. D.: A mutation in the amyloid precursor protein associated with hereditary Alzheimer's disease. *Science* 1991; 254:97-99.

Myers, R. D., Melchior, C. L.: Alcohol drinking: Abnormal intake caused by tetrahydropapaveroline in brain. *Science* 1977; 196:554-556.

Nader, R.: Introduction to *America, Inc.: Who Owns and Operates the United States*, by M. Mintz and J. S. Cohen, Dell Publishing Company, New York, 1971, pp. xi-xix.

National Institutes of Health Consensus Conference, *Journal of the American Medical Association* 1987; 258:3411.

National Research Council: *Environmental Neurotoxicology*. National Academy Press, Washington, D.C., 1991, p. 4.

National Soft Drink Association: Objections to a final rule permitting the use of aspartame in carbonated beverages and carbonated beverage syrup bases and request for a hearing on the objections. Docket No. 82F-0305, July 28, 1983.

National Soft Drink Association: *Congressional Record-Senate* May 7, 1985, S 5507-S 5511.

Nehmer v. United States Veterans Administration, F. Supp. WL 52821 (N.D. Cal. 1989).

Nelken, D.: Cited in *Lancet* 1998; 352:892.

Nelson, G.: Food Protection Act of 1972. *Congressional Record-Senate*. February 14, 1972, No. 18.

Neuberger, A.: The metabolism of D-amino acids in mammals. *Biochemical Society Symposium* 1948; 1:20-32.

Newberne, P. M., Conner, M. W.: Food additives and contaminants: An update. *Cancer* 1986; 58:1851-1862.

Nguyen, U. N., Dumoulin, G., Henriett, M., Regnard, J.: Aspartame ingestion increases urinary calcium, but not oxalate excretion, in healthy subjects. *Journal of Clinical Endocrinology and Metabolism* 1998; 83:165-168.

Nikfar, S., Abdollahi, M., Etemad, F., Sharifzadeh, M.: Effects of sweetening agents on morphine-induced analgesia in mice by formalin test. *General Pharmacology* 1997; 29:583-586.

Ninomiya, Y., Higashi, T., Mizukoshi, T., Funakoshi, M.: Genetics of the ability to perceive sweetness of D-phenylalanine in mice. In *Olfaction and Taste IX*, edited by Stephen D. Roper and Jelle Atema, *Annals of the New York Academy of Sciences* 1987; 510:527-529.

Nolley, K., Nolley, J.: Of science and ideology: A reply to Ephraim Kahn. *Journal of Pesticide Reform* 1987; 7:34-37.

Noren, C. J., Anthony-Cahill, S. J., Griffith, M. C., Schultz, P. T.: A general method for site-specific incorporation of unnatural amino acids in proteins. *Science* 1989; 244:182-188.

Norris, J. R., Meadows, G. G., Massey, L. K., et al.: Tryosine- and phenylalanine-restricted formula diet augments immunocompetence in health humans. *American Journal of Clinical Nutrition* 1990; 51:188-196.

Novick, N. L.: Aspartame-induced granulomatous panniculitis. *Annals of Internal Medicine* 1985; 102:206-207.

O'Donnell, M.: Evidence-based illiteracy: Time to rescue "the literature." *Lancet* 2000; 355:489-491.

Oliveira, M. C., Pizarro, C. B., Aleixo, C. B., et al.: Ki-67 antigen expression in tumoral prolactin cells. Presented at 81st Annual Meeting of the Endocrine Society, San Diego, June 12, 1999, P3-642.

Olney, J. W., Ho, O. L.: Brain damage in infant mice following oral intake of glutamate, aspartame or cysteine. *Nature* 1970; 227:609-611.

Olney, J. W., Ho, O. L., Rhee, V.: Brain-damaging potential of protein hydrolysates. *New England Journal of Medicine* 1973; 289:391-393.

Olney, J. W.: In *Glutamic Acid: Advances in Biochemistry and Physiology*, edited by L. J. Filer, Raven, New York, 1979, p. 287.

Olney, J. W., Labruyere, J., de Gubareff, T.: Brain damage in mice from voluntary ingestion of glutamate and aspartame. *Neurobehavioral Toxicology* 1980; 2:125-129.

Oster, K. A.: The egg controversy: Are eggs good or bad? *American Journal of Clinical Nutrition* 1982; 35:1259-1261.

Pardridge, W. M.: The safety of aspartame. *Journal of the American Medical Association*. 1986; 256:2678.

a. Pardridge, W. M.: The safety of aspartame. *Journal of the American Medical Association* 1987; 258:206.

b. Pardridge, W. M.: Phenylalanine transport at the human blood-brain barrier. In *Proceedings of the First International Meeting on Dietary Phenylalanine and Brain Function*, edited by R. J. Wurtman and E. Ritter-Walker, Washington, D.C., May 8-10, 1987, pp. 57-69.

Parker-Pope, T.: A common side effect, dry mouth, can cause serious tooth decay. *The Wall Street Journal* 2000; March 10: B-1.

Pasteur, L.: Untersuchungen über Asparaginäurer and Aepfelsäure. *Annals Chemistry* (German). 1952; 82:324-335.

Pearce, J. M. S.: Exploding head syndrome. *Lancet* 1988; 2:270-271.

Peacock, M. L., Warren, J. T., Jr., Murman, D. L., et al: Novel mutation in codon 665(Glu>Asp) in the amyloid precursor protein (APP) in a patient with late-onset Alzheimer's disease (AD). (Abstract). *Neurology* 1993; 43:A317.

Pellegrino, E.: Cited by *The Miami Herald* February 5, 1987, p. B-1.

Perry, B. K., et al.: Neurochemical activities in human temporal lobe related to aging and Alzheimer-type changes. *Neurobiology of Aging* 1981; 2:251-256.

Petsko, G. A., Ringe, D.: Blueprints for protein engineering. Presented at the annual meeting of the American Association for the Advancement of Science, Boston, February 13, 1988.

Phillip v. Kimwood Machine Co., 269 Or. 485, 525, P.2d 1033 (1974).

Pickford, J. C., McGale, E. H., Aber, G. M.: Studies on the metabolism of phenylalanine and tyrosine in patients with renal disease. *Clinica Chimica Acta* 1973; 48:77-83.

Pikkarainen, P. H., Raiha, N. C. R.: Development of alcohol dehydrogenase activity in the human liver. *Pediatrics Research* 1967; 1:165-168.

Pincus, J., Barry, K.: Feature in *Medical Tribune* August 27, 1986, p. 19.

Pincus, J. H., et al.: Plasma levels of amino acids correlate with motor fluctuations in Parkinsonism. *Archives of Neurology* 1987; 44:1006-1009.

Pi-Sunyer, F. X.: Testimony for the Committee on Labor and Human Resources, U.S. Senate, Hearing on *"NutraSweet"-Health and Safety Concerns* November 3, 1987. 83-178, U.S. Government Printing Office, Washington, 1988, pp. 390-392.

Pizzi, W. J., Barnhart, J. E., Fanslow, D. J.: Monosodium glutamate administration to the newborn reduces reproductive ability in female and male mice. *Science* 1977; 196:452-454.

Pittelkow, M. R., Benson, L. M., Naylor, S., Tomlinson, A.J.: Detection of corticosteroid in an over-the-counter product. *Journal of the American Medical Association* 1998; 280:327-328.

Podlisny, M. B., Lee, G., Selkoe, D. J.: Gene dosage of the amyloid β precursor protein in Alzheimer's disease. *Science* 238:669-671, 1987.

Poinar, H. N., Höss, M., Bada, J. L., Pääbo, S.: Amino acid racemization and the preservation of ancient DNA. *Science* 1996; 272:864-866.

Posner, H. S.: Biohazards of methanol in proposed new uses. *Journal of Toxicology and Environmental Health* 1975; 1:153-171.

Powley, T. L., Berthoud, H.: Diet and cephalic phase insulin responses. *American Journal of Clinical Nutrition* 1985; 42:991-1002.

Preston-Martin, S.: Descriptive epidemiology of primary tumors of the brain, cranial nerves and cranial meninges in Los Angeles County. *Neuroepidemiology* 1989; 8:2283-2295.

Price, J. M., Biava, C. G., Oser, B. L., et al.: Bladder tumors in rats fed cyclohexylamine or high doses of a mixture of cyclamate and saccharin. *Science* 1970; 167:1131.

Procter, A. W., Palmer, A. M., Stratmann, G. C., Bowen, D. M.: Glutamate/aspartame-releasing neurones in Alzheimer's disease. *New England Journal of Medicine* 1986; 314:1711-1712.

Proxmire, W.: Cited by Honorof (1975).

Publications Committee of the Endocrine Society: Ethical guidelines for publications of research. *Journal of Clinical Endocrinology and Metabolism* 1988; 66:1-2.

Randolph, T. G.: The descriptive features of food addiction: Addictive eating and drinking. *Quarterly Journal of Studies on Alcohol* 1956; 17:198-224.

Rao, K. R., Aurora, A. L., Mithaiyan, S., Remakrishnan, S.: Biochemical changes in brain in methanol poisoning – an experimental study. *Indian Journal of Medical Research* 1977; 65:285-292.

Rechtschaffen, A., Wolpert, E. A., Dement, W. C., Mitchell, S. A., Fischer, C.: Nocturnal sleep of narcoleptics. *Electroencephalography and Clinical Neurophysiology* 1963; 15:599.

Rechtschaffen, A., Maron, L.: The effect of amphetamine on the sleep cycle. *Electroencephalography Clinical Neurophysiology* 1964; 16:438.

Reeve, J. R., Jr., Eysselein, V., Solomon, T. E., Go, V. L. W.: *Cholecystokinin. Annals of the New York Academy of Sciences* 1994; Volume 713.

Reif-Lehrer, L.: Possible significance of adverse reactions to glutamate in humans. *Federation Proceedings* 1976; 35:2205-2211.

Reitano, G., Distefano, G., Vigo, R., et al.: Effect of priming of amino acids on insulin and growth hormone response in the premature infant. *Diabetes* 1978; 27:334-337.

Rennie, D., Knoll, E., Flanagin, A.: The international congress on peer review in biomedical publication. *Journal of the American Medical Association* 1989; 261:749.

Ribicoff, A. S.: *Chemicals and the Future of Man.* The U.S. Senate Subcommittee on Executive Reorganization and Government Research, Committee on Government Operations, April 6, 1971, pp. 1-2.

Roberts, H. J.: Long-term effective weight reduction: Experiences with Metrecal. *American Journal of Clinical Nutrition* 1960; 8:817.

Roberts, H. J.: Long-term weight reduction in cardiovascular disease. Experiences with hypocaloric food mixture (Metrecal) in 78 patients. *Journal of the American Geriatrics Society* 1962; 10:308-347.

a. Roberts, H. J.: The syndrome of narcolepsy and diabetogenic hyperinsulinism in the American Negro: Its relationship to diabetes mellitus, obesity, dysrhythmias and accelerated cardiovascular disease. *Journal of the National Medical Association* 1964; 56:18-42.

b. Roberts, H. J.: The syndrome of narcolepsy and diabetogenic ("functional") hyperinsulinism, with special reference to obesity, diabetes, idiopathic edema, cerebral dysrhythmias and multiple sclerosis (200 patients). *Journal of the American Geriatrics Society* 1964; 12:926-978.

c. Roberts, H. J.: Chronic refractory fatigue – an "organic" perspective: With emphasis upon the syndrome of narcolepsy and diabetogenic hyperinsulinism. *Medical Times* 1964; 92:1144-1161.

d. Roberts, H. J.: Afternoon glucose tolerance testing: A key to the pathogenesis, early diagnosis and prognosis of diabetogenic hyperinsulinism. *Journal of the American Geriatrics Society* 1964; 12:423-272.

e. Roberts, H. J.: Fatigue as an elusive organic problem. *Consultant* 1964; May 30.

a. Roberts, H. J.: Spontaneous leg cramps and "restless legs" due to diabetogenic hyperinsulinism: Observations on 131 patients. *Journal of the American Geriatrics Society* 1965; 13:602-638.

b. Roberts, H. J.: Diabetogenic hyperinsulinism – a major etiology of ischemic heart disease. *Clinical Research* 1965; 13:28.

c. Roberts, H. J.: Café-au-lait spots (CALS), localized hypomelanosis (LH), and the white forelock (WF) – clues to the syndrome of narcolepsy and diabetogenic hyperinsulinism. *Clinical Research* 1965; 13:267.

a. Roberts, H. J.: The role of diabetogenic hyperinsulinism in the pathogenesis of prostatic hyperplasia and malignancy. *Journal of the American Geriatrics Society* 1966; 14:795-825.

b. Roberts, H. J.: An inquiry into the pathogenesis, rational treatment and prevention of multiple sclerosis, with emphasis upon the combined role of diabetogenic hyperinsulinism and recurrent edema. *Journal of the American Geriatrics Society* 1966; 14:586-608.

c. Roberts, H. J.: On the etiology, rational treatment and prevention of multiple sclerosis. *Southern Medical Journal* 1966; 59:940-950.

a. Roberts, H. J.: The role of diabetogenic hyperinsulinism in nocturnal angina pectoris, with special reference to the etiology of ischemic heart disease. *Journal of the American Geriatrics Society* 1967; 15:545-555.

b. Roberts, H. J.: Obesity due to the syndrome of narcolepsy and diabetogenic hyperinsulinism: Clinical and therapeutic observations on 252 patients. *Journal of the American Geriatrics Society* 1967; 15:721.

c. Roberts, H. J.: Migraine and related vascular headaches due to diabetogenic hyperinsulinism: Observations on pathogenesis and rational treatment in 421 patients. *Headache* 1967; 7:41-62.

d. Roberts, H. J.: Pathogenesis of prostatic hyperplasia and neoplasia. *Geriatrics* 1967; 22:85-92.

a. Roberts, H. J.: The value of afternoon glucose tolerance testing in the diagnosis, prognosis and rational treatment of "early chemical diabetes": A 5-year experience. *Acta Diabetologica Latina* 1968; 5:532-565.

1010

b. Roberts, H. J.: Are the massive diet-fat-heart and coronary drug studies justified? A critical commentary. *Angiology* 1968; 19:652-664.

a. Roberts, H. J.: Hyperthyroidism and thyroiditis precipitated by severe caloric restriction: A report of 8 cases. Abstract 305. Program of the 51st meeting, Endocrine Society, New York, June 27, 1969.

b. Roberts, H. J.: A clinical and metabolic re-evaluation of reading disability. In *Selected Papers on Learning Disabilities. 5th annual conference, Association for Children with Learning Disabilities.* Academic Therapy Publications, San Raphael, California, 1969, p. 472-490.

c. Roberts, H. J.: Oral therapy in "early chemical diabetes." I. Serial glucose, cholesterol and uric acid responses to phenformin. *Acta Diabetologica Latina* 1969; 6:728-758.

Roberts, H. J.: Unrecognized narcolepsy and amphetamine abuse. *Medical Counterpoint* 1970; 2:28.

a. Roberts, H. J.: The role of pathologic drowsiness in traffic accidents: An epidemiologic study. *Tufts Medical Alumni Bulletin* 1971; 32:1-9.

b. Roberts, H. J.: *The Causes, Ecology and Prevention of Traffic Accidents.* Charles C Thomas, Springfield, 1971.

Roberts, H. J.: Spontaneous leg cramps and "restless legs" due to diabetogenic (functional) hyperinsulinism. *Journal of the Florida Medical Association* 1973; 60(5):29-31.

Roberts, H. J.: *Is Vasectomy Safe? Medical, Public Health and Legal Implications.* Sunshine Academic Press, 1979.

a. Roberts, H. J.: Perspective on Vitamin E as therapy. *Journal of the American Medical Association.* 1981; 246:129-131.

b. Roberts, H. J.: More on dolomite. (Letter) *New England Journal of Medicine* 1981; 340:1367.

Roberts, H. J.: Indoor air pollution. *Science* 223:6, 1984.

Roberts, H. J.: The hazards of very-low-calorie dieting. *American Journal of Clinical Nutrition* 1985; 41:171-172.

a. Roberts, H. J.: Respiratory hazards of anti-static clothes softeners. *Palm Beach County Medical Society Bulletin* 1986; January:24-31.

b. Roberts, H. J.: Exaerobic thrombophlebitis. *Palm Beach County Medical Society Bulletin* 1986; 13 (#3):30-31.

a. Roberts, H. J.: Is aspartame (NutraSweet®) safe? *On Call* (Palm Beach County Medical Society) 1987; January:16-20.

b. Roberts, H. J.: Neurologic, psychiatric and behavioral reactions to aspartame in 505 aspartame reactors. In *Proceedings of the First International Conference on Dietary Phenylalanine and Brain Function*, edited by R. J. Wurtman and E. Ritter-Walker, Washington, D. C., May 8-10, 1987, pp. 477-481.

a. Roberts, H. J.: Aspartame (NutraSweet®)-associated confusion and memory loss: A possible human model for early Alzheimer's disease. Abstract 306. Annual meeting of the American Association for the Advancement of Science, Boston, February 13, 1988.

b. Roberts, H. J.: Aspartame (NutraSweet®)-associated epilepsy. *Clinical Research* 1988; 36:349A.

c. Roberts, H. J.: Complications associated with aspartame (NutraSweet®) in diabetics. *Clinical Research* 1988; 3:489A.

d. Roberts, H. J.: The Aspartame Problem. Statement for Committee on Labor and Human Resources, U.S. Senate, Hearing on *"NutraSweet"-Health and Safety Concerns* November 3, 1987. 83-178, U.S. Government Printing Office, Washington, 1988, pp. 466-467.

e. Roberts, H. J.: Reactions attributed to aspartame-containing products: 551 cases. *Journal of Applied Nutrition* 1988; 40:85-94.

a. Roberts, H. J.: *Aspartame (NutraSweet®): Is It Safe?* Philadelphia, The Charles Press, 1989.

b. Roberts, H. J.: Endangered individualism in medicine: With emphasis upon the ongoing need for competent primary care. *Journal of the Florida Medical Association* 1989; 76:777-782.

c. Roberts, H. J.: The licensing of Simplesse®: An open letter to the FDA. *Journal of Applied Nutrition* 1989; 41:42-43.

a. Roberts, H. J.: Obstacles confronting consumer advocates: An overview of health-related issues. *Trauma* 1990; 31 (#5):55-63.

b. Roberts, H. J.: Pentachlorophenol-associated aplastic anemia, red cell aplasia, leukemia and other blood disorders. *Journal of the Florida Medical Association* 1990; 77:86-90.

c. Roberts, H. J.: Is Aspartame (NutraSweet®) Safe? Public Health and Legal Challenges. In *Proceedings for 30th Anniversary Conference on Legal Medicine*, Orlando, Florida, March 15-17, 1990, 64-84.

a. Roberts, H. J.: Does aspartame cause human brain cancer? *Journal of Advancement in Medicine* 1991; 4 (Winter):231-241.

b. Roberts, H. J.: Aspartame-associated confusion and memory loss. *Townsend Letter for Doctors* 1991; June:442-443.

c. Roberts, H. J.: Myasthenia gravis associated with aspartame use. *Townsend Letter for Doctors* 1991; August/September:699-700.

d. Roberts, H. J.: Joint pain associated with aspartame use. *Townsend Letter for Doctors* 1991; May:375-376.

a. Roberts, H. J.: *Sweet'ner Dearest: Bittersweet Vignettes About Aspartame (NutraSweet®).* West Palm Beach, Sunshine Sentinel Press, Inc., 1992.

b. Roberts, H. J.: Unexplained headaches and seizures. *Townsend Letter for Doctors* 1992; November:1001-1002.

c. Roberts, H. J.: Prostate cancer among black Americans. *Townsend Letter for Doctors* 1992; November:977.

d. Roberts, H. J.: Safety of aspartame. (Letter) *Townsend Letter for Doctors* 1992; November:977-978.

e. Roberts, H. J.: Aspartame: Is it safe? Interview with H. J. Roberts, M.D. *Mastering Food Allergies* 1992; 7 (#1), 3-6.

f. Roberts, H. J.: Toxicological Profile for Fluorides, Hydrogen Fluoride, and Fluorine: Critique submitted to the Agency for Toxic Substances and Disease Registry. Reprinted in *Townsend Letter for Doctors* 1992; July:623-624.

a. Roberts, H. J.: Testimony: Analysis of Adverse Reactions to Monosodium Glutamate. Federation of American Societies for Experimental Biology, Bethesda, April 8, 1993.

b. Roberts, H. J.: Aspartame (NutraSweet®). *NOHA News* 1993; Winter:5-6.

c. Roberts, H. J.: Aspartame-associated dry mouth (xerostomia). *Townsend Letter for Doctors* 1993; February/March:201-202.

d. Roberts, H. J.: *Is Vasectomy Worth the Risk? A Physician's Case Against Vasectomania* West Palm Beach, Sunshine Sentinel Press, 1993.

a. Roberts, H. J.: "Dry eyes" from use of aspartame (NutraSweet®). *Townsend Letter for Doctors* 1994; January:82-83.

b. Roberts, H. J.: Aspartame as a cause for diarrhea in diabetics. *Townsend Letter for Doctors* 1994; June:623-624.

c. Roberts, H. J.: *Mega Vitamin E: Is It Safe?* West Palm Beach, Sunshine Sentinel Press, 1994.

a. Roberts, H. J.: Aspartame and headache. *Neurology* 1995; 45:1631-1633.

b. Roberts, H. J.: *Defense Against Alzheimer's Disease: A Rational Blueprint for Prevention.* West Palm Beach, Sunshine Sentinel Press, 1995.

c. Roberts, H. J.: Lactose intolerance. (Letter) *New England Journal of Medicine* 1995; 333:1359.

d. Roberts, H. J.: Memory loss and aspartame. *Townsend Letter for Doctors* 1995; August/September:99-100.

a. Roberts, H. J.: Aspartame as a cause of allergic reactions, including anaphylaxis. *Archives of Internal Medicine.* 1996; 156:1027.

b. Roberts, H. J.: Chronic fatigue: A clue to evolving Alzheimer's disease? *Townsend Letter for Doctors & Patients* 1996; August/September:110-112.

c. Roberts, H. J.: Profile of Super Volunteer Activist: Betty Martini. *Townsend Letter for Doctors & Patients* 1996; May:106-110.

a. Roberts, H. J.: Critique of the Official Australia and New Zealand Food Authority (ANZFA) Position on Aspartame. *Soil & Health* 1997; July/September:15.

b. Roberts, H. J.: Preclinical Alzheimer's disease. (Letter) *Neurology* 1997; 48:549-55.

c. Roberts, H. J.: Aspartame effects during pregnancy and childhood. (Letter) *Latitudes* 1997; 3 (Number 1):3.

d. Roberts, H. J.: Effects of pentachlorophenol exposure. *Lancet* 1997; 349:1917.

a. Roberts, H. J.: "Dry eyes" from use of aspartame: Associated insights concerning the Sjögren syndrome. *Focus* (Information Forum For Retinal Degenerative Disorders) 1998: Volume 3 (No. 3):16-17.

b. Roberts, H. J.: Submission to FDA regarding Docket No. 981F-0052 (Food Additive Petition for Neotame), March 3, 1998.

c. Roberts, H. J.: What's blinding the world? *Focus* (Information Forum for Retinal Degenerative Disorders) 1998; Volume 3 (No. 3):15-16.

d. Roberts, H. J.: *Ignored Health Hazards for Pilots and Drivers: The A-B-C-D-E-F-G-H File* West Palm Beach, Sunshine Sentinel Press, 1998.

1012

e. Roberts, H. J.: Aspartame toxicity denied – Dr. Roberts responds. *Townsend Letter for Doctors & Patients* 1998; April:110-113.

f. Roberts, H. J.: *The CACOF Conspiracy: Lessons of the New Millennium.* West Palm Beach, Sunshine Sentinel Press, 1998.

g. Roberts, H. J.: Unrecognized aspartame disease in silicone breast implant patients. *Townsend Letter for Doctors & Patients* 1998; May:74-75.

h. Roberts, H. J.: Letter on proposed fluoridation of Pompano Beach municipal water. *The Pompano Pelican* June 1, 1998.

Roberts, H. J.: *Breast Implants or Aspartame (NutraSweet®) Disease? The Suppressed Opinion About a Perceived Medicolegal Travesty.* West Palm Beach, Sunshine Sentinel Press, 1999.

a. Roberts, H. J.: Aspartame (NutraSweet®) addiction. *Townsend Letter for Doctors & Patients* 2000; January (#198):52-57.

b. Roberts, H.J.: Carpal tunnel syndrome due to aspartame disease. *Townsend Letter for Doctors & Patients* 2000; November (#208): 82-84.

Roe, O.: Species differences in methanol poisoning. *CRC Critical Reviews in Toxicology* 1982; October:275-286.

Roelofs, R. I., Strickland, D., Goldman, L., Dolliff, G.: Epidemiologic study of association between dietary intake of excitatory amino acids and serum levels in ALS patients. (Abstract) *Neurology* 1991; 41 (Suppl. 1):393.

Rogers, P. J., Keedwell, P., Blundell, J. E.: Further analysis of the short-term inhibition of food intake in humans by the dipeptide L-aspartyl-L-phenylalanine methyl ester (aspartame). *Physiology & Behavior* 1991; 14:739-743.

Rogers, T. R., Leung, P. B. M.: The influence of amino acids on the neuroregulation of food intake. *Federation Proceedings* 1973; 32:1709-1719.

Rosenbaum, J. T.: Lessons from litigation over silicone breast implants: A call for activism by scientists. *Science* 1997; 276:1524-1525.

Rosenbaum, P. R.: Discussing hidden bias in observational studies. *Annals of Internal Medicine* 1991; 115:901-905.

Rosenberg, C. E.: *Explaining Epidemics and Other Studies in the History of Medicine.* New York: Cambridge University Press, 1992.

Rossi, A. C., Bosco, L., Faich, G. A., et al.: The importance of adverse reaction reporting by physicians. *Journal of the American Medical Association* 1988; 259:1203-1204.

Rothman, K. J.: Conflict of interest. *Journal of the American Medical Association* 1993; 269:2782-2784.

Roy-Byrne, P. P., Cowley, D. S.: Search for pathophychology of panic disorder. *Lancet* 1998; 252:1646-1647.

Roznoski, M. M., Huang, S., Burns, R.: Phenylalanine interferes with metabolism of exogenous L-dopa at the cell level. (Abstract). *Neurology* 1993; 43:A195.

Rubinstein, S., Caballero, B.: Is Miss America an undernourished role model? *Journal of the American Medical Association* 2000; 283:1569.

Rudgley R.: *The Alchemy of Culture: Intoxicants in Society.* London, British Museum Press, 1998.

Sabates, R. J.: *The Preventive Diet.* Hialeah, RSMDPA Corporation, 1996.

Sack, K. E., Criswell, L. A.: Eosinophilia-myalgia syndrome: The aftermath. *Southern Medical Journal* 1992; 85:878-882.

Sackett, D. L., Rosenberg, W. M., Gary, J. A., Haynes, R. B., Richardson, W. S.: Evidence-based medicine: What it is and what it isn't. *British Medical Journal* 1996; 312:71-72.

Salcman, M.: The morbidity and mortality of brain tumors. *Neurology Clinics* 1985; 3:229-257.

Samuels, A.: *MSG: A Review of the Literature and Critique of Industry Sponsored Research.* Private printing. July 1, 1991.

Samuels, A.: Excitatory amino acids in neurologic disorders. (Letter) *New England Journal of Medicine* 1994; 331:274-275.

Samuels, J. L.: Evaluation of the safety of amino acids and related products. Presented to Life Sciences Research Office, Federation of American Societies for Experimental Biology, Bethesda, Docket No. 90N-0379, February 4, 1991.

Samuels, S. W.: The fallacies of risk/benefit analysis. In *Public Control of Environmental Health Hazards*, edited by E. C. Hammond and I. J. Selikoff. *Annals of the New York Academy of Sciences* 1979; 329:267-273.

Sanchez-Guerrero, J., Colditz, G. A., Karlson, E. W., et al.: Silicone breast implants and the risk of connective-tissue disease and symptoms. *New England Journal of Medicine* 1995; 332:1666-1670.

Sapira, J. D.: Which will be the best medical school in ten years? *Southern Medical Journal* 1988; 81:1079.

Sardesai, V. M., Holliday, J. F., Kumar, G. K., Dunbar, J. C.: Effect of aspartame in diabetic rats. In *Proceedings of the First International Meeting on Dietary Phenylalanine and Brain Function*, edited by R. J. Wurtman and E. Ritter-Walker, Washington, D.C., May 8-10, 1987, pp. 482-487.

Scarborough, F. E.: Safety and testing of fat substitutes and replacements. Presented at 72nd Annual Meeting of the American Dietetic Association, Kansas City, Missouri, October 24, 1989.

Schafer, S., Giagounidis, A.A.N.,: Patents for intellectual property. *The Lancet* 2000; 356:2016.

Scher, A., Stewart, W. F., Liberman, J., Lipton, R. B.: Prevalence of frequent headache in a population sample. *Headache* 1998; 35 (5):404.

Scheer, R.: The great American breast-implant hoax. *Cosmopolitan* 1994; September:232-258.

Schiedermayer, D. L., and Siegler, M.: Believing what you read: Responsibilities of medical authors and editors. *Archives of Internal Medicine* 1986; 146:2043-2044.

Schiffman, S. S., Buckley, C. E., III, Sampson, H. A., et al.: Aspartame and susceptibility to headache. *New England Journal of Medicine* 1987; 317:1181-1185.

Schmid, R., Schusdziarra, V., Schulte-Frohlinde, E., Marer, V., Classen, M.: Circulating amino acids and pancreatic endocrine function after ingestion of a protein-rich meal in obese subjects. *Journal of Endocrinology and Metabolism* 1989; 68:1106-1110.

Schomer, D. L.: Monoamines and seizures in humans. In *Proceedings of the First International Meeting on Dietary Phenylalanine and Brain Function*, edited by R. J. Wurtman and E. Ritter-Walker, Washington, D.C., May 8-10, 1987, pp. 173-183.

Schrage, M.: Are ideas viruses of the mind? *The Miami Herald* November 13, 1988, pp. C-1, C-6.

Schuckit, M. A.: New findings in the genetics of alcoholism. *Journal of the American Medical Association* 1999; 281:1875-1876.

Schwartz, G. S.: Aspartame and cancer. (Letter) *Western Journal of Medicine* 1999; 171 (3):300-301.

Scott, I. C., Besag, F. M. C., Neville, B. G. R.: Buccal midazolam and rectal diazepam for treatment of prolonged seizures in childhood and adolescence: A randomised trial period. *Lancet* 1999; 353:623-626.

Sczuc, E. F., Barrett, K. E., Metcalfe, D. D.: The effects of aspartame on mast cells and basophils. *Food and Chemical Toxicology* 1986; 24:171-174.

Selkoe, D. J., Ihara, Y., Salazar, F. J.: Alzheimer's disease: Insolubility of partially purified paired helical filaments in sodium dodecyl sulfate and urea. *Science* 1982; 215:1243-1245.

Serdula, M. K., Mokdad, A. H., Williamson, D. F., et al.: Prevalence of attempting weight loss and strategies for controlling weight. *Journal of the American Medical Association* 1999; 282:1353-1358.

Shabin, H. M., Albert, M. L.: Aspartame: An evaluation of adverse effects. *Hospital Formulary* 1988; 23:543-546.

Shah, J., Carlson, H., Peters, M., Carr, J.: Differences in amino acid-induced insulin release between male and female. Abstract 308. 68th annual meeting of the Endocrine Society, Anaheim, California, June 24-27, 1986.

Shaham, J., Bomstein, Y., Melzer, A., Ribak, J.: DNA-protein crosslinks and sister chromatid exchanges as biomarkers of exposure to formaldehyde. *International Journal of Occupational and Environmental Health* 1997; 3:95-104.

Shaywitz, B. A., Novotny, E. J., Jr.: Aspartame and seizures. (Letter) *Neurology* 1993; 43:630.

Shephard, S. E., Wakabayashi, K., Magao, M.: Mutagenic activity of peptides and the artificial sweetener aspartame after nitrosation. *Food and Chemical Toxicology* 1993; 31:323-329.

Shipp, J. C., Matos, A. E., Knizley, H., Crevasse, L. E.: CO_2 formed from endogenous and exogenous substrates in perfused rat heart. *American Journal of Physiology* 1964; 207:1231.

Shoji, M., Golde, T. E., Chiso, J., et al.: Production of the Alzheimer amyloid β protein by normal proteolytic processing. *Science* 1992; 258:126-129.

Shomon, M.: Sticking out our necks. Issue #37, *The Thyroid News Report*. Cited on the Internet, March 31, 2000.

Sissons, J. G. P.: Superantigens and infectious diseases. *Lancet* 1993; 341:1627-1629.

Slaff, J.,Jacobson, D., Tillman, C. R., et al.: Protease-specific suppression of pancreatic exocrine secretion. *Gastroenterology* 1984; 87:44-52.

Smith v. E. R. Squibb and Sons Inc., 273 M.W. 2d 476 (Mich. 1979).

Smith, K. A., Fairburn, C. G., Cowen, P. J.: Relapse of depression after rapid depletion of tryptophan. *Lancet* 1997; 349:915-919.

Sokoloff, L.: Action of thyroid hormones and cerebral development. *American Journal of Diseases of Children* 1967; 114:498-506.

Solzhenitsyn, A. I.: Letter, *The New York Times* November 14, 1969.

Sommer, H.: The physiological fate of methyl alcohol released from pectin. *Industrielle Obst. Und Gemeseverwesting* 1962; 47:172-173.

Sood, V., Sobhy, T., Schade, D.S., Burge, M.R.: Low dose ethanol increases the glycemic threshold for epinephrine release during hypoglycemia. *Journal of Investigative Medicine* 2001; 49 (#1): Abstract 13.

Sorg, B. A., Willis, J. R., et al.: Repeated low-dose formaldehyde exposure produces cross-sensitization to cocaine; possible relevance to chemical sensitivity in humans. *Neuropsychopharmacology* 1998; 18:385-394.

Spellacy, W. N., Carlson, K. L.: Plasma insulin and blood glucose levels in patients taking oral contraceptives. *American Journal of Obstetrics and Gynecology* 1966; 95:474.

Spencer, P. S., et al.: Guam amyotrophic lateral sclerosis parkinsonism-dementia linked to a plant excitant neurotoxin. *Science* 1987; 237:517-522.

Spiegel, K., Leproult, R., Van Caruter, E.: Impact of sleep debt on metabolic and endocrine function. *Lancet* 1999; 354:1435-1439.

Spiers, P., Schomer, D., Sabounjian, L.: Aspartame and human behavior: Cognitive and behavioral observations. In *Proceedings of the First International Meeting on Dietary Phenylalanine and Brain Function*, R. J. Wurtman and E. Ritter-Walker (eds), Washington, D.C., May 8-10, 1987, pp. 193-206.

Spruill v. Boyle-Midway, Inc., 308 F.2d 79, 85 (4 Cir. 1962).

Spring, B., Bourgeois, M., Harden, M., et al.: Responses to carbohydrate consumption among juvenile-onset diabetics. In *Proceedings of the First International Meeting on Dietary Phenylalanine and Brain Function*, edited by R. J. Wurtman and E. Ritter-Walker, Washington, D.C., May 8-10, 1987, pp. 489-493.

Spyer, G., Hattersley, A.T., Macdinal, I.A., et al.: Hypoglycaemic counter-regulation at normal blood glucose concentrations in patients with well controlled type 2 diabetes. *The Lancet* 2000; 356: 1970-1974.

St. George-Hyslop, P. H., Tanzi, R. E., Polinsky, R. J., et al.: Absence of duplication of chromosome 21 genes in familial and sporadic Alzheimer's disease. *Science* 1987; 238:664-666.

Staamp, J.: *Some Economic Factors in Modern Life*. P. S. King & Son, Ltd., London, 1929, pp. 258-259.

Stacher, G.: Satiety effect of cholecystokinin and ceruletide in lean and obese men. In *Neuronal Cholecystokinin*, edited by J. Vanderhaegagn and J. N. Crawley, *Annals of the New York Academy of Sciences* 1985; 448:431-436.

Stancin, T., Link, D. L., Reuter, J. M.: Binge eating and purging in young women in IDDM. *Diabetes Care* 1989; 12:601-603.

Steginck, L. D., and Filer, L. J., Jr.: *Aspartame: Physiology and Biochemistry*, Marcel Dekker, Inc., New York, 1984.

Steginck, L. D. Filer, L. J., Jr., Bell, E. F., Ziegler, E. E.: Plasma amino acid concentrations in normal adults administered aspartame in capsules or solution: Lack of bioequivalence. *Metabolism* 1987; 36:507-512.

Stelfox, H. T., Chua, G., O'Rourke, K., Detsky, A. S.: Conflict of interest in the debate of calcium-channel antagonists. *New England Journal of Medicine* 1998; 338:101-106.

Stephen, L. J., Brodie, M. J.: Epilepsy in elderly people. *Lancet* 2000; 355:1441-1446.

Stewart, O.: Nutrition and the food technologist. (Editorial) *Food Technology* 1964; 18 (October):9.

Stingraber, S.: *Living Downstream: An Ecologist Looks at Cancer And The Environment*. Reading (Massachusetts), Addison-Wesley, 1997.

Stirrat, G. M.: Choice of treatment for menorrhagia. *Lancet* 1999; 353:2175-2176.

Stonier, C., McGale, E. H., Aber, G. M.: Studies of phenylalanine hydroxylase activity in patients with chronic renal failure: The effect of hemodialysis. *Clinica Chimica Acta* 1984; 143:115-122.

Strong, F. C.: Why do some dietary migraine patients claim they get headaches from placebos? *Clinical and Experimental Allergy* 2000; 30:739-743.

Sturtevant, F. M.: Aspartame – a new ingredient: Reply to the critical comments of Woodrow C. Monte. *Journal of Environmental Science and Health* 1985; 20:863-901.

Suarez, F. L., Savaiano, D. A., Levitt, M. D.: A comparison of symptoms after the consumption of milk or lactose-hydrolyzed milk by people with self-reported severe lactose intolerance. *New England Journal of Medicine* 1995; 333:1-4.

Swales, J. D.: Science and health care: An uneasy partnership. *Lancet* 2000; 355:1637-1640.

Swanson, J. M., Lerner, M., Williams, L.: More frequent diagnosis of attention deficit-hyperactivity disorder. *New England Journal of Medicine* 1995; 333:944.

Swartz, R. D., Millman, R. P., Billi, J. E., et al.: Epidemic methanol poisoning: Clinical and biochemical analysis of a recent episode. *Medicine* 1981; 60:373-382.

Sweeney, K. G., MacAulay, D., Gray, D. P.: Personal significance: The third dimension. *Lancet* 1998; 351:134-136.

Szasz, T.: Diagnoses are not diseases. *Lancet* 1991; 338:1574-1576.

Talal, N., Ansar Ahmed, S., Dauphine, M.: Hormonal approaches in immunotherapy of autoimmune disease. *Annals of the New York Academy of Sciences* 1985; 475:320-328.

Tallan, H. H.: Studies on the distribution of N-acetyl-L-aspartic acid in brain. *Journal of Biological Chemistry* 1957; 224:41-45.

Tamminga, C. A., Lucignani, G., Porrino, L. J., Chase, T. N.: Cholecystokinin octapeptide's effect on local cerebral glucose utilization in the laboratory rat. In *Neuronal Cholecystokinin*, edited by J. Vanderhaegagn and J. N. Crawley, *Annals of the New York Academy of Sciences* 1985; 448:663-665.

Taylor, K.: Liver toxicity linked to aspartame. *Townsend Letter for Doctors & Patients* 1996; June:120-122.

Taylor, L.: Testimony for Committee on Labor and Human Resources, U.S. Senate, Hearing on *"NutraSweet"-Health and Safety Concerns* November 3, 1987. 83-178, U.S. Government Printing Office, Washington, 1988, pp. 303-305.

Tendler, D. A., et al.: Effect of MK-801 on excitatory and inhibitory amino acids during hypoxia and seizure: In vivo cerebral microdialysis study. (Abstract) *Neurology* 1991; 41 (Suppl. 1):414.

Tephy, T. R., McMartin, K. E.: Methanol metabolism and toxicity. In *Aspartame: Physiology and Biochemistry*, edited by L. D. Stegink, J. L. Filer, Jr., Marcell Dekker, Inc., New York, 1984, pp. 111-140.

Thayer, A. M.: Use of specialty food additives to continue to grow. *Chemical & Engineering News* 1991; June 3:9-12.

Thomison, J. B.: Mens sana in corpore sano. *Southern Medical Journal* 1983:76:1-2.

Thompson, A. J., et al.: Magnetic resonance imaging changes in early treated patients with phenylketonuria. *Lancet* 1991; 337:1224.

Thrasher, J. F., Broughton, A., Micevich, P.: Antibodies and immune profiles of individuals occupationally exposed to formaldehyde. Six case reports. *American Journal of Industrial Medicine* 1988; 14:479-488.

Tieman, S. B., Butler, K., Neale, J. H.: N-acetylaspartylglutamate. *Journal of the American Medical Association* 1988; 259:2020.

Tilson, H. A., Zhao, D., Peterson, N. J., et al: Behavioral and neurological effects. In *Proceedings of the First International Meeting on Dietary Phenylalanine and Brain Function*, edited by R. J. Wurtman and E. Ritter-Walker, Washington, D.C., May 8-10, 1987, pp. 107-115.

Tocci, P. M., Beber, B.: Anomalous phenylalanine loading responses in relation to cleft lip and cleft palate. *Pediatrics* 1973; 52:109.

Tollefson, L., Barnard, R. J., Glinsmann, W. H.: Monitoring of adverse reactions to aspartame reported to the U.S. Food and Drug Administration. In *Proceedings of the First International Meeting on Dietary Phenylalanine and Brain Function*, edited by R. J. Wurtman and E. Ritter-Walker, Washington, D.C., May 8-10, 1987, 347-372.

Tordoff, M. G., Alleva, A. M.: Oral stimulation with aspartame increases hunger. *Physiology & Behavior* 1990; 47:555-559.

Tourian, A.: Control of phenylalanine hydroxylase synthesis and tissue culture by serum and insulin. *Journal of Cellular Physiology* 1975; 87:15-24.

Turski, L., Meldrum, D. S., Cavalheiro, E. A., et al.: Paradoxical anticonvulsant activity of the excitatory amino acid N-methyl-D-aspartate in the rat caudate-putamen. *Proceedings of the National Academy of Sciences USA* 1984; 64:1689-1693.

Unwin, C., Blatchley, N., Koker, W., et al.: Health of UK service men who served in Persian Gulf War. *Lancet* 1999;353:169-178.

Urakami, K., et al: Clinical biochemical evaluation of zeruletide in patients with dementia of the Alzheimer type. *Dementia* 1991; 2:35-38.

Uribe, M.: Potential toxicity of a new sugar substitute in patients with liver disease. *New England Journal of Medicine* 1982; 306:173.

Uzych, L.: Courtroom science. *Lancet* 1988; 1:361.

Valdovinos, M. A., Camilleri, M., Zimmerman, B. R.: Chronic diarrhea in diabetes mellitus: Mechanisms and an approach to diagnosis and treatment. *Mayo Clinic Proceedings* 1993; 68:691-702.

Vandenbroucke, J.P.: In defense of case reports and case series. *Annals of Internal Medicine* 2001; 134:330-334.

Vanderhaegagn, J., Crawley, J. N.: *Neuronal Cholecystokinin. Annals of the New York Academy of Sciences* 1985; Volume 448:315-333.

Van Den Eeden, S. K., Koepsell, T. D., Longstreth, W. T., Jr., et al.: Aspartame ingestion and headaches: A randomized crossover trial. *Neurology* 1994; 44:1787-1793.

van Loon, L.J.C., Saris, W.H.M., Verhagen, H., Wagenmakers, A.J.M.: Plasma insulin responses after ingestion of different amino acid or protein mixtures with carbohydrate. *American Journal of Clinical Nutrition* 2000; 72:96-105.

Vekrellis, K., Ye, Z., Qiu, W.Q., et al: Neurons regulate extracellular levels of amyloid β-protein via proteolysis by insulin-degrading enzyme. *Journal of Neuroscience* 2000; 20: 1657-1655/

Verrett, J.: Testimony for the Committee on Labor and Human Resources, U.S. Senate, Hearing on *"NutraSweet"-Health and Safety Concerns* November 3, 1987. 83-178, U.S. Government Printing Office, Washington, 1988, p. 385.

Vianna, N. J.: Hodgkin's disease. *Journal of the American Medical Association* 1975; 234:1133.

Vinters, H. V., Miller, B. L., Pardridge, W. M.: Brain amyloid and Alzheimer's disease. *Annals of Internal Medicine* 1988; 109:41-54.

Virkkunen, M.: Reactive hypoglycemic tendency among habitually violent offenders: A further study by means of the glucose tolerance test. *Neuropsychobiology* 1982; 8:35-40.

Virkkunen, M.: Insulin secretion during the glucose tolerance test in antisocial personality. *British Journal of Psychiatry* 1983; 142:598-604.

Virkkunen, M.: Reactive hypoglycemic tendency among arsonists. *Acta Psychiatry Scandinavica* 1984; 69:445-452.

Virkkunen, M., Nuutioa, A., Goodwin, F. K., Linnoila, M.: CSF monoamine metabolities in arsonists. *Archives of General Psychiatry* 1987; 44:241-247.

Volkow, N.: Cited in *Lancet* 1999; 354:924.

Wahren, J., Felig, P., Cerasi, E., Luft, R.: Splanchnic and peripheral glucose and amino acid metabolism in diabetes mellitus. *Journal of Clinical Investigation* 1972; 51:1870-1878.

Waisbren, S. E., Hanley, W., Levy, H. L., et al.: Outcome at age 4 years in offspring of women with maternal phenylketonuria. *Journal of the American Medical Association* 2000; 283:756-762.

Wallace, D. Wallace, F.: Cited in *People* Magazine, November 28, 1988, p. 159.

Walton, R. G.: Seizure and mania after high intake of aspartame. *Psychosomatics* 1986; 27:218-220.

Walton, R. G.: The possible role of aspartame in seizure induction. In *Proceedings of the First International Meeting on Dietary Phenylalanine and Brain Function*, edited by R. J. Wurtman and E. Ritter-Walker, Washington, D.C., May 8-10, 1987, pp. 495-499.

Walton, R. G., Hudak, R., Green-Waite, R. J.: Adverse reactions to aspartame: Double-blind challenge in patients from a vulnerable population. *Biological Psychiatry* 1993; 34:13-17.

Walton, R. G.: Survey of aspartame studies: Correlation of outcome and funding sources. Internet abstract, June 14, 1999.

Wang, G., Volkow, N.D., Logan, J., et al: Brain dopamine and obesity. *Lancet* 2001; 357:354-357.

Wang, H. L., Waisman, H. A.: Phenylalanine tolerance tests in patients with leukemia. *Journal of Laboratory and Clinical Medicine* 1961; 57:73-77.

Wannemacher, R. W., Klainer, A. S., Dinterman, R. E., Beisel, W. R.: The significance and mechanism of an increased serum phenylalanine-tyrosine ratio during infection. *American Journal of Clinical Nutrition* 1967; 29:997-1006.

Warner, K. E., Goldenhar, L. M., McLaughlin, C. G.: Cigarette advertising and magazine coverage of the hazards of smoking: A statistical analysis. *New England Journal of Medicine* 1992; 326:305-9.

Way, E. L., Hausman, R.: Effect of tetra-ethyl thiuramdisulfide (Antabuse) on toxicity of methyl alcohol. *Federation Proceedings* 1950; 9:324.

Weber, J. C. P., Griffin, J. P.: Adverse reactions in the elderly. *Lancet* 1986; 2:291.

Weiffenbach, J. M., Fox, P. C., Baum, B. J.: Taste and salivary gland dysfunction. In *Olfaction and Taste IX*, edited by Stephen D. Roper and Jelle Atema, *Annals of the New York Academy of Sciences* 510:698-699, 1987.

Weiss, J. H., Choi, D. W.: Beta-*N*-methylamino-L-alanine neurotoxicity: Requirement for bicarbonate as a cofactor. *Science* 1988; 241:973-975.

Weissler, A. M., Kruger, F. A.: Effect of glucose on the performance of the hypoxic isolated rat heart. (Abstract) *Circulation* 1964; 29:117.

Weidner, G., Istvan, J.: Dietary sources of caffeine. *New England Journal of Medicine* 1992 1985; 13:1421.

Weitzman, E. D., Schaumburg, H., Fishbein, W.: Plasma 17-hydroxycorticosteroid levels during sleep in man. *Journal of Clinical Endocrinology & Metabolism* 1966; 26:121.

Wells v. Ortho Pharmaceutical Corp., 788 F.2d 741, reh'g denied, 795 F.2d (11ᵗʰ Cir.), Cert. denied, 479 U.S. 950 (1986).

Wernicke, J. F.: The side effect profile and safety of fluoxetine. *Journal of Clinical Psychiatry* 1985; 46:59-67.

Wessely, S., Nimnuan, C., Sharpe, M.: Functional somatic syndromes: One or many? *Lancet* 1999; 354:936-939.

Widom, B., Simonson, D. C.: Glycemic control and neuropsychologic function during hypoglycemia in patients with insulin-dependent diabetes mellitus. *Annals of Internal Medicine* 190; 112:904-912.

Wilmshurst, P.: The code of silence. *Lancet.* 1997; 349:567-569.

Wilmshurst, P.: Academia and industry. (Editorial) *Lancet* 2000; 356:338-339.

Wilson, D. H., Gardner, W. J.: Benign intracranial hypertension with particular reference to its occurrence in fat young women. *Canadian Medical Association Journal* 1966; 95:102-103.

Wilson, E. O.: *Consilience: The Unity of Knowledge.* New York, Knopf, 1998: p. 59.

Wisconsin Alumni Research Foundation: *Long Term Saccharin Feeding in Rats. Final Report.* Madison, WARF, 1973.

Wokee, J. H. J.: Diseases that masquerade as motor neurone disease. *Lancet* 1996; 347:1347-1348.

Wolraich, M. L., Lindgren, S. D., Stumbo, P. J., et al.: Effects of diets high in sucrose or aspartame on the behavior and cognitive performance of children. *New England Journal of Medicine* 1994; 330:301-307.

Wurtman, R. J.: Aspartame: Possible effect on seizure susceptibility. *Lancet* 1985; 2:1060.

Wurtman, R. J.: Press conference on Cable News Network (CNN), July 17, 1986.

a. Wurtman, R. J.: Aspartame effects on brain serotonin. *American Journal of Clinical Nutrition* 1987; 45:799-801.

b. Wurtman, R. J.: Cited by *The Philadelphia Inquirer* February 22, 1987, p. H-9.

c. Wurtman, R. J., Maher, T. J.: Calculation of the aspartame dose for rodents that produces neurochemical effects comparable to those occurring in people. In *Proceedings of the First International Meeting on Dietary Phenylalanine and Brain Function*, edited by R. J. Wurtman and E. Ritter-Walker, Washington, D.C., May 8-10, 1987, pp. 207-213.

Wyshak, G.: Teenaged girls, carbonated beverage consumption, and bone fractures. *Archives of Pediatrics & Adolescent Medicine* 2000; 154:610-613.

Yamatsui, T., Matsui, T., Okamoto, T., et al.: G protein-mediated neuronal DNA fragmentation induced by familial Alzheimer's disease – associated mutants of APP. *Science* 1996; 272:1349-1352.

Yasaki, S., Dyck, P. J.: Effect of acute hypoglycemia on energy metabolism in rat peripheral nerve. (Abstract) *Neurology* 1991; 41 (Suppl. 1):206.

Yau, Y-H., O'Sullivan, M. G., Signorini, D., et al.: Primary lymphoma of central nervous system in immunocompetence in southeast Scotland. *Lancet* 1996; 348:890.

Yip, R. G. C., Bremer, A., Boyd, N. D., et al.: Photoaffinity labeling of the GIP receptor with a truncated GIP-benzoylphenylalanine. Presented at 81ˢᵗ Annual Meeting of the Endocrine Society, San Diego, June 12, 1999, P1-391.

Yokogoshi, H., Roberts, C. H., Caballero, B., Wurtman, R. J.: Effects of aspartame and glucose administration on brain and plasma levels of large neutral amino acids and brain 5-hydroxyindoles. *American Journal of Clinical Nutrition* 1984; 4:1-7.

Young, S. N.: Facts and myths related to the use and regulation of phenylalanine and other amino acids. *Proceedings of the First International Meeting on Dietary Phenylalanine and Brain Function*, edited by R. J. Wurtman and E. Ritter-Walker, Washington, D.C., May 8-10, 1987, pp. 327-335.

Young, V. R. Marchini, J. S.: Mechanisms and nutritional significance of metabolic responses to altered intakes of protein and amino acids, with reference to nutritional adaptation in humans. *American Journal of Clinical Nutrition* 1990; 51:270-289.

1018

Zametkin, A. J., et al.: Cerebral glucose metabolism in adults with hyperactivity of childhood onset. *New England Journal of Medicine* 1990; 323:1361-1366.

Zetinoglu, I. Y., Gherondache, C. N., Pincus, G.: The process of aging: Serum glucose and immunoreactive insulin levels during the oral glucose tolerance test. *Journal of the American Geriatrics Society* 1969; 17:1.

Zito, J. M., Safer, D. J., dosReis, S., et al.: Trends in the prescribing of psychotropic medications to preschoolers. *Journal of the American Medical Association.* 2000; 283:1025-1030.

INDEX